MAGNETIC RESONANCE IMAGING
of the SPINE

MAGNETIC RESONANCE IMAGING *of the* SPINE

SECOND EDITION

Michael T. Modic, M.D.

Chairman
Division of Radiology
The Cleveland Clinic Foundation
Cleveland, Ohio

Thomas J. Masaryk, M.D.

Head
Section of Neuroradiology
Department of Radiology
The Cleveland Clinic Foundation
Cleveland, Ohio

Jeffrey S. Ross, M.D.

Head
Section of Magnetic Resonance Imaging
Department of Radiology
The Cleveland Clinic Foundation
Cleveland, Ohio

With 1149 illustrations (38 in full color)

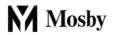 Mosby

St. Louis Baltimore Boston Chicago London Madrid Philadelphia Sydney Toronto

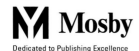

Publisher: George Stamathis
Editor: Anne S. Patterson
Developmental Editor: Carolyn A. Malik
Project Manager: John Rogers
Production Editor: George B. Stericker Jr.
Designer: Julie Taugner
Manufacturing Supervisor: Kathy Grone

Second Edition
Copyright © 1994 by Mosby–Year Book, Inc.

Printed in the United States of America
Composition by Clarinda Company
Printing/binding by Walsworth Publishing Company

Mosby–Year Book, Inc.
11830 Westline Industrial Drive
St. Louis, Missouri 63146

Library of Congress Cataloging in Publication Data

Modic, Michael T.
    Magnetic resonance imaging of the spine / Michael T. Modic, Thomas
J. Masaryk, Jeffrey S. Ross. — Ed. 2.
      p. cm.
    Includes bibliographical references and index.
    ISBN 0-8016-6838-7
    1. Spine—Diseases—Diagnosis. 2. Spine—Magnetic resonance
imaging. I. Masaryk, Thomas J. II. Ross, Jeffrey S. (Jeffrey
Stuart) III. Title.
    [DNLM: 1. Magnetic Resonance Imaging. 2. Spinal Diseases—
diagnosis. 3. Spine—anatomy & histology. WE 725 M692m 1993]
  RD768.M63   1993
  617.4′8207′548—dc20
  DNLM/DLC
  for Library of Congress   93-22424
                                  CIP

92 93 94 95 96 / 9 8 7 6 5 4 3 2 1

Contributors

Marilyn J. Goske, M.D.
Head, Section of Pediatric Radiology
Department of Radiology
The Cleveland Clinic Foundation
Cleveland, Ohio

Thomas J. Masaryk, M.D.
Head, Section of Neuroradiology
Department of Radiology
The Cleveland Clinic Foundation
Cleveland, Ohio

Michael T. Modic, M.D.
Chairman, Division of Radiology
The Cleveland Clinic Foundation
Cleveland, Ohio

Jeffrey S. Ross, M.D.
Head, Section of Magnetic Resonance Imaging
Department of Radiology
The Cleveland Clinic Foundation
Cleveland, Ohio

Paul M. Ruggieri, M.D.
Staff Neuroradiologist
Department of Radiology
The Cleveland Clinic Foundation
Cleveland, Ohio

Shiwei Yu, M.D.
Department of Radiology
NMR Research Laboratory
State University of New York
Syracuse, New York

*In memory of
William C. Strittmatter, M.D.,
for starting us all off.*

Preface to the Second Edition

Since the publication of the first edition of this book, MR has seen continued growth in its application to spinal diagnosis. The use of paramagnetic contrast agents has become well established in a variety of disorders, and three-dimensional acquisitions and postprocessing of data have become more commonplace. Coil design and sequence development continue unabated. Signal-to-noise, contrast, and speed have all been improved. Based on developments underway, we can look forward to further advancement in technique and in physiologic and functional studies that are in the early stages of implementation or design.

All of the above have resulted in a greater clinical experience with a methodology that continues to evolve. Toward that end, we have revised this text to be more reflective of the current state of the art. The initial chapters related to technical considerations have been completely revamped to present a more clinical approach, and chapter 9 (on the pediatric spine) has been completely rewritten. The remaining chapters have been expanded to reflect current knowledge.

It continues to be our opinion that MR is the best first test for the majority of clinical situations requiring spinal imaging. However, we freely admit that although well informed and well intentioned, this is "an opinion," and in many situations the role of MR has not been subjected to rigid scientific scrutiny and/or a critical cost efficacy analysis. There will always remain problems related to radiological research that are unique to diagnostic imaging. In particular, an approach that optimizes the attainment of diagnostic information may not readily provide simultaneous information on other indices such as patient treatment and patient outcomes. These differences in no way obviate or discredit MR's value but rather suggest where our efforts need to be directed over the next few years.

In addition, we need to concentrate more effort on determining the significance of the morphological changes we can now so exquisitely demonstrate. Clearly, there is a wide range of these derangements that can be identified in patients who are relatively asymptomatic. The identification of characteristics that separate them from the symptomatic group is not readily apparent. This underscores comments made in our original preface related to the relationship of anatomic derangements and symptom complexes. Again, we must emphasize that the management of patients with spinal disorders must begin and end with a thorough clinical assessment. Imaging is an intermediage test that must be integrated into, rather than isolated from, that assessment.

ACKNOWLEDGMENTS

We wish to continue thanking those whose contributions were critical to the first edition of this book. We would again especially like to recognize Ms. Helen Kurz, whose efforts were so important to the successful completion of both editions. In fact, if it were not for her viraginous personality, it is likely this project would never have been accomplished. We are also grateful to Bob Maynard for his photographic support, to all of our co-workers in MR, and especially to Mr. John Dillinger for creating the flexible environment where we could obtain many of the studies for this text. The people at Mosby–Year Book, Anne Patterson, Carolyn Malik, and George Stericker, deserve special credit as well. While they may have approached the line that separates attentive encouragement from insufferable nagging, they rarely crossed it. This is a tribute to their professionalism.

Lastly, and most importantly, we again thank our families for their support.

Michael T. Modic, M.D.
Thomas J. Masaryk, M.D.
Jeffrey S. Ross, M.D.

Preface to the First Edition

Since the introduction of MR, its potential for spinal imaging was obvious, but could not be immediately realized. The 15-mm thick, single-slice T_1 weighted images that took 8 minutes to acquire provided a glimpse into the multidimensional imaging world that MR would eventually achieve. T_2-weighted images provided the so-called CSF myelogram effect, but were time-consuming, talking between 20 and 40 minutes. Despite the cumbersome nature of the technique in the early days, the potential impact of MR provided a marked stimulus for development. Technical advances came rapidly in an effort to facilitate spinal exams. Multislice, multiecho techniques increased the area covered and improved the contrast available. Units with higher field strengths, surface coils, and sequence optimization increased signal-to-noise.This could be traded for smaller voxel elements and improved spatial resolution. Gradient-echo partial flip-angle imaging, cardiac gating, and refocusing pulses improved our control of contrast and intrinsic motion problems. Saturation pulses, half-Fourier imaging, and gradient-echo three-dimensional techniques provided artifact-free images in a shorter time with greater multidimensional reconstruction capability. Paramagnetic contrast agents have opened further avenues for both research and clinical applications by providing the ability to manipulate contrast in both normal and diseased tissues. Dispite this progress, the modality remains in an evolutionary stage, with almost unlimited room for improvement.

What has resulted from these improvements is not just an imaging exam with superb morphologic accuracy, but a procedure that has provided us a view of the biochemical and pathophysiological changes at the heart of disease processes.

In our opinion, it is already the best first test for the majority of clinical situations requiring spinal imaging. But while providing more information than more conventional studies, it demands more in terms of understanding from its user. It is all too easy for technical imaging options to be ordered in a "cook book" fashion. Nevertheless, we should strive to maintain a cognitive rather than Pavlovian attitude, and should made an effort to understand the technical options available. To optimize the technical considerations and imaging protocols requires an understanding of the pathogenesis, presentation, and potential treatment options in various disease processes, as well as the normal anatomy and basic science aspects of the modality.

Hopefully, this text will serve all clinical scientists whose interest is the spine, no matter which discipline they call home. We have attempted to impart the present status of MR, both in terms of technique and clinical applications, in a logical fashion. It is our intention to integrate normal anatomy, disease process, basic science, and technical considerations in the performance of the MR exam. The first chapter deals with the basic principles behind imaging stategies and is followed by a chapter on normal anatomy that consolidates the technical principles with the anatomic substrate of the MR signal. The remainder of the book concerns itself with pathological processes, again integrating technical considerations with clinical conditions and suggesting reasonable imaging strategies. In this fashion we hope to address the major questions of spinal imaging, not providing dogmatic answers, but allowing informed choices.

It must be emphasized that MRI represents a tool for morphologic and biochemical analysis. In certain situations there may only be a moderate correlation between the imaging evidence of morphologic alteration and the presence of symptoms. The jump from the indentification of an anatomic derangement to a symptom complex must be made with caution. The management of patients with spinal disorders must begin and end with a thorough clinical assessment, with imaging being an intermediate test that must be integrated into, rather than isolated from, that assessment.

Last, a critic might say that we do a disservice and perhaps even an injustice by focusing so strongly on MR as the primary diagnostic modality in the evaluation of the spine. That is their right, but this is our book.

Michael T. Modic, M.D.

Contents

The future's so bright
you gotta wear shades.

Tim Buk 3
The Future's So Bright

1

A Practical Approach to Magnetic Resonance Physics in Spinal Imaging

PAUL M. RUGGIERI

This chapter is intended not as a primer of general MR physics but as an overview of some of the basic principles necessary for routine spinal imaging in everyday practice. The principles it sets forth are particularly important to bear in mind when designing the clinical imaging protocols, choosing a coil for a particular examination, or altering the sequence parameters to meet a specific clinical need. An adjustment in any single parameter may have a profound impact on the signal-to-noise, contrast, and/or artifacts in the images. As a result the reader's ability to identify an abnormality on the clinical images may be significantly altered. For the most part, an improvement in any one aspect of the images will be costly and will demand compromises in other parameters to maintain similar image quality.

The radiologist must also be aware of the typical artifacts that arise in MR imaging of the spine so they are not misinterpreted as pathology. These artifacts may be related to the choice of sequence parameters, the patient, the system hardware, or extraneous factors such as foreign bodies or even the weather. A thorough knowledge of the underlying causes of these artifacts makes it possible to incorporate changes in the imaging protocols or the system's hardware to reduce, if not eliminate, the artifact.

What follows is a review of the basic MR concepts from a practical point of view and an introduction of new imaging methods that are expected to assume an increasingly important role in MR imaging of the spine. Various imaging protocols are also discussed with their underlying rationales as they have been introduced in the literature.[1-12]

PATIENT CONSIDERATIONS

Essential to any MR examination is patient comfort. Even subtle patient motion during the examination can severely degrade image quality and render the study uninterpretable. The key is to identify the underlying problem and manage it appropriately.

In some patients it may be necessary simply to provide an extra blanket to keep warm, use a softer cushion under the head, adjust the fan, turn on background music, or position a cushion under the knees to reduce strain on the lower back. In others the problem will be anxiety arising from confinement within the magnet bore of the conventional whole-body imaging system. Reassurance and a brief conversation between pulse sequences are often sufficient to relieve this. Some children may need just the familiar voice and touch of a parent in the scanning room to reduce their anxiety and avoid sedation.

When conservative measures fail to relieve a patient's anxieties, pharmacologic intervention is necessary. The choice of agents will vary depending on the experience of the individual physician. Intravenous midazolam hydrochloride (Versed) is generally an effective short-term anxiolytic in adults (1 to 2 mg) if their medical status permits. Although small doses of this benzodiazepine are relatively safe, one should always be wary of potential side effects (e.g., respiratory suppression) and the patient should always be monitored appropriately during the examination.[13,14] If significant problems arise, an intravenously administered antagonist, flumazenil (Mazicon), is now available; however, it is currently approved only for use in adults (0.2 mg, then 0.1 mg every 30 to 60 seconds as needed up to a total of 1 mg).

The choice of medications must always be tailored to the individual situation. For example, if a patient's respiratory status is severely compromised, an agent with relatively little respiratory suppressive effect would be preferable. In an older patient who is disoriented and whose mental status does not permit him or her to cooperate, haloperidol (Haldol) can be quite effective but a loading dose should be administered well before the imaging study to establish a therapeutic blood level. If pain is the reason that the patient cannot lie still (e.g., acute disk herniation), an anxiolytic is of little value. In this case the choice of pain relievers will depend on the examiner's familiarity with the agents, the level of patient discomfort, and the patient's medical condition.

In the very young or anxious child sedation may be necessary. A formal conscious sedation protocol should be arranged in conjunction with the anesthesiology department at each institution and should include standards for the following[15]: appropriateness of sedation; preanesthesia preparation (e.g., NPO status); preanesthesia medical evaluation (age, weight, past medical history, review of systems, baseline vital signs, physical examination [including an assessment of the airway], current medications, and history of prior sedation experience); parental consent; physiologic monitoring and documentation; a limited set of pharmacologic agents with which the radiologist and anesthesiologist are comfortable; a standard formula for dosage, route, and rate of administration of these agents, based on age and size of the child; and a set of fixed discharge criteria and outpatient follow-up measures. The necessary equipment must be available for monitoring, resuscitation, and (if necessary) general anesthesia.

The Joint Commission for Accreditation of Healthcare Organizations (JCAHO), the American Society of Anesthesiologists (ASA), and the American Academy of Pediatrics (AAP)[16,17] recommend appropriate physiologic monitoring for any patient undergoing conscious sedation. In a routine setting this should include direct observation, pulse oximetry for percent oxygen saturation, heart rate and rhythm, and respiration and blood pressure monitoring. Ideally, ECG monitoring could be included; but it is frequently difficult to maintain with the patient in the bore of the magnet and, besides, it is not vital in most children because of the nature of their medical problems. The respiratory belts conventionally installed in MR systems tend to be unreliable in small children; their respiration can be more effectively monitored by direct observation. Since this may at times be difficult, a capnometer that produces waveforms can be utilized to record the rate and pattern of respiration. (The measured CO_2 levels also are often erroneous because of the child's small tidal volumes and the large dead space that exists between the patient and the monitor.) A potential problem with monitoring blood pressure is that the blood pressure cuff may wake the child up if he

or she is only lightly sedated. Whereas blood pressure monitoring is currently recommended in children undergoing conscious sedation, continuous monitoring should not be as critical as following the other physiologic parameters. (A drop in blood pressure is generally a late finding when a child is getting into trouble and occurs long after a change in ventilation, CO_2 retention, and O_2 saturation.) In the MR facility monitoring may introduce significant problems. For example, the monitoring devices may cause a 60 Hz radiofrequency artifact and significantly degrade the S/N (signal-to-noise) of the images; additionally, the digital values on the monitor may be inaccurate or absent if enough of the magnet's radiofrequency power is transmitted to the monitoring unit itself, especially when the body coil is used as a transmitter and receiver. Fiber-optic technology seems to have eliminated these difficulties, since the fiber-optic cable does not serve as an effective antenna; but greater care must be taken with the cable, for it is significantly more fragile than conventional cables.

In children under 2 years of age chloral hydrate (75 to 100 mg/kg PO, 2 gm maximum) is generally quite effective for sedation, although on occasion it may be necessary to supplement this with 1 to 2 mg/kg of intravenous pentobarbital at 1 mg/kg increments.[15] In children over 2 years of age body weight may prohibit effective dosing with chloral hydrate. Intravenous pentobarbital (Nembutal) has proved to be quite reliable in this age group at the conventional dosage of 2 to 6 mg/kg.[18] On rare occasion a child may require as much as 8 mg/kg. The higher dosages can be avoided if an accurate record is maintained of previous sedations for each child who comes to the institution. For example, if a child was sedated with 4 mg/kg and requires an additional 2 mg/kg because he is beginning to wake up during the examination, starting out with 5 mg/kg for the follow-up examination may obviate the need for higher dosages. In some cases the child may appear asleep but will resist positioning or continue to move his legs after the pentobarbital has been administered. It may then be helpful to add 1 μg/kg of intravenous fentanyl (Sublimaze). However, it is important to remember that fentanyl must not be administered to children less than 2 years of age, because its respiratory suppressive effect persists longer than its sedative effect (age-dependent) and the child may become apneic in an unmonitored situation.[15] Children whose medical status is particularly guarded, who are known to be refractory to conventional medications, or who have had a previous adverse reaction to sedative agents should probably be sedated in a more controlled fashion, under general anesthesia.

CHOICE OF COILS

Surface coils continue to be the mainstay for imaging the thoracic and lumbosacral spine. Since the sensitive volume of a surface coil is roughly hemispherical in configuration and the S/N drops off relatively rapidly with distance, surface coils are well suited to spinal imaging (Fig. 1-1). As a result of this inherent nonuniformity, the S/N from the structures in the near field (spine) is maximized whereas the noise contribution from the rest of the body (chest, abdomen, pelvis) is minimized. The only potential pitfall with this design is that the signal intensity of the subcutaneous fat immediately overlying the coil may be so high as to obscure pathology in the region and make it difficult to adjust the window and center of the images for the tissues of interest anteriorly. This has led manufacturers to develop normalization algorithms for postprocessing the data so the technician can take advantage of a greater dynamic range of intensities when filming the region of interest (Fig. 1-2).

Because the normal cervical lordosis increases the distance between a flat surface coil and the spine, contoured coils have been designed to conform to the curvature of the neck and increase the S/N of the cervical spinal column (Fig. 1-3). Many of these contoured coils have also been fitted with anterior components to produce a Helmholtz-like volume coil configuration. This provides more uniform signal throughout the neck, allowing for

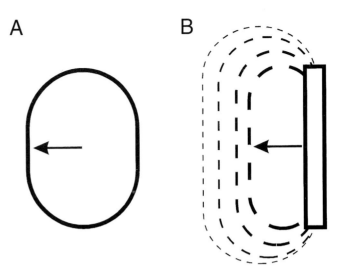

Fig. 1-1. A, In this frontal view of an elliptical surface coil the *arrow* defines the radius in the transverse dimensions. **B,** The usable, or sensitive, volume of the coil is in the shape of an elliptical hemisphere whose dimensions are roughly the length and transverse radius of the coil. The volume is inherently nonuniform, and the signal-to-noise (S/N) drops off rapidly with increasing distance from the coil.

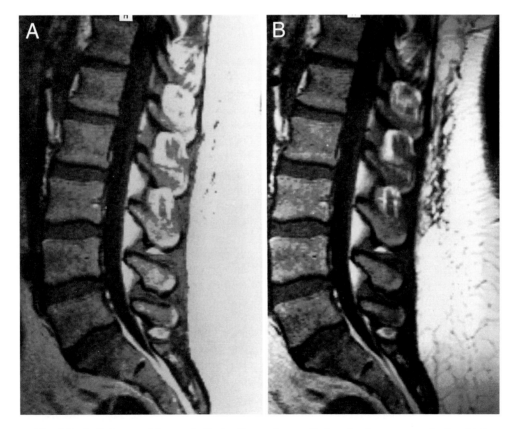

Fig. 1-2. A, Because of its proximity to the surface coil, dorsal subcutaneous fat has high signal intensity. **B,** The normalization algorithm reduces any discrepancy of signal intensities across the field of view so the adjacent lower-intensity tissues can be better visualized.

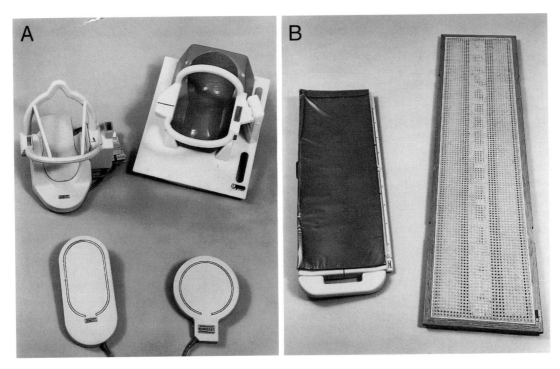

Fig. 1-3. A, Two Helmholtz-like neck coils are pictured at the *top.* In the smaller one *(left)* the anterior piece is detachable and the remainder can be used as a contoured surface coil. In the larger one the anterior piece is on a hinge. At the *bottom* are elliptical and round surface coils used in thoracic and lumbar spinal imaging. **B,** With the Bucky coil *(left)* and the "pizza" board the patient lies on the platforms shown here and the surface coil slides beneath the platform so it can be repositioned without moving the patient.

better visualization of the spine in patients with an accentuated cervical lordosis and better visualization of the prevertebral soft tissues in all patients (Fig. 1-4). However, the noise contribution from the anterior soft tissues can be detrimental to image quality (e.g., motion artifact from swallowing and respiration), and in routine cervical spinal imaging this is purposely suppressed with saturation pulses.

A surface coil is most efficient when its dimensions closely approximate the region of the spine to be studied. Ideally, the sensitive volume should have a large enough radius to include the superficial soft tissues, spinal canal, and bony spine; but the volume should be sufficiently well defined that little signal is derived from the tissues anterior to the vertebral column. In practice, no surface coil is this perfect and the sensitive volumes must penetrate more deeply to produce images with relatively uniform signal in the region of the spine. Additionally, if the coil is too small, it may not be able to visualize enough of the spine in the rostrocaudal dimension or detect signal as deeply as necessary in patients with a large body habitus. On the other hand, a coil that is too large with respect to the body part being studied will detect too much random noise from tissues outside the region

of interest and this will produce a lower S/N in the region of interest. In other words, to provide an appropriate "filling factor," the size of the coil must be suitable to the body part being examined.

Technical design factors are particularly important in determining the S/N of a coil. All spine coils rely on the body coil as a transmitter, and the surface coil acts as a detector for the signal emitted from the tissue (similar to an antenna). The conventional "receive-only" spine coils are linearly polarized and detect the signal from one set of antennae. New spine coils have been designed that are circularly polarized (quadrature coils). These coils contain two sets of perpendicularly oriented antennae and are able to produce a circular magnetic field; they thus are more efficient at collecting signal than linearly polarized coils. Because a greater component of the signal is detected, the S/N in the images from these coils is proportionately higher than from linearly polarized coils, typically on the order of 40% to 50% higher (Fig. 1-5).

Recent developments in the technology of spine coils have been directed toward solving such problems as field of view and examination time. Often it is necessary to evaluate more than one region of the spine, which can be very time consuming with conventional technology

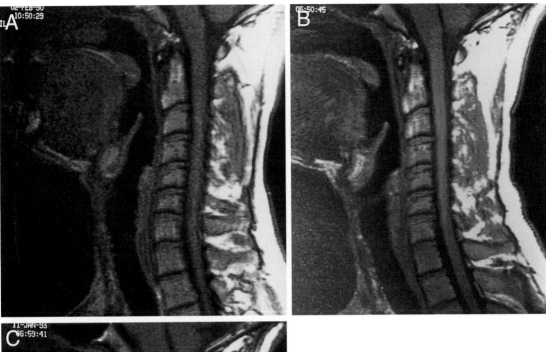

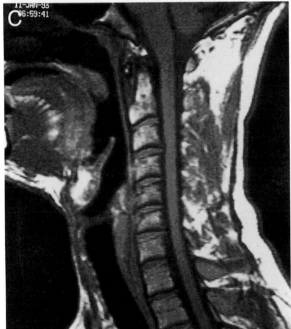

Fig. 1-4. Sagittal T$_1$-weighted images using, **A,** the flat round elliptical surface coil, **B,** the contoured surface coil, and, **C,** the Helmholtz-like volume coil. Because of the distance from the flat coil, the signal in the spine is relatively low. The contoured coil wraps partially around the neck, so the signal is improved. The signal is most uniform with the Helmholtz-like coil.

since it requires repositioning the coil and the patient between examinations. A simple answer is to place the conventional surface coil under the platform upon which the patient lies so it can be slid along the length of the patient and repositioned without moving the patient (Bucky coil or "pizza" board) (Fig. 1-3). It is somewhat more efficient to use a *phased-array* coil since this does not require any physical repositioning to evaluate several areas of the spine. The phased-array coil is a series of small coils linked in a ladderlike configuration, which allows

examination of a large area while taking advantage of the high S/N characteristics of the smaller coils. Although this option may seem particularly appealing, the phased-array technology has extensive hardware and software demands that, obviously, introduce an increased cost. Alternatively, the body coil can be used as the transmitter and receiver to examine contiguous areas of the spine; but this should be done only in survey examinations in which high spatial resolution and S/N are not so necessary (e.g., evaluation for cord compression

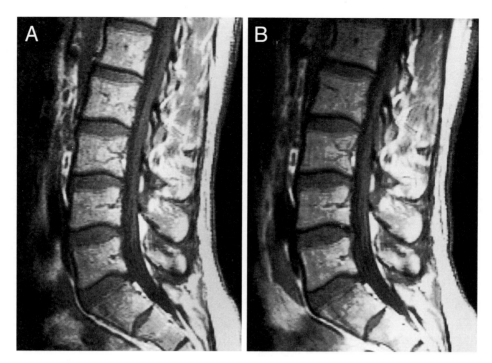

Fig. 1-5. Sagittal spin-echo images of the lumbar spine with a linearly polarized, **A**, and a circularly polarized (or quadrature), **B**, coil. The signal-to-noise of the image obtained with the circularly polarized coil is noticeably higher than that obtained with the linearly polarized coil.

from bony spinal metastases). Because of the expected discrepancy in image quality, appropriate changes in the pulse sequence parameters must be incorporated to compensate for the S/N lost by using the body coil as a receiver.[19]

PULSE SEQUENCE CONSIDERATIONS

When choosing the individual pulse sequences and pulse sequence parameters for a routine evaluation of the spine, one must maintain a careful balance between S/N, spatial resolution, contrast, examination time, and imaging artifacts. Adjusting the sequence parameters to enhance any of these factors will inevitably affect the others, often in a negative fashion. When any adjustment is made in the imaging protocol, all factors must be taken into consideration so diagnostic efficacy of the images will be maximized.

Among these considerations, S/N is perhaps the most important factor influencing one's judgment of image quality. The goal is to maximize the signal from the spins in each individual voxel in the volume of interest and to minimize the contribution of noise while maintaining the desired contrast. Since larger voxels contain more spins, an increase in the amount of signal per voxel can be achieved by merely increasing the size of the voxels. The primary problem with this strategy, however, is that

larger voxels reduce the spatial resolution of the images and, practically, MR can only approximate the high spatial resolution of CT under ideal circumstances. Alternatively, in some situations, spatial resolution may be sacrificed for the sake of contrast. Very small voxels will compromise the S/N, which, in turn, will have a direct effect on the contrast-to-noise ratio (C/N). When C/N is the primary consideration (e.g., intramedullary lesion), it may be desirable to increase the voxel size to improve C/N at the expense of spatial resolution.

Spatial resolution is thought of in terms of three-dimensional voxels. The in-plane spatial resolution is defined as the field of view (FOV) divided by the number of phase-encoding steps in one direction and the number of frequency-encoding steps in the other. Doubling the FOV or reducing the number of points along the phase-encoding and read directions by half will increase the voxel size fourfold but will significantly impair the in-plane resolution. Most surface coils are constructed to provide a 30 cm FOV maximum. With a matrix of 256 $\times$ 256 the in-plane resolution (voxel size) would be approximately 1.4 mm. A 23 to 25 cm FOV would produce an in-plane spatial resolution of 0.9 to 1 mm, which is more useful in most clinical situations. Because examination time is always a concern, many radiologists have chosen to use an intermediate matrix size of 192 phase-encoding steps while holding the frequency-

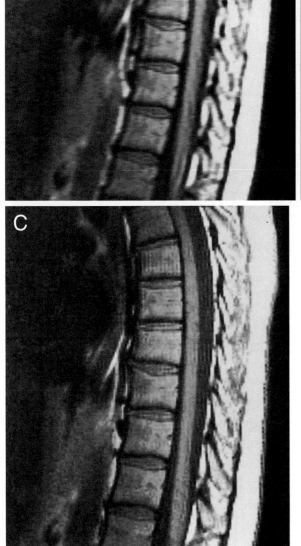

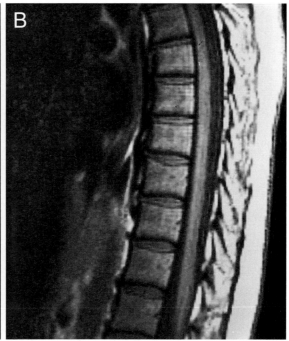

Fig. 1-6. Sagittal T$_1$-weighted images with matrices of 128×256, **A,** 192×256, **B,** and 256×256, **C.** As the number of phase-encoding steps is increased, the in-plane resolution increases. Whereas theory would predict a decline in signal-to-noise, the actual reduction is subtle; however, the improvement in spatial resolution is obvious as the number of phase-encoding steps increases and the field of view remains constant.

encoding steps constant at 256. This produces rectangular voxels with a larger volume and, hence, a higher signal-to-noise. Such an increase is not linear, as might be expected, since the number of phase-encoding steps is not held constant and the S/N is also proportionate to the square root of the number of times the data are sampled (number of phase-encoding steps) (Fig. 1-6).

In-plane resolution = FOV/Number of voxels

Through-plane resolution = Slice thickness

Through-plane resolution is defined by the slice thickness, but this is further compromised in conventional two-dimensional MR imaging by the interslice gap. Increasing slice thickness will also enlarge the voxels and improve the S/N but, as expected, the resolution will be compromised. The radiofrequency (RF) pulses conventionally used for excitation do not truly excite two-dimensional slices as rectangular slabs of tissue. The volume of excited tissue is always greater than the defined slice thickness, and the slice profiles are always of

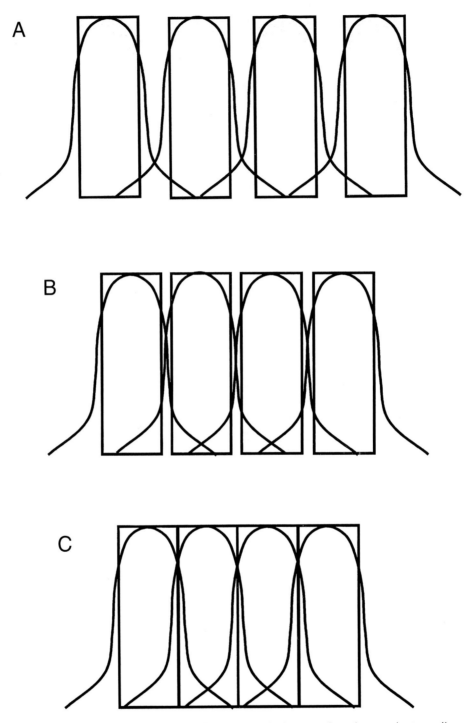

Fig. 1-7. The ideal slice profiles are defined by vertical rectangles whereas the true slice profiles are illustrated by parabolas. The overlap at the lower ends of the parabolic plots represents the regions of tissue excited by both of the adjacent radiofrequency pulses or the amount of cross talk. With a reduction in the interslice gap (**A** to **B** to **C**), there is increasing cross talk along with a lower signal-to-noise of the corresponding slices.

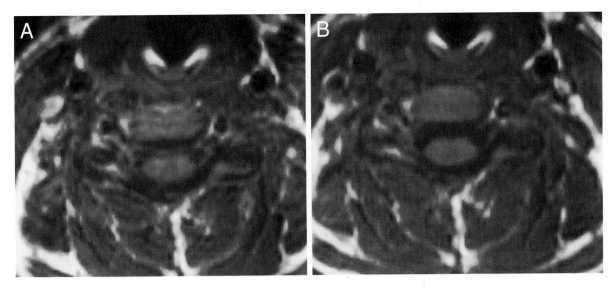

Fig. 1-8. There is a large amount of cross talk when the slices are contiguous, **A,** so the signal-to-noise is relatively low compared to the same images obtained with an interslice gap equal to the slice thickness (or full gap), **B.**

a somewhat parabolic configuration. The heels of these parabolas tend to overlap (cross talk), particularly if the edges of the defined slices are contiguous or very close together (Figs. 1-7 and 1-8). Since the tissue in these overlap regions is exposed to the RF pulses for each of the adjacent slices in the same TR interval, the spins in these regions are relatively saturated. If the slices are excited in a sequential fashion and have a narrow interslice gap, every slice except the first and last will be affected by three RF pulses during each TR interval. A significant proportion of the spins in the center slices will have less of a chance to regain their full longitudinal magnetization between excitations, and these slices will therefore have a lower S/N than the end slices.

Interleaving or manipulating the order of slice excitation within the TR interval (e.g., 1,3,5,7, . . . and then 2,4,6,8, . . . instead of 1,2,3,4, . . .) is automatically incorporated by some manufacturers. With this scheme the effective TR for the intervening tissue is prolonged but there is still a somewhat lower S/N for the second group of slices excited in the TR interval (2,4,6,8, . . .). The only way to eliminate such cross talk between slices is to incorporate a large interslice gap. This is not clinically practical, however, since a large gap may miss too much information or demand a second acquisition to include that tissue within the large gaps of the first acquisition. The best compromise is to add an interslice gap but keep it relatively small (33% to 50%), accept a small amount of cross talk, and adjust the parameters to compensate for the impaired S/N.

An alternative way to increase the S/N is simply to increase the number of acquisitions or excitations (NEX). This will improve the S/N in proportion to the square root of the number of acquisitions. Beyond four acquisitions, however, there is relatively little benefit in image quality despite the large increases in the time needed to acquire the data. Moreover, the longer acquisition time increases the likelihood that the patient will move during the examination. As a result two to four acquisitions are usually incorporated for conventional short TR two-dimensional imaging and one to two for long TR images (Fig. 1-9). This strategy is really effective only if the duration of one acquisition is relatively short (e.g., in a two-dimensional gradient echo, hybrid RARE, or T_1-weighted spin-echo sequence). The acquisition time of a conventional T_2-weighted spin-echo sequence would make the routine use of multiple excitations prohibitive.

Some improvement in S/N is possible with less compromise of the overall examination time. By convention, a T_1-weighted spin-echo sequence has a repetition time (TR) on the order of the T_1-relaxation time for the tissues of interest. Although the examination time is somewhat longer, increasing the TR will improve the S/N. A greater proportion of spins will be able to regain their longitudinal magnetization before the next RF pulse is applied and therefore contribute signal during the next TR interval. However, this will reduce the T_1 contrast and give the images more of a spin density appearance if the TR becomes too long. A short echo time (TE) is also desired for T_1-weighted spin-echo imaging. This will not only minimize the amount of T_2 decay and emphasize the T_1 influence, it will also increase the S/N of the images.

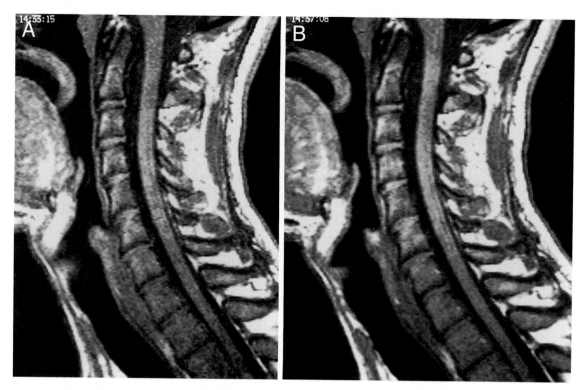

Fig. 1-9. As the number of acquisitions or excitations is doubled from two, **A**, to four, **B**, there is a $\sqrt{2}$ increase in the signal-to-noise.

In double-echo T_2-weighted sequences the TR must be long enough to avoid any T_1 influence in the images. Generally, to allow near-complete longitudinal recovery of the spins, the TR must be at least three times as long as the T_1 values for the tissues of interest. A short TE for the first echo will so limit the T_2 influence that the image is said to reflect the proton density of the tissues. Longer TEs for the second echo image will increase the T_2 weighting but decrease the S/N and decrease the number of slices that can be obtained for a given TR interval. There is an exponential decay in signal as the phases of the precessing spins randomly disperse over time, which accounts for the decline in S/N (for each image) as the echo time increases.

As the echo time is increased in gradient echo sequences, there is a reduction in S/N that exceeds that seen in spin-echo imaging. In gradient echo sequences the spins are refocused exclusively by inverting the gradients. In spin-echo imaging a 180-degree RF pulse is also applied at time ½ TE so any spin dephasing that is constant over time (e.g., that due to a local field inhomogeneity) will be corrected. The gradient and RF echoes occur simultaneously in spin-echo imaging whereas only the gradient echo is refocused at time TE in gradient echo imaging. This provides for more rapid spin dephasing than occurs because of the conventional T_2 de-

cay processes in spin-echo sequences and provides for the T_2^* contrast in gradient echo imaging. Consequently, it is even more important to keep the echo time as short as possible to maintain an adequate S/N in the gradient echo sequences. The only situations in which it might be helpful to prolong the echo time in these sequences would be when S/N can be sacrificed for T_2^* contrast or when small amounts of metal, calcium, or blood products need to be detected. For example, metal, calcium, or blood would be identified as sites of signal loss because the local field inhomogeneities created by these substances cause more rapid spin dephasing than in the adjacent tissue.

Most manufacturers have incorporated low bandwidth (BW) readout periods to improve S/N in sequences in which the S/N is particularly limiting (e.g., late echo T_2-weighted images). The low BW frequency-encoding gradient samples the field of view with a narrower frequency range and effectively reduces the sampled noise to increase the overall S/N (proportionate to the inverse of the square root of the BW) (Fig. 1-10). These lower gradients are longer in duration, which places restrictions on the minimum possible TE for a sequence. In a double echo T_2-weighted spin-echo sequence it is really only the second echo (very long TE) that is limiting with regard to the S/N so the low BW is generally applied only

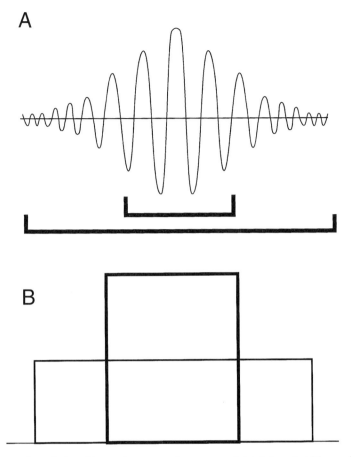

Fig. 1-10. A, Plot of signal intensity versus frequency. A high bandwidth readout period samples a broader frequency range that includes more of the signal but also more of the noise, resulting in a lower signal-to-noise. **B,** In a plot of gradient strength versus time the low bandwidth readout *(thin line)* is a weak gradient applied over a long period whereas the high bandwidth readout gradient *(bold line)* is applied as a strong gradient over a short time frame.

to this echo. In most other situations the lowest possible BW that can be accommodated by the sequence echo time should be incorporated. Another limitation of this modification is the chemical shift artifact, which is accentuated with low BW sequences, particularly at high field strengths.[20] Because the methylene protons of fat are more "protected" from the main magnetic field than the water protons, they will precess at a slightly different frequency from the water protons. Since differences in frequency are used to assign spatial position along the frequency-encoding direction, fat and water protons located at the same point in space will be assigned a different position in the image. With a low BW readout gradient, there is a lower gradient defining the points along the frequency-encoding axis and each voxel is represented by a smaller frequency range. This translates to a more obvious spatial misregistration between fat and

water, based on the difference in resonance frequencies at a given field strength (220 Hz at 1.5 T, 150 Hz at 1 T). Although this can be quite limiting in MR imaging of the orbit, it does not generally present a problem in spinal imaging.

Incorporating low BW readout periods into a sequence does not compromise the examination time, although many other schemes designed to improve image quality do significantly extend imaging times. A busy clinical practice does not allow excessive examination times. More important, patients cannot really be expected to remain still for extended periods. Generally, patients can easily remain still for 5 to 8 minutes and a cooperative patient may lie still as long as 10 to 12 minutes for an individual sequence. The number of sequences should be kept to an absolute minimum, and the duration of each sequence should be made as short as possible without

TABLE 1-1
Consequences of sequence manipulation in two-dimensional MR imaging

Change in parameters	Resolution	S/N	C/N	Examination time	T₁ contrast	T₂ contrast	Chemical shift	Truncation	Aliasing	Motion artifact	Field inhomogeneity
Decrease in field strength	↓ᵃ	↓	↓	←	→	←	→	-	-	→	→
Decrease in FOV	←	→	→	-ᵇ	-	-	→	→	-	-	→
Decrease in slice thickness	←	→	→	-ᵇ	-	-	-	-	-	↓ᵍ	→
Decrease in interslice gap	←	→	→	-ᵇ	-	-	-	-	-	-	-
Decrease in NEX	-	↓ᶜ	-/↑/↓ᵈ	→	←	→	-	-	-	→	→
Decrease in TR	-	↓	↑	→	←	→	←	-	-	-	←
Decrease in TE	-	←	←	-	-	→	-	-	-	→	←
Decrease in BW	→	↑ᶠ	←	→	-	-	←	←	-	↓ᵍ	→
Decrease in phase-encoding steps	→	←	←	-	-	-	←	←	-	↓ᵍ	←
Decrease in frequency encoding steps	-	→	→	→	-	-	-	-	-	-	-
Decrease in rectangular FOV	←	←	←	→	←	→	-	-	←	-	→
Decrease in inter-echo space	←	←	←	-	←	→	-	-	-	→	→
Decrease in echo train length	-	-	-	-	-	-	-	-	-	-	-

Code: *S/N*, Signal-to-noise; *C/N*, contrast-to-noise; *FOV*, field of view; *NEX*, number of excitations; *BW*, bandwidth; *SPGR*, spoiled GRASS; *ROI*, region of interest.

ᵃ Secondary to ↓ S/N
ᵇ ↑ if necessary to cover same through-plane ROI
ᶜ ↑ S/N with FISP/GRASS
ᵈ - with T₁, ↓ with T₂, ↑ with FISP/GRASS, ↓ with FLASH/SPGR
ᵉ ↑ with T₁, ↓ with T₂, ↑ with gradient echoes
ᶠ ↑ S/N with voxel size outweighs ↓ in S/N with number of sampling points
ᵍ ↑ intravoxel spin dephasing

compromising the information content in the images. (See Table 1-1.)

One of the first things to consider is the size of the volume to be assessed in the examination and the three-dimensional spatial resolution needed to answer the clinical question. Recall that examination time in a two-dimensional Fourier transform (2DFT) technique is defined as the repetition time multiplied by the number of acquisitions (or excitations) and the number of phase-encoding steps. If 4 mm through-plane resolution is thought to be necessary for the axial images and the chosen TR will not quite permit as many slices as needed, it is more efficient (in terms of S/N per unit time) to increase the TR to allow more slices than to perform concatenated sequences (two consecutive sequences) at a slightly shorter TR. Similarly, it is more efficient to incorporate a small interslice gap and take other steps to improve S/N (e.g., increase the number of excitations from two to three) than to acquire one sequence with a 100% interslice gap and repeat the sequence to cover the tissue in the gaps (concatenation).

Examination time = TR × Number of excitations
$\qquad$ × Number of phase-encoding steps

Number of slices = TR/(TE + Wait period*)

Another method of decreasing examination time is to reduce the number of phase-encoding steps. This produces rectangular voxels and accounts for a proportionate decrease in the examination time. It also compromises the in-plane spatial resolution, but this is not generally significant in routine spinal imaging. As mentioned previously, the larger voxel size compensates

---

*Varies with manufacturer.

for the decline in S/N attributable to the reduced number of sampling points along the phase-encoding gradient.

Another alternative is to center the reduced number of phase-encoding steps in the region of interest and incorporate a rectangular (asymmetric) field of view (FOV). Since surface coils will frequently include air anterior to the patient in the FOV, it is not efficient to spend time phase encoding space that contains no usable information. In these cases the FOV can be rectangular with the shorter axis oriented anteroposteriorly (Fig. 1-11). It is possible to maintain the same in-plane spatial resolution if the FOV in the phase-encoding direction is reduced proportionately to the reduction of phase-encoding steps. The examination time is reduced in proportion to the reduction in phase-encoding steps. The S/N is also reduced, and it is therefore necessary to increase the voxel size (e.g., make the in-plane voxel dimensions rectangular or increase the slice thickness) or adjust the acquisition parameters differently to compensate for the decline in S/N.

IMAGING ARTIFACTS

As discussed, many of the foregoing options may introduce artifacts in the images beyond the expected changes in spatial resolution, S/N, and/or contrast. The radiologist must be aware of these potential pitfalls and make adjustments in the pulse sequences to reduce if not eliminate them.

Truncation Artifact

If the FOV is held constant, reducing the number of phase-encoding steps shortens the examination time and increases the signal-to-noise. Beyond reducing the in-

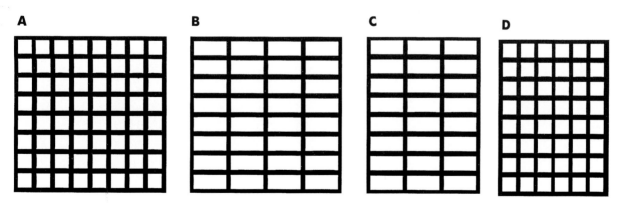

Fig. 1-11. A, Symmetric field of view with equivalent voxel dimensions in the frequency- and phase-encoding directions. **B,** Reducing the number of phase-encoding steps reduces examination time and increases the signal-to-noise but reduces in-plane spatial resolution. **C,** An asymmetric field of view eliminates the peripheral phase-encoding steps and reduces the examination time. **D,** Using square voxels in the asymmetric field of view compromises signal-to-noise because of voxel size while improving spatial resolution.

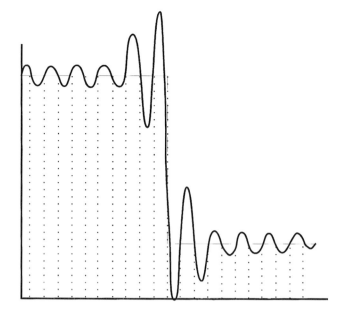

Fig. 1-12. The signal intensity in each pixel across the field of view is estimated by a series of sine and cosine waves. At the transition between two structures of high and low signal intensity, the sine integral function overshoots and undershoots the actual intensity until it eventually oscillates about the true intensity, which accounts for the ringing in the region of interface.

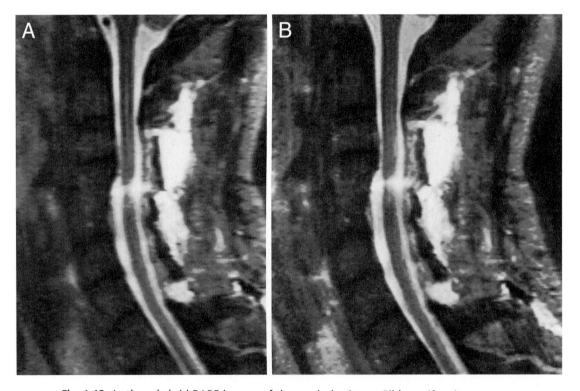

Fig. 1-13. In these hybrid RARE images of the cervical spine, a Gibbs artifact is represented by the *vertical linear band* paralleling the ventral surface of the cord in the image obtained with a 128×256 matrix, **A,** but much less apparent when the pixel dimensions in the phase-encoding direction (anterior-posterior) are reduced by incorporating a 256×256 matrix, **B.** The focal hyperintensity in the cord was due to metal artifact in this postoperative patient.

plane spatial resolution, larger voxels typically make the truncation artifact appear more obvious along interfaces perpendicular to the phase-encoding direction.[21-23] Effective spinal imaging relies on accurately visualizing various interfaces, and contrast between adjacent structures must be accentuated; it is along these linear contrasting interfaces that the truncation artifact is most obvious. Whereas the Fourier transform translates the two-dimensional MR signal into a finite number of sinusoidal components of different frequencies, the edge definition at tissue interfaces is composed of an infinite number of frequency components. Since the MR signal is incompletely sampled (truncated), edges cannot be precisely represented by the Fourier transform. The sum of the sampled sinusoidal waveforms is the sine integral function, which will overshoot and undershoot the actual intensities at regular intervals (integral multiples of the voxel dimension) on both sides of the interface. This oscillatory function decays and normalizes to the actual intensity with increasing distance from the interface (Fig. 1-12). The peaks and valleys of the integral function account for the lines of high and low intensity that parallel the interface and become less conspicuous with increasing distance from the interface. In a strict sense *Gibbs artifact* refers to the initial overshoot or undershoot on either side of the interface. In practice the term is generally applied to all overshoots and undershoots.

On sagittal and axial images the phase-encoding axis is typically oriented anteroposteriorly so the spinal cord is perpendicular to the phase-encoding direction. The truncation artifact is most commonly seen as a linear focus in the cord that parallels the ventral aspect of the cord and mimics syringohydromyelia (Fig. 1-13). It is most obvious in myelogram-like images because there is a large discrepancy in signal intensities between the bright CSF and low-intensity cord. Hence, the initial overshoot (9% of the difference in signal intensities) or Gibbs artifact is more noticeable, as are the adjacent parallel lines. This artifact is also evident on T_1-weighted images but less obvious (and hypointense) because there is a smaller difference in signal intensity between spinal cord and CSF than on the myelogram-like images. On axial myelogram-like images of the spine the phase-encoding direction is typically oriented anteroposteriorly so the truncation appears as bright line(s) in the spinal cord paralleling the ventral surface of the cord (Fig. 1-14).

A "ringing" appearance may also be seen along interfaces that are perpendicular to the frequency-encoding direction (e.g., lateral surface of the cord on an axial image). This is also a truncation artifact, but it is less obvious in the frequency-encoding direction if the resolution in this direction is higher than in the phase-encoding direction. It is generally less apparent since no additional examination time is needed to acquire more data points

in the frequency-encoding direction; thus the voxel dimensions are typically smaller along this axis. Ringing is usually seen in low-bandwidth sequences (long readout periods), which are positioned asymmetrically about the echo time in an effort to take advantage of a short TE as well as a low BW. When the center of the readout period is so shifted as to be more than 25% asym-

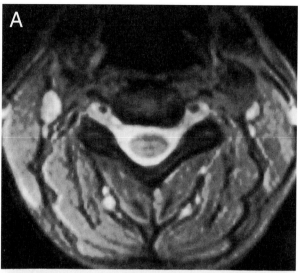

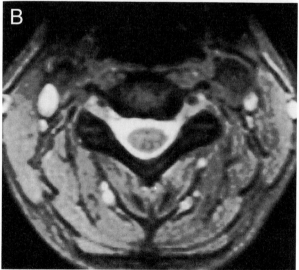

Fig. 1-14. Axial low–flip angle gradient echo images of the cervical spine with the phase-encoding direction oriented anteroposteriorly, **A,** and right to left, **B.** When the phase-encoding direction is perpendicular to the ventral surface of the cord and the same window and center for the images are used, a parallel bright line is evident within the cord and the margins are somewhat ill defined. Swapping the gradients decreases the voxel dimensions in the phase-encoding direction, eliminates the linear focus in the cord, and causes the entire cord to appear larger since the margins are no longer blurred.

metric, the ringing artifact becomes intolerable and one must then introduce half-Fourier reconstruction in the read direction to suppress it. The manufacturers take this into account when designing the short TE sequences, which limit the degree of asymmetry and minimize this problem.

Because it is not possible to sample data infinitely in the phase- and frequency-encoding directions, it is not really possible to eliminate the truncation artifact altogether. Even if infinite sampling were possible, the ringing would be effectively suppressed but the initial peak or Gibbs artifact would not be eliminated. It is possible, however, to reduce the conspicuousness of this artifact by reducing the voxel size along the phase-encoding (and frequency-encoding) direction either by reducing the FOV or increasing the matrix size. In either case the peaks are compressed into smaller voxels and therefore less obvious. If there are fewer points along the phase-encoding direction, switching the orientation of the frequency- and phase-encoding directions will have a similar effect on the artifact, because the voxel length will be reduced along the phase-encoding direction. Alternatively, filtering the raw data with a high-frequency filter (e.g., Hamming) will reduce the ringing, but not eliminate the Gibbs artifact, and will blur the normal interfaces since the high-frequency data lines are responsible for the edge definition in an image.[24,25]

The same artifact can broaden the interfaces and make the spinal cord appear fictitiously small in its anteroposterior dimensions, especially if there is strong contrast between the two adjacent tissues.[22,23] In a plot of intensity versus distance the sine integral function at the interface must slope up or down to some extent from one intensity to the other, and this sloping extends across one voxel in the phase-encoding direction. Again, reducing voxel dimensions in the phase-encoding direction will suppress the problem since the sloping line is now condensed into a smaller space. When the line is more vertical, the high-contrast edge is more sharply defined and the dimensions of the structure (e.g., spinal cord) are more correct (Fig. 1-14).

Aliasing

When the FOV is reduced to decrease the in-plane voxel dimensions, it must be remembered that this may be detrimental since it can introduce the problem of aliasing, wraparound, or overfolding. The same problem may be encountered when a rectangular FOV is used that is too small relative to the amount of tissue excited and detectable by the coil (Fig. 1-15). Aliasing may actually occur along the phase- and frequency-encoding axes in 2DFT imaging and along all three axes in three-dimensional imaging. Any spins excited by the RF pulses in the imaging sequence and detectable by the surface coil will be assigned a spatial location along the im-

aging gradients. Whenever the body coil is used as a transmitter (all currently available surface coils), a considerable amount of tissue may be excited along the imaging plane but outside the chosen FOV and beyond the physical limits of the surface coil. Tissues within the FOV assume positions in the image based on their individual phases and frequencies. Excited tissue outside the FOV will lie at higher spatial frequencies than the defined sampling interval. Since these frequencies are inadequately sampled and the signal from these tissues can still be detected by the coil, the peripheral tissues will be assigned phases or frequencies identical to those of tissues in the FOV and will therefore appear in the image. Ideally a surface coil with a well-defined sensitive volume will not detect signal from the peripheral tissues. Practically the coils are not constructed that precisely. One strategy to remedy the problem is simply to increase the FOV until the aliasing is eliminated. Alternatively,

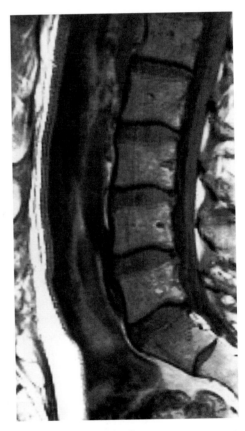

Fig. 1-15. There is prominent wraparound or aliasing, because one quarter of the phase-encoding steps were eliminated at each end to produce the rectangular field of view. When the length of the field of view in the phase-encoding direction is two thirds to three quarters that of the frequency-encoding direction, the aliasing should be reduced if not eliminated (depending on the patient's body habitus).

a commonly used strategy is to oversample the data (in the frequency- and phase-encoding directions) or acquire additional data at either end of the imaging gradients and then ignore this extra information at the time of image reconstruction. If aliasing still occurs, the redundant data are likely in those segments that were "trimmed off" before reconstruction and will not affect the final image. The acquisition of more data points along the frequency-encoding direction is effectively free, for it does not demand additional acquisition time, and some manufacturers automatically incorporate oversampling along this direction in all pulse sequences. Whereas oversampling is also possible in the phase-encoding direction, the examination time will increase proportionately. A corresponding reduction in the number of excitations will compensate for the increased examination time without affecting S/N. For example, increasing the phase-encoding steps from 256 to 512 and reducing the number of excitations from two to one will eliminate the overfolding, maintain the same S/N, and hold the examination time constant. Nevertheless, if there is physiologic motion in the region to be studied (e.g., CSF pulsations), the motion artifact in the image may be worse since the signal averaging that occurs with multiple excitations is reduced or eliminated.

Motion Artifact

Motion artifact presents a significant problem in routine spinal imaging, whether it arises from moving tissues outside the spine or from CSF pulsations. When the motion is periodic or nearly periodic, the moving tissues give rise to coherent ghosts that are produced across the image in the phase-encoding direction and obscure not only the moving tissue itself but also any other tissues through which the artifact is reflected. The regular motion causes view-to-view variation in both the average phase angle and the magnitude of signal from these voxels. The signal intensity adds coherently, but the net phase is shifted, which accounts for the mismapping across images.[26-29] The intensity of the moving tissue is reduced at its true location, and this signal is mismapped elsewhere as ghosts of the moving structure. Whereas the intensity of the artifact is dependent on the signal intensity of the moving structure and the amplitude of its motion, the absolute distance between ghosts varies with the frequency of motion, the time interval between phase-encoding steps, and the FOV in that direction. When the tissues move in a more random or aperiodic fashion, the resultant ghosting is less coherent and gives rise to a smeared appearance. Beyond the view-to-view variation, there is significant CSF motion within a single TR interval (between the initial RF pulse and the readout period) that causes intravoxel phase dispersion, ghosting, and blurring. Strategies have been implemented to suppress this artifact, which is due to motion

between the TR intervals and/or within the intervals.

If the tissues causing the motion artifact are outside the spine (regardless of the motion timing), the artifact is most effectively suppressed with saturation pulses.[29,30] Saturation pulses are spatially selective RF pulses that can be applied to any pulse sequence in any orientation to eliminate the signal from tissues causing the artifact (Fig. 1-16). The inherent inhomogeneity of a surface coil detects less signal from tissues moving anteriorly (e.g., anterior abdominal wall); but if these tissues are purposely saturated, there is no remaining signal to be mismapped into the region of interest. One limitation of these specialized pulses is that the minimum TR must be increased slightly to accommodate the same number of slices since the additional RF pulse must also fit within the TR interval. It should be recalled that the extra RF pulse will increase the power deposition of the sequence (specific absorption rate or SAR) but this does not generally present a significant problem in routine clinical imaging.

Alternative strategies must be incorporated if the image artifact is due to motion in the region of interest (pulsatile CSF). Motion artifact contributes to the overall

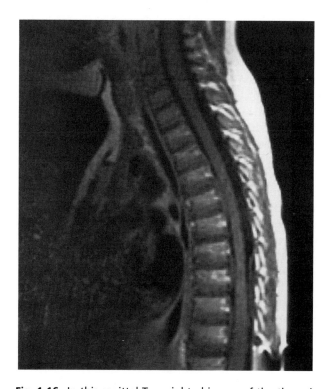

Fig. 1-16. In this sagittal T$_1$-weighted image of the thoracic spine the beating heart causes ghosting, which is reflected along the phase-encoding direction through the spinal canal. If a coronally oriented saturation pulse had been applied to cover the heart, the moving tissue would have had no signal and thus could not have been mismapped through the spine.

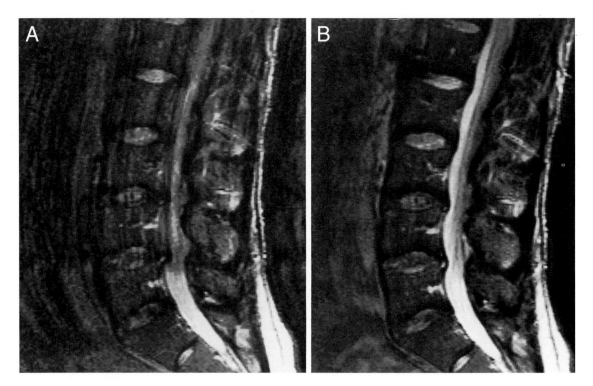

Fig. 1-17. Without flow-compensating gradients, **A,** the pulsatile CSF causes severe ghosting in the (anterior-posterior) phase-encoding direction and signal loss in the spinal canal, even in the lumbosacral region. These problems are essentially eliminated with the addition of flow compensating gradients, **B,** to the T_2-weighted pulse sequence.

noise in an image. Signal averaging (multiple acquisitions of each phase-encoding step) will reduce the inherent image noise by the square root of the number of acquisitions as well as reduce the signal intensity of the ghosts to the same degree by destructive interference or cancellation of the ghosts.[31] If the TR is shortened to make this more time efficient, there will be obvious consequences in contrast, S/N, and number of slices attainable.

Shortening the TE will also reduce the motion-related noise without compromising examination time. Whereas signal averaging serves to suppress the motion that occurs between TR intervals, the shorter TE suppresses all motion within a single TR interval (from the time of the initial RF pulse to the time of the readout period). The shorter echo time merely permits less time for intravoxel phase dispersion due to the pulsatile CSF, which in turn, limits the corresponding ghosting and signal loss. Beyond this, the short TE enhances T_1 and spin-density contrast; and it is also possible that it can increase the number of slices that might be obtained in a fixed TR interval.

The short echo times are sufficient to avoid motion artifacts in T_1 imaging of the spine since the CSF has a low signal intensity (long T_1 relaxation time) and therefore cannot cause significant motion artifact. In any pulse sequence that produces higher-intensity CSF (e.g., low–flip angle gradient echo, high–flip angle FISP/GRASS,* spin density), motion artifacts will be obvious without additional motion suppression schemes. Contrast considerations will prohibit significant reductions in the echo time for T_2-weighted spin-echo imaging. This has led to the use of flow-compensating gradients, which are typically incorporated in the read and slice-select directions to suppress or eliminate the motion artifact[32,33] (Fig. 1-17). These additional gradients compensate for the phase dispersion due to constant-velocity flow (first-order motion) of the CSF within the TE interval. This will reduce the ghosting and motion-induced spin dephasing (signal loss) but will have no effect on the blurring related to motion during the readout period (on-time for the analog-to-digital converter). The bipolar gradients do not alter the phase of the spins in stationary tissues, and they effectively reverse the phase shift of moving spins so their phase is zero at the time of the

---

*FISP, fast imaging with steady-state precession; GRASS, gradient recalled acquisition in the steady state.

echo (identical to stationary tissue). It is possible to compensate for higher orders of motion (e.g., acceleration); practically, however, there is little or no appreciable benefit in image quality, and this may make the motion artifact worse because of the necessarily longer TEs. It is also possible to compensate for velocity in the phase-encoding direction; but this, likewise, provides little if any noticeable improvement in the residual motion artifacts.

In cervical and thoracic spinal imaging the flow-compensating gradients may not be sufficient to eliminate flow artifacts. Not infrequently there are residual rounded or patchy areas of signal loss ventral or dorsal to the cord on T_2-weighted images (Fig. 1-18). This residual phase dispersion may relate to higher-order motion and pulsation of the CSF interacting with the dentate ligaments, dorsal and ventral nerve roots, and dorsal arachnoid septations.[34] Similarly, normal CSF motion may be altered by spinal pathology (e.g., large osteophytes) and the resultant complex motion will not be corrected by the flow-compensating gradients, which correct only for the phase dispersion caused by first-order motion. In cases with residual motion-induced signal loss and ghosting it may also be helpful to incorporate cardiac triggering or gating to synchronize the motion with the cardiac pulsations (which ultimately cause the CSF movement).[35,36] With no significant variation in the length of the cardiac cycle during an examination the data lines for each slice are obtained at a similar point in the cardiac cycle so the view-to-view variation is suppressed. In cardiac triggering the application of an RF pulse and the subsequent data acquisition begin after a user-defined delay from the R-wave on the ECG tracing. In cardiac gating the RF pulsing is constant but the data are acquired only within a preselected window during the cardiac cycle. Consequently the TR will vary with the heart rate in triggering whereas the TR will be constant in cardiac gating. These definitions vary with the manufacturer: some refer to prospective gating as "triggering" and to retrospective cardiac gating (continuous data and ECG acquisition with data lines that are correlated with the cardiac cycle during postprocessing) as "gating." Neither triggering nor gating is incorporated on a routine basis, since the gradient refocusing pulses are generally quite effective for suppressing motion artifact and, more important, both cardiac triggering and gating can significantly prolong the overall acquisition time (especially in a patient with a relatively slow heart rate).

The only other commonly encountered flow artifact that has not yet been discussed is flow-related enhancement. In the spine this is typically seen in the first and last slices of an axial acquisition. Fresh unsaturated spins wash into the end slices during each TR interval (view-

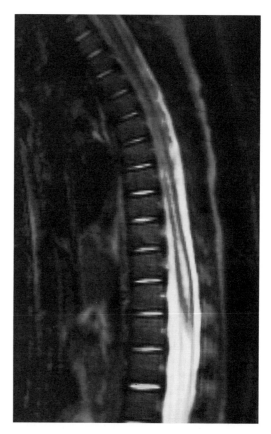

Fig. 1-18. In this sagittal T_2-weighted image there is a linear area of signal loss ventral to the cord with elliptical areas of low signal dorsal to the upper thoracic cord despite the flow compensation gradients. The central hyperintensity within the cord represents syringohydromyelia in this child.

to-view variation) as a result of the bidirectional, pulsatile, through-plane flow (Fig. 1-19). The TR does not allow the spins within the volume of excitation to relax fully, and they therefore become somewhat saturated relative to the CSF originating outside the imaging volume, which has not experienced previous RF pulses. If the TE is relatively short, the inflowing unsaturated spins will be affected by both RF pulses of a spin-echo sequence and will have higher signal than the tissue and CSF in the imaging volume. This is even more apparent in gradient echo imaging because of the shorter echo times, and all spins in the imaging volume need experience only one RF pulse to contribute to the signal. In routine spinal imaging this artifact is most frequently seen on axial T_1-weighted images (low-intensity CSF) as irregular areas of intermediate to high signal in the spinal subarachnoid space. It can easily be mistaken for an intradural extramedullary mass if one is not aware of the potential pitfall (Fig. 1-20).

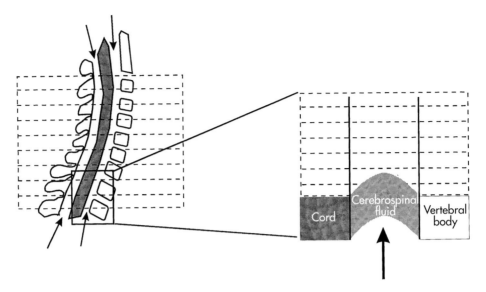

Fig. 1-19. Cerebrospinal fluid pulsates throughout the imaging volume; but the spins are relatively saturated in the middle, and the CSF (which has not been exposed to previous radiofrequency pulses) flows into the end slices during each TR period *(arrows)*. The spins therefore have a higher signal than the CSF already within the imaging volume (flow-related enhancement).

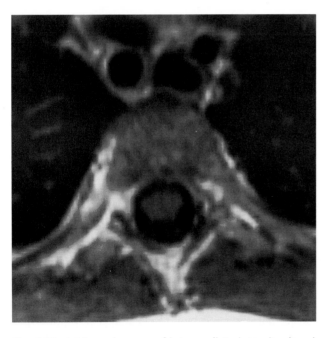

Fig. 1-20. A triangular area of intermediate intensity dorsal to the cord in the spinal subarachnoid space represents flow-related enhancement in the most superior slice of a series of axial T_1-weighted spin echo images. There was no evidence of an intradural mass on the sagittal T_1-weighted images.

Field Inhomogeneities

Another artifact to be aware of relates to distortions in the main magnetic field and in the applied gradients. Each manufacturer defines the inherent inhomogeneity of the imaging system that accounts for mild geometric distortion and signal variation in the periphery of the field. This is most noticeable at higher field strengths with a large FOV (e.g., 50 cm body coil) but is generally insignificant when using a small FOV with a surface coil. The applied gradients also tend to be somewhat nonlinear toward the edges of the gradient coil, which may cause spatial mismapping at the edges of the FOV. The patient's tissues themselves can introduce further inhomogeneities to affect the net magnetic field. A different level of magnetization is induced in each tissue, which is defined as that tissue's magnetic susceptibility. When two very different tissues are immediately apposed, they set up a localized gradient that disrupts the applied gradients to cause local image distortion or spatial misregistration and signal loss from spin dephasing. This dephasing is not recovered at all in gradient echo imaging and should be corrected by the 180-degree pulse in spin-echo imaging if the inhomogeneity is not too large. For example, bony osteophytes will typically appear larger on gradient echo images so the spinal canal or neural foramina appear narrower than on a corresponding T_1-weighted spin-echo or high-resolution axial CT image of the same region.[37] This same phenomenon accounts for the chemical shift artifact at a fat/water interface discussed earlier.

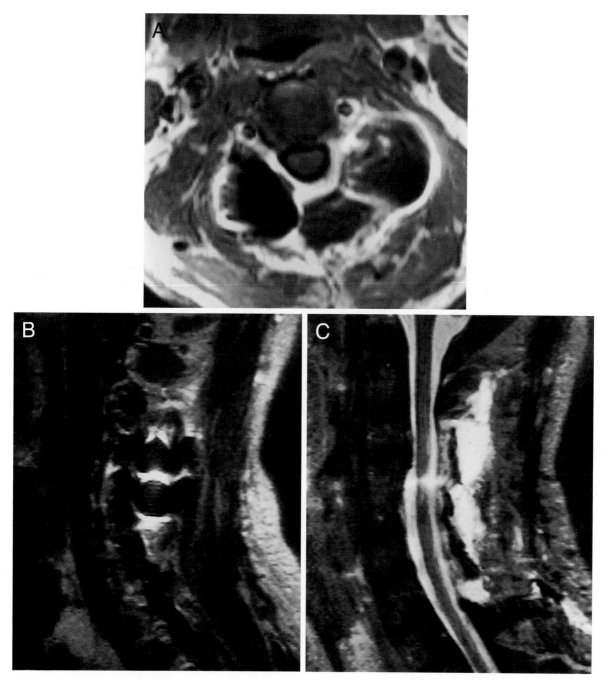

Fig. 1-21. A, Metallic screws and plates interconnecting the pedicles of two adjacent cervical vertebrae produce a prominent local field inhomogeneity. The regions of signal loss are much larger than the hardware itself, and some of the signal is compressed to the periphery as a rim of hyperintensity. **B,** The same phenomenon is evident in the sagittal hybrid RARE image. Despite the long echo time, the artifact is not that striking because of the series of 180-degree pulses applied for each echo space. A rim of hyperintensity is obvious in the parasagittal image; but, remember, the field distortion is three dimensional so the hyperintensity in the cord, **C,** represents this same phenomenon along the medial margin of the area of signal loss.

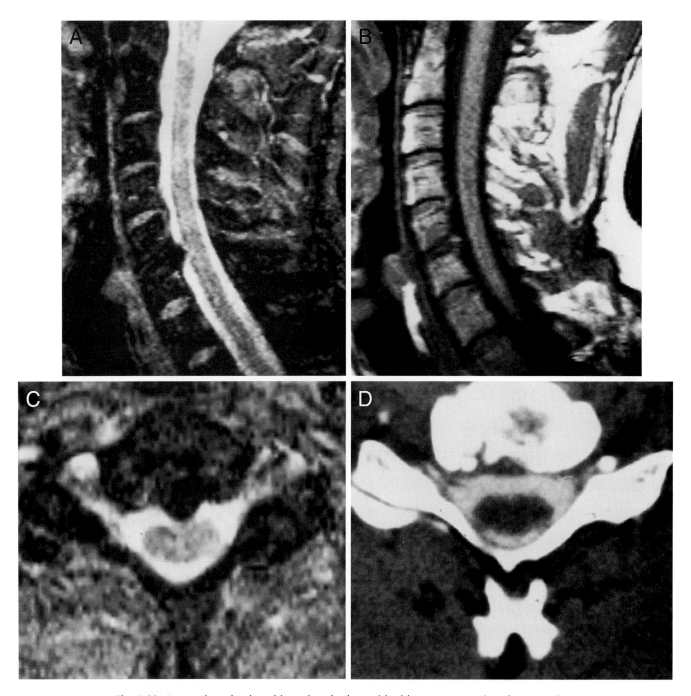

Fig. 1-22. It was thought that this patient had a residual bony spur causing the ventral extradural defect seen at the site of a previous anterior diskectomy. The local field inhomogeneities at the bone/CSF interface were thought to explain the larger apparent size on the gradient echo image, **A,** than on the spin-echo image, **B.** The extradural defect appears obvious on this three-dimensional gradient echo image, **C,** despite a 2 mm slice thickness and 7 msec TE. Since nothing was seen on the postmyelogram CT, **D,** the apparent defect was thought to be related to a small metal fragment(s) left at the site of the surgery.

The gradients are more obviously altered by ferromagnetic material within the body (e.g., stabilization plates, screws in the spine) or on the surface of the body (metallic snaps or skin staples). This metal causes a large local gradient that disrupts the imaging gradients. In the center of this region the local gradient is so strong that there is rapid spin dephasing with signal loss. The superimposed gradient is lower at the edges of the region. Along one edge an additive effect with the imaging gradient results in a localized pulling or stretched appearance of the adjacent tissues.[38] Along the opposite edge the superimposed gradient effectively reduces the imaging gradient, resulting in a peripheral rim of high signal intensity. Although this phenomenon is usually thought of in terms of its in-plane effects, the frequency selectivity of the slice-select RF pulses allows for image distortion in the slice-select direction (Fig. 1-21). In patients with a relatively large ferromagnetic implant (e.g., Harrington rod) there may be such a large amount of signal loss and image distortion that it is not possible to evaluate the region. The effect is not nearly so prominent if the implant is stainless steel instead of ferromagnetic material, and it is certainly less significant if the metal is spatially removed from the region of interest.

In a limited number of situations the presence of this artifact may even be helpful. The artifact can identify the site of the previous surgery by the focal signal loss due to metallic fragments of the drill bit,[39] distinguish the hypointense mass in the spinal subarachnoid space as air from a recent lumbar puncture, identify the hypointense extradural mass as a calcified disk fragment, or localize a focus of hemorrhage in the spinal cord at the site of an intramedullary mass. If the situation presents a problem on the scout images, certain adjustments can be incorporated into the sequences to limit the conspicuousness of the artifact—including use of high-bandwidth readout gradients, short echo times without resorting to partial Fourier reconstruction in the frequency-encoding direction, small voxels, and spin-echo instead of gradient echo sequences.[40] Because the local field inhomogeneities from tissues and implants cause constant dephasing over time, the 180-degree pulse of the spin-echo sequence should largely correct the spin dephasing seen in gradient echo imaging. If the echo time is reduced (especially in a gradient echo sequence), there is less time available for the inhomogeneity to impact on the spins in that immediate region, and hence less artifact. Smaller voxels will limit the problem by reducing the localized gradients per unit of tissue. Moreover, there will be less variation of phase across an individual voxel, merely because of its smaller size. This combination of factors accounts for more signal per unit of tissue and less image distortion (Fig. 1-22).

Data Handling

A separate group of artifacts not infrequently is seen in clinical imaging because of errors in the way the data are handled once acquired or because of the detection of extraneous signal by the receiver. Occasionally, images will have limited contrast and the FOV will be largely obscured by bandlike regions of prominent hyperintensity; it is then difficult to adjust the window and center of the images for filming (Fig. 1-23). This is the typical picture of data overflow, and it occurs when the receiver circuit converting the analog data to the digital image is saturated (e.g., when a relatively obese patient is scanned immediately after a small child). The normal automatic adjustment processes for the receiver set the attenuation values too high. Since this affects primarily the lower phase-encoding steps (data lines where the signal is greatest) and it is these data lines that primarily determine contrast, the contrast is severely impaired. If the sequence will not readjust itself, the easiest way to correct it is to adjust the receiver gain and image scale factor manually. Occasionally just the image scale factor for the sequence will be set inappropriately. This is but

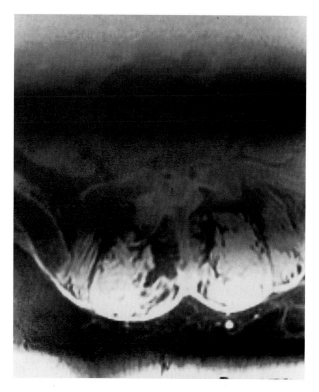

Fig. 1-23. Failure of the receiver circuit to adjust itself appropriately accounts for the data overflow, which is seen as alternating bands of hyperintensity that largely obscure the lumbar spinal canal on this axial T_1-weighted spin-echo image.

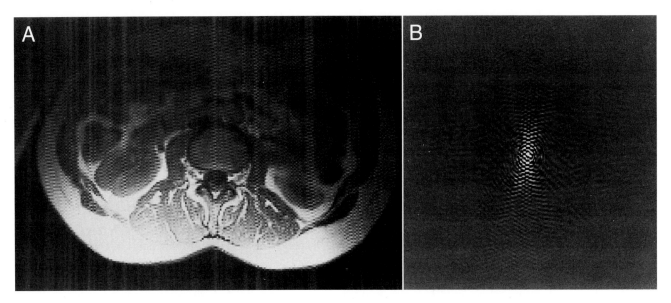

Fig. 1-24. A, Note the lines running vertically through the image. **B,** A severe artifact arises if the data spike is intense or occurs near the center of the K-space. In this case it is peripherally located (at the top of the image) but very strong.

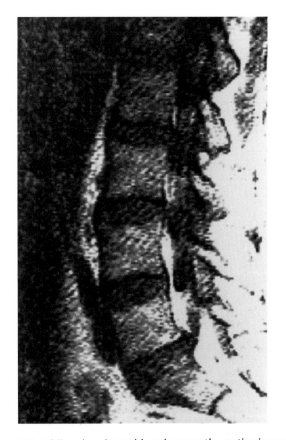

Fig. 1-25. Obliquely oriented bands cover the entire image of the lumbar spine. A malfunctioning air conditioning unit caused high humidity levels in the mobile MR unit. At the time of this image the hygrometer registered 85% humidity.

a multiplicative factor affecting the imaging data, so many of the pixel intensities will be set to high values. Not only will the object be more hyperintense, there will also frequently be a halo of hyperintensity surrounding the object.

When the receiver detects signal extraneous to the patient, this is generally manifested as a line or series of lines extending across the image. The data for each pixel across the image must be digitalized separately, and any data spike that occurs during this process can show up as a series of parallel lines across the entire image, giving it a corduroy appearance. The orientation of the lines is determined by the location of the data spike, and the severity of the artifact will depend on the timing of the event and intensity of the spike (Fig. 1-24). Such a digitalization error can arise because of static electricity from a patient's blanket or high humidity in the examination room[41] (Fig. 1-25). If these factors do not explain the problem and the artifact is persistent, malfunction of the system hardware should be suspected. Extraneous data can also be detected from electrical equipment operating in the area of the MR facility or within the examination room itself and will appear on the image as a series of lines extending across the FOV parallel to the frequency-encoding direction. The location in the FOV is dependent on the frequency at which the equipment is operating. This artifact can be diffuse if the electrical equipment operates both over a broad frequency range and throughout the acquisition (Fig. 1-26). It will be accentuated if the door of the MR facility is not closed during the scan or the RF shielding is in need of repair, if the patient is relatively tall (and thus serves as an effective antenna), if the line for the monitoring device extends out the magnet bore in such a way that it serves as an antenna and picks up extraneous signal, or if the machine itself is a high-field system.[41] The problem can be suppressed or eliminated by moving or shielding the equipment near the MR examination room, repairing the RF shielding in the examination room, using MR-compatible patient monitoring equipment (e.g., a pulse oximeter with fiber-optic technology), or repositioning the line for the monitoring device.

The aforementioned lines across the image should be distinguished from central artifacts, which have different underlying causes. Occasionally a central line will arise at the zero phase-encoding line parallel to the frequency-encoding axis. The tissue at the periphery of the two-dimensional slices is not excited by the expected 180-degree flip angle due to nonideal slice profiles of the RF pulses. As a result, these spins are influenced by intermediate flip angles, which cause a free induction decay in the case of a single echo sequence and stimulated echoes in the case of a multiecho sequence. The residual longitudinal magnetization of these spins is not typically phase encoded, thereby accounting for the central band of hyperintensity at the zero phase-encoding line. This artifact is determined primarily by the structure of the sequence. If an alternative sequence is not available, the artifact can be reduced by increasing the interslice gap or using an even number of acquisitions (excitations). A broader band can occur along the same direction in certain gradient echo imagings. FLASH (fast low-angle shot) imaging maintains only the equilibrium of longitudinal magnetization and purposely destroys any residual transverse magnetization.[42] With very short TRs and/or tissues with relatively long T_1 relaxation times the residual phase of the spins may not be effectively dispersed by the phase-encoding gradient in the center of the FOV (lowest phase-encoding steps), resulting in a bandlike area of hyperintensity. This artifact is suppressed by the routine incorporation of variable amplitude (or duration) gradient spoiler pulses after the readout period and before the next excitation pulse. RF spoiling has proved to be even more effective and can eliminate the artifact altogether.

SPECIALIZED TECHNIQUES
Hybrid RARE Imaging

T_2-weighted spin-echo imaging is generally the most time-consuming sequence in routine clinical examinations. Hybrid RARE (rapid acquisition with relaxation enhancement) or fast spin-echo imaging was introduced to shorten examination times while providing similar image quality and contrast[2-4] (Fig. 1-27). Consequently, it has effectively replaced the low-to-intermediate–flip-angle gradient echo imaging of the spine routinely used to create myelogram-like images. Conventional spin-echo imaging acquires one data line per TR interval and is quite a lengthy examination because of the long repetition times necessary for T_2-weighted imaging. By contrast, hybrid RARE imaging acquires multiple data lines per excitation and the acquisition time is reduced nearly in proportion to this value. A 90-degree RF pulse initially excites the spins, which are then exposed to a series of 180-degree pulses to refocus multiple echoes (echo train) separated by a predetermined delay time or interecho spacing. The data in each echo of the echo train are collected at a different phase-encoding step. Because the central data lines are primarily responsible for the contrast in the image, they are collected at about the chosen effective echo time for the sequence and the higher frequency data lines are collected at the other echo intervals. For example, in a double echo sequence with an interecho spacing of 18 msec, an echo train of 8, and effective echo times of 18 and 90 msec, the data for the first echo image are collected at 18, 36, 54, and 72 msec while data for the second echo image are collected at 90, 108, 126, and 144 msec. The central 25% of the data lines would be preferentially collected at 18 and 90 msec for the first and second echo images respectively.

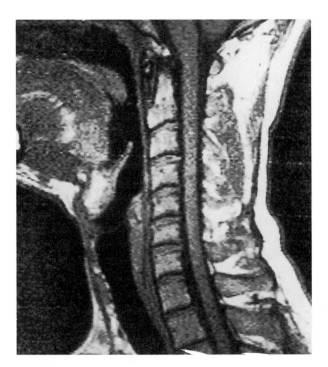

Fig. 1-26. An older pulse oximeter was monitoring the patient during the acquisition of this sagittal T_1-weighted image of the cervical spine. The extraneous radiofrequency signal is detected as several distinct horizontal lines as well as diffuse interference throughout the image, reminiscent of poor signal-to-noise.

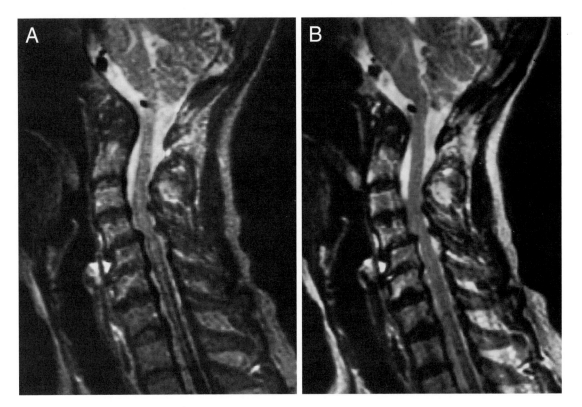

Fig. 1-27. Comparison of a conventional spin-echo image, **A,** and a hybrid RARE image, **B,** in a patient with severe cervical spondylosis. At the same effective echo time (90 msec) the contrast between tissues is similar, although the fat is more hyperintense in the hybrid RARE image. The S/N in the hybrid RARE study is higher, probably because of the discrepancy in number of acquisitions (two vs one).

Beyond the obvious advantage in time, using multiple 180-degree pulses provides for a certain amount of motion compensation, reduced susceptibility artifact due to local field inhomogeneities (e.g., less signal loss in the region of a metallic implant), and higher signal from fat on the late echo image compared to the conventional pulse sequence (Fig. 1-27). The sequence also introduces some edge enhancement in T_2-weighted images and a component of natural magnetization transfer contrast.[43] The motion artifact, however, is not completely eliminated, which has led some manufacturers to add motion-compensating gradients to suppress it further. In addition, the sampling of data lines at different times across the K-space introduces a new variable to be considered—T_2 filtering. This phenomenon accounts for the edge enhancement of T_2 contrast images but causes diffuse blurring of spin density images, even in the absence of motion. T_2 filtering varies somewhat spatially, since it is dependent on the T_2 of the tissue (being most severe with short-T_2 tissues). The blurring is especially evident on the first echo image because T_2 decay is exponential over time, causing a greater variation in signal sampled at the earlier echo times than at later echo times

(Fig. 1-28). Additionally, the collection of higher spatial frequencies at the later echo times suppresses these data in a manner similar to the way the Hamming filter does. The T_2 filtering is accentuated, with longer echo trains, longer interecho spacing, and later effective echo times.[44] The best way to reduce this artifact while maintaining the significant time advantage over conventional spin-echo sequences is to incorporate shorter interecho spacing. To date, the interecho spacing has been reduced to 6 msec; but this has been possible only at the expense of suboptimal slice profile, larger minimum slice thickness, increased signal bandwidth, and greater power deposition for a given TR.[45]

The contrast is also somewhat different from that of conventional T_2-weighted spin-echo sequences. A longer repetition time would be helpful to increase the number of slices possible for a given echo train, but this would introduce stronger T_2 contrast. The T_2 influence is also accentuated by collecting data at echo times later than the effective echo time (even though only the higher frequency data lines are collected at these alternative echo times). This compromise in image contrast is most apparent on spin density images because the CSF may be-

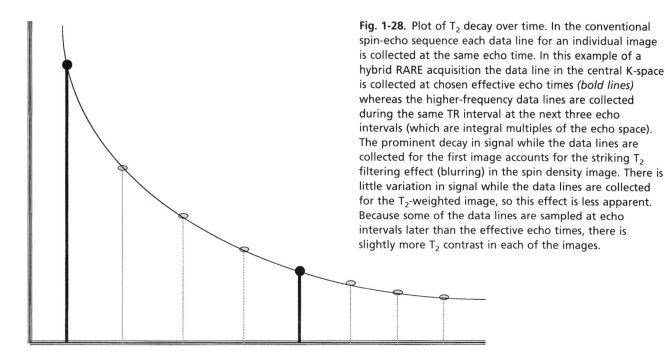

Fig. 1-28. Plot of T_2 decay over time. In the conventional spin-echo sequence each data line for an individual image is collected at the same echo time. In this example of a hybrid RARE acquisition the data line in the central K-space is collected at chosen effective echo times *(bold lines)* whereas the higher-frequency data lines are collected during the same TR interval at the next three echo intervals (which are integral multiples of the echo space). The prominent decay in signal while the data lines are collected for the first image accounts for the striking T_2 filtering effect (blurring) in the spin density image. There is little variation in signal while the data lines are collected for the T_2-weighted image, so this effect is less apparent. Because some of the data lines are sampled at echo intervals later than the effective echo times, there is slightly more T_2 contrast in each of the images.

come bright, thereby limiting the detection of an intramedullary lesion at the periphery of the spinal cord. As a result some investigators now acquire a single echo sequence with a shorter TR (e.g., 2000 msec) to ensure contrast that will more nearly approximate the contrast of conventional spin density images (since a large number of slices is not necessary to cover the spine sagittally). A longer TR is used for the T_2-weighted images to enhance the T_2 contrast and permit more data lines to be acquired per TR interval (shorter examination time).

Three-Dimensional Gradient Echo Imaging

Compared to computed tomography, two-dimensional (2D) MR imaging is limited in terms of minimum slice thickness and the need for an interslice gap to maintain adequate S/N in the images. In three-dimensional (3D) imaging a large slab of tissue is excited and a second phase-encoding gradient is added in the slice-select direction to define the individual slices within the larger slab. The relatively long TRs of spin-echo imaging would make examination times prohibitively long, so these studies are performed only with the much shorter TRs of gradient echo sequences. Since the entire slab of tissue is excited during each TR interval and the number of excitations of that volume is increased by the number of slices in the overall volume (number of points along the second phase-encoding gradient), there is a proportionate increase in the S/N compared to 2D gradient echo images with the same slice thickness. The phase-encoding gradient used to define the slices not only eliminates the interslice gaps that would normally separate

2D slices but also provides for slice profiles that are more nearly rectangular than in 2D imaging. Finally, the relatively large slab of tissue excited with each RF pulse places lower demands on the slice-select gradient, which can be exploited to incorporate shorter echo times in the 3D sequences. Compared to conventional 2D gradient echo imaging, this combination of factors permits thin contiguous slices with higher through-plane spatial resolution, higher S/N, less difficulty due to volume averaging problems, and less motion artifact and artifact related to local field inhomogeneities.

Since 3D imaging permits high resolution in all three directions, it provides the capability of reconstructing the data along planes that are different from the original plane of acquisition. When this is attempted with 2D images, the thick slices and interslice gaps demand such a large amount of interpolation by the reconstruction algorithm that the reconstructed images are blurred and the physical dimensions distorted. If the 3D imaging parameters are chosen so the imaging voxels are isotropic (equal dimensions in all three planes) or nearly isotropic, the reconstructed images should be identical in quality to the original data. Currently reconstruction algorithms provide good-quality reconstructions so long as one voxel dimension is less than twice the length of the other two dimensions. Ideally, if the physical dimensions in the reconstructed images are important clinically, the dimensions of the voxels should be identical. Not infrequently, however, the data are acquired anisotropically to reduce imaging time and improve the S/N.

Although the profile of the individual 3D slices is significantly better than in 2D imaging, the 3D technique is somewhat limited by the profiles of the selective RF pulses defining the large slabs. Whenever a large slab is excited, the flip angle will fall off in the peripheral slices, which obviously compromises the contrast and S/N in these regions. In addition, the RF pulses may excite tissue outside the chosen volume because the slice profile is not truly rectangular. Since there is now a phase-encoding gradient in the slice-select direction, this tissue may now be aliased into the peripheral slices at the opposite ends of the volume, thereby reducing the number of clinically useful slices in the volume. The second phase-encoding gradient also means that motion artifacts will be reflected along the in-plane and slice-select phase-encoding gradients and truncation artifact will be a problem in a second direction. All these factors must be taken into consideration when choosing the sequence parameters and the size and orientation of the volume.

Because of the high demands for spatial resolution, 3D imaging has been used most frequently in cervical spinal examinations.[46-48] It has also been attempted in the thoracic and lumbar regions, but high spatial resolution is not as necessary here and the existing surface coils cannot routinely provide the S/N necessary for the relatively small voxels in 3D imaging. For the cervical spine, axial low–flip angle gradient echo images are routinely used to complement sagittal T_1-weighted spin-echo and 2D sagittal hybrid RARE images. The myelogram-like images increase the conspicuousness of extradural disease impinging on the spinal canal and demonstrate the nerve root sleeves much better than axial T_1-weighted spin-echo images do. Because there is very little epidural fat to provide contrast between bone and the CSF space in the cervical spine, T_1 images are limited not only by spatial resolution but also by contrast.

The low flip angle for excitation in gradient echo imaging accounts for the high-intensity myelogram-like images but is still somewhat limiting in terms of S/N. In the low–flip angle range (below the optimum flip angle or Ernst angle for the given tissue and TR) the S/N increases almost linearly with the flip angle. Whereas it would be preferable to use a flip angle higher than the conventional 5 to 10 degrees, the CSF intensity changes too dramatically with small increments in the flip angle to allow it.

High flip angles (e.g., 70 degrees) may be used with conventional 3D FISP or GRASS sequences to produce high-intensity CSF if there is little or no CSF motion. Despite flow-compensating gradients, CSF motion occurs between the time of the echo and the application of the next RF pulse. This disrupts the steady-state equilibrium necessary to maintain the high intensity of the CSF. The gradient structure of true FISP is perfectly balanced over each TR interval to compensate for this motion and maintain the steady-state equilibrium.[48] However, the balanced gradients make the contrast dependent on local field inhomogeneities, which introduces bandlike areas of signal loss extending across the image. It is possible to overcome these difficulties by using consecutive 3D sequences performed with 180-degree phase-alternated and non–phase-alternated RF pulses. Through postprocessing, the data of these two 3D sequences are compared on a pixel-by-pixel basis and the pixels with the maximum intensity are used for the final image. There is such strong contrast in this image between the high-intensity CSF and the low-intensity stationary tissues that further postprocessing with a maximum intensity projection algorithm may be incorporated to produce a 3D myelogram that can be viewed on rotating axes[49] (Fig. 1-29).

If the 3D technique is performed with an intermediate flip angle using a FLASH* (or spoiled GRASS) technique, the signal intensity of CSF will be so reduced that it appears T_1-like. This obviously reduces the contrast between bone and CSF, and the sequence has therefore been performed after the administration of intravenous gadolinium.[50] This enhances the epidural venous plexus in the neural foramina and along the dorsal aspect of the disk spaces to serve a function similar to that of epidural fat in the lumbar spine. An alternative sequence incorporates a preparatory inversion pulse, a short wait period (inversion time), and very short TRs and TEs in a FLASH sequence. A single data line for each of the slice-select phase-encoding steps in the volume is acquired after each preparatory pulse.[51] This variation on the standard 3D technique makes it possible to acquire many more 3D slices in a shorter period and to increase the S/N for each of the slices (more phase-encoding steps in the slice-select direction). Although this sequence provides a stronger T_1 contrast than standard FLASH imaging, the preparatory inversion pulse and inversion time do not appear to be necessary in the evaluation of degenerative disk disease and the contrast will be similar if it is performed as a very fast (very low flip angle, very short TR) FLASH sequence.[52] This single sequence could potentially replace all sequences in the cervical spine since the images can be acquired axially and reformatted in the sagittal plane. Oblique images may also be reconstructed along the plane of the individual disk spaces or perpendicular to the orientation of the neural foramina to better assess bony compromise–disk compromise of the thecal sac and neural foramina.

Fat-Water Imaging

T_1-weighted spin-echo sequences have been used in routine imaging of the spine to obtain information about

---

*Fast low-angle shot.

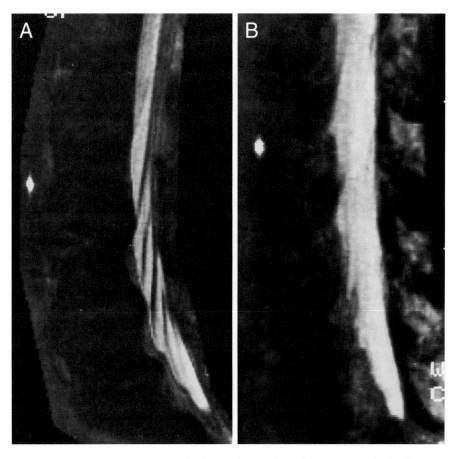

Fig. 1-29. A, The final true FISP acquisition in this patient demonstrates the high contrast between CSF, nerve roots, and extradural tissues for easy identification of extradural defects. **B,** The final data sets were submitted to a maximum-intensity projection postprocessing algorithm, which reproduced three-dimensional myelogram images that could be rotated to show the exiting nerve root sleeves.

the bone marrow. T_1 contrast is quite sensitive for the presence of infiltrative processes such as metastases of a primary malignancy, vertebral body edema in early disk space infection, and reactive changes related to degenerative disease in the adjacent intervertebral disks.[53-62] T_2-weighted imaging has been incorporated to increase the specificity of MR in the evaluation of degenerative and infectious disk disease.[58,62] In most cases of neoplastic infiltrative processes, T_2 imaging does little to increase the sensitivity or specificity of the study.[53,63] The most significant problem in the MR imaging of marrow is that the hypointensity of the marrow compartment on T_1-weighted images indicates only some sort of replacement process.[64-66] Although specificity continues to be a problem, investigators[67,68] have suggested that chemical shift imaging (selectively imaging the fat or water components of a tissue such as marrow) improves the ability to distinguish marrow that is primarily fat-replaced from marrow that is infiltrated by abnormal tissue (e.g., tumor cells).

Chemical shift imaging, in any form, takes advantage of the differing precession frequencies of fat and water protons in a magnetic field.[69] Based on the Larmor equation, the frequency of precession depends on the gyromagnetic ratio of the nucleus and the field strength of the system. The local magnetic field of a nucleus varies from the main magnetic field because of the local chemical environment of the nucleus. The methylene protons of fat will not process as quickly as the protons in water molecules, the actual difference being 3.3 parts per million. This translates to 220 Hz at 63 MHz (or 1.5 T) and 150 Hz at 43 MHz (or 1 T). The larger difference in frequency for these nuclei makes it easier to perform selective imaging at higher field strengths. A stronger magnet is also preferred for purposes of signal-to-noise. If only one of the two major species is represented in an image, the signal-to-noise in the final image will be decreased proportionately.

Chemical shift techniques can be divided basically into those that selectively excite the species of interest and those that selectively suppress the signal of the unwanted species.[70-76] In a water-only image the areas with tumor infiltration in the vertebrae will appear hyperintense because of their high water content whereas the normal marrow will be hypointense because of its higher fatty component (especially with increasing age). The converse is true for the fat-only images.

The *Dixon technique* or a modified version of it has been used clinically to evaluate marrow disease[67,68] in the spine. It relies on the fact that water protons precess slightly more rapidly than methylene protons of fat do. A graph of phase versus time will produce sinusoidal plots of the precessing spins. The vector sum of the phases of the fat and water spins within a voxel will be additive if two maxima overlap (in phase) and will detract from each another if the data are sampled at a different time when a maximum from water overlaps with a minimum from fat. In the Dixon technique the position of the 180-degree pulse is varied in the spin-echo sequence so the data are sampled when the spins are in phase (fat and water contributing to the signal) or out of phase (water minus fat). Addition and subtraction of the individual images will produce water and fat images. Quantitative analysis of the different images has allowed two groups of investigators[67,68] to calculate fat and water signal fractions in the marrow. The changes in relative fractions of the two components were thought to be a more sensitive indicator of tumor replacement than visual assessment of the signal intensity changes on T_1-weighted images. This was also thought to provide an objective means of following patients that would not be affected by the window and center settings for filming.

A *short time-to-inversion recovery* (STIR) sequence has been used to study bone marrow.[68] In this sequence an initial nonselective 180-degree inversion pulse is applied and a 90-degree excitation pulse is then applied after a delay period or inversion time. Since fat has a short T_1 relaxation time relative to water, the longitudinal magnetization of the fat protons will regrow more quickly and reach zero magnetization when the water spins still have a nonzero net longitudinal magnetization. If an inversion time is chosen (approximately 150 msec at 1.5 T) so the fat spins have essentially no net magnetization at the time of the 90-degree excitation pulse, the fat will have little or no transverse magnetization and hence no signal at the time of readout. Although the TE is short, the TR must be relatively long to allow complete regrowth of all spins between inversion pulses (and allow for multiple slices). The longer T_1 of the tumor infiltration will not be suppressed by this scheme, so the tumor cells remain hyperintense and well contrasted against the low-intensity (suppressed) fatty marrow. One prob-

lem described with this technique is that the size of the lesions may be exaggerated since the surrounding edema may not be distinguishable from the tumor cells.[68]

Neither of these schemes has been implemented on a routine basis since both are quite time consuming. In the Dixon technique one slice is obtained at a time and the described clinical implementation requires significant postprocessing. In STIR imaging a long TR is necessary, which increases the examination time. The sequence is especially limited at high field strengths because of the longer TRs needed as well as the greater problem with motion artifact.

A more efficient method of fat suppression utilizes a *frequency-selective RF pulse* to excite the fat protons preferentially and a subsequent spoiler gradient to dephase the spins. As a result the fat spins have no net longitudinal or transverse magnetization when the excitation pulse is applied for the conventional pulse sequence.[76] These specialized pulses are typically applied before the normal excitation pulse in a conventional sequence. They have a relatively narrow bandwidth and are offset in the frequency range; thus only the fat spins are affected while the water spins remain unchanged.

This scheme is difficult to implement in a routine clinical setting. The additional RF pulse has no special temporal relation to the subsequent 180-degree pulse of the spin-echo sequence and is therefore significantly impaired by inhomogeneities in the local and main magnetic fields.[77,78] Every imaging system has intrinsic inhomogeneities in the main magnetic field, particularly with a large FOV. These inhomogeneities can be somewhat reduced by localized shimming, but the process is time consuming and gradients set up by the local tissue inhomogeneities cannot be eliminated. Local susceptibility differences will exist at an air/soft tissue interface anterior to the spine (bowel) or a bone/soft tissue interface that cause a local distortion in the main magnetic field and will shift the resonance frequency of the spins in this region. As a result the frequency-selective pulse will not effectively saturate the intended fat protons in this region and may even preferentially suppress the water protons. Inhomogeneities in the RF will also contribute to variability of the fat suppression across the FOV. Recent developments[78-80] have introduced methods to limit the problems related to these field inhomogeneities, including a modification of the Dixon method that acquires three images (three-point Dixon technique) and a new type of RF pulse that is both spatially selective and frequency selective.

FLAIR Imaging

An appropriate inversion time can be selected to nullify the signal of fat and create water-only STIR images.

Similarly, an inversion time can be selected to nullify the signal intensity of CSF. This has recently been combined with relatively long echo times to produce T_2-like contrast without hyperintense CSF in fluid-attenuated inversion recovery (FLAIR) sequences.[81] In theory this single image appears similar to the spin density image as regards CSF signal intensity although the other tissues have a stronger T_2 influence. Since pulsatile CSF is primarily responsible for image degradation in the cervical and thoracic spine, reducing its intensity in T_2-weighted imaging can improve image quality and might even replace the conventional double echo sequence in evaluating intramedullary disease. Preliminary clinical results in the head and spine[82-84] appear promising. Use of this sequence in the head, however, is particularly limiting because of the long acquisition times and limited number of slices available despite a relatively long TR. A large number of slices is not necessary for sagittal imaging of the spine, and the acquisition time for head and spinal imaging can be markedly reduced if this strategy is combined with the hybrid RARE pulse sequences.[85] The reliability of these new pulse sequences for identifying spinal intramedullary and brain parenchymal lesions remains to be tested in a large-scale clinical trial.

CSF Flow Imaging

The same phenomena that cause motion artifact in routine spinal imaging can be exploited for the evaluation of CSF motion in the spinal canal. Preliminary studies of CSF motion using pneumoencephalography and Pantopaque myelography[86-88] provided some insight into normal CSF movement in the spine, but these were invasive studies and their information was limited. Other techniques have since been designed in MR that confirm the findings of these earlier studies and have a number of obvious advantages over them—including the absence of extraneous contrast agents (which may alter CSF dynamics), the ability to study multiple areas of the spine in different imaging planes, and the capability to make flow-velocity measurements. Studies conducted in volunteers and patients[86-91] have demonstrated the normal flow patterns within the spinal subarachnoid space. CSF movement in the spinal subarachnoid space is thought to be transmitted largely from intracranial CSF motion. The intracranial arterial compartment expands with the influx of blood and compresses the brain parenchyma to pump CSF out of the ventricular system (CSF systole). Bulk cranial flow occurs shortly thereafter (CSF diastole). However, the net flow is out of the ventricles; for CSF, which is produced in the ventricles, must be circulated throughout the neuraxis. Its ejection from the ventricles, in combination with downward movement of the brain stem, provides a pumping action that forces CSF out of the head and into the spinal canal.[92] Flow is most rapid in the cervical and upper thoracic region, faster caudally than rostrally (toward the cranium), and of increased velocity at sites of narrowing. The CSF moves caudally at a peak velocity nearly coincident with the carotid upstroke whereas the peak diastolic velocity (which is rostral) occurs after a short additional delay. These predominantly rostrocaudal movements tend to be delayed in the thoracic spine relative to the cervical spine. Flow has been found to be most prominent in the wider subarachnoid spaces (usually ventral to the cervical cord) and somewhat compartmentalized by the nerve roots, dentate ligaments, and dorsal arachnoid septations.

It is hoped that CSF flow studies can be implemented with routine spin-echo imaging of the spine to improve their specificity and possibly have an impact on patient management. For example, the presence of pulsatile or turbulent CSF within intramedullary cystic lesions should distinguish hydromyelia from posttraumatic myelomalacia. The presence of such prominent flow in the hydromyelic cavity of a symptomatic patient may predict the success of a syringopleural shunt for relieving symptoms.[91] Studying the flow patterns in syringohydromyelia may also help in understanding the mechanism of formation and growth of these cavities.

Initially flow studies[91-94] were based on the demonstration of signal loss in hyperintense CSF caused by motion or flow-related enhancement from the inflow of unsaturated spins into the imaging plane. These techniques have been replaced by others that are more reliable, more sensitive to variations in flow patterns, and more capable of making quantitative measurements.

A few investigators[95-97] have studied motion using a bolus-tracking technique that incorporates in-plane saturation band(s) to tag moving spins selectively and follow them over time to confirm the direction and measure the velocity of flow. The simplest approach is to apply a single saturation band across the FOV perpendicular to the direction of flow. The hyperintense blood/CSF then moves into the saturated region, and the distance it moves can be correlated with the time over which the images are obtained to determine the velocity of movement.[98] When a grid of saturation bands is applied across a FOV, motion within the FOV causes deformation of the grid pattern over time and this can also be quantitated.[97] The quantitative measurements may be difficult if it becomes necessary to measure movement in a very small structure relative to the FOV or the saturation band becomes somewhat ill-defined over the course of the measurement.

Phase-sensitive techniques[89,91,99-105] are more popular for measuring CSF flow since they can be made extremely sensitive to slow flow and have the capability for quantification. They are based primarily on modified gradient echo sequences synchronized with the cardiac cycle (peripheral pulse or cardiac gating/triggering), and multiple sequential images are obtained in the same plane across the cardiac cycle. Many of these methods incorporate paired or interleaved sequences in which bipolar gradients are designed with different velocity encodings along a preselected direction (e.g., rostrocaudal and caudorostral flow in the sagittal plane). When the data from corresponding pixels and points in the cardiac cycle are combined, the phase of the stationary tissue is equal to zero. Spins moving along a gradient cause a phase shift that is not corrected or is accentuated by the additional bipolar pulses. As a result there is a nonzero phase difference in pixels containing spins that are moving along the chosen direction and this phase difference is calculated to be proportionate to velocity. The strength and duration of the bipolar gradients in these sequences determine the range of velocities over which the acquisition is sensitive. If multiple images are acquired across the cardiac cycle, the variation in direction and velocity of the CSF motion in that imaging slice can be studied over time.

One variation on the phase contrast technique is Fourier velocity encoding, in which phase encoding is replaced by velocity encoding to produce velocity spectra.[101,102] Although this version has proved effective in evaluating CSF flow, the velocity resolution and in-plane spatial resolution are somewhat lower than with other methods and the in-plane resolution is only one dimensional.[101,103] Another variation uses a single gradient echo sequence in which the bipolar gradients are designed to produce a phase change that is directly proportionate to the velocity of flow.[105] The average phase change over the cardiac cycle at any point in the ventricular system is assumed to be zero and can therefore be subtracted from these data to derive final values for each pixel. (This method omits the factor of CSF production, thereby causing an 8% velocity offset relative to the mean, peak, systolic CSF velocity.) The technique also incorporates retrospective cardiac gating, which permits the acquisition of data points throughout the cardiac cycle instead of a fraction of the cycle as in conventional gating.[106] In addition, retrospective gating eliminates the error caused by eddy currents, which complicate the data from other cine phase contrast techniques.

IMAGING PROTOCOLS AND THEORY

The imaging protocols for extradural, intradural-extramedullary, and intramedullary disease are lists of suggested sequences for routine spinal imaging based on the compartment in the spine in which the pathology is suspected clinically. We recognize that individual radiologists will have their own preferences. The proposed sequences often represent a compromise between diagnostic capability and examination time. The individual

sequence parameters are designed for a field strength between 1 and 1.5 T. Adjustments may be necessary in certain sequence parameters depending on the capability of individual coils, the shorter T_1-relaxation times, and the inherently lower signal-to-noise of systems with lower field strengths.

The protocols are listed at this point in the discussion since they refer to prior explanations of the physics involved in routine MR imaging of the spine. Adjustments may be necessary to answer specialized questions (e.g., disk space infection with epidural abscess), but such refinements are discussed in later chapters of this text.

Extradural Disease

Pathology in the extradural compartment is the most common reason for requesting an MR examination of the spine. Degenerative disease accounts for the overwhelming majority of spinal disorders whereas malignancy, infection, and trauma account for a smaller (but still significant) percentage. The T_1-weighted spin-echo (T1WSE) pulse sequence is essential in all regions of the spine, primarily to demonstrate anatomy but also to provide information about the marrow space. Sagittal gradient echo imaging (e.g., FISP, GRASS*) has been used to provide additional contrast between bony structures, soft tissue, intervertebral disks, and CSF to create myelogram-like images, thereby increasing the conspicuousness of extradural defects.[1] In the past, the choice of gradient echo images over T_2-weighted spin-echo (T2WSE) images was made primarily in the interest of imaging time. Hybrid RARE† or fast spin-echo imaging can now be performed in a significantly shorter time.[2-4] Because hybrid RARE imaging can be manipulated to demonstrate strong T_2 contrast (and is not reliant on a combination of T_1 and spin density contrast as in the low–flip angle gradient echo images), it may provide more information about the vertebral body marrow, integrity of the intervertebral disks, and nature of the adjacent soft tissues.[5-10] Sagittal and axial images should have spatial resolution similar to that in axial computed tomography of the cervical and thoracic spine. Although the contrast will be high in axial T2WSE imaging, the signal-to-noise will be a limiting factor if the similar spatial resolution is maintained. Hybrid RARE or low–flip angle gradient-echo images can provide the contrast, spatial resolution, and signal-to-noise (within a reasonable examination time) that are needed in the axial examinations of the cervical and thoracic spine. Regardless of the sequence used, obtaining the same large number of axial slices as in CT would be very time consuming with MR. The sagittal images, however, iden-

---

*Fast imaging with steady-state precession. Gradient recalled acquisition in the steady state.
†Rapid acquisition with relaxation enhancement.

tify abnormal levels and limit the size of the area to be covered on the axial images. Axial T1WSE images are preferred in the lumbar spine since they have a significantly higher signal-to-noise and there is relatively more epidural fat in this region, which supplies the necessary contrast between the thecal sac and the adjacent disks or bony structures.

1. Sagittal T1WSE scout (to assess patient positioning, midline slice, and location of anterior saturation pulse to be used in each of the following sequences):

    TR 200 msec, TE 15 msec, slice 10 mm, gap 5 mm, FOV 300 mm, matrix 128×256, NEX 1

2. Sagittal T1WSE:

    TR 500 msec, TE 15 msec, slice 3 mm, gap 1.0 mm, rectangular FOV 250 mm, matrix 192×256, NEX 4

3. Sagittal hybrid RARE:

    TR 2000 msec, TE 120 msec, echo space minimum, echo train length 16, slice 4 mm, gap 2 mm, FOV 250 mm, matrix 192×256, NEX 2

4. Lumbar: Axial T1WSE

    TR 600 msec, TE 15 msec, slice 4 mm, gap 2 mm, rectangular FOV 250 mm, matrix 192×256, NEX 4

    Thoracic: Axial GRASS or FISP with flow compensation

    TR 600 msec, TE minimum, flip angle 10 degrees, slice 4 mm, gap 2 mm, rectangular FOV 250 mm, matrix 192×256, NEX 4

    Cervical: Axial 3D GRASS or FISP with flow compensation

    TR 40 msec, TE minimum, flip angle 5 degrees, slice 2 to 3 mm (64 slices), rectangular FOV 250 mm, matrix 192×256, NEX 1

Intradural-Extramedullary Disease

Pathology in the intradural-extramedullary compartment (within the thecal sac but extrinsic to the spinal cord) is far less common than extradural disease and is usually attributable to meningiomas and schwannomas or neurofibromas (and possibly to drop metastases, depending on the referral base). Since the diagnosis is based largely on clinical history, morphology, location, and presence of coexistent masses, it is important to identify the anatomy of the mass(es) with T1WSE images in the sagittal and axial planes. T2WSE images may, occasionally, be helpful but generally provide little additional information since the signal intensity characteristics of the masses in this compartment are quite variable. Enhancement with intravenous gadolinium is generally far more helpful since it increases the conspicuousness of the mass, better demonstrates the relationship of adjacent normal structures (e.g., spinal cord), may identify additional smaller masses not seen on the unenhanced images, and provides information about the vascularity of the mass to refine the differential diagnosis.

1. Sagittal T1WSE scout (to assess patient positioning, midline slice, and location of the anterior saturation pulse to be used in each of the following sequences):

    TR 200 msec, TE 15 msec, slice 10 mm, gap 5 mm, FOV 300 mm, matrix 128×256, NEX 1

2. Sagittal T1WSE:

    TR 500 msec, TE 15 msec, slice 3 mm, gap 1.0 mm, rectangular FOV 250 mm, matrix 192×256, NEX 4

3. Axial T1WSE:

    TR 600 msec, TE 15 msec, slice 4 mm, gap 2 mm, rectangular FOV 250 mm, matrix 192×256, NEX 4

4. Sagittal T1WSE with gadolinium:

    TR 500 msec, TE 15 msec, slice 3 mm, gap 1.0 mm, rectangular FOV 250 mm, matrix 192×256, NEX 4

5. Axial T1WSE with gadolinium:

    TR 600 msec, TE 14 msec, slice 4 mm, gap 2 mm, rectangular FOV 250 mm, matrix 192×256, NEX 4

Intramedullary Disease

Intramedullary disease, or a lesion within the spinal cord itself, most commonly includes entities such as demyelination, edema related to trauma or ischemic disease, vascular lesions, and neoplasms. Because it is important to localize the lesion accurately, quantify the associated cord enlargement if present, and evaluate the adjacent bony and soft tissue structures for related pathology (e.g., vertebral fracture and epidural hematoma), it is important to begin the study with a sagittal T1WSE sequence. Moreover, severe extradural disease (e.g., osteoarthritis, bony vertebral metastases) is far more common in the population as a whole and may mimic an intramedullary process clinically if there is significant cord compression. Most cord lesions will increase the water content in that region of the cord and thus be more sensitively detected by a T2WSE (or T_2-weighted hybrid RARE) study, particularly if there is no associated cord enlargement (e.g., chronic multiple sclerosis). Unless the diagnosis is obvious, the intramedullary lesion should be further characterized with intravenous gadolinium. In patients with an intramedullary neoplasm the edema and cord enlargement may be extensive despite a relatively small mass (e.g., hemangioblastoma) and gadolinium enhancement is essential to identify the site of breakdown in the spinal cord blood/brain barrier.[11,12] The diagnosis may be obvious, as in a young woman with known MS and a nonexpansile intramedullary lesion or hemorrhagic contusion at the level of an acute vertebral body fracture. In such cases it may be necessary only to confirm the presence of the lesion, evaluate for hemorrhage (in the case of a contusion), and identify the specific location within the cord at that level. This can be done with an axial gradient echo image with prolonged echo time and repetition time, low flip angle, and large voxels to increase the T_2* influence. Similarly, in a patient with a syrinx and known Chiari II malformation it is necessary only to confirm the presence and extent of the syrinx cavity with T1WSE images. If there is no known explanation for the syringohydromyelia, the patient should also be studied with T2WSE and gadolinium-enhanced T1WSE sequences to improve the sensitivity for detecting an underlying mass lesion.

1. Sagittal T1WSE scout (to assess patient positioning, midline slice, and location of anterior saturation pulse to be used in each of the following sequences):

    TR 200 msec, TE 15 msec, slice 10 mm, gap 5 mm, FOV 300 mm, matrix 128×256, NEX 1

2. Sagittal T1WSE:

    TR 500 msec, TE 15 msec, slice 3 mm, gap 1.0 mm, rectangular FOV 250 mm, matrix 192×256, NEX 4

3. Sagittal hybrid RARE (spin density and T_2 weighted):

    TR 2000, TE minimum, echo space minimum, echo train length 4, slice 4 mm, gap 2 mm, FOV 250 mm, matrix 192×256, NEX 2

    TR 2000, TE 120, echo space minimum, echo train length 16, slice 4 mm, gap 2 mm, FOV 250 mm, matrix 192×256, NEX 2

4. Sagittal T1WSE with gadolinium:

    TR 500 msec, TE 15 msec, slice 3 mm, gap 1.0 mm, rectangular FOV 250 mm, matrix 192×256, NEX 4

5. Axial T1WSE with gadolinium:

    TR 600 msec, TE 15 msec, slice 4 mm, gap 2 mm, rectangular FOV 250 mm, matrix 192×256, NEX 4

6. Optional axial GRASS or FISP with flow compensation:

    TR 600 msec, TE 20 msec, flip angle 10 degrees, slice 4 mm, gap 2 mm, rectangular FOV 250 mm, matrix 192×256, NEX 4

REFERENCES

1. Enzmann DR, Rubin JB: Cervical spine: MR imaging with a partial flip angle, gradient-refocused pulse sequence. I. General considerations and disk disease. *Radiology* 1988;166:467-472.

2. Hennig J, Nauerth A, Friedburg H: RARE imaging: a fast imaging method for clinical MR. *Magn Reson Med* 1986;3:823-833.

3. Hennig J, Friedburg H, Ott D: Fast three-dimensional imaging of cerebrospinal fluid. *Magn Reson Med* 1987;5:380-383.

4. Mulkern RV, Wong STS, Winalski C, Jolesz FA: Contrast manipulation and artifact assessment of 2D and 3D RARE sequences. *Magn Reson Imaging* 1990;8:557-566.

5. Moulopoulos LA, Varma DGK, Dimopoulos MA, et al: Multiple myeloma: spinal MR imaging in patients with untreated newly diagnosed disease. *Radiology* 1992;185:833-840.

6. Modic MT, Pavlicek W, Weinstein MA, et al: Magnetic resonance imaging of intervertebral disk disease: clinical and pulse sequence considerations. *Radiology* 1984;152:103-111.

7. Yu S, Ho PS, Sether LM, et al: Nucleus pulposus degeneration: MR imaging. *Radiology* 1987;165(P):77.

8. Haughton VM: MR imaging of the spine. *Radiology* 1988:166:297-301.

9. Yu S, Sether LA, Ho PS, et al: Tears of the anulus fibrosus: correlation between MR and pathologic findings in cadavers. *AJNR* 1988;9:367-370.

10. Modic MT, Feiglin DH, Piraino DW, et al: Vertebral osteomyelitis: assessment using MR. *Radiology* 1985;157:157-166.

11. Solomon RA, Stein BM: Unusual spinal cord enlargement related to intramedullary hemangioblastoma. *J Neurosurg* 1988;68:550-553.

12. Parizel PM, Baleriaux D, Rodesch G, et al: Gd-DTPA-enhanced MR imaging of spinal tumors. *AJNR* 1989;10:249-262.

13. Keeter S, Benator RM, Weiberg SM, Hartenberg MA: Sedation in pediatric CT: national survey of current practice. *Radiology* 1990;175:745-752.

14. Kanal E, Shellock FG: Patient monitoring during clinical MR imaging. *Radiology* 1992;185:623-629.

15. Ball WS, Bisset GS: Proper sedation essential to MR imaging in children. *Diagnost Imaging* 1990;12:108-112.

16. American Academy of Pediatrics, Committee on Drugs: Guidelines for monitoring and management of pediatric patients during and after sedation for diagnostic and therapeutic procedures. *Pediatrics* 1992;89:1110-1115.

17. American Society of Anesthesiologists, House of Delegates: *Standards for basic intraoperative monitoring. Directory of members*. Park Ridge Ill, The Society, 1992, pp 675-676.

18. Strain JD, Campbell JB, Harvey LA, Foley LC: IV Nembutal: safe sedation for children undergoing CT. *AJR* 1988;151:975-979.

19. Anderson CM, Lee R: Large FOV spine screening with 512 matrix and body coil: contrast to noise comparison with surface coil imaging. In Society of Magnetic Resonance in Medicine: *Book of abstracts*, Berkeley Calif, The Society, 1990, p 1104.

20. Smith AS, Weinstein MA, Hurst GC, et al: Intracranial chemical-shift artifacts on MR images of the brain: observations and relation to sampling bandwidth. *AJR* 1990;154:1275-1283.

21. Levy LM, DiChiro G, Brooks RA, et al: Spinal cord artifacts from truncation errors during MR imaging. *Radiology* 1988;166:479-483.

22. Czervionke LF, Czervionke JM, Daniels DL, Haughton VM: Characteristic features of MR truncation artifacts. *AJR* 1988;151:1219-1228.

23. Yousem DM, Janick PA, Atlas SW, et al: Pseudoatrophy of the spinal cord on MR images: a manifestation of the truncation artifact? *AJR* 1990;154:1069-1073.

24. Norton RH, Beer R: New apodizing functions for Fourier spectrometry. *J Opt Soc Am* 1976;66:259-264.

25. McVeigh ER, Henkelman RM, Bronskill MJ: Noise and filtration in magnetic resonance imaging. *Med Phys* 1985;122:586-591.

26. Ehman RL, McNamara MT, Brasch RC, et al: Influence of physiologic motion on the appearance of tissue in MR images. *Radiology* 1986;159:777-782.

27. Perman WH, Moran PR, Moran RA, Bernstein MA: Artifacts from pulsatile flow in MR imaging. *J Comput Assist Tomogr* 1986;10:473-483.

28. Ehman RL, Felmlee JP, Houston DS, et al: Nondispersive phase shifts caused by bulk motion and flow: significance

for MR imaging (abstr). In Society of Magnetic Resonance in Medicine: *Book of abstracts,* Berkeley Calif, The Society, 1986, vol 4, pp 1099-1100.

29. Felmlee JP, Ehman RL: Spatial presaturation: a method for suppressing flow artifacts and improving depiction of vascular anatomy in MR imaging. *Radiology* 1987;164:559-564.

30. Edelman RR, Atkinson DJ, Silver MS, et al: FRODO pulse sequences: a new means of eliminating motion, flow, and wraparound artifacts. *Radiology* 1988;166:231-236.

31. Wood ML, Henkelman RM: Suppression of respiratory motion artifacts in magnetic resonance imaging. *Med Phys* 1986;13:794-805.

32. Moran PR: A flow velocity zeugmatographic interlace for NMR imaging in humans. *Magn Reson Imaging* 1982;1:197-203.

33. Haacke EM, Lenz GW: Improving MR image quality in the presence of motion by using rephasing gradients. *AJR* 1987;148:1251-1258.

34. Lenz GW, Haacke EM, White RD: Retrospective cardiac gating: a review of technical aspects and future directions. *Magn Reson Imaging* 1989;7:445-455.

35. White RD, VanRossum AC: Introduction to the use of magnetic resonance imaging. In Elliott LP (ed): *Cardiac imaging in infants, children, and adults.* Philadelphia, Lippincott, 1991, pp 63-83.

36. Enzmann DR, Pelc NJ: Normal flow patterns of intracranial and spinal cerebrospinal fluid defined with phase-contrast cine MR imaging. *Radiology* 1991;178:467-474.

37. Tsuruda JS, Remley K: Effects of magnetic susceptibility artifacts and motion in evaluation the cervical neural foramina on 3DFT gradient-echo MR imaging. *AJNR* 1991;12:237-241.

38. Ludeke K, Roschmann P, Tischler R: Susceptibility artifacts in NMR imaging. *Magn Reson Imaging* 1985;3:329-343.

39. Ross JS, Masaryk TJ, Modic MT: Postoperative cervical spine: MR assessment. *J Comput Assist Tomogr* 1987;11:955-962.

40. Haacke EM, Tkach JA, Parrish TB: Reduction of T2* dephasing in gradient field echo imaging. *Radiology* 1989;170:457-462.

41. Henkelman RM, Bronskill MJ: Artifacts in magnetic resonance imaging. *Rev Magn Reson Med* 1987;2:1-126.

42. Haase A, Frahm J, Matthaei D, et al: FLASH imaging: rapid NMR imaging using low flip-angle pulses. *J Magn Reson* 1986;67:258-266.

43. Melki PS, Mulkern RV: Magnetization transfer effects in multislice RARE sequences. *Magn Reson Med* 1992;24:189-195.

44. Ross JS, Ruggieri P, Tkach J, et al: Lumbar degenerative disk disease: prospective comparison of conventional T2-weighted spin echo imaging and T2-weighted RARE. *AJNR.* (In press.)

45. Vinitski S, Mitchell DG, Rao VM, et al: Ultrashort-TE conventional and fast spin-echo imaging. *J Magn Reson Imaging* 2(P):54, 1992.

46. Tsuruda JS, Norman D, Dillon W, et al: Three-dimensional gradient-recalled MR imaging as a screening tool for the diagnosis of cervical radiculopathy. *AJNR* 1989;10:1263-1271.

47. Tsuruda JS, Remley K: Effects of magnetic susceptibility artifacts and motion in evaluating the cervical neural foramina on 3DFT gradient-echo MR imaging. *AJNR* 1991;12:237-241.

48. Ross JS, Modic MT, Masaryk TJ, et al: Assessment of extradural degenerative disease with Gd-DTPA-enhanced MR imaging: correlation with surgical and pathologic findings. *AJNR* 1989;10:1243-1249.

49. Mugler JP III, Brookeman JR: Three-dimensional magnetization-prepared rapid gradient-echo imaging (3D MP RAGE). *Magn Reson Med* 1990;15:152-157.

50. Haacke EM, Wielpolski PA, Tkach JA, Modic MT: Steady state free precession imaging in the presence of motion: applications for improved visualization of the cerebrospinal fluid. *Radiology* 1990;175:545-552.

51. VanDyke C, Modic MT, Beale S, et al: 3D MR myelography. *J Comput Assist Tomogr* 1992;16:497-500.

52. Ross JS, Tkach J, Masaryk TJ, et al: Optimization of 3D T1 weighted MP RAGE for cervical degenerative disease. *Radiology* 1991;181(P):193.

53. Smoker WRK, Godersky JC, Knutzon RK, et al: The role of MR imaging in evaluating metastatic spinal disease. *AJNR* 1987;8:901-908.

54. Colman IK, Porter BA, Redmond J III, et al: Early diagnosis of spinal metastases by CT and MR studies. *J Comput Assist Tomogr* 1988;12:423-426.

55. Avrahami E, Tadmor R, Dally O, et al: Early MR demonstration of spinal metastases in patients with normal radiographs and CT and radionuclide bone scans. *J Comput Assist Tomogr* 1989;13:598-602.

56. Mehta RC, Wilson MA, Perlman SB: False-negative bone scan in extensive metastatic disease: CT and MR findings. *J Comput Assist Tomogr* 1989;13:717.

57. Carmody RF, Yang PJ, Seeley GW, et al: Spinal cord compression due to metastatic disease: diagnosis with MR imaging versus myelography. *Radiology* 1989;173:225-229.

58. Modic MT, Feiglin DH, Piraino DW, et al: Vertebral osteomyelitis: assessment using MR. *Radiology* 1985;157:157-166.

59. Masaryk TJ, Boumphrey F, Modic MT, et al: effects of chemonucleosysis demonstrated by MR imaging. *J Comput Assist Tomogr* 1986;10:917-923.

60. Aoki J, Yamamoto I, Kitamura N, et al: End plate of the discovertebral joint: degenerative change in the elderly adult. *Radiology* 1987;164:411-414.

61. DeRoos A, Kressel H, Spritzer C, et al: MR imaging of marrow changes adjacent to end plates in degenerative lumbar disc disease. *AJR* 1987;149:531-534.

62. Modic MT, Steinberg PM, Ross JS, et al: Degenerative disk disease: assessment of changes in vertebral body marrow with MR imaging. *Radiology* 1988;166:193-199.

63. Libshitz HI, Malthouse SR, Cunningham D, et al: Multiple myeloma: appearance at MR imaging. *Radiology* 1992;182:833-837.

64. Porter BA, Shields AF, Alson DO: Magnetic resonance imaging of bone marrow disorders. *Radiol Clin North Am* 1986;24:269-289.

65. Vogler JB III, Murphy WA: Bone marrow imaging. *Radiology* 1988;168:679-693.

66. Smith SR, Williams CE, Davies JM, Edwards RHT: Bone marrow disorders: characterization with quantitative MR imaging. *Radiology* 1989;172:805-810.

67. Rosen BR, Fleming DM, Kushner DC, et al: Hematologic bone marrow disorders: quantitative chemical shift MR imaging. *Radiology* 1988;169:799-804.

68. Guckel F, Brix G, Semmler W, et al: Systemic bone marrow disorders: characterization with proton chemical shift imaging. *J Comput Assist Tomogr* 1990;14:633-642.

69. Brateman L: Chemical shift imaging: a review. *AJR* 1986;146:971-980.

70. Pukett IL, Rosen BR: Nuclear magnetic resonance: in vivo proton chemical shift imaging. *Radiology* 1983;149:197-201.

71. Sepponen RE, Sipponen JT, Tanttu JI: A method for chemical shift imaging: demonstration of bone marrow involvement with proton chemical shift imaging. *J Comput Assist Tomogr* 1984;8:585-587.

72. Rosen BR, Wedeen VJ, Brady TJ: Selective saturation NMR imaging. *J Comput Assist Tomogr* 1984;8:813-818.

73. Dixon WT: Simple proton spectroscopic imaging. *Radiology* 1984;153:189-194.

74. Axel L, Glover G, Pelc N: Chemical-shift magnetic resonance imaging of two-line spectra by gradient reversal. *Magn Reson Med* 1985;2:428-436.

75. Haase A, Frahm J, Hanicke W, Matthaei D: 1H NMR chemical shift selective (CHESS) imaging. *Phys Med Biol* 1985;30:341-344.

76. Joseph PM: A spin echo chemical shift MR imaging technique. *J Comput Assist Tomogr* 1985;9:651-658.

77. Keller PJ, Hunter WW, Schmalbrock P: Multisection fat-water imaging with chemical shift selective presaturation. *Radiology* 1987;164:539-541.

78. Pope JM, Walker RR, Kron T: Artifacts in chemical shift selective imaging. *Magn Reson Imaging* 1992;10:695-698.

79. Lodes CC, Felmlee JP, Ehman RL, et al: Proton MR chemical shift imaging using double and triple phase contrast acquisition methods. *J Comput Assist Tomogr* 1989;13:855.

80. Glover GH, Schneider E: Three-point Dixon technique for true water/fat decomposition with Bo inhomogeneity correction. *Magn Reson Med* 1991;18:371-383.

81. Meyer CH, Pauly JM, Macovski A, Nishimura DG: Simultaneous spatial and spectral selective excitation. *Magn Reson Med* 1990;15:287-304.

82. DeCoene B, Hajnal JV, Gatehouse P, et al: MR of the brain using fluid-attenuated inversion recovery (FLAIR) pulse sequences. *AJNR* 1992;13:1555-1564.

83. Bydder, GM, Hajnal JV, Young IR: Comparison of FLAIR pulse sequences with heavily T2-weighted SE sequences in MR imaging of the brain. *Radiology* 1992;185(P):151.

84. White SJ, Hajnal JV, Bydder GM: Use of FLAIR sequences in MR imaging of the spinal cord and nerve roots. *Radiology* 1992;185(P):151.

85. Hajnal JV, DeCoene B, Lewis PD, et al: High signal regions in normal white matter shown by heavily T2-weighted CSF nulled IR sequences. *J Comput Assist Tomogr* 1992;16:506-513.

86. DuBoulay GH: Pulsatile movements in the CSF pathways. *Br J Radiol* 1966;39:255-262.

87. DuBoulay GH, O'Connell J, Currie J, et al: Further investigations on pulsatile movements in the cerebrospinal fluid pathways. *Acta Radiol* 1972;13:496-523.

88. Lane B, Kricheff II: Cerebrospinal fluid pulsations at myelography: a videodensitometric study. *Radiology* 1974;110:579-587.

89. Enzmann DR, Pelc NJ: Normal flow patterns of intracranial and spinal cerebrospinal fluid defined with phase-contrast cine MR imaging. *Radiology* 1991;178:467-474.

90. Itabashi T, Arai S, Kitahura H, et al: Quantitative analysis of cervical cerebrospinal fluid pulsation. *Radiology* 1988;169(P):198.

91. Quencer RM, Donovan Post MJ, Hinks RS: Cine MR in the evaluation of normal and abnormal CSF flow: intracranial and intraspinal studies. *Neuroradiology* 1990;32:371-391.

92. Feinberg DA: Modern concepts of brain motion and cerebrospinal fluid flow. (Editorial.) *Radiology* 1992;185:630-632.

93. Bergstrand G, Bergstrom M, Nordell B, et al: Cardiac gated MR imaging of cerebrospinal fluid flow. *J Comput Assist Tomogr* 1985;9:1003-1006.

94. Sherman JL, Citrin CM: Magnetic resonance demonstration of normal CSF flow. *AJNR* 1986;7:3-6.

95. Sherman JL, Citrin CM, Bowen BJ, Gangarowa RE: MR demonstration of altered cerebrospinal fluid flow by obstructive lesions. *AJNR* 1986;7:571-579.

96. Kemp SS, Zimmerman RA, Bilaniuk LT, et al: Magnetic resonance imaging of the cerebral aqueduct. *Neuroradiology* 1987;29:431-436.

97. Atlas SW, Mark AS, Fram EK: Aqueductal stenosis: evaluation with gradient echo rapid MR imaging. *Radiology* 1988;169:449-453.

98. Edelman RR, Mattle H, Kleefield J, Silver MS: Quantification of blood flow with dynamic MR imaging and presaturation bolus tracking. *Radiology* 1989;171:551-556.

99. Axel L, Dougherty L: Heart wall motion: improved method of spatial modulation of magnetization for MR imaging. *Radiology* 1989;172:349-350.

100. Edelman RR, Wedeen VJ, Davis KR, et al: Multiphasic MR imaging: a new method for direct imaging of pulsatile CSF flow. *Radiology* 1986;161:779-783.

101. Thomsen C, Ståahlberg F, Stubgaard M, Nordell B: Fourier analysis of cerebrospinal fluid flow velocities: MR imaging study. The Scandinavian Flow Group. *Radiology* 1990;177:659-665.

102. Levy LM, DiChiro G: MR phase imaging and cerebrospinal fluid flow in the head and spine. *Neuroradiology* 1990;32:399-406.

103. Feinberg D, Mark AS: Human brain motion and cerebrospinal fluid circulation demonstrated with MR velocity imaging. *Radiology* 1987;163:793-799.

104. Wendt RE III, Nitz WR, Murphy PH, Bryan RN: Characterization of fluid flow using low-spatial-resolution velocity spectra from NMR images. *Magn Reson Med* 1989;10:71-88.

105. Nitz WR, Bradley WG, Watanabe AS, et al: Flow dynamics of cerebrospinal fluid: assessment with phase-contrast velocity MR imaging performed with retrospective cardiac gating. *Radiology* 1992;183:395-405.

106. Spraggins TA: Wireless retrospective gating: application to cine cardiac imaging. *Magn Reson Imaging* 1990;8:675-681.

2

Normal Anatomy

MICHAEL T. MODIC
SHIWEI YU

LUMBAR SPINE
Osteology

The lumbosacral spine—composed of vertebral bodies, lateral and posterior elements, and adjacent soft tissues—serves to carry the load of the upper body and transfer it to the lower limbs.

The bony lumbar spinal canal is formed by the vertebral bodies anteriorly, the pedicles laterally, and the laminae and bases of the spinous processes posteriorly (Figs. 2-1 to 2-3). On T_1-weighted spin-echo (SE) sequences (short repetition time [TR]/short echo time [TE]), the cancellous hematopoietic portion of the osseous structures is of an intermediate signal intensity between paraspinal fat and muscle. The signal intensity is primarily a reflection of the marrow space with its lipid and hematopoietic elements. The relative signal intensity becomes brighter (diffusely, or in a focal spotty fashion) with increasing age secondary to an increase in the lipid component of the marrow space[1,2] (Fig. 2-4). Occasionally, single focal areas of high signal intensity on T_1-weighted images with an intermediate signal intensity on T_2-weighted images will be noted secondary to regions of focal yellow marrow. Whereas these can be normal findings, they have also been related to age and the presence of pathologic changes such as spondylitis, kyphoscoliosis, and spondylosis.[3] The osseous structures are outlined by a thin low signal intensity from cortical bone. There is often a discrepant appearance of the superior and inferior endplates secondary to chemical shift (Fig. 2-2).

The superior lumbar spinal canal is usually round or oval in shape with a transverse diameter equal to or greater than the anterior-posterior dimension. In the midlumbar and lower lumbar regions the spinal canal takes on a more triangular configuration with the base pro-

jected anteriorly. Again, the transverse diameter is usually equal to or greater than the anterior-posterior dimension.

The transverse diameter of the lumbar vertebral body is larger than the anterior-posterior diameter. The vertebral bodies have a convex anterior and lateral margin with a flat or concave posterior margin. The superior and inferior vertebral body margins are flat or slightly concave. The venous drainage of the vertebral endplate capillary bed is via a plexus of postcapillary venules in the subchondral region that drains into a horizontal subarticular collecting vein. This vein then joins the anterior internal vertebral venous plexus. There are also anastomotic connections through the vertical tributaries and the basivertebral system of veins. On MR occasionally one will see slow-flowing venous blood in the endplate venous plexus as a line of high signal intensity parallel to the endplate against the low signal of the red marrow. They are more clearly seen following enhancement with gadolinium. They can be differentiated from chemical shift artifacts in that they are seen on both sides of the disk and persist despite reversal of the phase-encoding gradients.[4] Basivertebral channels are usually present in the midportion of the vertebral body. These regions often have a high signal intensity on T_1-weighted images that is due to fat surrounding the basivertebral plexus and/or slow flow of venous blood (Fig. 2-5).

The pedicles are bony pillars that project posteriorly and laterally from the superior aspect of the vertebral body and form the superior and inferior margins of the neural foramen. They are composed primarily of dense cortical bone but still contain enough marrow to approximate the signal intensity of the vertebral body on T_1-

weighted sequences. The laminae are angled bony projections extending from the pedicles to the base of the spinous process and forming a sort of arch over the spinal canal. Their superior aspects lie anterior to their inferior margins.

The spinous process extends posteriorly and slightly inferiorly from the vertebral arch. The transverse processes extend laterally and slightly posteriorly from the junction of the pedicle with the lamina and are composed primarily of cancellous bone. The articular pillars include the bone at the junction of the lamina and pedicles. In normals the marrow signal in the pars is usually uninterrupted, extending from the superior to the inferior articular facet in the parasagittal plane. The superior and inferior articular processes arise from the articular pillars and in the transverse plane appear at the midlevel of the intervertebral foramen. The concave surface of the superior articular process and convex surface of the inferior articular process form the diarthrodial facet joints. The superior articular facet of the body below lies anterior and lateral and faces posteromedial to the inferior articular facet of the body above. At the inferior aspect of the intervertebral foramen the superior articular facet becomes contiguous with the pedicle below and forms the posterior border of the lateral recess where the traversing nerve root lies medial to the pedi-

cle, anterior to the superior articular facet, and posterior to the vertebral body and disk.[5-8]

Facet Joints

Hyaline cartilage covers each facet and varies in thickness from 2 to 4 mm. Medial and lateral fibroelastic capsules enclose the joint. On the medial surface the capsule is reinforced by the anterolateral attachment of the ligamentum flavum. The superior and inferior aspects of the capsule contain synovium and fat, both of which can extend between the facets, even in normal subjects.[9-12] The facets and intervening joints, though seen in the sagittal plane, are best visualized in the axial plane. The cartilage can be identified on spin-echo images but is better seen on gradient echo scans, where its increased signal stands out sharply against the decreased signal of adjacent cortical bone. Depending on the direction of the readout gradient, a chemical shift artifact can cause apparent asymmetry of the cortical thickness[9] (Fig. 2-6). There is a variable appearance to the ventral and dorsal aspects of the lumbar facet joint on MR images because the synovium and joint space extend beyond the articular surface of the joint in most adults. Extensions of the synovium and joint space along the superior and inferior articular processes under the ligamentum flavum and into the ligamentum have also been recognized.[13]

Text continued on p. 45.

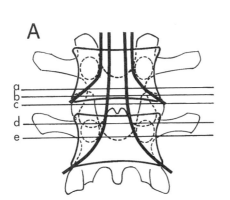
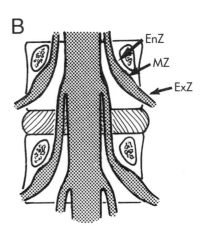

Fig. 2-1. Coronal plane of the lower lumbar spine. **A** and **B,** Schematics (horizontal lines *a* to *e* correspond to Fig. 2-3, *A*), **C,** a cryomicrotome anatomic section, and **D** to **F,** T$_1$-weighted coronal MR images (500/17). *DRG,* Dorsal root ganglion; *ef,* epidural fat; *enr,* exiting nerve root; *EnZ (enz),* entrance zone; *ExZ (exz),* exit zone; *if,* inferior facet; *LF,* ligamentum flavum; *MZ (mz),* midzone; *p,* pedicle; *s,* sacrum; *sf,* superior facet; *TNR (tnr),* traversing nerve root.

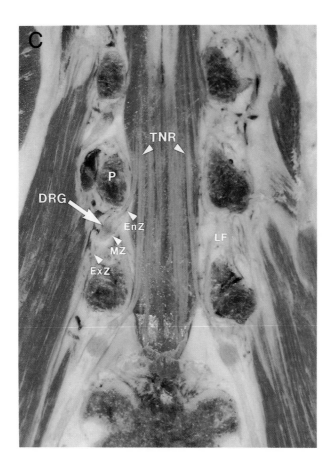

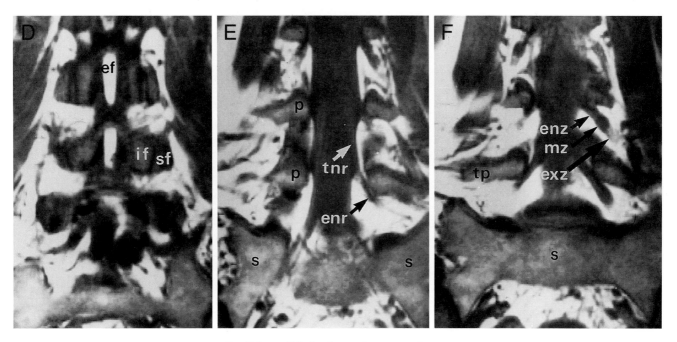

Fig. 2-1, cont'd. For legend see opposite page.

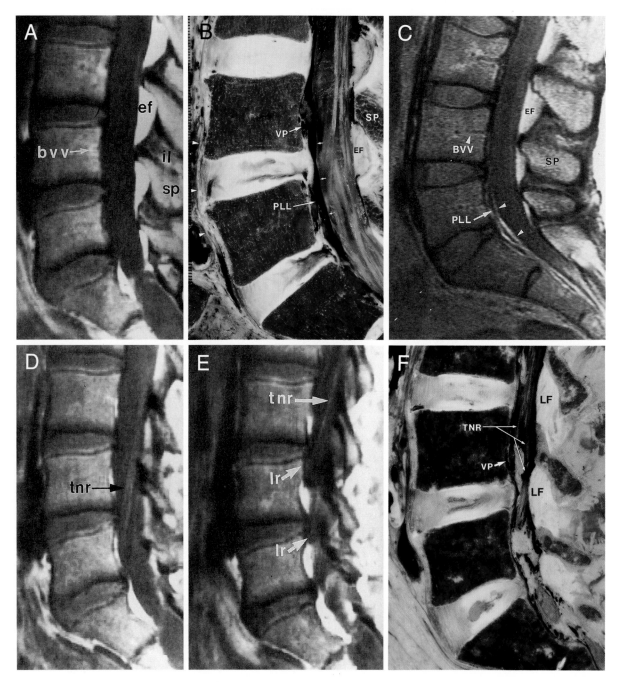

Fig. 2-2. For legend see opposite page.

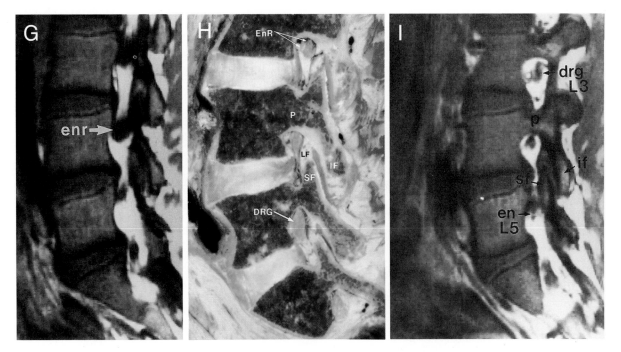

Fig. 2-2. Sagittal plane of the lumbar spine. Cryomicrotome anatomic sections, **B, D, F,** and **H,** with T$_1$-weighted MR images (500/17), **A, C, E, G,** and **I.** (The sagittal proton density, **C,** shows the posterior longitudinal ligament *[PLL]* separated from cortical bone of the vertebral bodies and the dura mater *[arrowheads]* in the lower lumbar region. See also **B.**) *Arrowheads* point to the anterior longitudinal ligament. *A,* Articular process; *BVV (bvv),* basivertebral vein(s); *D,* disk; *DRG (drg),* dorsal root ganglion; *EF (ef),* epidural fat; *EnR (enr),* exiting nerve root; *IF,* inferior facet; *IL,* intraspinal ligament; *LF,* ligamentum flavum; *lr,* lateral recess; *P,* pedicle; *small arrows,* dura mater; *SF,* superior facet; *SP,* spinous process; *TNR (tnr),* traversing nerve root; *VP,* venous plexus; *VSR,* ventral spinal root.

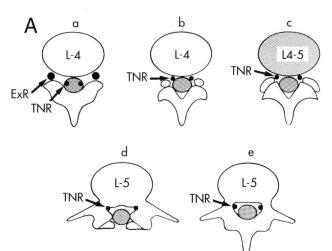

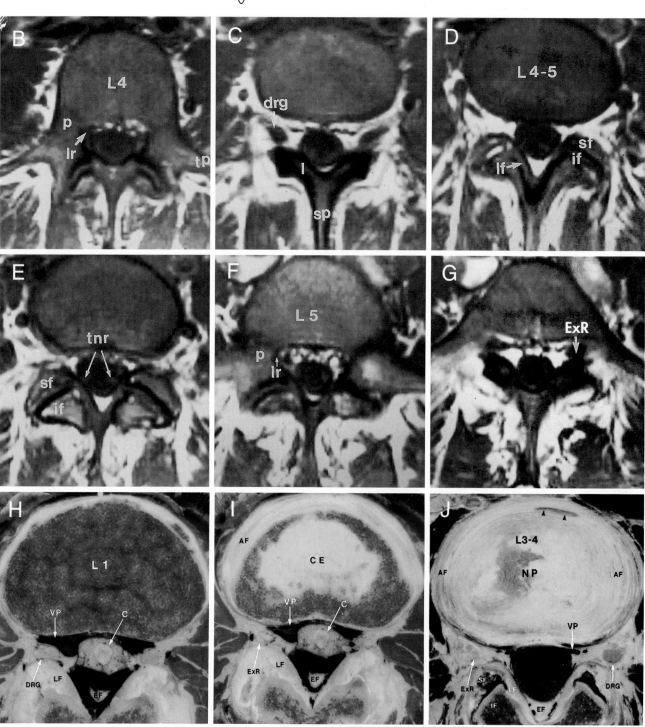

Fig. 2-3. Axial plane of the lumbar spine. **A** is a schematic of the T$_1$-weighted MR images (500/17) through L4-5, **B** to **G**. Cryomicrotome anatomic sections are through the L1 body, L1-2 disk level, and L3-4 disk level, **H** to **J**. (*Arrowheads* in **J** point to a concentric tear.) *AF,* Anulus fibrosus; *C,* spinal cord; *CE,* cartilaginous endplate; *DRG (drg),* dorsal root ganglion; *EF,* epidural fat; *ExR,* exiting nerve root; *IF (if),* inferior facet; *l,* lamina; *LF (lf),* ligamentum flavum; *lr,* lateral recess; *NP,* nucleus pulposus; *p,* pedicle; *SF (sf),* superior facet; *sp,* spinous process; *TNR (tnr),* traversing nerve root; *tp,* transverse process; *VP,* venous plexus.

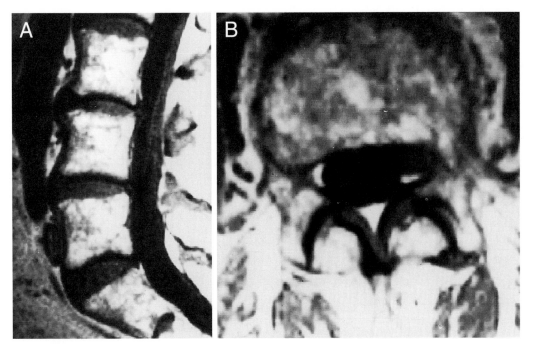

Fig. 2-4. Sagittal, **A,** and axial, **B,** T$_1$-weighted spin-echo (500/17) images through the lumbar spine. The "spotty" high signal intensity of the vertebral body marrow is secondary to an increased lipid content that is common with advancing age.

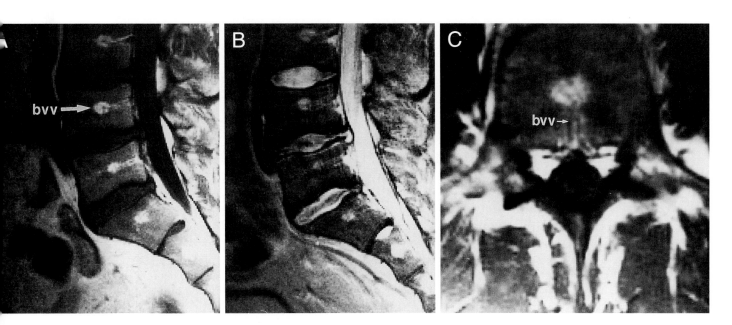

Fig. 2-5. Basivertebral vein *(bvv).* **A,** Sagittal T$_1$-weighted SE (500/17). **B,** Sagittal T$_2$-weighted SE (2000/90). **C,** Axial T$_1$-weighted SE (500/17). Note the high signal intensity secondary to increased lipid content and/or slow flow *(arrows).*

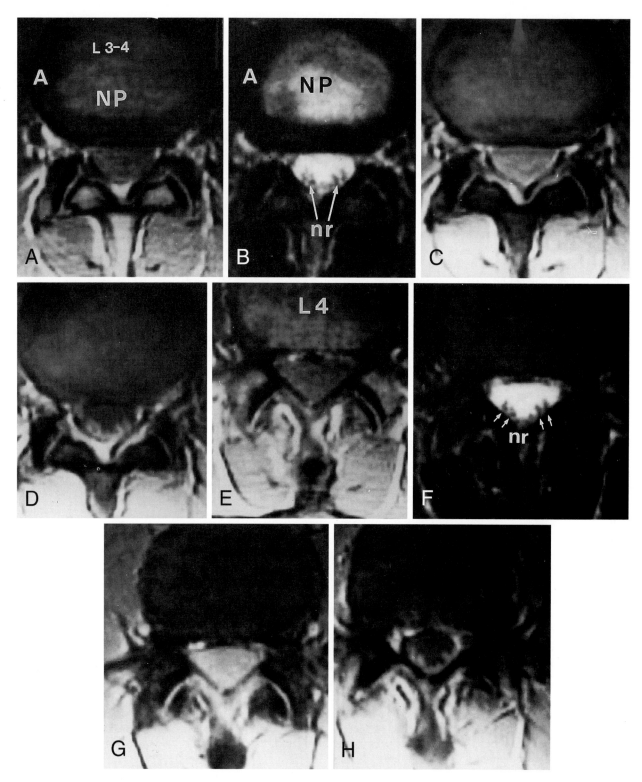

Fig. 2-6. L3-4 disk and L4 vertebral body. **A** and **E** are normal axial T_1-weighted SE (500/17), **B** and **F** are T_2-weighted SE (2000/90), **C** and **G** are FLASH 50/13/10 degree, and **D** and **H** are FLASH 50/13/60 degree images. Note the high signal intensity of the articular cartilage within the facet joints on the FLASH* images. *Arrows* indicate nerve roots within the thecal sac. *A,* Anulus fibrosus; *NP,* nucleus pulposus; *nr,* nerve root.

*FLASH, fast low-angle shot.

Epidural Space and Ligaments

The epidural space lies between the dura and the bony confines of the spinal canal. Its contents include epidural fat, ligaments, nerves, and blood vessels. The epidural fat has a high signal intensity on T_1-weighted sequences and lies anterior and anterolateral to the dura and posterior and medial between the ligamenta flava. Epidural fat is usually not seen in this latter region at the L5-S1 level, where the dural sac enlarges and usually lies in direct contact posteriorly with the ligamentum flavum and intraspinal ligament. The fat anterior to the dura at the L_5-S_1 level, however, is usually abundant compared to that in the superior lumbar spine. The signal intensity of the ligamentum flavum on T_1-weighted sequences is slightly higher than that of other spinal ligaments and adjacent osseous elements (Fig. 2-3). It also is higher on fast gradient echo, low–flip angle, scans similar to that of articular cartilage within the facet joints (Fig. 2-6). This increased signal has been speculated to be secondary to its high elastin (80%) and low type I collagen (20%) content. Conversely, the low signal of other ligaments may be due to their higher type I collagen content.[9] The ligamentum flavum forms the anterior lining of the interlaminal interval. It inserts on the anterior surface of the lower edge of the superior lamina and the posterior surface of the inferior lamina and is usually 3 to 5 mm thick. The anterolateral extension of the ligamentum flavum serves to reinforce the medial portion of the facet joint capsule with which it fuses laterally. Its thickness in the axial plane in normal subjects has been measured at 4.5 ± 0.97 mm.[9]

The posterior longitudinal ligament is a fibrous structure that is continuous from the base of the skull to the sacrum.[14] On sagittal views of the lumbar spine it appears as a very thin band that is separable from the posterior cortical bone of the vertebral bodies anteriorly (Fig. 2-2, *B*). In this area it stretches across the concave posterior osseous surface of the vertebral body, allowing vascular structures to enter and leave. It is tightly adherent to the posterior midsurface of the outer anulus of the intervertebral disk. Posteriorly it is closely juxtaposed to the dura in the upper lumbar region; in the lower lumbar region it may separate from the dura if a large amount of fat is present in the epidural space posterior to the ligament. Viewed posteriorly, the posterior longitudinal ligament is a segmental structure. Its retrovertebral segments are narrow bands that fan out laterally at the disk level and terminate at the medial borders of the neural foramen.

In a review of imaging studies and cadaveric spines[15] a sagittal midline septum spanning the posterior longitudinal ligament and dorsum of the vertebral body has been identified. It is most apparent in the lower lumbar spine, where it is largest. Histopathologic review of this septum demonstrates it to be a lamella of compact collagen connected dorsally with the posterior longitudinal ligament and ventrally with the thickened periosteum of the vertebrae. The posterior longitudinal ligament and this midline septum form a T-shaped complex that creates a left and a right compartment within the anterior epidural space. It is present only posterior to the vertebral bodies and not at the disk space, where the posterior longitudinal ligament attaches firmly to the anulus.[15]

The anterior longitudinal ligament is a strong band of fibers that is continuous from the occipital bone to the first sacral segment and provides a wide covering of the anterior vertebral body and disk. It is relatively narrower in the cervical region and expands in the thoracic and lumbar regions. It consists of three sets of fibers: (1) deep, spanning one intervertebral articulation; (2) intermediate, uniting two or three levels; and (3) superficial, connecting four or five vertebral bodies. Although the anterior longitudinal ligament is loosely attached to the connective tissue band that encircles the anulus, it is firmly bound to the osseous surface of the vertebral body itself above and below the diskovertebral junction.[14,16] Both the anterior and the posterior longitudinal ligament have a decreased signal intensity on magnetic resonance imaging. In the upper lumbar region the posterior longitudinal ligament is not readily separable from the dura or the cortical bone of the vertebral bodies on MR images. In the lower lumbar region the decreased signal intensity of the posterior longitudinal ligament blends with the decreased signal intensity of the peripheral portion of the anulus of the intervertebral disk. The retrovertebral portions of the posterior longitudinal ligament, however, may be detectable on T_1-weighted sagittal MR images as a linear low signal intensity due to the high signal intensity contrast of fat on both sides (Fig. 2-2, *C*). The posterior longitudinal ligament can also be identified on coronal images.

The dura is a dense fibrous tissue extending distally to the S2 segment. Its lateral outpouching at the level of the nerve roots also contains arachnoid, which forms the neural sheath. The arachnoid is loosely attached to but separated from the dura by a normally small subdural space. These structures are usually indiscernible from the underlying cerebrospinal fluid.

Spinal Cord and Nerve Roots

The spinal cord lies within the subarachnoid space, with its terminal portion (the conus medullaris) at the level of L1-2 (Fig. 2-7). The conus medullaris has a variable appearance at the T11-12 level. It can be oval, or less commonly, round, occasionally with a rounded eminence posteriorly. At the mid-T12 level the posterolateral margins are often linear. At the T12-L1 level two constant features are noted: the anterior median fissure (seen as a small groove on the central aspect of the cord) and a small conical projection present on the dorsal aspect.[17,18] These are often effaced by intramedullary tumors. The neural elements within the subarachnoid space have an intermediate signal intensity similar to that of

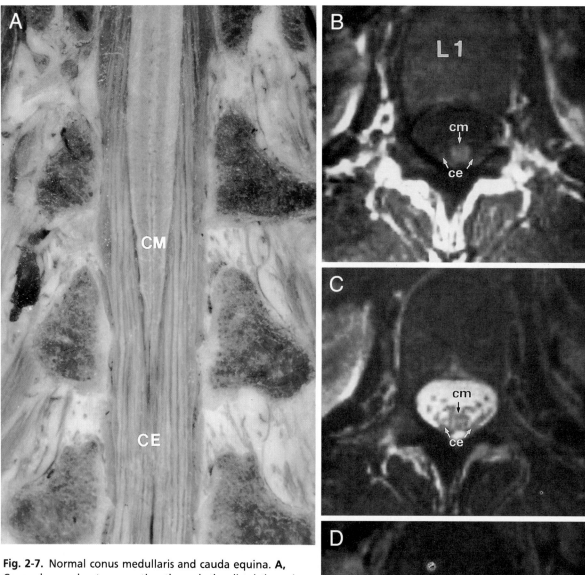

Fig. 2-7. Normal conus medullaris and cauda equina. **A,** Coronal cryomicrotome section through the distal thoracic cord, conus medullaris, and proximal cauda equina. **B,** Axial T$_1$-weighted SE (500/17). **C,** Axial T$_2$-weighted SE (2000/90). **D,** Axial FLASH (50/13/10 degree). *CM (cm),* Conus medullaris; *CE (ce),* cauda equina.

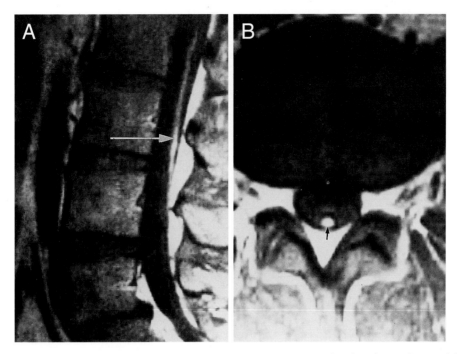

Fig. 2-8. Fat in the filum terminale. **A,** Sagittal midline T$_1$-weighted SE (500/17). **B,** Axial T$_1$-weighted SE (500/17) through the L3 level. *Arrows* denote the high signal intensity of the fat.

the intervertebral disk on T$_1$-weighted sequences but are decreased in signal intensity relative to the disk and CSF on more T$_2$-weighted examinations (Fig. 2-7). The filum terminale is the fibrous filament that extends inferiorly from the conus to the distal sac. Although its signal intensity is similar to or less than that of the neural elements, in approximately 5% of normal cases it can contain variable amounts of fat that stand out as a high signal intensity (Fig. 2-8). The cauda equina is the downward-passing lumbar and sacral nerve roots at the level of the conus.

The nerve roots of the cauda equina descend alongside the conus medullaris and are more densely packed into ventrolateral and dorsolateral bundles. The appearance of these roots at the conus—whence they descend inferiorly—is often described as "spiderlike" on axial sections[18] (Fig. 2-7). At the L2 level they are seen as a mass of soft tissue signal in the dependent portion of the thecal sac. They assume a smooth crescentic appearance following the curvature of the thecal sac. Their most common pattern at the L3 level is as a group of fibers that mass posteriorly (dependent position) in a crescentic and smooth or globular and irregular arrangement. The roots about to exit the dural tube are located anterolaterally in a symmetric pattern. At the L4 level they are often dispersed enough to be seen as separate delicate entities, arranged symmetrically within the CSF. By the L5 level the few roots present are equally spaced within the thecal sac. Conglomeration within the center

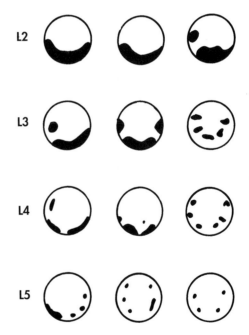

Fig. 2-9. Variations in the MR axial appearance of lumbar nerve roots.

of the thecal sac is notably lacking at this level[19] (Fig. 2-9). Midline sagittal images show the roots as a single linear area of intermediate signal intensity following the posterior thecal sac. The roots gradually taper from the conus to the L4 level. More parasagittal images demonstrate them fanning out as they travel in a posterior-

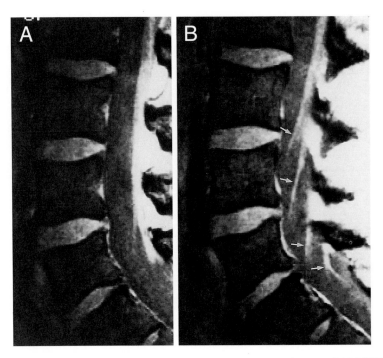

Fig. 2-10. Traversing nerve roots in the sagittal plane on FLASH images (200/13/60 degrees). **A,** Midline and, **B,** parasagittal 1 cm to the left of midline. Note the high signal intensity of the roots within the thecal sac in **B** *(arrows).*

superior to anterior-inferior direction (Fig. 2-2). The appearance of the neural elements relative to the CSF differs on fast gradient echo, variable–flip angle scans, depending on the flip angle employed. At lower flip angles the signal intensity of the nerve roots is less than that of the surrounding CSF, but it gradually increases as the flip angle approaches 90 degrees (Fig. 2-10).

The traversing portions of the nerve roots pass downward from the conus within the dural sac (Figs. 2-1 to 2-3), extending anteriorly and laterally at the level of the disk above. The traversing portions at the level below lie in the lateral recess formed where the superior articular facet becomes contiguous with the pedicle below. The nerve root sleeves usually end ventrally near the medial border of the superior articular facet at the inferior portion of the neural foramina of the level above. This area is also referred to as the "entrance zone." The traversing nerves become exiting nerves when they pass laterally underneath the pedicle and into the foramen. There they enlarge and become the dorsal root ganglion in a region referred to as the "midzone." From here the peripheral nerves distal to the ganglion pass laterally out the foramen, known as the "exit zone." The boundaries of the neural foramen are (1) the pedicles above and below, (2) the posterolateral aspect of the vertebral body laterally, (3) the intervertebral disk anteriorly and medially, and (4) the superior articular facet joint posteriorly and laterally[5,6] (Figs. 2-1 to 2-5). On both axial and

parasagittal T$_1$-weighted SE images the nerve roots appear as areas of decreased signal intensity surrounded by epidural fat beneath the pedicle. Occasionally two or more nerve roots will join and exit from the same foramen (Fig. 2-11). Epidural veins appear as areas of decreased signal intensity, usually located superior and anterior to the nerves (Figs. 2-1 to 2-3).

Disk

The intervertebral disk consists of three distinct parts[20-23]: the cartilaginous endplate, the anulus fibrosus, and the nucleus pulposus. As a structural unit it is designed to alleviate shock and transmit forces applied to the spine from every conceivable combination of vectors. The lumbar disks are reniform, and the lumbar lordosis is due to the equivalent increase in differential between the anterior and posterior thicknesses of the disks, a situation that makes the lumbosacral disk the most wedge shaped.[16] On axial sections the first four lumbar disks have a slightly concave or flat posterior border, conforming to the adjacent vertebral bodies; the L5 disk has a flatter slightly convex posterior border. In the literature descriptions of the blood supply vary.[21,24-27] The endplate contains numerous blood vessels at birth, which persist up to 20 years of age. There are small blood vessels present in the posterior-lateral aspect of the anulus, running mainly concentrically among the lamellae, but the normal nucleus pulposus remains

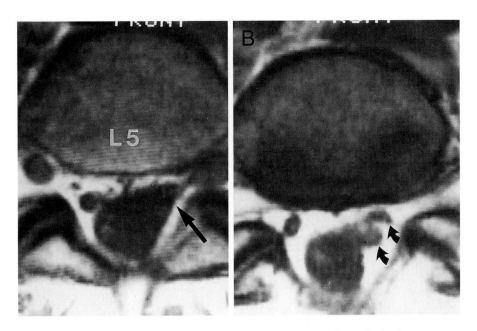

Fig. 2-11. Conjoined nerve roots. Axial T$_1$-weighted SE images through the lower L5 vertebral body, **A**, and the L5-S1 superior endplate, **B**. *Arrows* point to asymmetry of the thecal sac on the left.

avascular throughout life. The innervation of the intervertebral disk remains controversial.

The cartilaginous endplate is composed of hyaline cartilage that covers the inferior and superior vertebral body surfaces central to the site of fusion of the previous epiphyseal ring (Fig. 2-12, *A*). Although the endplate in the adult lumbar spine is avascular, it serves as a biomechanical and metabolic interface between the vertebral body and nucleus pulposus, where it becomes the major site of diffusion in the vertebral body spongiosa. The cartilaginous endplate is indiscernible from the nucleus pulposus or cortical bone of the vertebral bodies on MR images.[28]

The anulus fibrosus is the limiting capsule of the nucleus pulposus (Fig. 2-12, *B*). Its collagenous fibers are short and stout, providing greater strength anteriorly than posteriorly (where they are thinner, fewer in number, and more closely packed). The anulus is completely circular, attached superiorly and inferiorly to the vertebral body at the site of the fused epiphyseal ring by Sharpey fibers as well as to the longitudinal ligaments anteriorly and posteriorly. Its purpose is to resist radial tension induced by axial loading of the disk, through confinement of the nucleus pulposus, as well as to resist stresses from torsion and flexion.[20-23] Transverse and concentric tears in the anulus are shown on cryomicrotomy studies as common incidental findings in adult disks.[28] Whether the transverse tear and concentric tear are symptom-producing lesions is unknown. The hydration of the anulus is approximately 80% in children. Type I collagen predominates in the peripheral anulus, and type II collagen in the inner anulus and nucleus pulposus. The tensile strength of the anulus is attributed to the type I collagen fibers, as found in tendons elsewhere in the body. The type II collagen fibers in the inner anulus and nucleus pulposus provide compressive protection and are abundant in hyaline articular cartilage, which covers the surfaces where compressive forces are high.[29] Examination of the collagen within the disk suggests that the type II collagen fibers may be more hydrated than type I fibers, with covalent cross-linking perhaps determining their behavior.[30]

The nucleus pulposus represents the definitive remnant of embryonal notochord and is normally composed of well-hydrated, loose, delicate fibrous strands forming an incompressible gelatinous matrix (Fig. 2-12, *A*). Although a sharp demarcation between the nucleus pulposus and anulus fibrosus can occasionally be seen on cryomicrotome sections in adults, it usually blends imperceptibly with the anulus with no clear demarcation between the two (Fig. 2-12, *C*). Collagen and proteoglycans comprise the major macromolecular constituents of the nucleus pulposus and anulus fibrosus. The nucleus is richer in proteoglycans than the anulus; chondroitin-6-sulfate, keratan sulfate, hyaluronic acid, and chondroitin-4-sulfate have all been noted.[31,32] The hydrostatic properties of the disk arise from its high state of hydration. The nucleus consists of 85% to 90% water and the anulus 80% water. The hydrophilia of the disk is not strictly biochemical, since diurnal variations in disk height indicate that water can be expressed via pressure.[30]

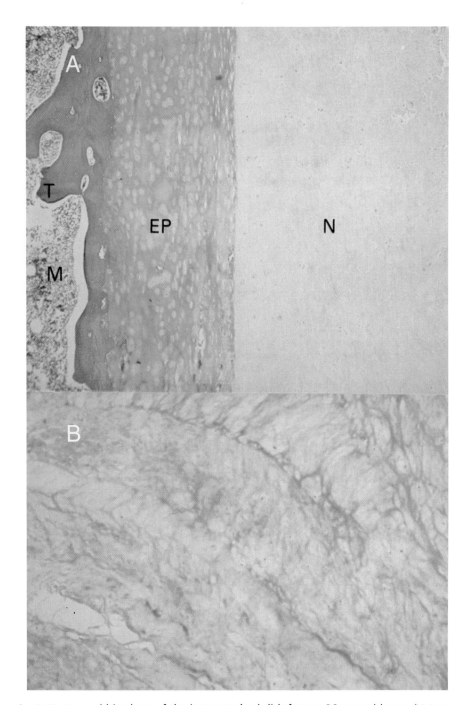

Fig. 2-12. Normal histology of the intervertebral disk from a 36-year-old man (H & E stain). **A,** Low power of the endplate at its junction with the nucleus pulposus in the central portion of the disk. *EP* is the endplate, *M* the subcortical vertebral body marrow, *N* the nucleus, and *T* trabeculae. **B,** High power of the anulus fibrosus. The anulus is composed of pink-staining collagenous fibers that ascend both obliquely and spirally.

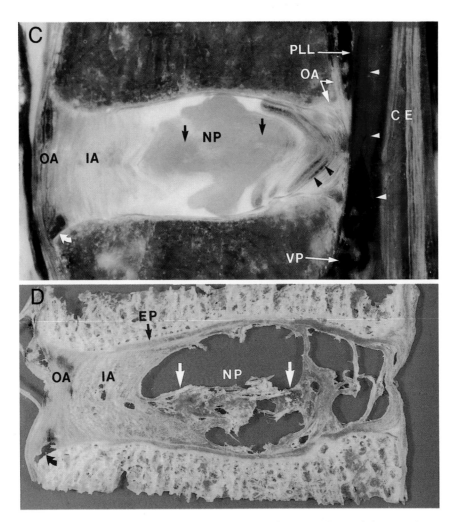

Fig. 2-12, cont'd. C, Sagittal cryomicrotome section of a normal L4-5 disk. *CE* is the cauda equina, *IA* the inner anulus, *NP* the nucleus pulposus, *OA* the outer anulus, *PLL* the posterior longitudinal ligament, and *VP* the venous plexus. Note the attachments of the outermost layers of the anulus fibrosus. In the middle brown-colored region of the nucleus *(NP)* a darker brown zone *(arrows)* can be seen. Concentric tears *(black arrowheads)* and a transverse tear *(curved arrow)* are also demonstrated. *White arrowheads* point to the dura mater. **D,** Dehydrated sagittal section of the same specimen showing the central fibrous structure *(arrows)* within the nucleus pulposus *(NP)*. *EP* is the endplate cartilage, *OA* the outer anulus, and *IA* the inner anulus. *Curved arrow* points to a transverse tear.

The central region of the disk is usually stained with lipofuscin, which gives it a brown color (Fig. 2-12, *C*). The staining, however, is not necessarily confined to the borders of the nucleus pulposus. Fissures filled with fluid are common findings within these pigmented areas in adults. A much darker zone is identified in the midportion of this lipofuscin-stained area and represents a plate of fibrous tissue. This fibrous plate in the equator of the disk most likely represents a normal progressive aging change of the intervertebral disk.[33] It consists of collagenous, reticular, and elastic fibers. These fibrous bands begin to develop in adolescence, with an accurate appearance in either the anterior or the posterior aspect of the nucleus. In adults it becomes denser and forms a transverse band through the entire nucleus (Fig. 2-12, *D*).

On T_1-weighted images the central portion of the disk has a slightly decreased signal intensity when compared to the peripheral portion, which then blends with an area of even greater decreased signal intensity, representing the outer layers of the anulus fibrosus at its confluence with the longitudinal ligament[34] (Figs. 2-1 and 2-3). A

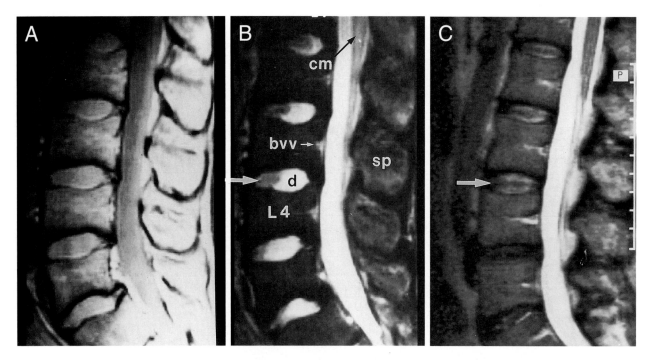

Fig. 2-13. A, Intermediate 2000/20 msec SE and, **B,** T$_2$-weighted SE (2000/90 msec) sagittal images through the lumbar spine. Note the normal high signal intensity of the central portion of the disk *(d)* on the 90 msec TE image. Anteriorly an area of decreased signal intensity bisects the disk *(arrow)*. This appearance is typical of a young disk. **C,** More mature or older disk. The decreased signal traverses the entire nucleus pulposus *(arrow)*. There is also decreased signal intensity in the L4-5 and L5-S1 disk consistent with degeneration. *bvv,* Basivertebral vein; *cm,* conus medullaris; *sp,* spinous process.

Fig. 2-14. Spin-echo and gradient echo sagittal images. **A,** Intermediate SE (2000/20). **B,** T$_2$-weighted SE (2000/90). **C,** FLASH (50/13/10 degrees). **D,** FLASH (50/13/60 degrees). **B** shows decreased signal in the L4-5 and L5-S1 disk, consistent with degeneration. **A** and **B** were performed with refocusing gradients that eliminated virtually all CSF ghosting artifacts (compare with Figure 2-15). Note the high signal intensity of CSF on the 10-degree flip-angle images compared with the 60-degree. **E** and **F,** Conventional T$_2$-weighted spin-echo (2000/90) and T$_2$-weighted turbo-SE (5000/100). Whereas **E** required 10 minutes of acquisition time, **F** required less than 2. The contrast in the two images is similar.

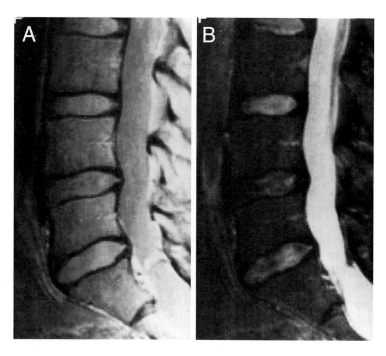

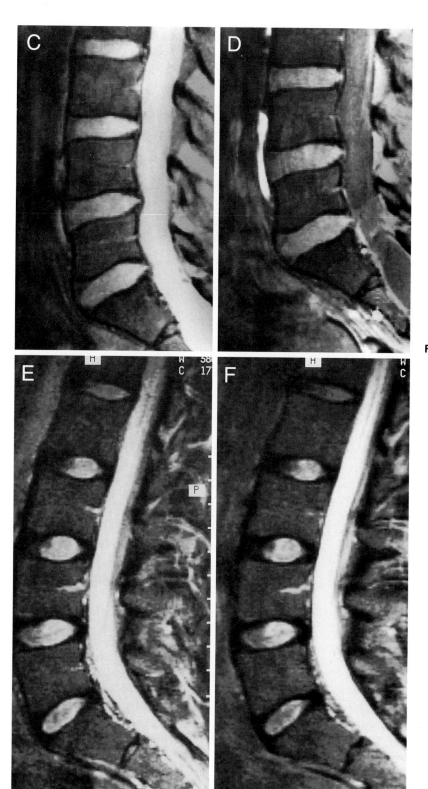

Fig. 2-14, cont'd. For legend see opposite page.

similar appearance is also noted on T_2-weighted images, although the signal intensities are reversed: on T_2-weighted spin-echo sequences the normal disk has a central portion of high signal intensity and a peripheral portion of decreased signal intensity (Figs. 2-6 and 2-13). Anatomic correlation suggests that there is no clear separation of the nucleus pulposus and anulus fibrosus; rather an inner region represents the nucleus as well as the inner portion of the anulus, and a more peripheral region represents the outer layers of the anulus and its confluence with the longitudinal ligament.[35] It is tempting to suggest that the signal intensity differences are related to the differences in hydration between the inner nuclear anulus and the outer complex, reflecting a longer T_1 and T_2 centrally and shorter relaxation times peripherally. How this relates to the degree of hydration of type I and type II collagen, proteoglycan distribution, and aggregation is as yet not understood.

On more T_2-weighted images there is often a decreased-signal zone within the central increased-signal portion of the disk, which we have referred to as the intranuclear cleft.[36] This creates a notched biconcave appearance of the disk similar to that seen at diskography. Although not immediately apparent on gross inspection, it corresponds on histologic studies and dehydrated sections to the fibrous plate just mentioned within the nucleus pulposus.[26,33,36] It is almost universally seen after 30 years of age (Fig. 2-13) as a decreased-signal zone, usually thick and with a slightly irregular contour. It can also be seen in the thoracic region of the spine. If seen in the thoracic region, however, it should be differentiated from a truncation artifact, which is a uniform, straight, low-signal line located in the midportion of the disk. This artifact will also disappear with changes in the imaging matrix and/or phase-encoding direction.

The appearance of the disk and vertebral body on gradient echo images will vary depending on whether lipid and water components are in phase or opposed (dependent on TE) and on whether the TR and flip angle are employed.[37] The signal intensity of the normal disk is usually higher than that of the adjacent vertebral body and quite homogeneous (Fig. 2-14).

Cerebrospinal Fluid

The signal intensity of the CSF is decreased relative to the extradural elements on T_1-weighted images secondary to its long T_1 and T_2 (Fig. 2-2). With increasing TE and TR, the signal intensity will increase. In gradient echo images the signal intensity is highest relative to extradural structures with low flip angles (Fig. 2-14). Its appearance, however, is variable depending on the degree of CSF pulsations and the pulse sequence parameter employed.[38,39] In the lumbar region the problem most often encountered on T_1-weighted sequences is a variable signal intensity masquerading as an intradural mass

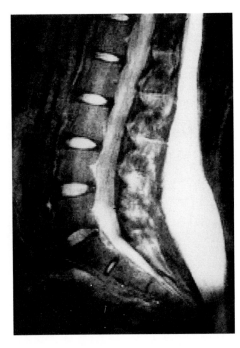

Fig. 2-15. CSF ghosting artifacts. Sagittal T_1-weighted SE (2000/90) without cardiac gating or refocusing. Note the prominent ghosting artifacts secondary to CSF pulsations (compare with Figure 2-14, *B*).

or arachnoiditis. This is presumably secondary to either slow flow or variable flow in different portions of the CSF. On T_2-weighted images a loss of signal due to spin dephasing and ghosting artifacts may also occur.[19] Ghosting artifacts can be projected not only outside the spine from the CSF but also over the spine from the adjacent abdominal vessels or secondary to excessive abdominal breathing (Fig. 2-15). A more in-depth discussion of the variability of signal intensity and its causes appears in Chapter 1.

Vascular Anatomy

The blood supply of the lumbar spine consists of paired segmental lumbar arteries that arise from the posterior aspect of the abdominal aorta at the first four lumbar levels. The fifth lumbar arteries are of more variable origin and often arise from the sacral artery. The arterial supply of the dural sac and its contents is provided by segmental radiculomedullary branches of the segmental lumbar arteries (Fig. 2-16), the most important of which is the artery of Adamkiewicz, which usually arises from the intercostal branches of the lower thoracic aorta (typically T9 on the left) and less frequently the upper lumbar arteries.[16]

The venous anatomy consists of spinal radicular veins (intervertebral veins) that interconnect the anterior internal vertebral veins and the ascending lumbar veins. The intervertebral veins course laterally through the neural

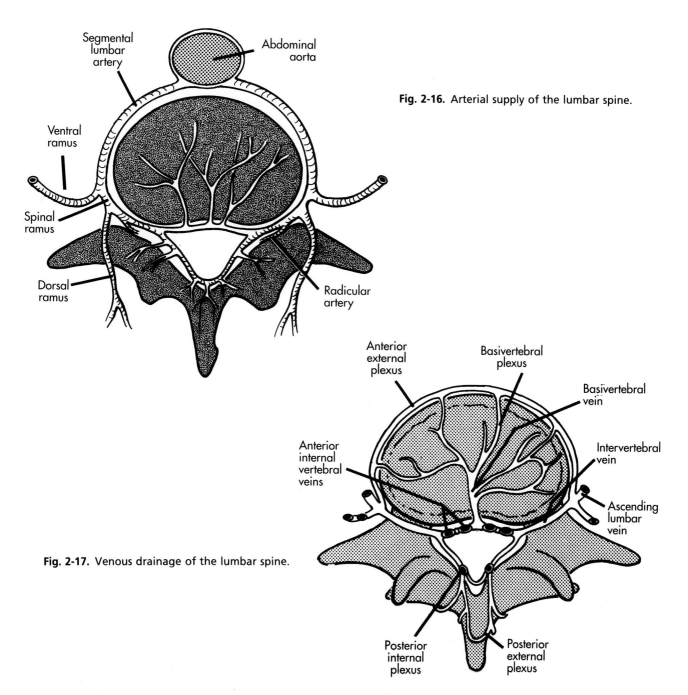

Fig. 2-16. Arterial supply of the lumbar spine.

Fig. 2-17. Venous drainage of the lumbar spine.

foramen above or below the pedicle to join the segmental lumbar veins. From here the venous drainage extends anteriorly through the anterior external plexus into the common iliac vein. The posterior-inferior venous plexus also communicates with the intervertebral veins. The basivertebral veins (single or paired) are formed by radiating venous channels within the vertebral body. They communicate posteriorly with the anterior internal vertebral veins in the midportion of the vertebral body. The anterior internal vertebral veins are usually paired and lie on both sides of the midline, coursing longitudinally behind the vertebral bodies and intervertebral disks in the epidural space[16] (Fig. 2-17). Inferiorly they begin in the

sacral canal and pass superiorly the entire length of the spinal canal to become continuous with the clival venous plexus at the craniovertebral junction. Their size and appearance are inconstant and may occasionally be represented by a plexus of smaller venous channels rather than by the usual paired structures. They anastomose extensively with the posterior internal venous plexus and ascending lumbar veins via the intervertebral veins. They are most prominent on transverse imaging at the L5-S1 level, and less so at the L4-5 level.

Whereas the signal intensity of arterial structures is usually decreased due to the velocity of blood flow, the appearance of epidural venous structures is more variable and the full gamut of signal intensities may be seen (reflecting the often slower velocities and potential for even echo rephasing on certain sequences). As on computed tomography, when prominent on MR they may blend their signal intensity with that of the adjacent intervertebral disks, especially at the L5-S1 level.

Innervation

The classically described patterns of peripheral nerve distribution have been based on the segmental aspects of vertebral development.[16] Clinical observation, however, has shown substantial individual variation from the expected system of innervation, particularly in the lumbosacral region. These atypical neurologic patterns are attributed to peculiarities in plexus formation, intrathecal alterations in the level of spinal nerve origins and vertebral exits, and anomalous connections between adjacent nerve roots. In addition, more recently, a previously described[40] intersegmental system of axons has been observed on the ventrolateral surface of the conus medullaris. Although these axons usually unite with rootlets of a more caudal spinal nerve, they have been seen combining with others to form grossly visible ectopic rootlets that can be traced to where they join a typical spinal nerve root one to several segments caudal to their level of origin.[40]

Classically, innervation of the lumbar canal has been ascribed to the sinu-vertebral nerve, a branch of each spinal nerve that passes back through the intervertebral foramen and supplies fibers to the articular connective tissue, periosteum, meninges, and vascular structures associated with the vertebral canal. The nerve originates distal to the dorsal root ganglion (Fig. 2-18) and passes backward through the foramen, curving upward around the base of the pedicle and dividing to give a superior and an inferior branch that approach the posterior longitudinal ligament. Branches are distributed to the periosteum, posterior longitudinal ligament, and dural and epidural vessels in a pattern that roughly corresponds to the arterial distribution. The posterior primary ramus innervates the facet joints at this same level, and usually the level above, as well as the soft tissues in the first three lumbar segments. Anatomic work[16] has revealed anastomotic connections at each level. The existence of such connections with adjacent segments provides an explanation for the mutual overlapping of segmental sensory nerve distribution and suggests that diskogenic pain from a single level may involve more than one recurrent branch of the spinal nerve. Free nerve endings and complex unencapsulated pain terminations are demonstrable in the posterior and anterior longitudinal ligaments, the periosteum of the vertebral body, and the synovial capsules of the articular facets. The lack of neural elements within the nucleus pulposus and inner lamella of the anulus is accepted, but the presence of nerve endings

within the outer lamella has been both demonstrated and denied by various investigators. The point is moot, however, since the relationship of this structure to well-documented innervated areas is clearly verifiable, particularly as regards the posterior longitudinal ligament and central disk herniation.[16]

THORACIC SPINE

The MR signal intensity of the osseous, soft tissue, and fluid structures of the thoracic spine is similar to that in the lumbar region (Figs. 2-19 to 2-21).

Osteology

The thoracic spinal canal is defined by the vertebral bodies and disks anteriorly, the pedicles laterally, and the lamina and base of the spinous processes posteriorly.[6-8,41] The thoracic spinal canal has a relatively constant size throughout its length, with equal transverse and anterior-posterior dimensions and a rounded configuration.

The bodies are convex anteriorly and concave posteriorly with an approximately equal transverse and anterior-posterior dimension. There is a progressive increase in the size of the thoracic vertebral bodies moving rostral to caudal.

The pedicles arise from the upper half of each vertebral body and pass posterolaterally and slightly inferiorly to the articular pillar and posterior neural arch. They form the upper and lower boundaries of the intervertebral foramen. The laminae are broad and short, passing from the articular pillars in a medial and posterior direction and overlapping. The spinous process is longer and more slender than in the lumbar region and again passes downward and posteriorly. The transverse processes extend outward, upward, and posteriorly from the articular pillars. They are closely related to the heads, necks, and tubercles of the corresponding ribs.

The superior articular processes project superiorly from the junctions of the pedicles and the lamina on each side. The facets are directed posteriorly and slightly laterally. The portion of the neural arch at the junction of the pedicle and lamina and between the articular facets is called the articular pillar. At the lateral portion of the lamina, the inferior articular process projects inferiorly and anteriorly.

The intervertebral foramen is directed laterally at the inferior half of the vertebral body. Its superior and inferior margins are formed by the pedicles with the neck of the rib anterolaterally, the vertebral body anteriorly, and the facet joints posteriorly. The foramina for the thoracic spinal nerves lie in a higher position relative to the intervertebral disk than do those of the cervical vertebral bodies.

Text continued on p. 62.

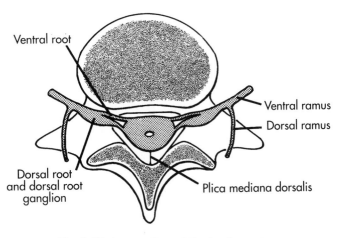

Fig. 2-18. Innervation of the lumbar spine.

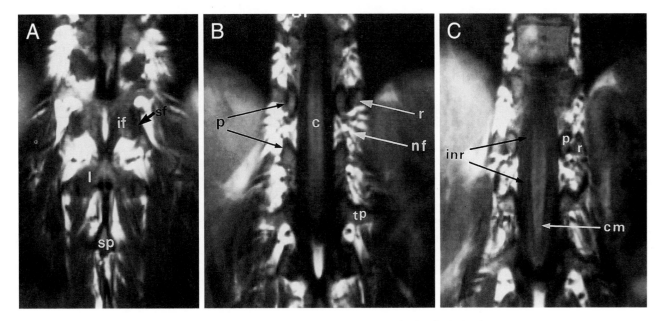

Fig. 2-19. Normal thoracic T$_1$-weighted SE MR anatomy (500/17). *C*, Cord; *cm*, conus medullaris; *if*, inferior facet; *inr*, intradural nerve root; *l*, lamina; *nf*, neural foramen; *p*, pedicle; *r*, rib; *sf*, superior facet; *sp*, spinous process; *tp*, transverse process.

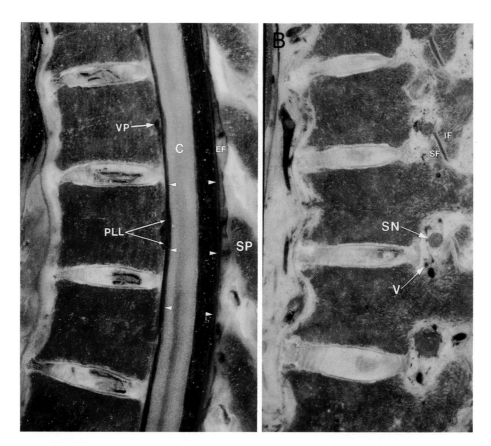

Fig. 2-20. Normal sagittal thoracic cryomicrotome and MR anatomy. **A,** Midline cryomicrotome section in the sagittal plane through the upper thoracic cord. **B,** Parasagittal cryomicrotome section through the neural foramina at the same level. *AF,* Anulus fibrosus; *bvv,* basivertebral vein; *C,* cord; *CE (ce),* cauda equina; *CM (cm),* conus medullaris; *d,* disk; *EF,* epidural fat; *IF (if),* inferior facet; *nf,* neural foramen; *NP,* nucleus pulposus; *p,* pedicle; *PLL,* posterior longitudinal ligament; *SF (sf),* superior facet; *SN,* spinal nerve; *SP (sp),* spinous process; *V,* vein; *VP,* venous plexus. *Arrowheads* point to the dura mater.

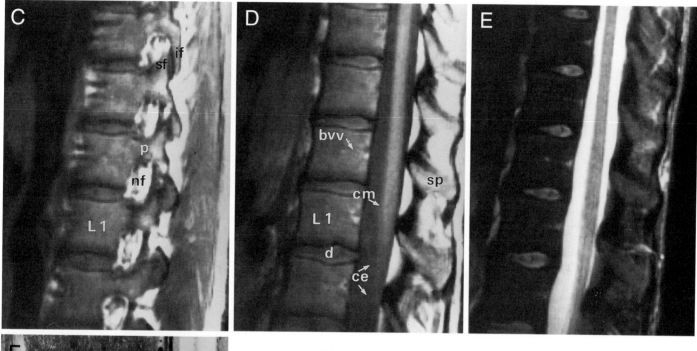

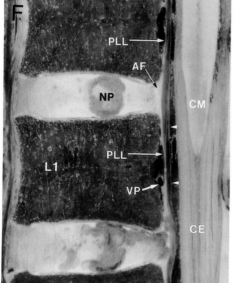

Fig. 2-20 cont'd. C, Parasagittal T$_1$-weighted SE (500/17) through the neural foramina. **D,** Midline sagittal T$_1$-weighted SE (500/17) through the distal thoracic cord and conus medullaris. **E,** Midline sagittal T$_2$-weighted SE (2000/90) through the same plane. **F,** Midline cryomicrotome section through the distal thoracic cord and conus medullaris.

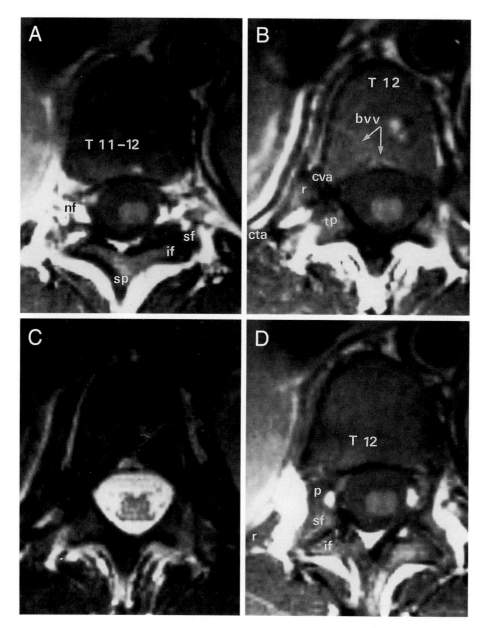

Fig. 2-21. Normal axial T$_1$-weighted (500/17) and T$_2$-weighted SE (2000/90) images of T11-12 through the T12-L1 disk. **A, B, D, F,** and **H** are T$_1$-weighted. **C, E, G,** and **I** are T$_2$-weighted. *bvv*, Basivertebral vein; *cta*, costotransverse articulation; *cva*, costovertebral articulation; *dr*, dorsal root; *if*, inferior facet; *nf*, neural foramen; *p*, pedicle; *r*, rib; *sf*, superior facet; *sp*, spinous process; *tp*, transverse process; *vr*, ventral root.

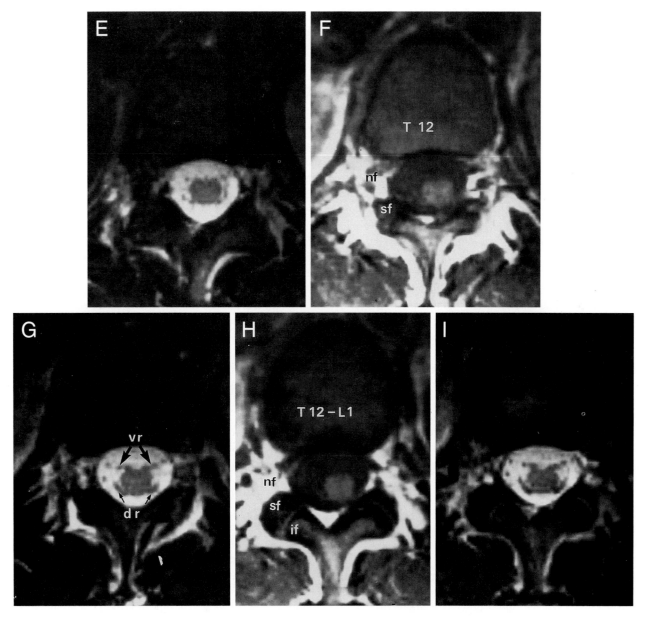

Fig. 2-21, cont'd. For legend see opposite page.

The ribs of the 12 thoracic vertebral bodies are apposed posteriorly to the transverse process and vertebral body of the same number. There is a smaller articulation with the lower aspect of the next higher body. The crest of the head of each rib is joined at the intervertebral disk by an intraarticular ligament and lies parallel to the plane of the intervertebral disk.

Epidural Space and Ligaments

The epidural space and contents are similar to those in the cervical and lumbar regions. There is abundant epidural fat posteriorly between the neural arch and the dura and laterally in the intervertebral foramen, but less fat in the anterior half of the epidural space than in the lumbosacral region. The anterior longitudinal ligament is thicker in the thoracic region than in the cervical or lumbar region and is more prominent opposite the bodies. The posterior longitudinal ligament extends along the posterior aspect of the vertebral bodies and, again, is thicker than in the cervical or lumbar region.

Cord and Nerve Roots

The thoracic dural sheath is significantly larger than the spinal cord and extends along the nerves for a shorter distance than in the lumbar region. The thoracic cord, dorsal and ventral thoracic nerve roots, radicular veins, and spinal arteries are surrounded by CSF and occupy the intradural compartment. The thoracic cord is more rounded than the usual elliptic appearance of the cervical cord. An anterior median fissure indents its ventral surface. The posterior intermediate and posterolateral sulci on the dorsal surface of the cord are shallow. In the upper thoracic spine the number of the cord segment is two levels lower than the number of the corresponding vertebra (e.g., cord segment 4 lies at the level of the vertebral canal of thoracic vertebra 2). In the lower thoracic spine there is a difference of three levels between the cord and vertebra. Thus, depending on location, the dorsal and ventral thoracic nerve roots must descend two to three vertebral body segments in the subarachnoid space to exit through the appropriate intervertebral foramen. The upper six pairs are larger than their caudal counterparts. Both groups, however, are significantly smaller than their cervical, lumbar, or sacral counterparts.[6-8,41]

Disk

The thoracic disks are somewhat heart shaped on section, and the nuclei pulposi are more centrally located than in the lumbar region. The thoracic disks are also thinner vertically than their cervical or lumbar counterparts but of larger volume than the cervical disks. The endplates of the vertebral bodies are flat. Both the thickness and the horizontal dimensions of thoracic disks increase caudally with the corresponding increase in size

of the vertebral bodies. The normal thoracic kyphosis results from a disparity between the anterior and posterior heights of the vertebral bodies, for the disks are of uniform thickness.[16] The disks are confined anteriorly and posteriorly by the longitudinal ligaments, with an attachment to the crest of the ribs posterolaterally. The area of decreased signal intensity seen within the high signal intensity of the disk on T_2-weighted sequences is not as constant as in the lumbar region.

Cerebrospinal Fluid

The CSF signal intensity is more variable in the thoracic than in the lumbar region because of more prominent CSF pulsations. On T_1-weighted axial images this may be manifested as areas of relatively intermediate signal that are curvilinear or oval and appear both anterolaterally and posteriorly to the cord. On T_2-weighted images oval areas of decreased signal intensity may be noted (Fig. 2-22). Again, these most likely reflect differences in the velocity of the CSF in different portions of the canal and are, to some degree, produced by the exiting nerve roots and the septum posticum.

Problems with signal loss and ghosting of the CSF on T_2-weighted images are also more prominent in the thoracic than the lumbar region secondary to the greater pulsatile flow. In addition, overlying cardiac and respiratory motion may severely obscure the extradural, intradural, and intramedullary interfaces. This latter problem can usually be addressed with saturation pulses placed so the signal intensity of these artifacts is decreased.[38]

The arteries and veins in the thoracic region are similar to those in the cervical and lumbar regions.

CERVICAL SPINE
Osteology

In the sagittal plane the cervical spine has a slightly lordotic curvature, the bodies becoming broader and gradually increasing in size from C3 to C7[5,6,42] (Figs. 2-23 to 2-26). The first and second cervical vertebrae are unique in their configuration. C1 (the atlas) is devoid of a body and spinous process; it consists of a posterior arch joined by two lateral masses that support the weight of the skull. C2 (the axis) has a bony protuberance that projects rostrally from the body—the dens or odontoid process. Unlike the remaining portions of the cervical spine, the dens can demonstrate a decreased signal relative to other vertebral bodies, presumably due to partial volume averaging. A persistent remnant of the subdental synchondrosis is often recognized on sagittal MRI as a horizontal dark band at the base of the odontoid process; this is a normal feature and should not be mistaken for a fracture. Approximately midway between the end-

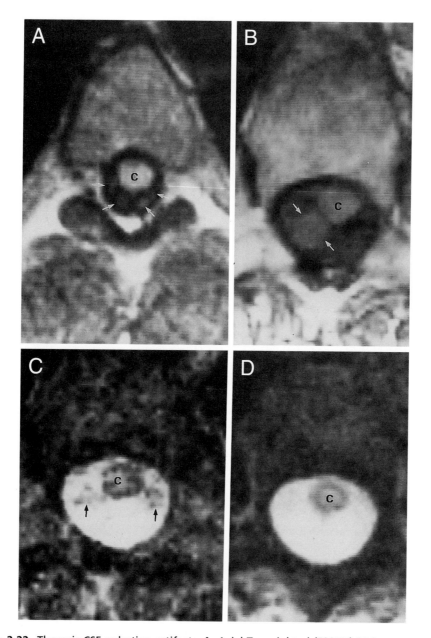

Fig. 2-22. Thoracic CSF pulsation artifacts. **A,** Axial T_1-weighted (500/17) SE image through the midthoracic spine. Note the small ovoid areas of increased signal intensity compared to the adjacent CSF surrounding the posterior and lateral aspect of the cord *(white arrows)*. These represent areas of relatively slower CSF flow and pulsations and should not be mistaken for intradural masses. **B,** T_1-weighted SE (500/17) image through the midthoracic spine. An ovoid area of signal intensity similar to that of the adjacent cord *(c)* is visible posteriorly and laterally on the right. **C,** Axial T_2-weighted SE (2000/90) ungated or refocused image. Note the two areas of relatively decreased signal intensity, approaching that of the adjacent cord laterally and posteriorly *(black arrows)*. This is at the same level as **B.** The fluctuations in signal intensity on both T_1- and T_2-weighted SE images are secondary to variations in the CSF flow and, as seen in **D,** are not evident on an axial FLASH (200/13/10 degree) image.

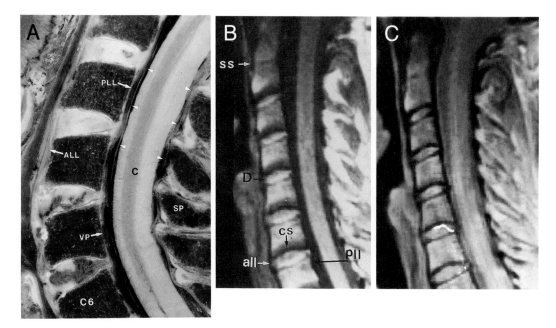

Fig. 2-23. Normal cervical spinal anatomy. **A,** Midline cryomicrotome section through the cervical spine. **B,** Midline sagittal T₁-weighted SE (500/17). **C,** Midline sagittal intermediate SE (2000/20). *ALL (all),* anterior longitudinal ligament; *bvv,* basivertebral vein; *C,* spinal cord; *CS,* chemical shift; *D,* disk; *nl,* nuchal ligament; *PLL (pll),* posterior longitudinal ligament; *SP (sp),* spinous process; *SS,* subdental synchondrosis; *VP (vp),* venous plexus. *Arrowheads* point to the dura mater. **D,** Sagittal midline T₂-weighted (2000/90) refocused image. **E,** Sagittal midline FLASH (200/13/10 degree) image. **F,** Sagittal midline FLASH (200/13/60 degree) image. **G,** Sagittal midline T₁-weighted SE (500/17) before administration of Gd-DTPA. **H,** Sagittal midline T₁-weighted SE (500/17) following the intravenous administration of 0.1 mmol/kg of Gd-DTPA. Note that there is some enhancement of the basivertebral veins but little in the midline posterior to the vertebral bodies. **I,** Parasagittal T₁-weighted SE (500/17) following the administration of 0.1 mmol/kg of Gd-DTPA. Note that there is now enhancement in the anterior longitudinal epidural venous plexus. **J,** Sagittal midline T₂-weighted turbo-SE (5000/100).

plates the cervical vertebral bodies are penetrated by the basivertebral veins, as are the thoracic and lumbar vertebrae.

The cervical pedicles are paired, short, cylindric structures filled with cancellous bone marrow and surrounded by a compact cortical bone rim. They connect the vertebral body to the articular pillars midway between the superior and inferior articular processes. Axial sections through the pedicles reveal the spinal canal completely surrounded by bone. The laminae (originating from the articular pillars) are two struts of bone that join in the midline at an obtuse angle to form the spinous process. The cervical vertebrae are characterized by a foramen within each transverse process (foramen transversarium) that transmits the vertebral artery and small veins. The transverse foramina of C2 through C6 are round or oval and slightly larger on the left than on the right.

The uncinate processes are short bony ridges that project superiorly from the lateral margins of C3 to C7 and fit into corresponding notches laterally and posterolaterally in the lower endplates of C2 to C6. Although in the same plane as the disk superiorly, they can usually be discerned by the increased signal from the vertebral marrow. Oblique clefts in the disk following the medial contour of the uncinate process give the impression of true articulations, commonly referred to as the uncovertebral joints of Luschka.

The configuration of the cervical spinal canal is triangular with the apex posterior. The spinal canal decreases in size from C1 to C3 and has a fairly uniform dimension from C3 through C7. The anterior-posterior diameter of the normal cervical canal has a lower limit of 12 mm in the lower cervical spine, 15 mm at C2, and 16 mm at C1 in both males and females. C7 is a transitional vertebra, whose spinous process is longer, thicker, and

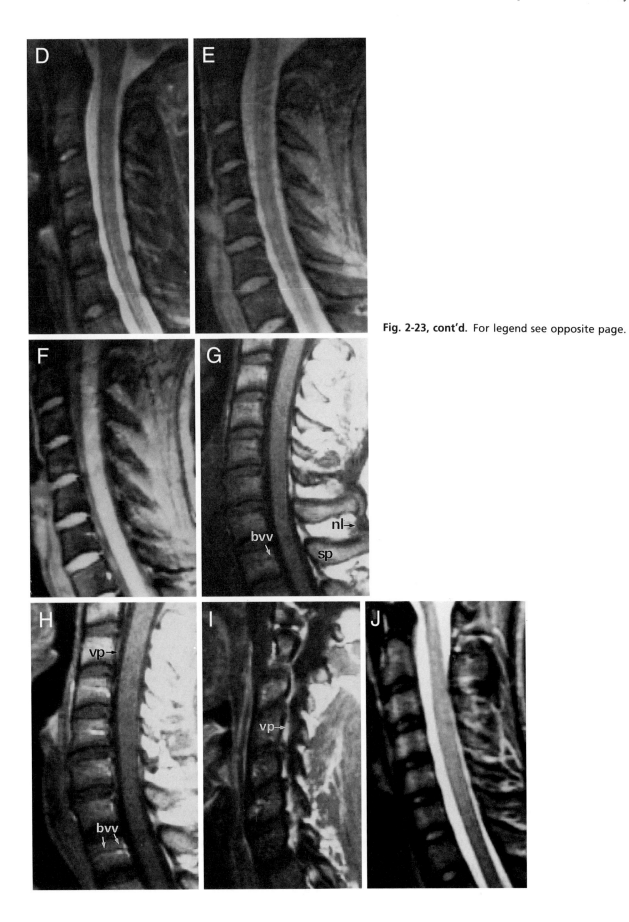

Fig. 2-23, cont'd. For legend see opposite page.

has a more inferior tilt than the more rostral cervical spinous process.

Facet Joints

The facets form diarthrodial joints between the superior and inferior articular processes of adjacent neural arches. They are more oblique in the cervical than in the thoracic and lumbar spine, with capsules that are more lax than at other levels to allow a gliding motion. They lie approximately halfway between the axial and coronal planes. The lining of each joint surface is articular cartilage. Menisci are present within the cervical facets and have a variable appearance depending on the level and the subject's age. Their purpose is the uniform distribution of pressure.[43] In adults they are usually small and triangular but in children may be large and flat. Surrounding each joint is a fibrous capsule with a synovial membrane on its inner aspect.

The facets between the dens and atlas, the occipital condyles and atlas, and the atlas and axis form synovial joints. The pivot facets between the odontoid process and the atlas and axis usually contain two small synovial cavities, one anteriorly between the anterior arch and the dens and the other between the dens and the transverse ligament. The more posterior one, together with the transverse ligament and prominent venous structures, forms a small protuberance of intermediate signal intensity.

Epidural Space and Ligaments

The cervical epidural space that surrounds the thecal sac contains neurovascular and connective tissue elements. The cervical vertebrae are connected by the anterior and posterior longitudinal ligaments. The anterior longitudinal ligament covers the anterior-lateral aspect of the disks and vertebral bodies from the anterior margin of the foramen magnum to the sacrum. The posterior longitudinal ligament extends over the posterior aspect of the vertebral bodies from the posterior surface of C2 to the sacrum. Its fibers diverge at each disk level and blend with the anulus fibrosus and adjacent margins of the vertebral bodies. At the midvertebral level the ligament is narrower and lies 1 to 2 mm behind the bodies posterior to the retrovertebral venous plexus. A rostral extension, the tectorial membrane, extends to the foramen magnum and merges into the basiocciput at the level of the hypoglossal canal inside the skull.

The supraspinous ligament connects the tips of the spinous processes, and the intraspinous ligament extends between them. The ligamentum flavum is situated in the posterior aspect of the spinal canal and attaches to the laminae of the adjacent neural arches. The elastic fibers within it impart a yellow color on anatomic sections. The signal intensity of the ligamentum flavum on T_1-weighted spin-echo images is less than that of fat and equal to or slightly greater than that of muscle.

Beneath the tectorial membrane lies the cruciform ligament of the atlas. The most important component of this structure is the transverse ligament, crossing the ring of the atlas to enclose the odontoid process. The inferior and superior longitudinal bundles extend from the transverse ligament respectively down to the body of the axis and up to the basiocciput. The accessory atlantoaxial ligaments extend from the bases of the lateral masses at the atlas to merge into the base of the dens and the body of the axis. These ligaments may be significant because of the arteries they support (i.e., branches of the vertebral artery that provide the dens with a portion of its blood supply). At the apex of the dens is the small apical ligament, which attaches to the anterior rim of the foramen magnum. It is flanked by two alar ligaments that pass out to the lateral margin of the foramen magnum.[5,6,42]

Cord and Nerve Roots

The cervical spinal cord is nearly elliptic in cross section, and the vertically oriented dentate ligaments tether it laterally. The dentate ligaments take the form of a serrated ribbon attached along the lateral surface of the cord midway between the dorsal and ventral roots. The spinal cord is enlarged in two regions for innervation of the limbs. The rostral enlargement extends from C4 through T1. The corresponding spinal nerves join in the brachial plexus to supply the upper extremities. Eight pairs of spinal nerves arise from the cervical cord. Each consists of a dorsal (sensory) and a ventral (motor) root. The nerve roots fuse just beyond or lateral to the dural sheath to form the spinal nerves. The dorsal root ganglion is located in the neural foramen just proximal to the point of union of the dorsal and ventral roots. The roots of each spinal nerve from C1 through C7 leave the spinal canal through the intervertebral foramina above the corresponding vertebrae. There are eight cervical cord segments and seven cervical vertebrae.[5,6,42] The first and second cranial nerves lie respectively on the vertebral arches of the atlas and axis. The eighth cervical nerve passes through the foramen between the seventh cervical and first thoracic vertebrae.[5,6,42]

The size and contour of the spinal cord are well depicted on T_1-weighted images, where the cord has a higher signal intensity than the CSF, allowing maximum cord-CSF contrast. On fast gradient echo scans the cord has a decreased signal intensity, with flip angles of 5 to 15 degrees relative to the signal intensity of the CSF and an isointense crossover at approximately 20 degrees (Fig. 2-23). With increasing flip angles the CSF loses signal intensity relative to the cord. On T_2-weighted spin-echo images with refocusing or cardiac gating the signal intensity of the CSF, again, is high relative to that of the cervical cord[39] (Fig. 2-23).

Sagittal images through the cervical cord often reveal linear regions of altered signal intensity that can cause problems by obscuring the anatomy and simulating pathologic conditions (e.g., syrinx formation). The signal may be decreased on T_1-weighted but increased on more T_2-weighted images. This appearance is created by sampling-related effects (truncation errors), which can be predicted to occur at high-contrast anatomic boundaries. It is possible to reduce or eliminate them by increasing the number of phase-encoded steps, interchanging the phase-encoded direction with frequency direction or filtering. They are usually not a problem when a 256×256 matrix or smaller field of view is used.[44,45] (See Chapter 1.)

Axial sections through the cervical cord often reveal internal structure (e.g., gray-white architecture) as well as external surface anatomy (Figs. 2-24 and 2-25). The ventral and dorsal nerve roots are identified coursing through the subarachnoid space en route through their respective neural foramina. In the anterior-lateral recesses of the neural foramina a high signal intensity is often visualized surrounding the nerve roots that represents the extensive venous network in the anterior cervical epidural space and foramina.[46] In contrast to the lumbar region, there is a paucity of fat in the cervical epidural region.

Cross-sectional imaging is best performed with acquisitions oriented parallel and orthogonally to the area of interest. This allows complete evaluation by means of two views differing by 90 degrees. In the cervical spine transverse and sagittal views are complementary in the central portion of the neural canal and obviate some of the disadvantages of partial volume averaging. The routine parasagittal images, however, are not optimally oriented for the neural foramina, which forces reliance on the axial image. The additional acquisition of oblique MR images oriented perpendicular to the true course of the neural foramina facilitates the identification of disease laterally by providing a second, orthogonal, imaging plane relative to the diseased area.[47-49] This can be acquired either directly or, more commonly, with multiplanar reformations from three-dimensional datasets (Fig. 2-26). Anatomic studies have described the cervical neural foramen as a 4 to 5 mm long bony canal through which the cervical nerve roots pass anterolaterally 45 degrees to the coronal plane and inferiorly 10 degrees to the axial plane. This is best depicted by oblique T_1-weighted images in which the ventral and dorsal nerves are identified in the inferior portion of the neural foramen at or below the disk level.[47] Each foramen is outlined by a dark line corresponding to the compact cortical bone of the inferior pedicle superiorly, the superior pedicle inferiorly, the posterior vertebral bodies anteriorly, and the posterior elements posteriorly. The uncinate process appears as a small triangular osseous projection.[47] The visual integration of oblique and axial images decreases the problem of partial volume averag-

ing and the potential problem created by an interspace gap; it also allows one to distinguish disk from bone accurately and to determine the relationship of both the neural structures. The oblique plane can be oriented to include all the cervical neural foramina but must be interpreted on contiguous images since the foramina do not lie in the same superoinferior plane.

Disk

The cervical intervertebral disks are similar in composition to but smaller than the thoracic and lumbar disks. Their lateral extent is less than that of the corresponding vertebral body because of the uncinate processes on the vertebrae. In the cervical, as in the lumbar, spine the disks are wedge shaped, the greater width being anterior. This produces the normal cervical lordosis.[16] Their signal intensity on various pulse sequences is, again, similar to that in the lumbar region but not as well appreciated because of their smaller volume.

Cerebrospinal Fluid

The effect of physiologic parameters on the MR behavior of CSF is greatest in the cervical region. Here again changes in the signal intensity may be related to flow-related enhancement, ghosting, and/or spin dephasing. Flow-related enhancement is most obvious in the cervical region, where it usually occurs at the entry slice secondary to a wash-in of the unsaturated spins produced by the pulsatile motion of CSF[39] (Fig. 2-27, *A*). It is less commonly seen as an exit slice phenomenon secondary to the pulsatile to-and-fro nature of the CSF motion. Ghosting and spin dephasing can also degrade the quality of the examination—especially at higher field strengths, where one excitation is the rule (Fig. 2-27, *B*) and thus refocusing and/or gating are usually employed (Fig. 2-27, *C* and *D*). As mentioned, an additional trick to reduce ghosting artifacts is to exchange the read and phase direction so they are oriented away from the area of interest[38] (Fig. 2-27, *E* and *F*).

Vascular Anatomy

The transverse foramina contain the vertebral arteries and veins in a plexus of sympathetic nerve fibers. The arteries usually enter the foramina at the C6 level, but may enter at C5 or C7, and exit the foramina in the area of the transverse process of the atlas; they wind around the lateral masses, passing in a group just posterior to the superior articular facet, from the cranial surface to the posterior arch. Blood for the spinal cord is from branches of the vertebral, thyrocervical, and costocervical arteries, which enter the canal through the intervertebral foramina.[46]

The cervical epidural venous plexus, an extensive sinusoidal network in the cervical epidural space[46] (Figs.

Text continued on p. 77.

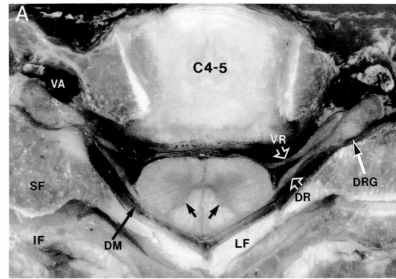

Fig. 2-24. For legend see opposite page.

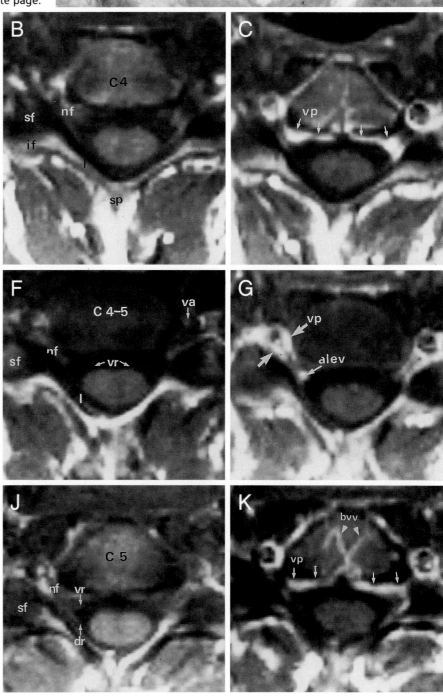

Fig. 2-24. Normal axial anatomic sections and MR images (T$_1$-weighted and FLASH) before and after administration of Gd-DTPA at the C4 through C5 levels. **A,** Cryomicrotome section through the C4-5 disk. **B, C, F, G, J,** and **K,** T$_1$-weighted SE (500/17) images before and after administration of Gd-DTPA through the L4-5 disk and adjacent vertebral bodies. **D, E, H, I, L,** and **M,** FLASH (200/13/60) before and after Gd-DTPA through the same locations. *alev,* Anterior longitudinal epidural vein; *bvv,* basivertebral vein; *cfp,* communicating foraminal plexus; *DM,* dura mater; *DR (dr),* dorsal root; *DRG,* dorsal root ganglion; *IF (if),* inferior facet; *I,* lamina; *LF,* ligamentum flavum; *nf,* neural foramen; *SF (sf),* superior facet; *sp,* spinal process; *VA (va),* vertebral artery; *vp,* venous plexus; *VR (vr),* ventral root. *Arrows* point to the gray matter. **B, C, D,** and **E** are through C4. **F, G, H,** and **I** are through the L4-5 disk. **J, K, L,** and **M** are through the C5 body.

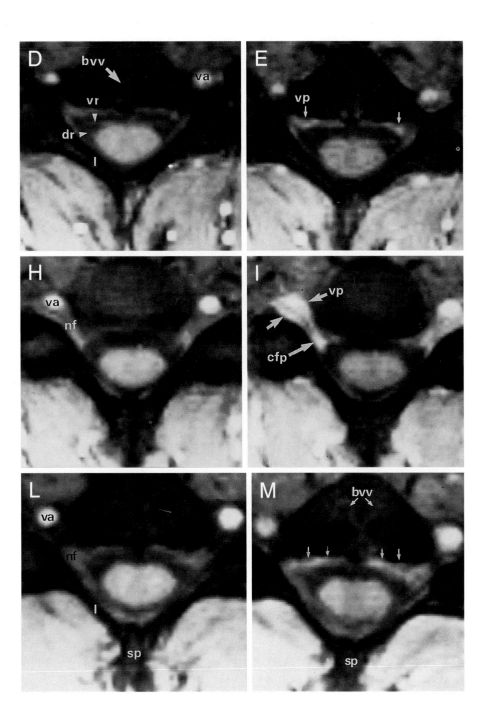

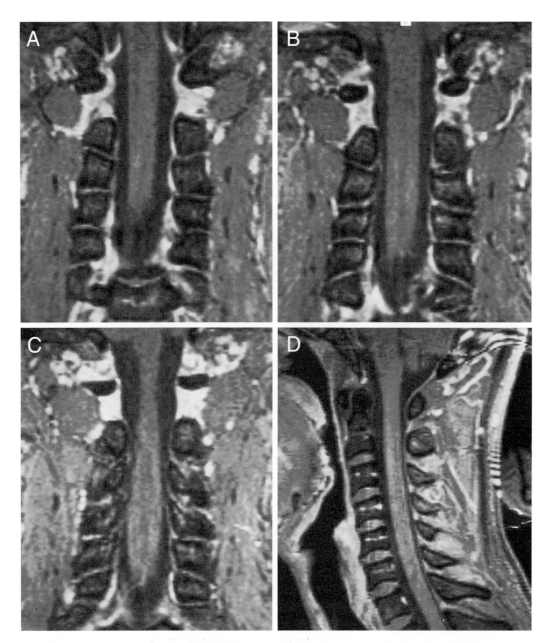

Fig. 2-25. Three-dimensional MPRAGE* dataset following the administration of Gd-DTPA. **A, B,** and **C** are 1.2 mm coronal partitions from anterior to posterior through the cervical cord. **D** is a 1.2 mm midline reformatted sagittal image from the three-dimensional coronal partition dataset. **E, F, G,** and **H** are 1 mm axial reformations through the C4-5 disk space from the coronal partition dataset. There is a high signal intensity within the epidural venous plexus from the gadolinium, which is useful for increasing the conspicuousness of extradural disease.

*Magnetization-prepared rapid-acquisition gradient echo.

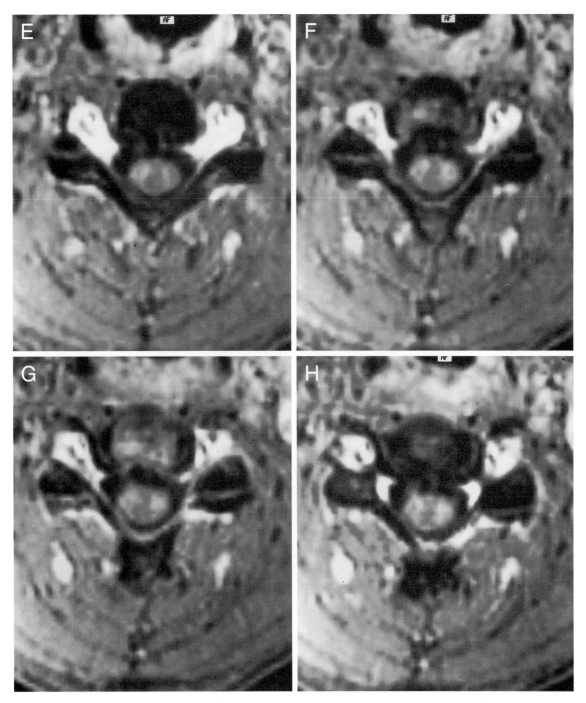

Fig. 2-25, cont'd. For legend see opposite page.

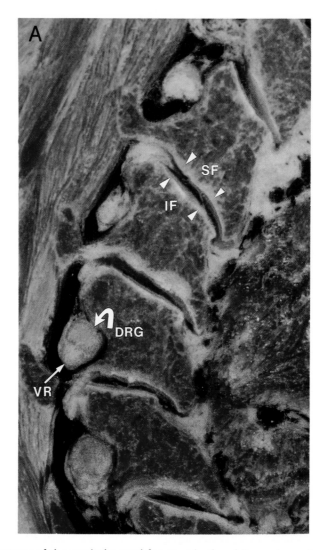

Fig. 2-26. Anatomy of the cervical neural foramen in the oblique plane. **A,** Cryomicrotome section through the cervical neural foramen. *IF (if),* Inferior facet; *SF (sf),* superior facet; *DRG,* dorsal root ganglion; *VR,* ventral root; *nf,* neural foramen; *up,* uncinate process; *p,* pedicle; *va,* vertebral artery. **B** and **C,** Contiguous T$_1$-weighted spin echo (500/17) 4 mm oblique images through the neural foramen. **D, E,** and **F,** 1 mm oblique reformatted images from a coronal three-dimensional MPRAGE dataset (see Figure 2-25).

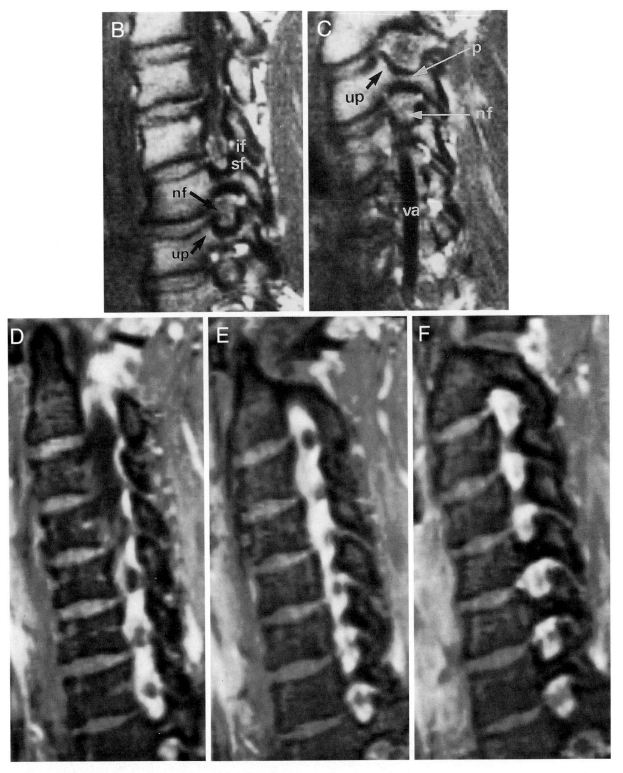

Fig. 2-26, cont'd. For legend see opposite page.

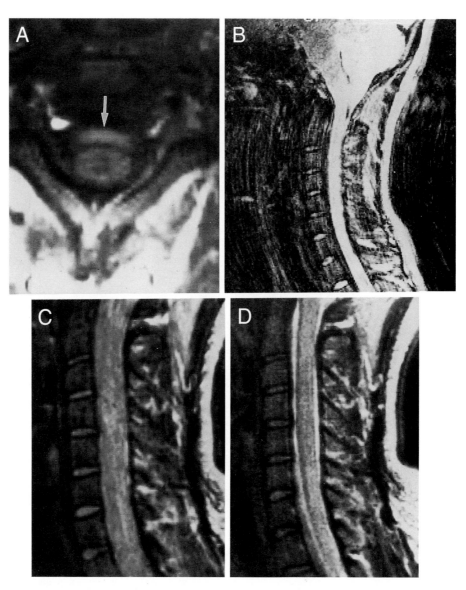

Fig. 2-27. CSF pulsations and refocusing. **A,** An axial T$_1$-weighted SE (500/17) image that is the first of a multislice series shows increased signal intensity anterior to the cord (demarcated by the *arrow*) representing the entry slice phenomenon that is secondary to entry of unsaturated CSF into the imaging volume. **B,** Midline sagittal T$_2$-weighted SE (2000/90) unrefocused or gated image. Note the extensive CSF ghosting artifacts on this long TE image with only one excitation without gating or refocusing. **C,** Sagittal midline T$_2$-weighted SE (2000/90) partially refocused image. Even with one excitation, this long TE image shows little if any CSF ghosting. The refocusing, however, is partial, with no clear separation between CSF and cord, indicating that there is still some blurring of the margins. **D,** Midline sagittal T$_2$-weighted SE (2000/90) image with more carefully calibrated refocusing in the same plane as **C.** With better-calibrated refocusing there is now a clear separation of the CSF/cord interface as well as elimination of CSF ghosting artifacts.

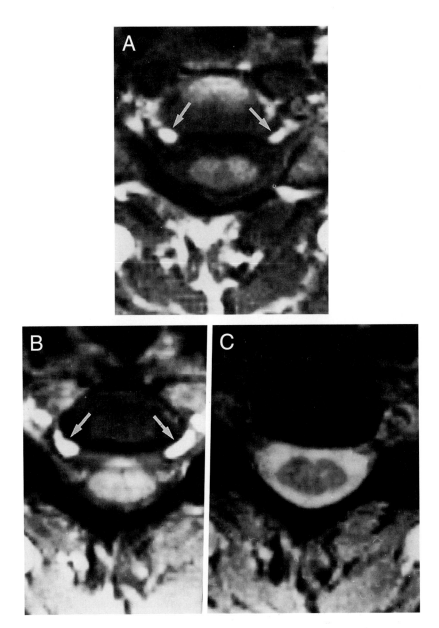

Fig. 2-28. Variable epidural venous signal. **A,** Axial T_1-weighted SE (500/17) image through the region of the neural foramina at C4-5. Note the high signal intensity of the epidural veins and proximal portion of the neural foramen (as outlined by the *arrows*). **B,** Axial FLASH 200/13/60 degrees. Again, note the high signal intensity of the epidural venous plexus, lateral aspect of the neural canal, and proximal portion of the neural foramen. **C,** An axial FLASH (200/13/10 degree) image shows no increased signal intensity of the epidural venous plexus in the same plane as **A** and **B.** This variation in signal intensity is related to multiple factors—which include pseudogating, the TR, and the velocity of blood within the venous plexus and epidural veins. Signal intensity of the blood within the epidural veins and plexus is related to the TE, TR, and slice position as well as to any physiologic gating.

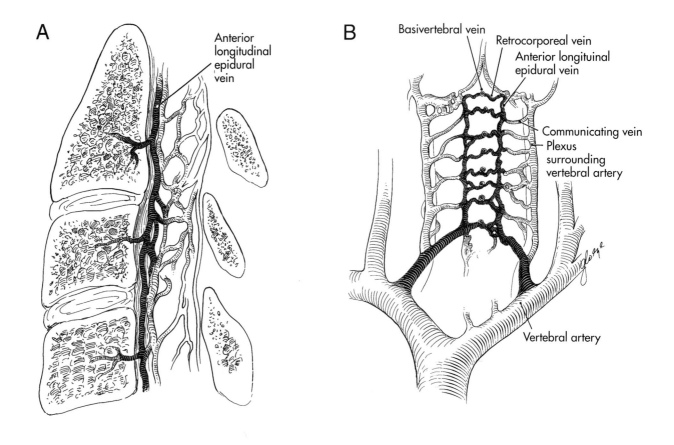

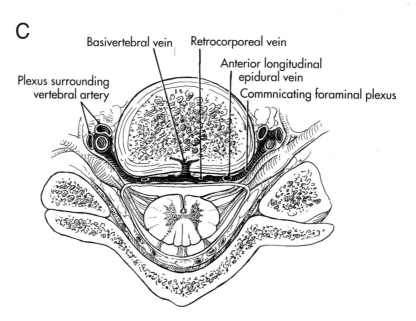

Fig. 2-29. Cervical vertebral venous anatomy in the sagittal, **A,** coronal, **B,** and axial, **C,** planes. **D, E,** and **F** represent maximum intensity pixel-projected magnetic resonance venographic images of the epidural venous plexus. These images were obtained from a 3D MPRAGE dataset following the administration of Gd-DTPA. (**A** to **C** from Flanagan BD, Lufkin RB, McGlade C, et al: *AJNR* 1987;8:27-32.)

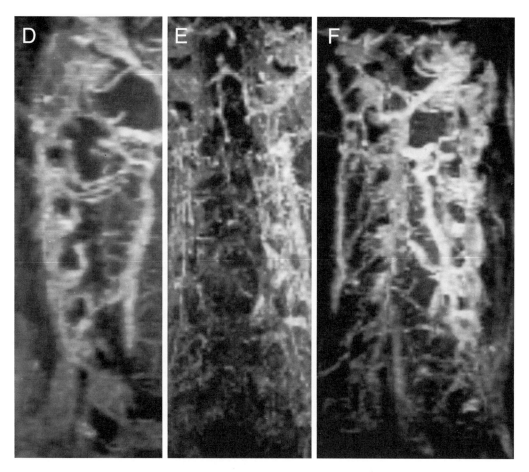

Fig. 2-29, cont'd. For legend see opposite page.

2-23, 2-24, 2-28, and 2-29), is especially prominent at the level of C2. It consists of medial and lateral longitudinal channels in the anterolateral portion of the epidural space connected behind each vertebral body by retrocorporeal veins (like rungs on a ladder) that communicate with the basivertebral venous system at the midportion of each vertebral body. Posterior internal veins lie ventral to the vertebral arches and ligamenta flava and receive veins from these structures. The anterior internal veins lie behind the vertebral bodies and receive veins from the ventral dura and vertebral bodies. The external venous plexus lies outside the vertebral channel along the surfaces of the vertebral bodies and communicates with the internal plexus through veins in the neural foramina. The longitudinal channels communicate with the foraminal venous plexus, which extends anteriorly to surround the vertebral artery on each side. This system is an intricate latticelike network composed of slowly flowing blood. The veins can be seen on both sagittal and axial images as areas of increased signal intensity. Parasagittal views demonstrate them best in the anterior-lateral recess of the cervical spinal canal (Fig. 2-23). Increased intensity denotes slow to stagnant venous flow. Axial sections show these segmented longitudinal bandlike channels as areas of high signal intensity in the anterolateral recess of the spinal canal (Fig. 2-28). Though often seen on nonenhanced contrast studies, the epidural venous plexus can appear confusing depending on the direction and velocity of blood flow. It is more consistently and accurately depicted following the administration of gadolinium diethylenetriamine pentaacetic acid (Gd-DTPA), which produces a uniform high signal intensity of the epidural venous structures outside the extradural space along the anterolateral aspects of the spinal canal and neural foramina (Figs. 2-23 and 2-24).

REFERENCES

1. Kricun ME: Red-yellow marrow conversion: Its effect on the location of some solitary bone lesions. *Skeletal Radiol* 1985;14:10-19.
2. Ricci C, Cova M, Kang YS, et al: Normal age related patterns of cellular and fatty bone marrow distribution in the axial skeleton: MR imaging study. *Radiology* 1990;177:83-88.
3. Hajek PC, Baker LL, Goobarg JE, et al: Focal fat deposition axial bone marrow: MR characteristics. *Radiology* 1987;162:245-249.
4. Saywell WR, Crock HV, England JPS, Steiner RE: Demonstration of vertebral body end plate veins by magnetic resonance imaging. *Br J Radiol* 62:290-292, 1989.
5. Dorwart RH, Sauerland EK, Haughton VM, et al: Normal lumbar spine. In Newton TH, Potts DG (eds): *Computed tomography of the spine and spinal cord.* San Anselmo Calif, Clavadel, 1983, pp 93-114.
6. Latchaw R, Taylor S: CT of the normal and abnormal spine. In Latchaw R (ed): *Computed tomography of the head, neck, and spine.* Chicago, Year Book, 1985, pp 595-618.
7. Daniels DL, Haughton VM, Williams AL: *Cranial and spinal magnetic resonance imaging.* New York, Raven, 1987.
8. Schnitzlein HN, Murtagh FR: *Imaging anatomy of the head and spine.* Baltimore, Urban & Schwarzenberg, 1985.
9. Grenier N, Kressel HY, Schielber ML, et al: Normal and degenerative posterior spinal structures: MR imaging. *Radiology* 1987;165:517-525.
10. Lewin T, Moffet B, Viidik A: The morphology of the lumbar synovial intervertebral joints. *Acta Morphol Neerl Scand* 1962;4:299-319.
11. Schellinger D, Wener L, Ragsdale BD, et al: Facet joint disorders and their role in the production of back pain and sciatica. *Radiographics* 1987;7:923-944.
12. Harris RI, McNab I: Structural changes in the lumbar intervertebral disks: their relationship to low back pain and sciatica. *J Bone Joint Surg (Br)* 1954;36:304-322.
13. Xu GL, Haughton VM, Carrera GF: Lumbar facet joint capsule: appearance at MR imaging and CT. *Radiology* 1990;177:415-420.
14. Resnick D: Degenerative diseases of the vertebral column. *Radiology* 1985;156:3-14.
15. Schellinger D, Manz HJ, Vidic B, et al: Disk fragment migration. *Radiology* 1990;175:831-836.
16. Parke WW, Schiff DCM: The applied anatomy of the intervertebral disc. *Orthop Clin North Am* 1971;2:309-324.
17. Grogan JP, Daniels DL, Williams AL, et al: The normal conus medullaris: CT criteria for recognition. *Radiology* 1984;151:661-664.
18. Monajati A, Wayne WS, Rauschning W, et al: MR of the cauda equina. *AJNR* 1987;8:893-900.
19. Ross JS, Masaryk TJ, Modic MT, et al: MR imaging of lumbar arachnoiditis. *AJNR* 1987;8:885-892.
20. Coventry MB, Ghormley RK, Kernohan JW: The intervertebral disc: its microscopic anatomy and pathology. I. Anatomy, development, and physiology. *J Bone Joint Surg [Am]* 1945;27:105-112.
21. Coventry MB, Ghormley RK, Kernohan JW: The intervertebral disc: its microscopic anatomy and pathology. II. Changes in the intervertebral disc concomitant with age. *J Bone Joint Surg [Am]* 1945;27:233-247.
22. Coventry MB, Ghormley RK, Kernohan JW: The intervertebral disc: its microscopic anatomy and pathology. III. Pathological changes in the intervertebral disc. *J Bone Joint Surg [Am]* 1945;27:460-474.
23. Coventry MB: Anatomy of the intervertebral disk. *Clin Orthop* 1969;67:9-15.
24. Uebermuth H: Über die Altersveränderungen der menschlichen Zwischenwirbelscheibe und ihre Beziehung zu den chronischen Gelenkleiden der Wirbelsäule. *Ber Sachs Ges Akad Wiss* 1929;81:111-170.
25. Uebermuth H: Die Bedeutung der Altersveränderungen der menschlichen Bandscheiben für die Pathologie der Wirbelsäule. *Arch Klin Chir* 1930;156:567-577.
26. Luschka HV: Die Altersveränderungen der Zwischenwirbelknorpel. *Virchows Arch* 1856;9:311-327.
27. Peacock A: Observations on the postnatal structure of the intervertebral disc in man. *J Anat* 1952;86:162-178.
28. Yu S, Sether LA, Ho PSP, et al: Tears of the annulus fibrosus: correlation between MR and pathologic findings in cadavers. *AJNR* 1988;9:367-370.
29. Adams P, Eyre DR, Muir H: Biochemical aspects of development and aging of human lumbar intervertebral discs. *Rheumatol Rehabil* 1977;16:22-29.
30. White AA, Gordon SL: Synopsis: Workshop on idiopathic low-back pain. *Spine* 1982;7:141-149.
31. Lipson SJ, Muir H: Experimental intervertebral disc degeneration: morphological and proteoglycan changes over time. *Arthritis Rheum* 1981;24(1):12-21.
32. Lipson SJ, Muir H: Proteoglycans in experimental intervertebral disc degeneration. *Spine* 1984;6, No. 3.
33. Yu S, Haughton VM, Ho PSP, et al: Progressive and regressive changes in the nucleus pulposus. II. The adult. *Radiology* 1988;169:93-97.
34. Modic MT, Pavlicek W, Weinstein MA, et al: Magnetic resonance imaging of intervertebral disc disease. *Radiology* 1984;152:103-111.
35. Pech P, Haughton VM: Lumbar intervertebral disk: correlative MR and anatomic study. *Radiology* 1985;156:699-701.
36. Aguila LA, Piraino DW, Modic MT, et al: The intranuclear cleft of the intervertebral disk: magnetic resonance imaging. *Radiology* 1985;155:155-158.
37. Winkler ML, Ortendahl DA, Mills TC, et al: Characteristics of partial flip angle and gradient reversal MR imaging. *Radiology* 1988;166:17-26.
38. Edelman RR, Modic MT: New spinal strategies to overcome motion artifacts. *Diagnost Imag* 1987, pp 86-92, Dec.
39. Rubin JB, Enzmann DR: Imaging of spinal CSF pulsation by 2D FTMR: significance during clinical imaging. *AJNR* 1987;8:297-306.
40. Parke WW, Watanabi R: Lumbosacral intersegmental epispinal axons and ectopic ventral nerve root outlets. *J Neurosurg* 1987;67(2):269-277.

41. McMasters DL, deGroot J, Haughton VM, et al: Normal thoracic spine. In Newton TH, Potts DG (eds): *Computed tomography of the spine and spinal cord.* San Anselmo Calif, Clavadel, 1983, pp 79-92.

42. McMasters DL, deGroot J, Haughton VM, et al: Normal cervical spine. In Newton TH, Potts DG (eds): *Computed tomography of the spine and spinal cord.* San Anselmo Calif, Clavadel, 1983, pp 53-78.

43. Yu S, Sether L, Haughton VM: Facet joint menisci of the cervical spine: correlative MR imaging and cryomicrotomy study. *Radiology* 1987;164:79-82.

44. Levy LM, Di Chiro G, Brooks RA, et al: Spinal cord artifacts from truncation errors during MR imaging. *Radiology* 1988;166:479-483.

45. Bronskill MG, McVigh ER, Kucharczyk W, et al: Syrinx-like artifacts on MR images of the spinal cord. *Radiology* 1988;166:485-488.

46. Flanagan BD, Lufkin RB, McGlade C, et al: MR imaging of the cervical spine: neural vascular anatomy. *AJNR* 1987;8:27-32.

47. Daniels DL, Hyde JS, Kneelon KN, et al: The cervical nerves and foramina: local coil MR imaging. *AJNR* 1986;7:129-133.

48. Modic MT, Masaryk TJ, Ross JS, et al: Cervical radiculopathy: value of oblique MR imaging. *Radiology* 1987;163:227-231.

49. Daniels DL, Grogan JP, Johansen JG, et al: Cervical radiculopathy: computed tomography and myelography compared. *Radiology* 1984;151:109-113.

3

Degenerative Disorders of the Spine

MICHAEL T. MODIC

Degenerative disorders of the spine are one of the most common causes of impairment in both men and women and are among the leading causes of disability in the working years.[1-3] Foremost among the disorders attributed to degenerative disease is low back pain. It is estimated[4] that low back pain affects 5% of the adult population each year and that the lifetime incidence of low back pain in American adults is 70% to 80%. Fortunately, the natural history of back pain is such that the majority of sufferers improve with little or no medical intervention. An estimated 60% recover within 1 month, 80% in 2 months, and 90% by 3 months. Some 10% remain disabled after 3 months, and approximately 3% (286,000) have surgery. Nevertheless, despite the self-limited nature of most low back pain, the total societal cost in the United States is estimated at 16 to 60 billion dollars annually[5] and, since back pain is the second leading cause of physician visits among American adults, it is believed that more than 10 billion dollars is spent on direct medical care each year.[6] Much of the direct cost of treating patients with low back pain is related to diagnostic tests.[7] In fact, if one considers the number of MR scanners in the United States, the average cost per examination, and the percentage of the total studies related to the lumbar spine, a figure of 2 billion dollars a year for MR of the lower back alone is a distinct possibility.

Deterioration of the osseous and soft tissue structures of the spine is a normal consequence of the aging process and can be predisposed to or accelerated by a variety of developmental and/or acquired factors. The manner of degeneration of the various components of the spine is mediated and manifested by the specific structure involved. The consequences and symptom complex with which patients present usually involve instability and malalignment abnormalities, intervertebral disk degeneration, and/or herniation, spinal stenosis, and facet disease.[8]

Of the multitude of symptoms that may result from degenerative diseases of the spine, the three most important for attempting to localize a lesion and develop an etiologic differential are pain, sensory changes, and weakness.

Pain is the most important symptom, by virtue of its frequency and the fact that it usually causes debilitation. It may be divided into local, referred, radicular, and secondary (arising from muscular spasm).

Local pain is usually caused by a process that involves the sensory nerve endings. This therefore requires innervation of a structure. For instance, a large amount of vertebral body destruction can occur without pain whereas small lesions involving the periosteum, anulus fibrosus, ligaments, or facet joint capsule lead to extreme pain.

Referred pain is projected from or to the spine and into or from other structures lying within the same dermatome. Pain from diseases of the upper lumbar spine is usually referred to the anterior thighs, legs, or lower back. Pain produced in the lower lumbar spine is usually referred to the lower buttocks because of irritation to the lower spinal nerves, which also activate regions in the posterior thighs and calves. Conversely, pain in the abdominal or pelvic bursae may be referred to the spine.

Radicular pain is similar to referred pain but is usually of greater intensity, with the distal radiation confined to the territory of the irritated nerve root. Radiculopathy refers to pain, weakness, or dysesthesias in the distribution of the spinal nerve with or without reflex changes caused by compression of a nerve root. In the lumbar region the symptom is often called sciatica—that is, pain radiating in the distribution of the sciatic nerve. Radicular pain nearly always emanates from a central position near the spine to some part of the lower extremity and is usually superimposed on a dull referred ache.

Pain from muscular spasm usually occurs in relation to local pain and is reflexive to guard the diseased portions against motion.

Although the pattern of pain can often be described, the pathophysiology of pain in the degenerative spine is not well understood.[9,10] Poor localization of pain caused by disk disease may be related to the multilevel distribution of a single sinu-vertebral nerve.[11] Experimental compression of normal nerve roots induces well-defined functional changes in terms of motor and sensory impairment, but not pain.[12] If the same stimuli are applied to edematous and irritated nerve roots with fibrosis and segmental demyelination, however, significant pain can result.[13-15] Furthermore, compression or displacement of nerve roots is likely to be associated with the release of neurogenic inflammatory agents such as substance P for mediation of nociperception,[16] although this relationship has yet to be fully established. A unifying theory to explain these variables in pain is not yet within our grasp.

In addition to pain, other symptoms of spinal degenerative disease, especially when the cord itself is involved, include weakness of the extremities, spasticity, and/or a sensory deficit. Myelopathic symptoms such as these, particularly in the cervical and thoracic regions, can be caused by extrinsic spinal cord compression from degenerative or neoplastic disease or by intrinsic causes such as cysts, neoplasms, multiple sclerosis, amyotrophic lateral sclerosis, and myelitis.[17] The role of imaging is to sort out these differential considerations, a task for which magnetic resonance is well designed.

The gaps in our knowledge regarding the true causes of back pain in no way invalidate the sensitivity and specificity of MR imaging with respect to anatomic accuracy. They merely show that the depiction of anatomic change by means of MR imaging is but a limited factor in the evaluation of symptomatic patients. Which patients should be watched and rested and which should undergo invasive therapy will continue to be a complex clinical decision. For instance, a patient likely to have a favorable result from lumbar disk excision would have the following: a clear history of sciatica, straight leg raising of less than 30 degrees reproducing sciatica, objective neurologic signs such as reflex sensory or motor loss, and imaging evidence of a disk herniation that corresponded with the appropriate anatomic area. Similar results could be expected in patients with neurogenic claudication, degenerative spondylolisthesis, or complete myelographic blocks. By contrast, the results for

surgical intervention are poor for less well-defined pathology such as disk disruption syndrome, degenerative segmental instability, and bulging lumbar disks, wherein the confirmatory clinical symptoms, signs, and radiographic images are less certain. Therapeutic results are much poorer for pain alone, especially with less well-defined pathologic conditions.[5]

It is also important at the outset to emphasize that just because there is a morphologic abnormality does not mean that it is necessarily responsible for the patient's symptomatology or that the patient must be symptomatic.[18,19]

MALALIGNMENT

Traditionally the evaluation of malalignment abnormalities has consisted of a combination of plain radiographs and tomography with flexion and extension films for the evaluation of abnormal motion. This may still provide the most rapid and cost-effective way of evaluating the bony spinal canal for malalignment. Whereas MR can be used with both flexion and extension views, its major role has been in the evaluation of overall spinal canal contour and alignment in the sagittal, coronal, and axial planes as well as in appraisals of the intervertebral disks, ligaments, and neural foramina. This can best be accomplished by a T_1-weighted spin-echo (SE) sequence or fast variable–flip-angle gradient echo scan in the axial and sagittal planes. Oblique views may be necessary for assessing the pars interarticularis and the cervical neural foramina.

Various types of alignment abnormalities can exist alone or in combination, but the two most frequent are segmental instability and spondylolisthesis.

Segmental instability. Degenerative changes involving the intervertebral disk, vertebral bodies, and facet joints can impair the usual pattern of spinal movement, producing motion that is irregular, excessive, or restricted.

Spondylolisthesis. This condition results when one vertebral body becomes displaced relative to the next most inferior vertebral body (Fig. 3-1). The most common types include degenerative, isthmic, iatrogenic, and traumatic. *Degenerative* spondylolisthesis is seen usually with an intact pars interarticularis, is related primarily to degenerative changes of the apophyseal joints, and is most common at the L4-5 vertebral level presumably because the more sagittal orientation of the facet joints makes them increasingly prone to anterior displacement. Degenerative disk disease may predispose to or exacerbate this condition secondary to narrowing of the disk space, which can produce subsequent malalignment of the articular processes and lead to rostrocaudal subluxation. Retrolisthesis is more common in the cervical and lumbar regions, which are more mobile. *Isthmic* spondylolisthesis occurs secondary to a defect in the pars interarticularis that results in subluxation of the vertebral bodies. *Iatrogenic* spondylolisthesis can occur second-

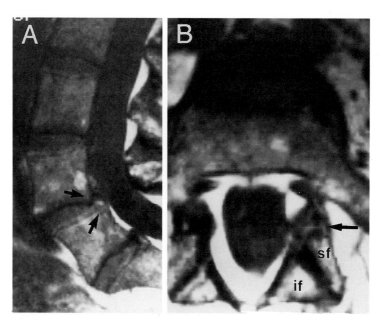

Fig. 3-1. Spondylolisthesis. **A,** This sagittal midline T$_1$-weighted spin-echo (500/17) image demonstrates a grade I spondylolisthesis of L4 on L5 *(arrows).* **B,** This axial T$_1$-weighted spin-echo (500/17) was obtained through the pars of L5. *Black arrow* denotes the region of spondylolysis. *sf,* Superior facet; *if,* inferior facet.

ary to surgery, especially with concomitant facetectomy that produces a loss of stability. This may also occur above levels of fusion secondary to stress fractures because of abnormal motion. *Traumatic* spondylolisthesis can result from fractures of the neural arch and/or facet dislocation. It is more common in the lower thoracic and cervical regions but has been identified in the lower lumbar spine. Various and miscellaneous entities can also result in spondylolisthesis—including rare congenital abnormalities, such as dysplastic spondylolisthesis, and certain pathologic bone states, such as Paget's or metastatic disease, that can result in changes predisposing to abnormal motion.[20]

Sagittal T$_1$-weighted images provide the most accurate means of identifying the spondylolisthesis, but axial and oblique images are needed to define elements of the motion complex as well as the facet joint, pars, and neural arches. There is a decreased signal on all pulsing sequences in the pars resulting from marginal sclerosis at the site of the break. Occasionally there will be increased signal within the gap secondary to the presence of soft tissues. This defect is best appreciated on parasagittal gradient echo images (Fig. 3-2). There are four situations in which the uninterrupted pars can simulate spondylosis on sagittal MR imaging[21]: The first is sclerosis of the neck of the pars. The second is partial volume imaging of a degenerative spur of the superior facet, which may simulate a break. The third is a partial facetectomy. The fourth is osteoblastic metastatic replacement of the marrow of the pars.

DEGENERATIVE DISK DISEASE

Degeneration of the intervertebral disk complex is a process that begins early in life and is a consequence of a variety of environmental factors as well as normal aging. The pathophysiology of this disorder is complicated and poorly understood. It has been stated[22] that *degeneration* as commonly applied to the intervertebral disk covers such a wide variety of clinical, radiologic, and pathologic manifestations as to be really "only a symbol of our ignorance."

The sequelae of disk degeneration remain among the leading causes of functional incapacity in both sexes and are an all too common source of chronic disability in the working years. In accordance with its incidence, morbidity, and socioeconomic impact, degenerative disk disease has given rise to extensive research efforts into its epidemiology, anatomy, biomechanics, biochemistry, and neuromechanisms[23]; and, correspondingly, in an effort to facilitate understanding of its causes as well as their impact on clinical symptomatology and therapy, advances in imaging have been applied both in vivo and in vitro. Again, it is important to stress that imaging studies traditionally have been tools for morphologic analysis.[18,19] A study of 39 children 15 years of age with low back pain[24] showed disk degeneration present in 15 (38%) and in 10 (26%) of normal age-matched controls. Lumbar degeneration was most frequently associated with disk protrusion in Scheuermann-type changes. Tho-

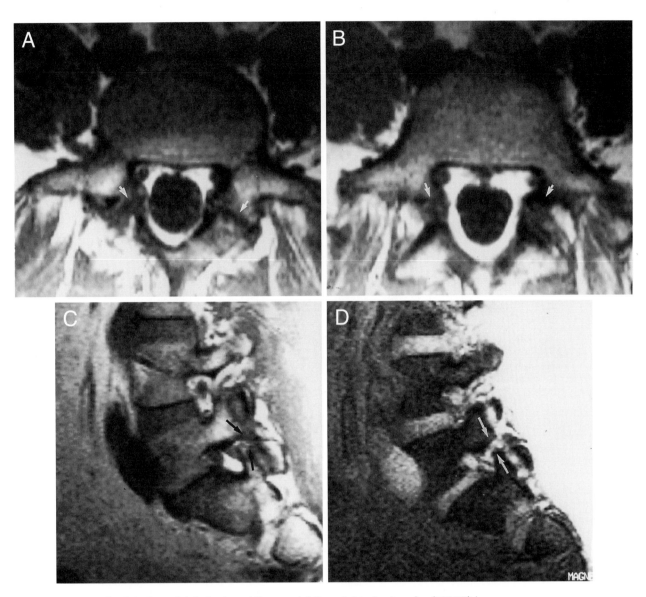

Fig. 3-2. Spondylolysis. **A** and **B** are axial T$_1$-weighted spin-echo (500/17) images demonstrating a defect in the pars bilaterally. **C** and **D** are parasagittal T$_1$ and gradient echo images. *Arrows* identify the pars defect.

racolumbar disk degeneration is enhanced in 20-year-olds with low back pain who have radiologic evidence of Scheuermann disease.[25] By the age of 50 years, 85% to 95% of adults show evidence of degenerative disk disease at autopsy[26]; and thus the jump from identifying an anatomic derangement to proposing a symptom complex must be made with caution, since to date only a moderate correlation has been found between imaging evidence of disk degeneration and symptomatology.[23]

A variety of biochemical and structural changes take place during the processes of aging and degeneration that are so similar as to cause the process of degeneration itself to be thought of as a normal phenomenon of senescence over time.

During aging the cartilaginous endplate becomes thinner and more hyalinized. Fissuring, chondrocyte regeneration, and granulation tissue formation may be noted within the endplate of a severely degenerated disk (Fig. 3-3, *A*) as well as in the anulus fibrosus and nucleus pulposus, indicating attempts at healing.[27]

With degeneration and aging, type II collagen increases outwardly in the anulus and there is a greater water loss from the nucleus pulposus than from the anulus. This results in a loss of the hydrostatic properties of the disk, with an overall reduction of the hydration in both areas to about 70%. The individual chemical structures of the proteoglycans are not changed with degeneration, but their relative composition is. The ratio of keratan sul-

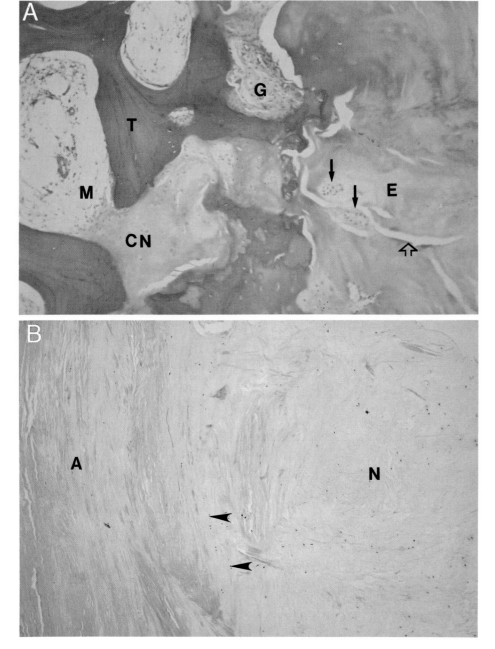

Fig. 3-3. Histology of a degenerated intervertebral disk. **A,** The endplate *(E)* shows cracks and fissures *(open arrow)* as well as areas of pale staining. Packets of chondrocytes *(black arrows)* and granulation tissue *(G)* are characteristic of regeneration and degeneration. A cartilaginous node *(CN)* protrudes between thickened trabeculae *(T).* The adjacent marrow space *(M)* shows an increase in lipid elements. (H&E, low power.) **B,** The transition zone between degenerated nucleus pulposus *(N)* and anulus fibrosus *(A)* shows evidence of fragmentation, fissuring, and sequestration of collagen in both regions, with a loss of normal architecture. Several multinucleated chondrocytes *(arrow)* are indicative of regeneration. (H&E, low power.)

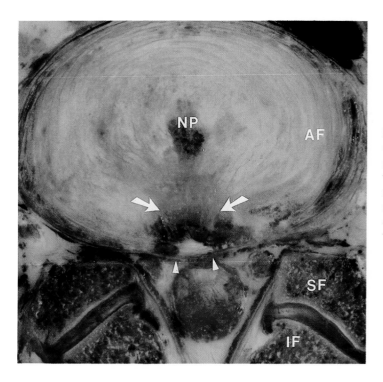

Fig. 3-4. Protruding disk in a 63-year-old woman. On this axial cryomicrotome section of L4-5 the nucleus pulposus *(NP)* protrudes into the anulus fibrosus *(AF)* posteriorly through a radial tear *(arrows)*, producing a focal extension of the disk margin. The outermost layers *(arrowheads)* of the anulus are intact. *SF,* Superior facet; *IF,* inferior facet. (From Yu S, et al: *Radiology* 1988; 169:761-763.)

fate to chondroitin sulfate increases, and there is a diminished association with collagen that may reduce its tensile strength. The decrease in water-binding capacity of the nucleus pulposus is thought to be related to the decreased molecular weight of its nuclear proteoglycan complexes (aggregates). Aggregating proteoglycans, then, may be a sign of health since they are seen to decrease with both aging and degeneration. The disk becomes progressively more fibrous and disorganized, with the end stage represented by amorphous fibrocartilage and no clear distinction between nucleus and anulus[28-31] (Fig. 3-3, *B*).

The etiology of disk degeneration is as yet unknown. Multiple factors have been implicated—autoimmune reaction, genetic makeup, resorption, biomechanics. The immunology of collagen has been studied in some detail, and at least ten different types of collagen have been noted. Some investigators[32-34] have demonstrated the ability of disk tissue to stimulate lymphocytes in regional lymph nodes, but there is no evidence of circulating antibodies or inflammatory infiltrates in the disk itself. Although this issue is by no means resolved, autoimmune reaction has been discounted as a major factor in disk degeneration.[23] In a study of identical twins,[35] data analysis revealed 18% greater mean disk degeneration scores in the lumbar spine of smokers as compared to nonsmokers. The effect was present across the entire lumbar spine, implicating a mechanism acting systemically. Genetic predisposition has been suggested by animal models that consistently develop degenerative disk disease at

an early age (36) as well as by reports of familial osteoarthritis and lumbar canal stenosis in humans.

Cryomicrotome studies have led some workers[37,38] to suggest that the intervertebral disk normally progresses from an immature form through a transitional state to the adult form of nucleus and anulus. As described in the previous chapter, transverse and concentric tears in the anulus fibrosus of normal adult disks are common incidental findings. Whether these are related to symptoms is not yet understood. A study of intervertebral disks based on 160 postmortem examinations[39] showed that anular radial tears often occur early in the process of degeneration and can be followed by prolapse of disk tissue through the fissure. This type of tear may produce instability. Again, whether these are necessarily symptomatic remains controversial. Radial tears begin to develop in the inner and middle portions of the anulus fibrosus. Nuclear material can protrude into a tear and yet be contained within the disk by the intact outer layers of the anulus (Fig. 3-4). These tears may be in the anterior anulus or located centrally or laterally in the posterior anulus as part of a focal bulge of the disk contour. Consequently, the convexly oriented inner layers on the side opposite the radial tear begin to reverse inwardly (Fig. 3-6). At this stage the disk height may still be in the normal range or slightly reduced. As degeneration progresses, the internal structures of the disk become increasingly disarranged and more dense amorphous fibrous tissue with cystic spaces forms within it. A complete disruption may eventually develop in the outermost

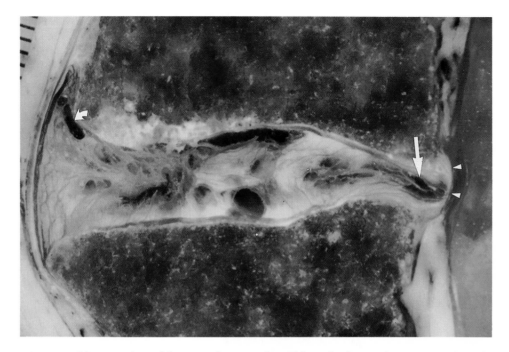

Fig. 3-5. Disk protrusion with severe degeneration. This sagittal cryomicrotome section of the L5-S1 disk in a 60-year-old woman shows the derangement of internal structures. The disk is replaced by cystic spaces and fibrous tissue. A small transverse tear *(curved arrow)* and a radial tear *(arrow)* are evident. Note that the outermost layers of the anulus are intact *(arrowheads)* around the bulge. (From Yu S, et al: *Radiology* 1988; 169:761-763.)

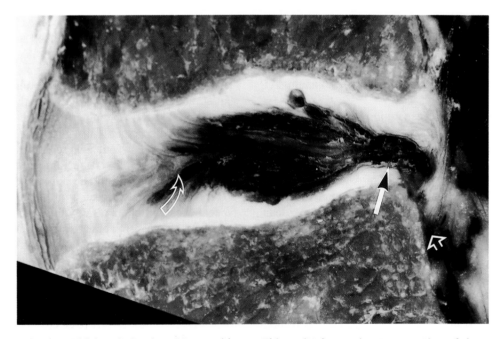

Fig. 3-6. Disk herniation in a 54-year-old man. This sagittal cryomicrotome section of the L5-S1 disk shows a radial tear *(arrow)* with disruption of the outermost anulus *(open arrow)*. The anterior inner anulus reverses inwardly *(curved open arrow)*. (From Yu S, et al: *Radiology* 1988; 169:761-763.)

layers of the anulus, and the nucleus may extrude into the epidural space (Fig. 3-6). At this stage, the disk height is severely reduced and there may be changes in the adjacent endplate and underlying marrow. It is known that the volume of the intervertebral disk tissue decreases with degeneration. The lumbar disk may decrease in volume from 15 to 1 cc, and disk herniation explains only a minor part of this process. In some situations the interior of the disk may be completely replaced by cystic spaces and dense fibrous tissue while the outer layers of the anulus remain intact (Fig. 3-5).

Failure of the lumbar intervertebral disk occurs more frequently in that part of the spine, which is generally subjected to the heaviest mechanical stresses. In studies of high vertical loads on postmortem disks,[40-42] the specimens burst superiorly or inferiorly whereas radial rupture of the anulus was uncommon. Torsional or flexion stresses appear to be more damaging to the anulus fibrosus.[40,41,43]

Results of animal studies suggest that degeneration takes place in response to a loss of the confined fluid state rather than to a primary defect in the proteoglycans. The anulus may begin to fragment, resulting in radial and concentrically oriented fissures that can predispose to degeneration and subsequent herniation of the nucleus both into and through the anulus. Degeneration always follows herniation. It seems likely, then, that the anulus fibrosus may determine the fate of the disk, allowing it to adapt to axial loading or to decompensate, resulting in biochemical changes within the disk itself.[30,31]

This concept, however, is not universally accepted. There are those who believe that the cartilaginous endplate is the critical structure.[22] Others believe that degeneration occurs because as the diskovertebral complex ages its ability to remove cellular catabolites and extracellular matrix degradation products decreases, resulting in abnormal and detrimental biomechanical and biophysical tissue properties.[44,45]

The contrast sensitivity and multiplanar imaging capability of proton MR place this modality in a position to provide a unique noninvasive means of imaging intervertebral disks. The implementation of surface coil technology,[46] cardiac gating,[47] gradient refocusing[48] with paramagnetic contrast agents,[49] saturation pulses,[50] gradient echo volume imaging, turbo (fast)–T_2-weighted spin-echo, and magnetization transfer techniques is likely to refine further the utility of MR imaging for degenerative disk disease.

When a combination of imaging planes and pulse sequence parameters is used, the anatomy of the intervertebral disk, spinal nerves, dural sac, and adjacent structures can be clearly depicted. From a morphologic aspect, MR imaging may be the most accurate means of evaluating the intervertebral disk. Accordingly, most research to date has been directed clinically toward optimizing anatomic image display in a fashion similar to that of CT for the assessment of disk contour.[51-57] Unlike CT and conventional radiography, however, which are dependent on information related to electron density, proton MR signals are influenced by the T_1 and T_2 relaxation times and by proton density, providing greater tissue contrast. Thus its role may go beyond gross anatomic appraisal, to actual tissue characterization of pathology and biochemical change.[58]

The relationship among the vertebral body, endplate, and disk has been studied[59-62] using both degenerated and chymopapain-treated disks as models. Signal intensity changes in vertebral body marrow adjacent to the endplates of degenerated disks are a common observation in MR imaging, appearing to take three main forms:

Type I changes demonstrate decreased signal intensity on T_1-weighted images and increased signal on T_2-weighted images and have been identified in approximately 4% of patients scanned for lumbar disease (Fig. 3-7). They are also seen in approximately 30% of chymopapain-treated disks, which may be viewed as a model of acute disk degeneration.[62]

Type II changes are represented by increased signal on T_1-weighted images and isointense or slightly hyperintense signal on T_2-weighted images (Fig. 3-8) and have been identified in approximately 16% of cases.

In both types there is always evidence of associated degenerative disk disease at the level of involvement.[60] Mild enhancement of type I vertebral body marrow changes is seen with Gd-DTPA that at times extends to involve the disk itself and is presumably related to the vascularized fibrous tissue within adjacent marrow (Fig. 3-9).

Histopathologic sections of disks with type I changes show disruption and fissuring of the endplate and vascularized fibrous tissues within the adjacent marrow, prolonging T_1 and T_2 (Fig. 3-10). Disks with type II changes also show evidence of endplate disruption, with yellow marrow replacement in the adjacent vertebral body resulting in a shorter T_1 (Fig. 3-10). There appears to be a relationship between these, for type I changes have been observed to convert to type II with time but type II changes seem to remain stable. To date no attempt has been made to correlate the marrow changes with clinical symptoms or to determine whether they are related to specific biomechanical derangements such as instability.

Type III changes are represented by a decreased signal intensity on both T_1- and T_2-weighted images that appears to correlate with extensive bony sclerosis on plain radiographs.

Type I and type II changes show no definite correlation with sclerosis seen at radiography (which is not

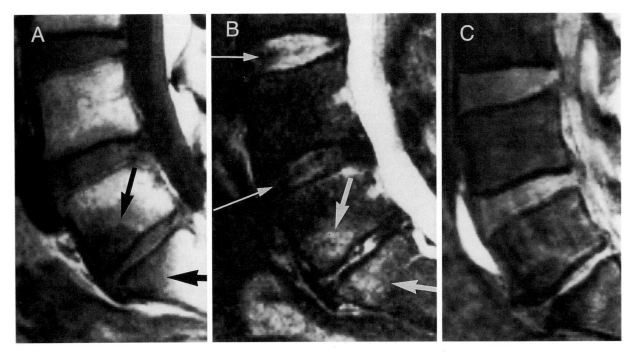

Fig. 3-7. Degenerated lumbar disk and type I marrow change in a 38-year-old woman. **A,** T₁-weighted sagittal (500/17) 4 mm midline section. There is mild narrowing at the L4-5 interspace with moderate narrowing at L5-S1. Note the decreased signal intensity of the adjacent anterior portion of L5 and S1 *(arrows)*, indicative of this type of change. **B,** T₂-weighted sagittal (2000/90) 4 mm midline section. The L3-4 disk has a normal configuration and signal intensity. There is decreased signal of the degenerated L4-5 disk with increased signal of the adjacent portions of L5 and S1 *(large white arrows)*. Note the linear regions of decreased signal bisecting the L3-4 and L4-5 disk *(arrows)*. The high signal intensity within the disk space at L5-S1 is presumably due to fluid within the cracked and fissured L5-S1 disk. **C,** FLASH sagittal (50/13/50 degrees) 4 mm section. The signal difference between the normal L3-4 and degenerated L4-5 disk spaces is reduced compared to that in **B.**

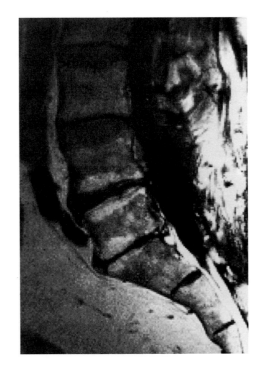

Fig. 3-8. Type II vertebral body change in a 56-year-old man. T₁-weighted sagittal (500/17) 4 mm midline section. Note the high signal intensity within the vertebral body marrow at the L4-5 and L5-S1 disk spaces *(small black arrows)*.

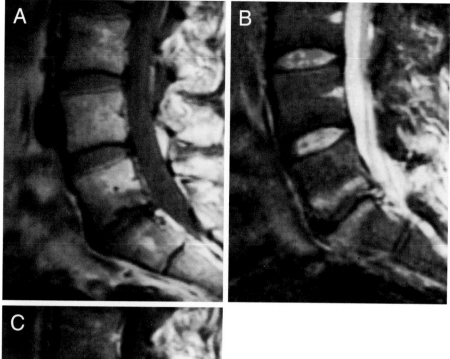

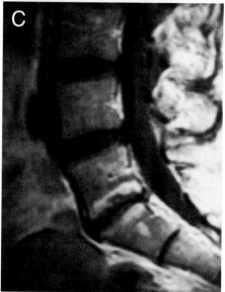

Fig. 3-9. Degenerated lumbar disk with type I marrow change in a 42-year-old woman. **A,** T_1-weighted sagittal (500/17) 4 mm midline section. There is narrowing of the L5-S1 disk space with irregularity of the inferior margin of L5. Note the decreased signal intensity of the adjacent portions of L5 and S1, indicative of this type of change. **B,** T_2-weighted sagittal (200/90) midline section. Note the high signal intensity of the adjacent L5 and S1 vertebral bodies. **C,** T_1-weighted sagittal (500/17) midline section following the administration of Gd-DTPA. There is now enhancement of the decreased signal L5 and S1 in the region of the marrow change.

surprising when one considers the histology); the sclerosis seen on plain radiographs is a reflection of dense woven bone within the vertebral body rather than of the marrow elements. The MR signal intensity is more a reflection of the marrow elements, normal hematopoietic tissue, fibrovascular tissue, and lipid (or lack thereof) between trabeculae.

The lack of signal in the type III change no doubt reflects the relative absence of marrow in areas of advanced sclerosis. Whereas the signal intensity changes of type I may be similar to those seen in vertebral osteomyelitis, the distinguishing factor (at least in adults) is involvement of the intervertebral disk, which shows an abnormal high signal inten-

sity and abnormal configuration on T_2-weighted images of infection.[63] Diskovertebral destruction in ankylosing spondylitis will also cause abnormal signal intensity of the adjacent endplates but will usually show decreased signal in the disk region itself on T_2-weighted images. Increased signal from the disk may suggest an active inflammatory process.[64]

Disk narrowing, sclerosis, and vertebral endplate irregularity suggestive of osteomyelitis have also been demonstrated in long-term hemodialysis and calcium pyrophosphate disease. Classically, in the patient with hemodialysis spondyloarthropathy, the intervertebral disk maintains a low signal intensity on both T_1- and T_2-weighted sequences. Crystal

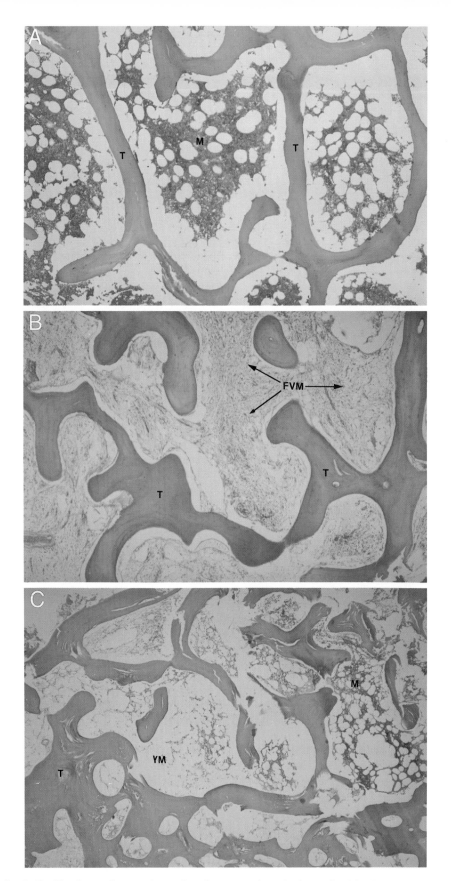

Fig. 3-10. Histology of normal type I and type II subcortical vertebral body marrow changes adjacent to the endplate. **A,** Normal marrow consists of both hematopoietic and lipid elements *(M)*. The bony trabeculae *(T)* are of normal thickness. **B,** In the type I change fibrovascular tissue has entirely replaced normal marrow *(FVM)* between thickened bony trabeculae *(T)*. **C,** In the type II change there is increased lipid content *(YM)* of the marrow space compared to the normal distribution of lipid and hematopoietic elements *(M)*. Note also the thickened woven bony trabeculae *(T)*.

disorders should show increased signal intensity on long TE/TR sequences.[65] Exceptions have been noted, however, when noninfectious spondyloarthropathy demonstrated increased signal within the involved interspace.

Work using T_2-weighted spin-echo sequences[58] further suggests that MR is capable of detecting changes in the nucleus pulposus and anulus fibrosus relative to degeneration and aging based on a loss of signal presumed to be secondary to known changes of hydration that occur within the intervertebral disk (Fig. 3-7). However, the correlation is not straightforward since differences in signal intensity appear to be somewhat exaggerated for the degree of water loss noted with degeneration (about 15%).[17] At present the role that specific biochemical changes (proteoglycan ratios, aggregating of complexes) play in the altered signal intensity is not well understood. In fact, it may be not the total quantity of water but the state that the water is in. Sodium images suggest that the T_2 signal intensity in the disk tracks the concentration and regions of high GAG percentages. Thus it seems likely that the health and status of the proteoglycans determine the signal intensity.

In the case of a severely degenerated disk whose overall signal intensity is decreased there may be linear areas of high signal on T_2-weighted spin-echo images that are thought to represent free fluid within cracks or fissures of the degenerated complex[66] (Fig. 3-7). However, gradient echo images are not so sensitive to the signal-intensity changes within the disk or to T_1 and T_2 changes noted in the adjacent vertebral body with degeneration (Fig. 3-7).

Conventional theory would imply that degeneration and aging are very similar processes, albeit occurring at different rates. Some investigators,[37,68,69,69a] however, have suggested that they can be distinguished by examining the signal intensity on T_2-weighted images. The hypothesis is that normal signal of the intervertebral disk indicates a normally aging disk and decreased signal indicates a radial tear with degeneration.[67] The contention, then, is that anular disruption is the critical factor in degeneration and, when a radial tear develops in the anulus, there is shrinkage with disorganization of the fibrous cartilage of the nucleus pulposus and replacement of the disk by dense fibrous tissue with cystic spaces.[37,68,69,69a]

Although it has certainly been verified that anular disruption is a sequela of degeneration, and certainly is often associated, its role as the causal agent of disk degeneration has certainly not been proved. There is no unifying theory regarding the cause of disk degeneration. It is likely that degeneration and aging are multifactorial processes that encompass a wide spectrum of changes and sequelae, of which the radial tear is but one. In light of the existing controversy and lack of longitudinal studies, to imply that radial tears are anything more than a manifestation of advanced degeneration is unwarranted.

The vacuum phenomenon within a degenerated disk is represented on spin-echo images as areas of signal void[70]; it may not be seen with the same sensitivity as on plain films or CT. Gradient echo sequences demonstrate it better than conventional spin-echo sequences do and as well as plain radiographs and CT (Fig. 3-11). This is due to the magnetic susceptibility effects caused by the intradiskal gas collection and the nature of the gradient echo technique. Magnetic susceptibility effects have been shown[71] to exaggerate the interface between air and blood or bone in other tissues. At these boundaries the susceptibility effect manifests itself as a localized static field inhomogeneity that may have a spatial extent ranging over many pixels. Spin-echo and gradient echo sequences differ in their ability to control this inhomogeneity-produced artifact, which dephases the MR signal intensity locally. The gradient echo sequences lack the spin refocusing pulse of spin-echo sequences, and spin dephasing leads to focal MR signal loss in the vicinity of the susceptibility interface. The longer the TE and the gradient echo sequence, the greater is the dephasing of parent signal loss.[71] Whereas the presence of gas within the disk is usually suggestive of degenerative disease rather than an infected process, spinal infection may (rarely) be accompanied by intradiskal or intraosseous gas.[72]

A gas density cleft within a transverse separation of the vertebral body appearing in extension and disappearing in flexion is characteristic of the vacuum phenomenon within a region of ischemic vertebral collapse. The region of intraosseous gas may be accompanied by high signal intensity on T_2 and is presumably related to fluid within the cleft; it can change with position and time. Rarely the phenomenon has been identified with vertebral body neoplasms such as multiple myeloma.[73-77]

Hyperintense intervertebral disks are a not infrequent finding on T_1-weighted MR images of the spine, and it has been suggested[78] that the relatively "bright" intervertebral disk may reflect diffuse abnormality and loss of normal signal in the marrow of the adjacent vertebral bodies. In the child there is a greater amount of hematopoietic marrow and this results in a lower vertebral body signal intensity versus the disk. As one ages, the lipid to hematopoietic ratio increases and there is a greater difference in signal between body and disk.

Calcification has usually been described on MR as a region of decreased or absent signal. The loss of signal is attributed to a low mobile proton density as well as, in the case of gradient echo imaging, to its sensitivity to the heterogeneous magnetic susceptibility found in cal-

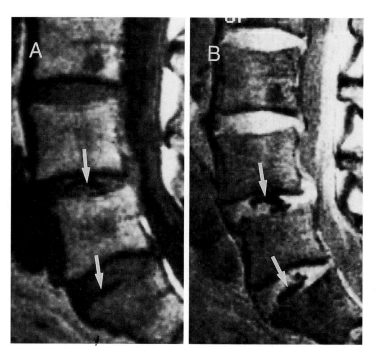

Fig. 3-11. The vacuum phenomenon. **A,** T_1-weighted sagittal (500/17) spin-echo 4 mm midline section. Linear areas of decreased signal are evident in the L4-5 and L5-S1 disks consistent with intradiskal gas or calcification *(arrows).* Note also the herniation at L4-5. **B,** FLASH sagittal (200/13/50 degrees) 4 mm midline section. The areas of decreased signal are more conspicuous on this gradient echo image compared to **A.**

cified tissue. Several causes for calcification in the intervertebral disk have been proposed—trauma, infection, congenital malformation, metabolic disorder, and degenerative change. Ossification of the embryonic disk cartilage has also been observed. In addition, an association has been reported[79-82] between calcification of the nucleus pulposus and patent ductus arteriosus, spina bifida, congenital cataracts, mongolism, ventricular septal defects, pulmonary stenosis, renal hypoplasia, adrenal hyperplasia, and fatty metamorphosis of the liver. Calcification and ossification have been noted in the supporting ligaments.

There is, however, variability of signal intensity of calcium on various sequences; and the type and concentration of calcification are probably important factors. Multiple examples of a hyperintense signal on T_1-weighted spin-echo images in areas that contain calcification on CT have been reported in the literature. These hyperintensities have been attributed to the paramagnetic effects of methemoglobin,[83-85] melanin,[86] and trace elements[87,88] as well as to the T_1-shortening effects of lipids and cholesterol,[89] proteins,[90,91] and laminar necrosis associated with infarction and calcification.[92-96] Focal or diffuse areas of hyperintensity on T_1-weighted spin-echo sequences may also be encountered in the intervertebral disk. A retrospective study of 27 patients who had anecdotally been noted to have one or more hyperintense disks on T_1-weighted images[97] demonstrated that there

was calcification on plain films and/or CT correlating with the hyperintense MR signal intensity at 26 of 31 levels. The converse was not necessarily true. At some levels calcification on plain films and CT corresponded to isointense or decreased signal on T_1-weighted images. In a subsequent analysis there was a significant association between signal on T_1-weighted images and the degree of calcification on plain films, suggesting that heavily calcified disks result in an iso- or hypointense signal intensity.[97] These data correspond nicely to another reported finding that particulate calcium can reduce T_1 relaxation times by a surface-relaxation mechanism. Calcium particles with greater surface areas had greater T_1 relaxation times; and reduced proton density with reduced T_2 tended to diminish the signal intensity, but reduced T_1 increased the signal intensity. For concentrations of calcium particulate up to 30% by weight, the signal intensity on standard T_1-weighted images increased but then subsequently decreased.[92,93] The regions of high signal on T_1 were unaffected by fat suppression, suggesting that it is a T_1-shortening effect rather than the presence of lipid (Fig. 3-12).

Hyperintensities that are affected by fat-suppression techniques have also been noted within intervertebral disks.[97] These are presumably related to areas of ossification with formation of a lipid marrow in the ossified disk space; they also appear calcified on conventional studies (Fig. 3-13).

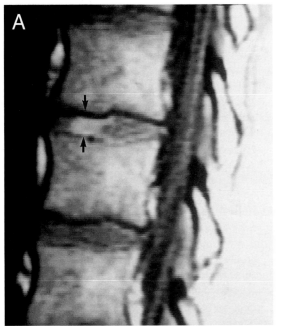

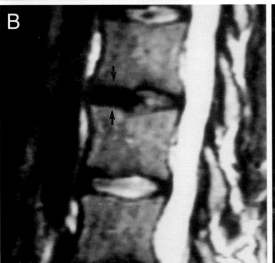

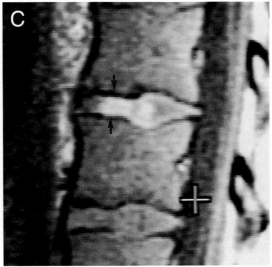

Fig. 3-12. Calcified intervertebral disk in a 28-year-old woman with nonspecific low back pain. **A** is a midline T₁-weighted spin-echo sagittal image (500/17), **B** a midline sagittal T₂-weighted spin-echo (2000/90), and **C** a midline fat-suppressed T₁-weighted spin-echo. The *arrows* point to an area of signal alteration on the anterior aspect of the L2-3 disk. In **A** and **C** there is increased signal intensity that corresponds to the area of decreased signal in **B**. This does not suppress with fat suppression. On CT a faint calcification was identified here.

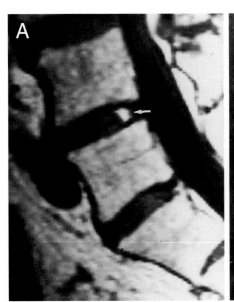

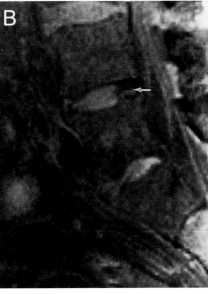

Fig. 3-13. Ossification and marrow formation. **A** is a sagittal T₁-weighted spin-echo image (500/17), and **B** a fat-suppressed T₁-weighted spin-echo. Note the area of high signal in **A** at the posterior aspect of the L4-5 disk *(arrow)*, which is suppressed in **B**. This presumably represents a lipid component within an area of ossification. Calcification was noted here on plain radiographs.

SEQUELAE OF DISK DEGENERATION

Disk herniation, especially in the lumbar and thoracic regions, is probably better depicted by MR imaging than by other modalities.[52-57,98,99] Although degeneration may be seen without herniation, most herniated disks appear degenerated. Notable exceptions are the uncommon juvenile disk herniation and the acute disk herniation as may be noted with spinal trauma. It is, again, important to bear in mind that not all morphologic changes are a cause of symptoms. In a prospective study of individuals who had never had low back pain, sciatica, or neurogenic claudication,[100] one third of the subjects were found to have substantial abnormalities. In patients who were less than 60 years of age 20% had a herniated nucleus pulposus. In the group that was 60 years or older findings were abnormal on 57% of the scans. Thirty-six percent of the subjects had a herniated nucleus pulposus, and 21% had spinal stenosis. There was degeneration or bulging of a disk at at least one lumbar level in 35% of the subjects between 20 and 39 years of age and in all but one of the 60-to-80-year-old subjects.[100] More recent studies[101,102] have confirmed the observation that disk bulges and protrusions are common findings in the asymptomatic population. These latter studies, however, suggest that frank disk extrusion is rare; a disk bulge was observed to be age related, but disk protrusion was not. Anular defects were seen in 13% of asymptomatic individuals. These authors have underscored the point that standardization of nomenclature would be desirable in terms of the accuracy of anatomic description and might provide better correlation of symptomatic versus asymptomatic morphologic changes.[101,102]

Multidimensional imaging allows the direct acquisition of orthogonal views covering long segments of the spine without requiring secondary reconstructions. Alternatively, three-dimensional datasets can be acquired with or without contrast, which allows multiplanar reformation from partition thicknesses for improved overall spatial resolution and reduced examination times. The outer anulus–posterior longitudinal ligament (PLL) complex can usually be seen as an area of decreased signal relative to the inner anulus–nucleus pulposus, which helps in characterizing the type of herniation (protrusion, extrusion, sequestration).[103] This ability to characterize and differentiate the various subgroups of disk herniations has certain diagnostic and therapeutic ramifications, particularly in the lumbar region.

The ensuing categories, which are not universally accepted, have been adapted from the classification scheme utilized by the surgical services at our institution and are similar to those reported by McNab and co-workers. Abnormal disks can be classified as an anular bulge or herniation (protruded, extruded, or free fragment). Concurrently, herniated disk disease should be described by contour, size, location, and presence or absence of enhancement.

The distinction between a bulging anulus and a herniated disk has been thought to be important inasmuch as the bulging disk is less often associated with sciatica than the herniated disk is.

Bulge. An anular bulge is the result of disk degeneration with a grossly intact, albeit lax, anulus, usually recognized as a generalized extension of the disk margin beyond the margins of the adjacent vertebral endplates, regardless of the signal of the interspace. The margin is smooth, symmetric (although occasionally more prominent bilaterally), and without evidence of focal protrusion (Figs. 3-14 and 3-15). An index of disk bulging using sagittal anatomic sections from 149 lumbar disks[104] has been studied. The largest disk bulgings were always associated with radial tears of the anulus, which contradicts the previously held concept that the anulus fibrosus remains intact with a bulging disk.

Some investigators would recognize the anular tear as an intermediate category between bulge and herniation. The significance of the anular tear, however, remains extremely unclear; and it is perhaps best considered as a sequela of disk degeneration rather than as a discrete category that may imply some type of clinical significance.

As mentioned previously, three types of anular tears have been identified: *concentric,* characterized by fluid-filled spaces between adjacent lamellae; *radial,* characterized by rupture of all layers in the anulus between the nucleus and the surface of the disk; and *transverse,* characterized by rupture of Sharpey's fibers of the periphery of the anulus, near the ring apophysis. In a study by Yu et al.[105] T_2-weighted MR images had a 67% sensitivity for the identification of radial anular tears when cryomicrotome anatomic sectioning was used as a comparison. On nonenhanced T_2-weighted MR images anular tears were best appreciated as an area of high signal extending into the area of decreased signal of the anulus-ligamentous complex (Fig. 3-16). Anular tears also can enhance, and a characteristic configuration may be identified on T_1-weighted images after contrast (Figs. 3-17 and 3-18).

Lumbar disk herniations. Obviously some degree of anular disruption is an intrinsic component of any disk herniation.

A protrusion represents herniation of nuclear material through a defect in the anulus, producing a focal or broad-based extension of the disk margin (Fig. 3-19). The extension is less than occurs with an extrusion. At least some fibers of the overlying anulus and PLL remain intact, and the disk is described as "contained." Orthogonal images are critical in evaluating the contour and separating a bulge from a protrusion, a distinction that may not be as apparent on sagittal images alone. The signal intensity of the parent nucleus is usually decreased, as is the extradural defect, particularly on T_2-weighted images. On sagittal T_2-weighted or spin density acquisitions a decreased–signal intensity line

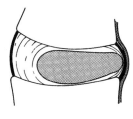
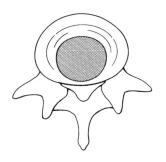

Fig. 3-14. Bulging intervertebral disk. The bulging of the anulus fibrosus is recognized as a generalized extension of the disk margin beyond the boundaries of the adjacent vertebral body endplates, regardless of the signal from the interspace on a T$_2$-weighted image.

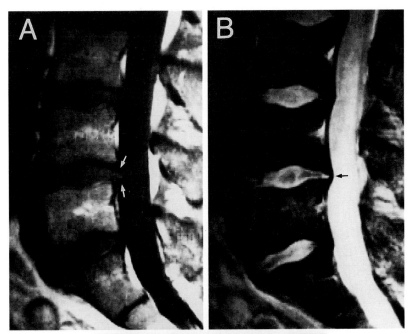

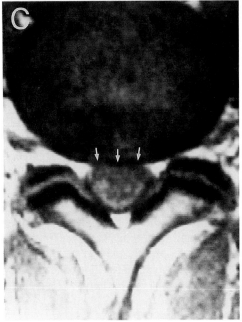

Fig. 3-15. Bulging intervertebral disk. **A,** This midline sagittal T$_1$-weighted spin-echo (500/17) image of the lower lumbar spine demonstrates an extradural defect at the L4-5 level. **B,** A midline sagittal T$_2$-weighted spin-echo (2000/90) of the lower lumbar spine, again, shows a mild anterior extradural defect at the L4-5 level. Note that there is no focal extension of the high-signal disk material beyond the interspace *(arrow)*. **C,** An axial T$_1$-weighted (500/17) spin-echo image through the L4-5 disk demonstrating smooth symmetric extension of the anulus beyond the margins of the adjacent endplate *(arrows)*.

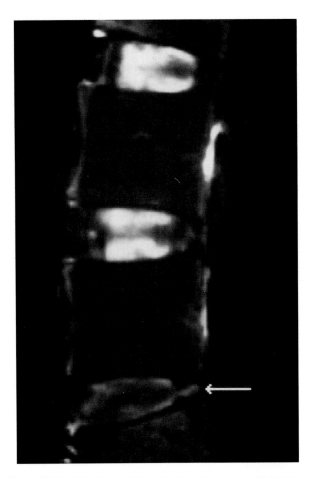

Fig. 3-16. Sagittal T_2-weighted spin-echo image (2000/90) through a cadaveric spine. Note the loss of signal intensity at the L4-5 disk and the region of high signal extending into the anulus-ligament complex. This represents an anular tear.

containing the disk protrusion is often evident. These defects can be central or lateral (Figs. 3-20 to 3-22).

The next two categories, extrusion and sequestration, represent herniations that are no longer contained by the overlying anulus and ligament. In an extrusion nuclear material becomes an anterior extradural mass that remains attached to the nucleus of origin, often via a high-signal pedicle on T_2-weighted images (Fig. 3-23). The signal intensity of the extruded portion may be increased or decreased. The disk usually appears contained by the PLL and remaining contiguous portions of the anulus, which show up as curvilinear areas of decreased signal (Figs. 3-24 and 3-25). All disk herniations, whether small or large, can be associated with enhancement and, as will be discussed later, this enhancement may constitute a large portion of the extradural mass (Fig. 3-26).

The term *free fragment* or *sequestrated disk* refers to disk material external to the anulus fibrosus and no longer contiguous with the parent nucleus (Fig. 3-27). A free fragment can lie anterior to the PLL, especially

if it has migrated behind a vertebral body, where the ligament is not in direct apposition (Figs. 3-28 and 3-29), posterior to the PLL (Figs. 3-30 and 3-31), and even rarely within the dura (Fig. 3-32). Nevertheless, there is almost invariably penetration through the PLL, either posteriorly (at the point of fusion with the anulus) or superiorly or inferiorly (at the point of fusion with the vertebral body margin). Again, contained portions of the anulus and PLL may be seen as curvilinear areas of decreased signal surrounding the disk fragment.

In the majority of patients in whom a free disk fragment has migrated behind the vertebral body it will lateralize, pushing disk material across the midline with its leading edge smoothly capped. It has been postulated[106] that this shape is imposed by a midline septum in the anterior epidural space, which is largest in the lower lumbar region, delineated posteriorly by the PLL and laterally attached membranes and anteriorly by the vertebral body. It is thus divided into two compartments by the sagittally aligned septum.[106]

Free disk fragments within the lateral recess and the neural foramen have been shown to erode cortical bone and expand those spaces and thus should be considered in the differential diagnosis of a mass arising within and expanding the neural foramen and lateral recess. Free fragments may also (uncommonly) migrate posteriorly in relation to the thecal sac and even intradurally. Intradural disk herniation is rare, with only 52 cases reported (Fig. 3-32). It seems more frequent in the lower lumbar spine, where its incidence varies between 0.04% and 0.33%, and it may be related to the development of a chronic inflammation with adhesions between the dura and PLL.[107,108] As the herniated disk pushes outward, the ligament extends through the dura instead of pushing it aside. Other possible causes are congenital connections between the ligament and the dura[107] or previous surgery.[108]

A frequent finding with both extruded and free fragments is the presence of a high–signal intensity extradural defect often surrounded by a curvilinear area of decreased signal that is distinct from the interspace of origin. This separation is best appreciated on sagittal T_2-weighted images, in which the contrast between extradural defect and interspace is greatest. It should again be emphasized that visual integration of orthogonal planes is important in the characterization and localization of herniated disk disease.

These distinctions may be important, especially in the recognition of an extruded and sequestrated disk, because such disks (1) may produce misleading localizing signs and symptoms, (2) are a contraindication to the use of chymopapain and percutaneous diskectomy techniques, (3) can cause postoperative back pain, and (4) may require a more extensive surgical approach for complete removal.

Text continued on p. 108.

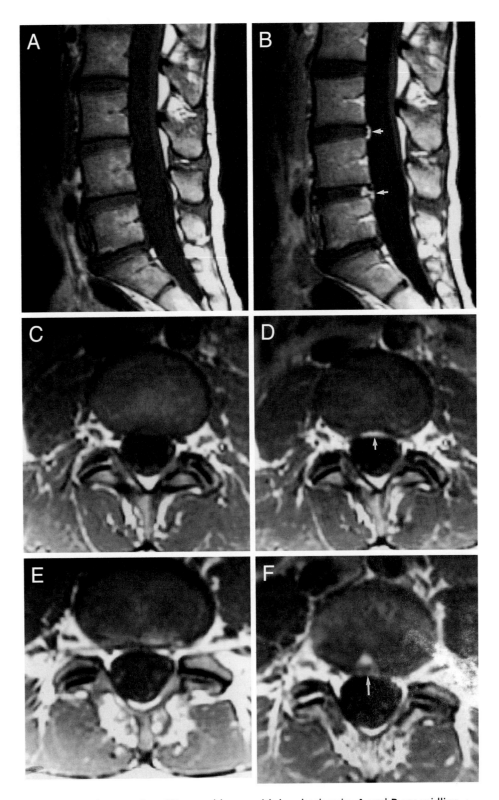

Fig. 3-17. Anular tears in a 28-year-old man with low back pain. **A** and **B** are midline sagittal T$_1$-weighted spin-echo images before and after Gd-DTPA, and **C** to **F** are axial T$_1$-weighted spin-echos (500/17) before and after the contrast. There is enhancement of the posterior portions of the L3-4 and L4-5 disks consistent with anular tearing *(arrows)*. The enhancement is presumably related to granulation tissue that has formed as an attempted reparative response.

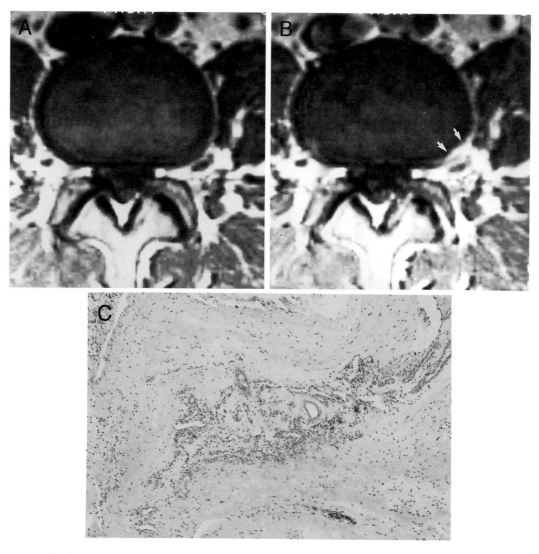

Fig. 3-18. Lateral anular tear. **A** and **B** are axial T$_1$-weighted spin-echo images (500/17) before and after gadolinium. **C** is a low power H&E stain of the surgical specimen obtained. The region of enhancement is denoted by the *arrows* in **B**. There is fibrovascular granulation tissue interspersed between the avascular anular and ligamentous tissue fibers.

Fig. 3-19. Disk protrusion. When a disk protrudes, there is focal extension of the margin, with nuclear material herniating through a defect in the anulus *(black line)*. The anulus, though cracked and/or fissured, remains intact, as does the posterior longitudinal ligament. Herniated material is contiguous with the parent nucleus and may or may not have high signal on T$_2$-weighted images.

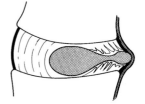
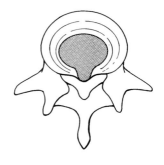

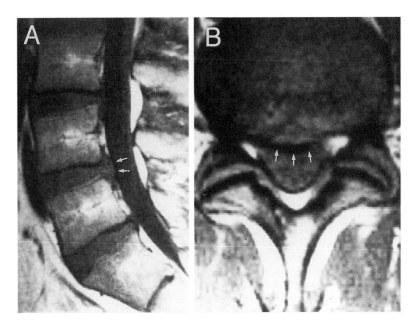

Fig. 3-20. Protruding L4-5 disk. **A** is a sagittal midline T_1-weighted (500/17) spin-echo image. The *arrows* denote protrusion of disk material beyond the margin of the adjacent vertebral endplates. **B** is an axial T_1-weighted (500/17) spin-echo through the disk. There is focal asymmetry of the posterior disk margin centrally, indicative of protrusion *(arrows).*

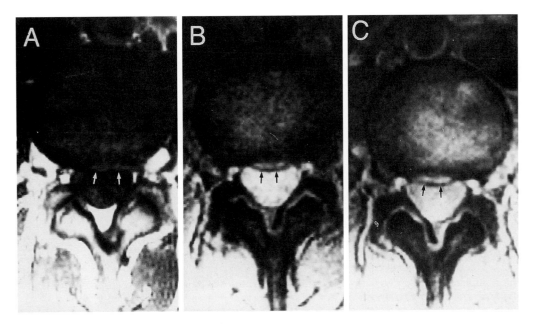

Fig. 3-21. Protrusion of the L3-4 disk *(arrows).* **A,** An axial T_1-weighted (500/17) spin-echo image through the disk shows focal bulging of the posterior central portion. **B** and **C** are axial FLASH (200/13/10 and 40 degree) images. Note the high signal intensity of the protruding segment on these gradient echo studies.

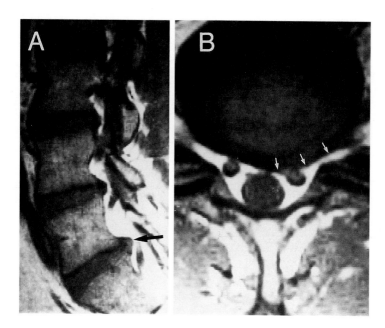

Fig. 3-22. Lateral L5-S1 disk protrusion. **A,** Parasagittal T_1-weighted (500/17) spin-echo image through the lumbar spine. The *black arrow* denotes the bulging. There is also a milder degree of protrusion of the L4-5 disk. **B,** An axial T_1-weighted (500/17) spin-echo image shows the asymmetric protrusion to the left *(arrows).* In addition, there is mild posterior displacement of the S1 nerve root.

Fig. 3-23. An extruded lumbar disk results in a subligamentous mass of nuclear material that remains contiguous with the interspace of origin. The mass may have increased or decreased signal on T_2-weighted images. The extrusion ruptures the anulus fibrosus *(heavy black line)* but is usually contained to some degree by the posterior longitudinal ligament *(dotted gray line).*

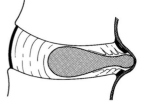

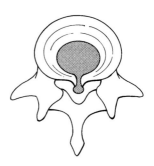

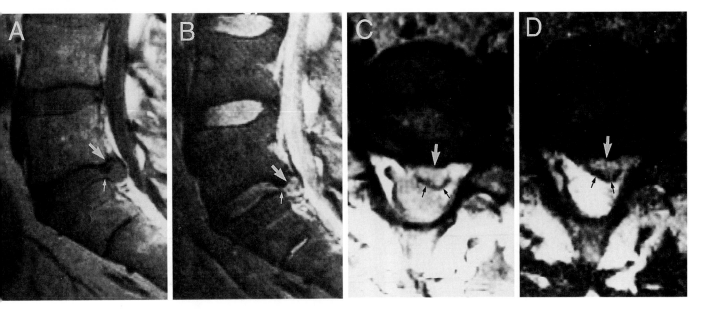

Fig. 3-24. Extruded L5-S1 disk. **A,** Sagittal T_1-weighted spin-echo (500/17). There is subligamentous herniation *(large white arrow)*. The disk fragment itself, however, remains connected by a thin pedicle *(small white arrow)* to the parent disk. **B,** Sagittal T_2-weighted spin-echo (2000/90). The extruded disk fragment has high signal intensity *(large white arrow)*, greater than the parent disk. Again, a thin pedicle connecting the fragment to the parent disk is evident *(small white arrow)*. **C** and **D,** Intermediate (2000/20) and T_2-weighted (2000/90) spin-echo axial images through the herniation. Note the high signal on both sequences *(large white arrow)*. A curvilinear area of decreased signal outlines the herniated disk segment *(small black arrows)*. This area is thought to represent portions of the anulus fibrosus carried with the herniation as well as confluence of the anulus with the stretched posterior longitudinal ligament.

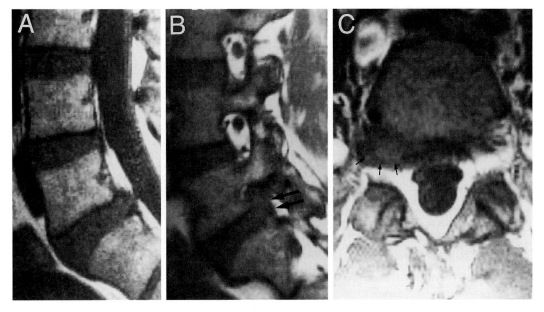

Fig. 3-25. Lateral extrusion of the L5-S1 disk. **A,** Sagittal T_1-weighted (500/17) spin-echo image through the lower lumbar spine. There is a mild herniation on the posterior aspect of the disk. **B,** Parasagittal T_1-weighted (500/17) spin-echo image through the right neural foramen. Note the obliteration of normal epidural fat signal within the foramen and the inability to separate the dorsal nerve root ganglion from the large soft tissue mass contiguous with the disk *(arrows)*. **C,** Axial T_1-weighted (500/17) spin-echo image through the neural foramen. The soft tissue mass represents laterally extruded disk material *(small arrows)* within the neural foramen on the right.

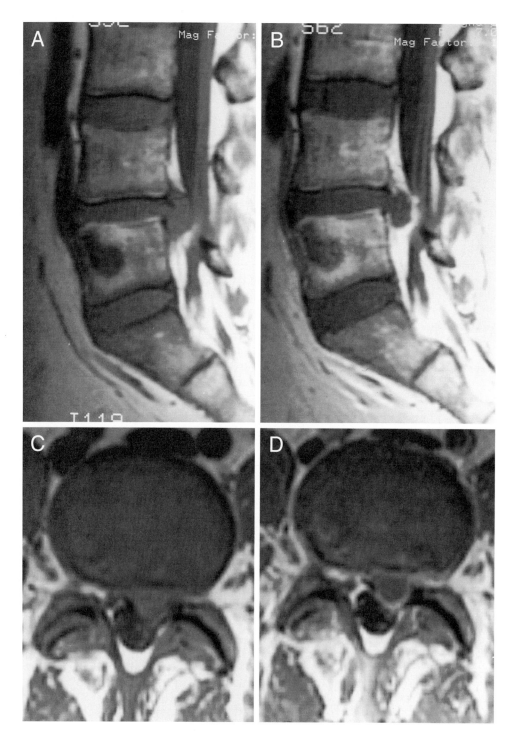

Fig. 3-26. L4-5 disk herniation. **A** and **B,** Pre- and postcontrast sagittal T_1-weighted spin-echo images demonstrate an extradural mass at the disk level. **C** and **D,** Axial T_1-weighted spin-echo (500/17) images before and after contrast show the peripheral enhancement of disk material, which can be better appreciated on the sagittal images. The enhancing areas of granulation tissue contribute to the overall size of the mass.

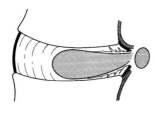
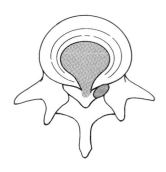

Fig. 3-27. A free (sequestered) fragment of lumbar disk is best appreciated on sagittal T$_2$-weighted images, where it appears to lie either anterior or posterior to the posterior longitudinal ligament and inferior or superior to the adjacent interspace. In this diagram it has disrupted both the anulus *(heavy black line)* and the posterior longitudinal ligament *(dotted gray line).*

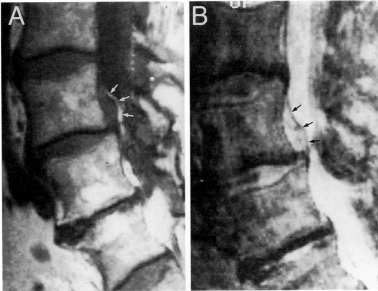

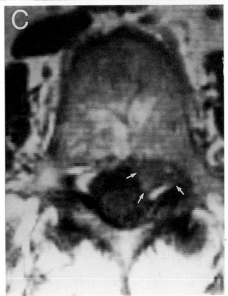

Fig. 3-28. Migrated free fragment from the L4-5 disk. **A,** This sagittal T$_1$-weighted (500/17) spin-echo image through the lower lumbar spine shows narrowing of the L4-5 and L5-S1 disk spaces with type II vertebral body changes at the latter level. There is a soft tissue–density fragment posterior to the inferior aspect of L3 *(arrows).* The high signal intensity surrounding it most likely represents epidural fat. At surgery it was found to be posterior to the vertebral body but anterior to the posterior longitudinal ligament. **B** and **C,** Sagittal T$_2$-weighted (2000/90) spin-echo and axial T$_1$-weighted (500/17) spin-echo images. The migrated fragment is, again, demarcated by the *small arrows.*

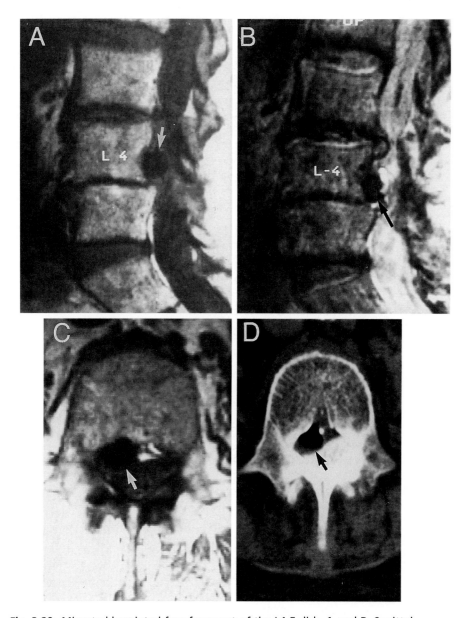

Fig. 3-29. Migrated herniated free fragment of the L4-5 disk. **A** and **B,** Sagittal T$_1$-weighted (500/17) and T$_2$-weighted (2000/90) spin-echo images through the lower lumbar spine. There is an ovoid area of decreased signal posterior to the inferior aspect of L4, with moderate to severe narrowing of the L3-4 and severe narrowing of the L4-5 disk. Note the central disk herniation at L3-4. At surgery this ovoid area of decreased signal intensity represented a large migrated extruded fragment containing gas (vacuum phenomenon). **C** and **D,** Axial T$_1$-weighted (500/17) spin-echo and high-resolution CT with intrathecal contrast through the inferior aspect of L4. *Arrow* denotes the herniated migrated free fragment, complete with its own vacuum phenomenon.

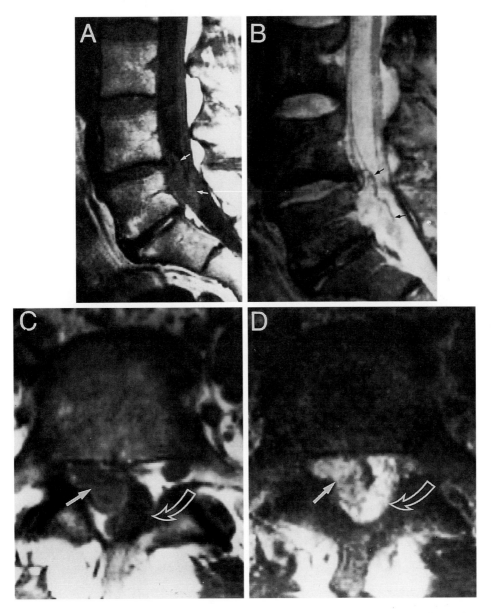

Fig. 3-30. Free fragment of the L4-5 disk. **A** is a sagittal midline T_1-weighted (500/17) spin-echo image, and **B** a T_2-weighted (200/90) spin-echo. *Arrows* point to a soft tissue mass (with high signal intensity in **B**) occupying a large portion of the spinal canal posterior to L5. At surgery this was found to be a free fragment that had ruptured through the posterior longitudinal ligament. **C** and **D** are axial T_1-weighted (500/17) and T_2-weighted (2000/90) spin-echos through L5. The fragment *(solid arrow)* has high signal on the T_2-weighted sequence. *Open arrow* denotes the markedly displaced and compressed thecal sac at this level.

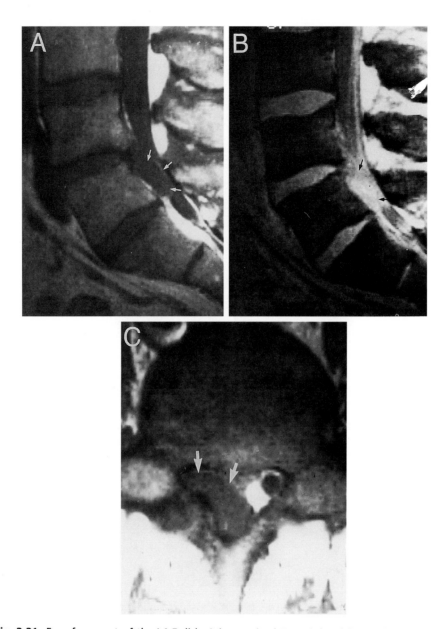

Fig. 3-31. Free fragment of the L4-5 disk. **A** is a sagittal T_1-weighted (500/17) spin-echo image just to the right of midline. *Arrows* denote an ill-defined soft tissue mass lying posterior to L5. Differentiation of this large free fragment is not as clear in this sequence as it is in **B,** which is a FLASH (200/13/60 degree) showing the free disk fragment with a high signal relative to the adjacent CSF *(arrows).* **C,** The axial T_1-weighted (500/17) spin-echo image demonstrates a large free fragment *(arrows)* obscuring the region of the S1 nerve root and both distorting and displacing the thecal sac posteriorly.

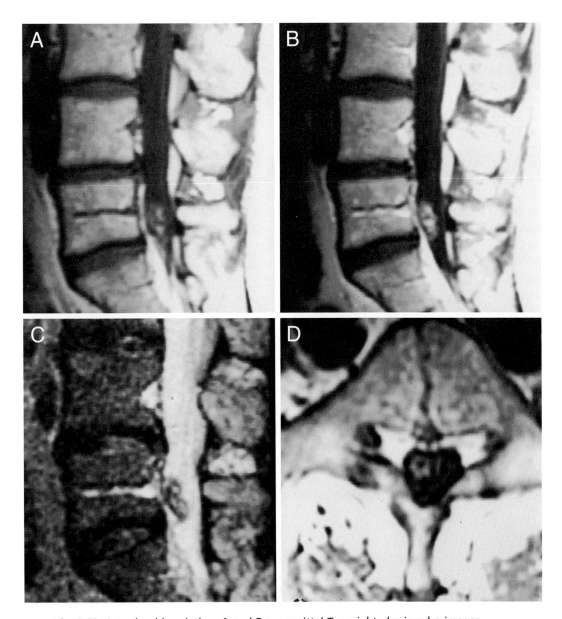

Fig. 3-32. Intradural herniation. **A** and **B** are sagittal T$_1$-weighted spin-echo images before and after Gd-DTPA, **C** is a sagittal midline T$_2$-weighted image, and **D** is an axial T$_1$-weighted spin-echo. Note the irregular mass in **A** just above the L5-S1 disk space within the thecal sac and slightly to the right. It shows some enhancement following contrast **(B)** and decreased signal on the T$_2$-weighted sequence **(C)**. The lesion was thought to represent an intradural calcified disk herniation.

Whereas all of the foregoing has become a part of our clinical lore, it is not at all clear whether these findings are clinically relevant. It has been proposed, for example, that differentiating between various degrees of herniation is critically important; and yet the reality of the situation is that any disk herniation most likely represents a spectrum or continuum rather than a discrete entity with specific clinical relationships. One may view the continuum of herniated disk disease as starting with anular disruption, proceeding to a small focal herniation that does not break through the anulus-ligamentous complex, and winding up as a frank herniation (extrusion) that does indeed dissect through the anulus–posterior ligamentous complex. These stages may show variable degrees of containment, with a line of decreased signal being reported around free fragments and large extruded disks where there has clearly been disruption of the anulus and PLL. This is thought to be secondary to anular and ligamentous fibers that were carried away with the herniation. The anulus fibrosus and PLL are so inter-

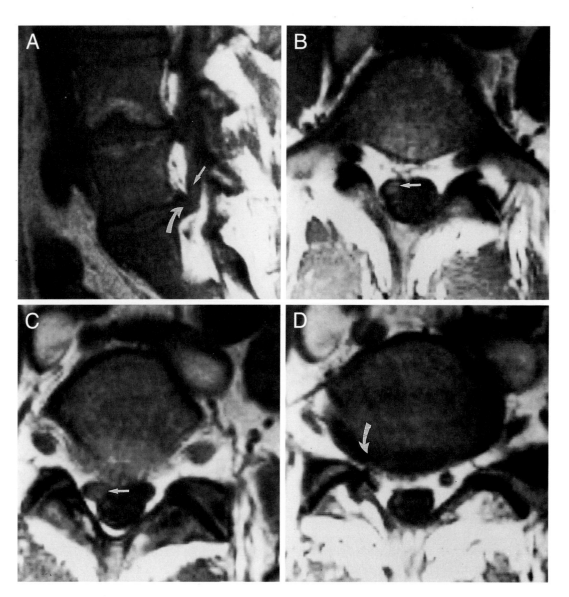

Fig. 3-33. Swollen right S1 nerve root. **A,** A right parasagittal T_1-weighted (500/17) spin-echo image and, **B** to **D,** axial T_1-weighted (500/17) spin-echos through L5-S1 show the traversing portion of the nerve root *(straight arrow)* to be thickened and of higher intensity than the contralateral root. There is impingement from an osteophyte and from the disk on the right at the L5-S1 level (which can be better appreciated in **A** and **D,** *curved arrow).*

twined at the level of the disk that a distinction between the two structures may be impossible and, for that matter, irrelevant.

High signal intensity on T_2-weighted images has been identified in both extruded disks and free fragments.[103] It has been hypothesized[109] that some disk fragments have a higher water content that causes a prolongation of the T_2 signal. The reason for the high signal intensity of extruded disks or free fragments, however, is not clear. Peck and Haughton[110] have suggested that gross degeneration of intervertebral disks may be present despite their high signal on long TR/TE images. It may be reasonable to assume that such large fragments become symptomatic early in their clinical course, bringing the patient to seek medical attention (and a diagnostic workup) soon after the onset of symptoms, that is, large extruded and sequestered disks, which present earlier, may have a higher water content than smaller herniations, which present later.

An alternative explanation for the same finding[30,31] takes into consideration the fact that with rupture and loss of the confined fluid from the disk there is initially a reparative process that leads to a transient gain in water content of the disk. Again, assuming an acute clinical presentation, this may present as a high signal intensity on more T_2-weighted images. There are also vascular correlations between disk changes and the number and location of vessels surrounding the penetrating areas of disk pathology.

Traversing nerve roots within the thecal sac above a particular level of impingement from a herniated disk or stenosis have been noted to be enlarged compared to the contralateral side. This may be a reflection of nerve root edema (Fig. 3-33). Enhancement of traversing nerve roots within the thecal sac has also been reported[111] on MR, the majority of which were associated with focally protruding disk pathology (Fig. 3-34). A significant number of these patients, however, had isolated enhancement of multiple nerve roots without significant associated anatomic pathology. The mechanism of such enhancement may be related to the blood/nerve barrier of this spinal nerve root, which is altered by compression.[112]

Despite the fact that disks appear more often to herniate laterally, presumably because of the absence of PLL fibers and the thinness of the anulus in that region, they can herniate both centrally and peripherally in the neural foramina, where they may be confused with neurogenic tumors. When a fragment is adjacent to the interspace, it may have a somewhat rounded configuration; but if it migrates superior or inferiorly to the interspace, it frequently appears oval or oblong.

In a prospective evaluation of surface coil MR, CT, and myelography for lumbar herniated disk disease and canal stenosis,[54] there was 82.6% agreement between

MR and surgical findings regarding type and location of disease, 83% agreement between CT and surgical findings, and 71.8% agreement between myelography and surgical findings. There was a 92.5% agreement when MR and CT were used jointly and an 89.4% agreement when CT and myelography were used jointly. In another study[113] the accuracy of CT, myelography, CT-myelography, and MRI for lumbar herniated nucleus pulposus was compared prospectively in 59 patients, all of whom underwent surgical CT-myelographic exploration. Magnetic resonance was the most accurate (76.5%), CT-myelography next (76%), and then CT (73%) and myelography (71%). The false-positive rate was lowest for MR, at 13%, followed by myelography and CT.[113] Similar data from a carefully controlled prospective study in Wisconsin[114] suggest the same equivalence for plain CT, CT-myelography, and MRI. These

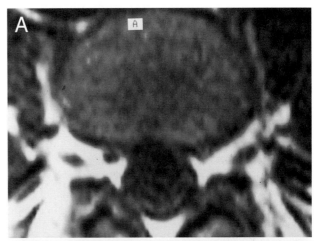

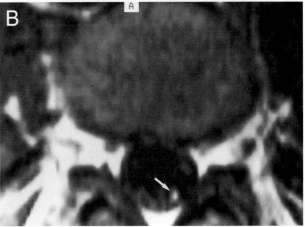

Fig. 3-34. Enhancing L5 nerve root. T_1-weighted axial spin-echo pairs (500/17), **A,** precontrast and, **B,** postcontrast through L4 in a patient who has a large L4-5 disk herniation. The traversing portion of the left nerve root is well enhanced in **B** *(arrow).*

data, then, suggest that MR and CT are equivalent tests for herni-ated disk disease. Unfortunately, one does not have an a priori diagnosis that herniated disk disease is the cause of a patient's symptoms; and the argument could be made that MR has a greater advantage because of its larger field of view, greater tissue contrast sensitivity, and an increased ability to identify differential considerations such as infection, neoplasm, and scarring, which may not be as apparent on CT.

The natural history of lumbar disk herniation has recently engendered increased interest, and MR has been an excellent tool for these investigations. Multiple studies[115-119] have demonstrated that the size of a herniation can change with time, and studies of patients treated conservatively have shown that the majority experienced a reduction in size of 30% to 100%. The larger herniations had the most significant size decrease. However, correlation of disk changes with time and symptom resolution has not yet been carefully worked out.[115-119] In a prospective study underway at our institution[120] it seems that symptom resolution often takes place before the extradural mass changes. (See Figs. 3-40 to 3-42.) Most patients with acute radiculopathy have complete resolution of their symptoms with conservative management by 6 weeks. The majority show no significant change in the size of the extradural mass although some show a dramatic decrease in size. No good correlation has been drawn, then, between the response to conservative management in terms of symptom resolution and herniated disk size during the first 6 weeks after symptoms.

As part of a long-term natural history study[120] patients with acute radiculopathy were evaluated clinically and with contrast-enhanced MR to determine whether there was a correlation between presenting symptoms and the type, size, location, and enhancement of disk herniation presentations. Among the patients with acute radiculopathy 72% had a herniated nucleus pulposus. There was excellent agreement between the MR and clinical findings for level and size but no correlation of pain and disability with disk size or type. Enhancement of the herniated nucleus pulposus was a constant feature even in this acute phase. The degree of enhancement was variable and probably related to granulation tissue that developed around and through the herniated disk. This granulation response is presumably an in vivo reparative process secondary to disruption of tissue. The granulation tissue response itself may comprise a fair percentage of the herniated disk mass. One possible explanation for the change of a disk with time then is that the granulation tissue undergoes cicatrization and retraction, a normal phenomenon for reparative tissue.[120,121] At pathology, closely connected with necrotic degenerated portions of disk tissue, loose granulation tissue is sometimes noted, providing a potential mechanism of absorption or retraction. Whether this is an etiologic factor or a secondary phenomenon in disk degeneration is as yet unclear.[122]

Differential considerations. The differential diagnosis for the MR findings of sequestered lumbar disks includes epidural abscess, extradural neoplasm (e.g., neurofibroma), and postoperative epidural fibrosis or fluid collection. Epidural abscesses are usually associated with disk space infection and can be distinguished from free fragments by the characteristic signal changes seen at the infected interspace and adjacent endplates. Extradural or intradural tumors may be more difficult to exclude, although the multiplicity of lesions and/or the presence of bone marrow changes should help narrow the differential (Fig. 3-35). Postoperative scars in the lumbar spine are typically identified as a loss of signal intensity from the epidural fat on T_1-weighted images; but they often demonstrate high signal on T_2-weighted images, particularly anteriorly and laterally, and may be difficult to separate from a disk fragment (Fig. 3-36). The presence or absence of mass effect on the thecal sac can help distinguish the two. In any event, the utilization of gadolinium diethylenetriamine pentaacetic acid (Gd-DTPA) has proved to be a highly efficient means of differentiating among the various considerations. Tumor and epidural fibrosis usually enhance diffusely whereas cysts and recurrent herniations generally have peripheral enhancement (Fig. 3-37). Postoperative changes may also mimic high–signal intensity extradural defects such as free fragments on T_2-weighted images, but they usually resolve within 4 to 6 weeks following surgery.

Another differential consideration for an extradural mass is synovial cyst (Figs. 3-38 and 3-39). Intraspinal synovial or ganglion cysts are relatively uncommon. A review of 54 reported cases[123] revealed a female predominance in the age range 30 to 76 years, with a mean of 58 years at presentation. Most patients were symptomatic at the time of diagnosis. Although the origin of synovial cysts remains controversial, most are thought to develop as a consequence of degenerative joint disease or trauma. This is supported by the frequency of these cysts at the L4-5 and L5-S1 levels, which represents the most mobile segment of the lumbar spine and is the usual location of degenerative disease.[123] Synovial cysts are distinguished by some investigators[114,115] from ganglion cysts by differences in their lining and content. The classic synovial cyst is lined by synovium and attaches to the adjacent articular cavity. The typical ganglion cyst does not have a synovial lining, and there is no direct communication with the joint cavity. The distinction may be arbitrary, however, because of transitional forms.[124,125]

Text continued on p. 119.

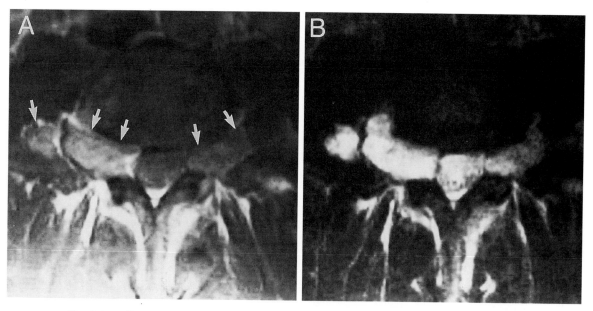

Fig. 3-35. Bilateral L3-4 neurofibromas. Axial intermediate (2000/20) and T$_2$-weighted (2000/90) spin-echo images through the L3-4 neural foramen show ovoid masses of high signal intensity occupying the neural foramen bilaterally *(arrows)*. At surgery and pathology these were found to be neurofibromas.

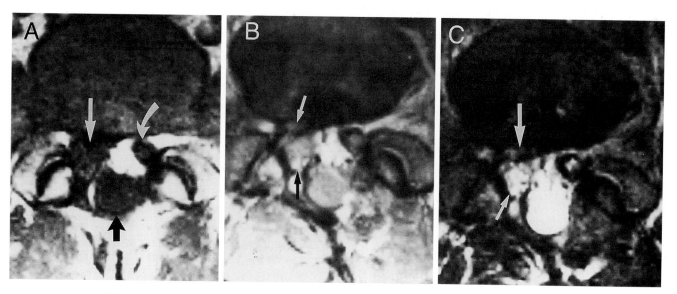

Fig. 3-36. Epidural fibrosis. **A** to **C** are T$_1$-weighted (500/17), intermediate (2000/30), and T$_2$-weighted (2000/90) spin-echo images through the L5-S1 disk. A soft tissue mass in **A** surrounds the region of the S1 nerve root on the right *(straight white arrow)*. The S1 nerve root on the left is shown by the *curved white arrow.* The *black arrow* points to the thecal sac. Note the laminectomy defect posteriorly on the left. The soft tissue mass in **B** and **C** has high signal intensity *(small black arrow* and *small white arrow)*. Anteriorly there is a disk herniation *(white arrow* in **B**, *large white arrow* in **C**). At surgery a mass of epidural fibrosis was documented, but the region where the herniated disk was noted anteriorly on MR could not be visualized.

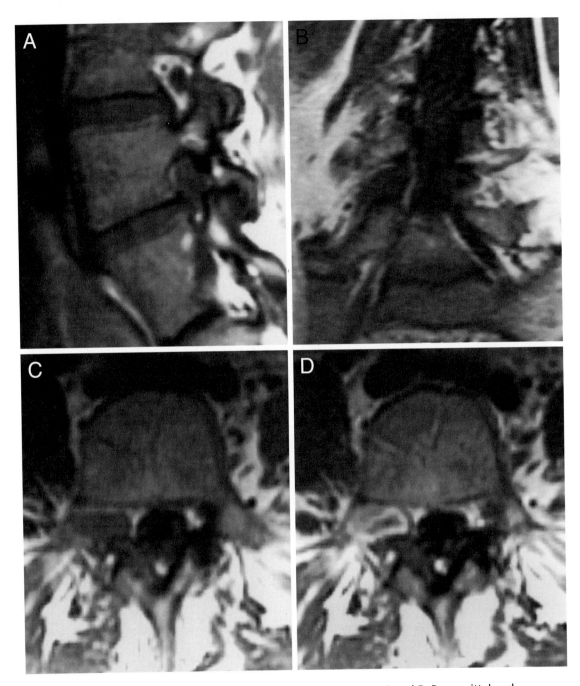

Fig. 3-37. Right-sided L4 radiculopathy in a 36-year-old man. **A** and **B,** Parasagittal and coronal T$_1$-weighted spin-echo images (500/17). There is a large soft tissue mass in the right L4-5 neural foramen. **C** and **D,** Axial T$_1$-weighted spin echos before and after gadolinium. The mass is seen to enhance peripherally, with an area of nonenhancement centrally, suggesting a large disk herniation. A neoplasm would be expected to enhance diffusely.

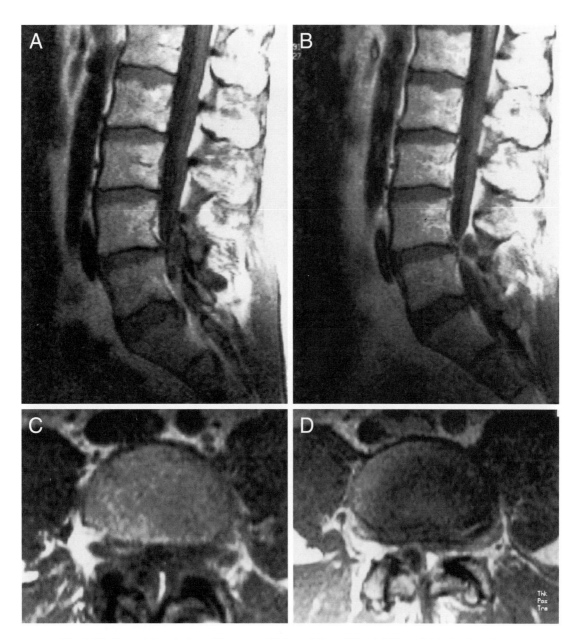

Fig. 3-38. Synovial cyst. **A** and **B** are sagittal, and **C** and **D** axial, T$_1$-weighted spin-echo pre- and postgadolinium pairs. There is a posterolateral extradural mass at the L4-5 level, which shows peripheral enhancement following Gd-DTPA. This is characteristic of a synovial cyst. Note the degenerative changes in the adjacent facet joint as well as the proximity of the cyst to the joint capsule.

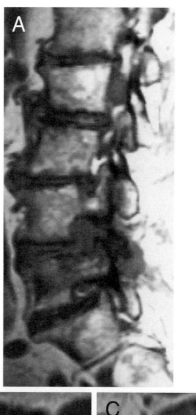

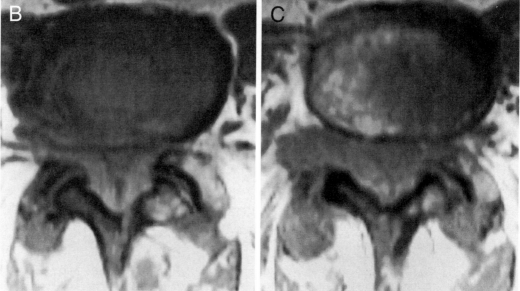

Fig. 3-39. Degenerative synovial cysts. **A** is a parasagittal T₁-weighted spin-echo, and **B** and **C** are axial T₁-weighted spin-echo sequences. Note the large ovoid soft tissue masses contiguous with the facet joints. There is marked ligamentum thickening as well as central and foraminal stenosis.

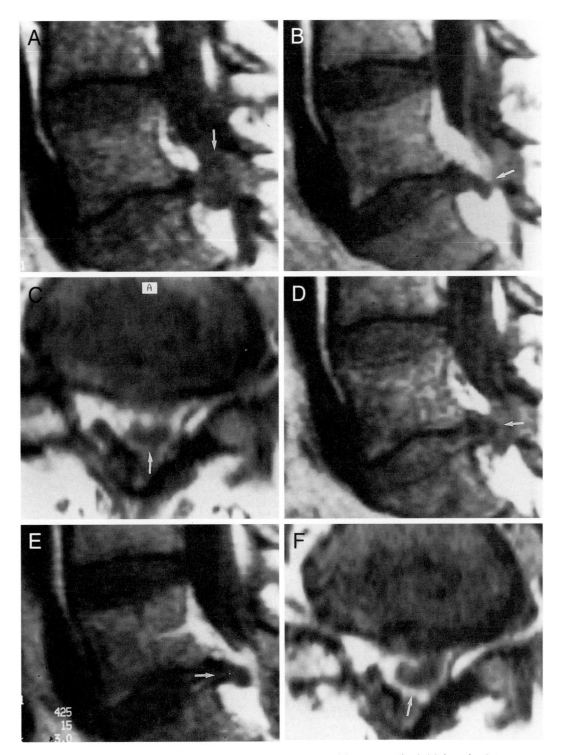

Fig. 3-40. Acute left-sided radiculopathy in a 43-year-old woman. The initial study, **A** to **C**, was acquired within 6 days of the onset of symptoms. **A** and **B** are T$_1$-weighted sagittal pre- and postgadolinium images, and **C** an axial T$_1$-weighted postgadolinium image. In the follow-up study at 6 weeks, when the patient was virtually symptom free, **D** to **F**, the overall size of the herniation is essentially unchanged. **D** and **E** are T$_1$ sagittals before and after contrast, and **F** is an axial postcontrast image. There is a large amount of enhancement surrounding the herniation *(arrows)*.

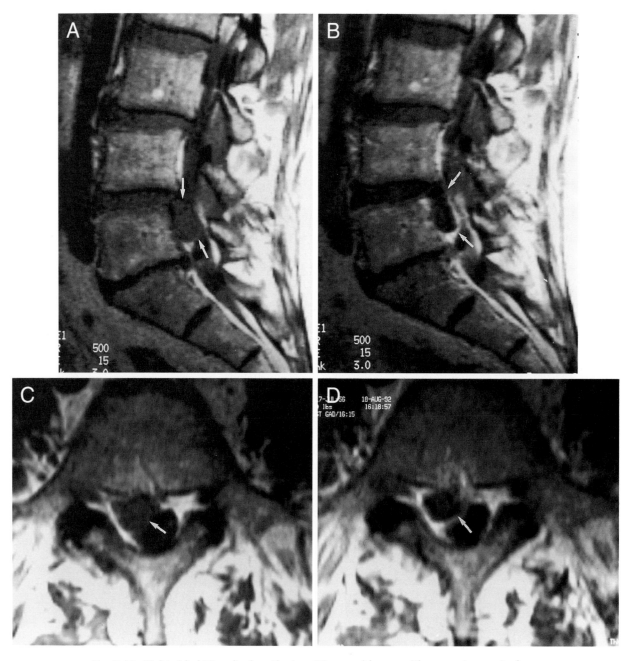

Fig. 3-41. Right-sided L5 radiculopathy in a 52-year-old man with an acute onset of symptoms. In the presenting study, **A** to **D**, which are T$_1$-weighted sagittal and axial pre- and postgadolinium pairs, there is a large free fragment behind L5 on the right. The enhanced studies (**B** and **D**) show peripheral uptake of contrast.

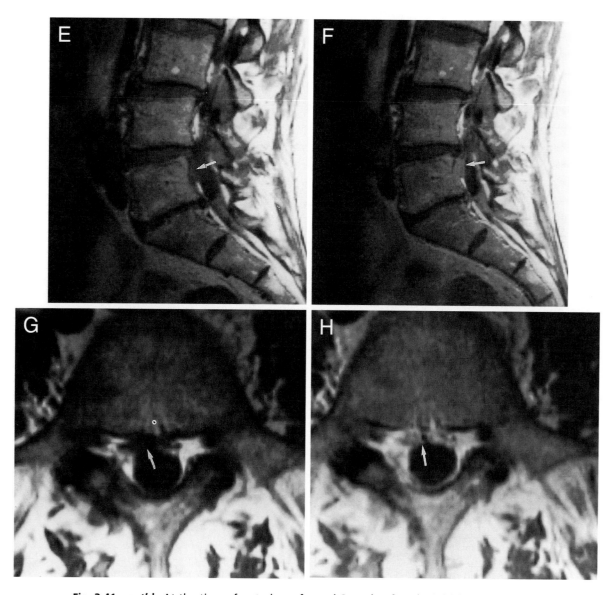

Fig. 3-41, cont'd. At the time of a study performed 6 weeks after the initial episode, **E** to **H,** with the patient virtually symptom free, there has been almost complete resorption or retraction of the herniation. These sagittal and axial pre- and postgadolinium T_1-weighted spin-echo pairs show only a small aberrant soft tissue mass remaining.

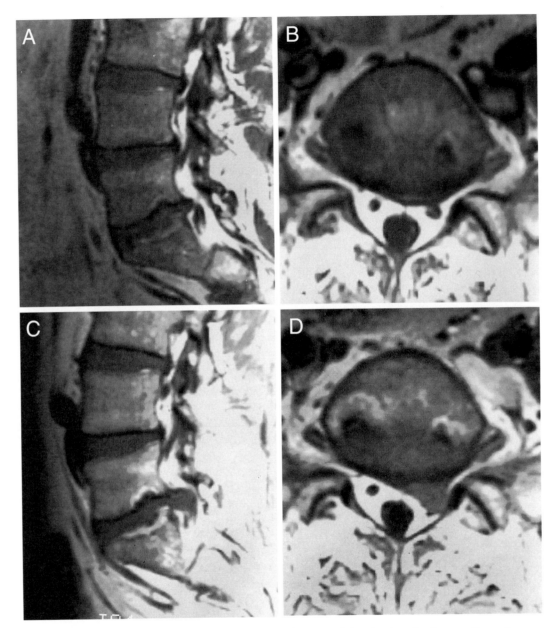

Fig. 3-42. Asymptomatic disk herniation. **A** and **B,** T_1-weighted spin-echo images through the L5-S1 interspace in a patient with central and right-sided low back pain. Note the asymmetric bulging, or perhaps a broad-based protrusion of the L5-S1 disk, on the left. This patient was followed conservatively. He returned 6 months later, at which time **C** and **D** images were obtained. There is now a large herniation on the left at L5-S1 seen on these sagittal and axial T_1-weighted spin-echo sequences. The patient's symptoms were unchanged despite this defect.

The presenting symptoms of a synovial cyst are usually those of radiculopathy. A mass is invariably identified posterolaterally within the spinal canal and continuous with the facet joints. Increased intensity may be noted in the adjacent apophyseal joint secondary to an inflammatory or traumatic joint effusion. The adjacent ligament may be thickened as well.[126]

The MR findings of synovial cysts have been variable. True synovial cysts contain a clear serous fluid showing an isointense T_1 and hyperintense T_2 pattern. A cyst with more viscous contents may show a hyperintense pattern relative to CSF on all pulse sequences. A cyst containing blood may show marked hyperintensity on all pulse sequences or marked hyperintensity on T_1 and mixed on T_2. Since the wall of a synovial cyst can vary from a thin synovial lining to a thick fibrous sheath and occasionally a calcified capsule, the rim may show variable thickness of low signal intensity. Enhancement of the border (periphery) of the mass has been reported on contrast-enhanced studies.

Thoracic disk herniations. Although less common than lumbar or cervical herniations, thoracic herniations have been noted more frequently with the advancement of imaging techniques[57] (Figs. 3-43 to 3-45). A higher prevalence of asymptomatic morphologic change is also present in the thoracic spine. In one series[127] 15% of patients without thoracic back pain or radiculopathy had a herniated disk. It has been postulated[128,129] that the relatively low incidence of disk herniations in the thoracic spinal canal is due to the fact that the weight-bearing axis of the thoracic spine does not intersect the posterior margins of the vertebral bodies and thus the thoracic spine is not as mobile (because of the restraining ribs and sternum). The higher incidence of herniations at T11 and T12 has been explained[130] by the increased mobility of the spine at that level, which arises from the fact that the ribs there are free ending.

Paresthesias below the level of the lesion, a loss of sensation both deep and superficial, and paraparesis or paraplegia are the usual clinical manifestations. The symptom complex, however, may be difficult to interpret. Retrospective studies with surface coil MR[131] have shown that it is highly accurate. Over a 2-year period 63 patients who had symptoms in which thoracic disk herniation was part of the initial differential underwent thoracic examinations. Magnetic resonance identified 20 thoracic disk herniations in 17 of these patients. Sixteen suspected herniations in 13 patients had a confirmatory imaging study (plain film myelography–computed tomography with metrizamide [PFM-CTM]) and/or surgical verification (8 patients with surgery at ten levels, including 6 with PFM-CTM at eight levels and 5 with PFM-CTM at six levels without surgery). The result with CTM-PFM was positive at all eight surgical levels and

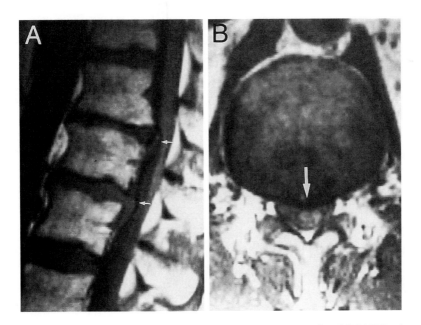

Fig. 3-43. Thoracic disk herniations. **A,** A sagittal midline T_1-weighted (500/17) spin-echo image of the lower thoracic spine shows anterior extradural soft tissue masses at the T9-10 and 10-11 levels (arrows). **B,** An axial T_1-weighted (500/17) spin-echo through the T9-10 disk also shows a central protrusion. The normal CSF space within the thecal sac anterior to the spinal cord has been obliterated, and the posterior margin of the disk is in direct contact with the spinal cord.

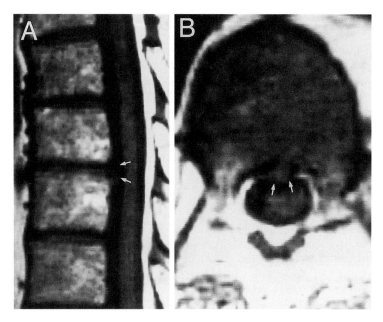

Fig. 3-44. Thoracic disk herniation. **A,** A sagittal midline T$_1$-weighted (500/17) spin-echo image demonstrates protrusion of the T8-9 disk *(arrows)*. **B,** An axial T$_1$-weighted (500/17) spin-echo also shows the defect.

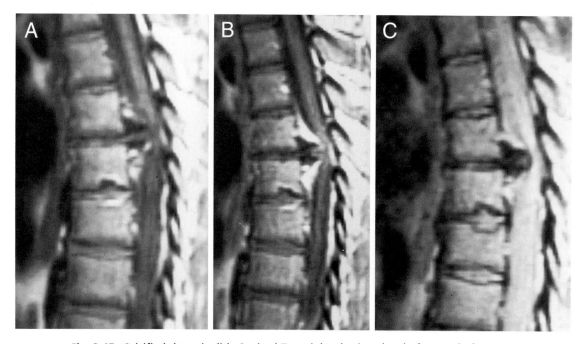

Fig. 3-45. Calcified thoracic disk. Sagittal T$_1$-weighted spin-echos before and after gadolinium, **A** and **B,** and a T$_2$-weighted midline sagittal section, **C,** show the extradural defect with marked cord compression at T6-7. On all pulse sequences there is a rim of decreased signal intensity with the central core of intermediate signal. This was thought to represent calcification of the disk, which was confirmed by CT. Note the enhancement surrounding the herniation.

at six levels without surgery (14/14). When considered alone, PFM showed extradural defects at nine of fourteen levels. If sagittal and axial images on MR were considered together, MR defined 16 of 16 abnormal thoracic levels (surgical verification at ten). Thin slices are critical for adequate evaluation. The configuration of the herniation is similar to that seen in the lumbar and cervical regions, although the extradural defect is usually not so large. Indentation and rotation of the cord are ancillary signs that can be utilized. Caution must be taken, however, in evaluating thoracic disk herniations when the usual orientation of phase-encoded and frequency direction has been reversed to compensate for cardiac and respiratory ghosting. In these situations the chemical shift artifact will now appear in an anterior to posterior direction and can obscure disk herniation on the sagittal view.[131]

Cervical disk herniations. Symptomatic cervical disk herniations are most common in young patients (third and fourth decades) and frequently occur without recognized trauma. In a prospective study of patients with no symptoms of cervical disease,[132] 10% of subjects less than 40 years of age had a herniated nucleus pulposus and 4% had foraminal stenosis. Of the subjects who were older than 40 years of age, 5% had a herniated nucleus pulposus, 3% a bulging disk, and 20% foraminal stenosis. Narrowing of the disk space, degeneration of a disk, spurs, or compression of the cord were noted at one or more levels in 25% of the subjects less than 40 years of age and in almost 60% of those who were older than 40.

The nerve roots are more likely to be compressed with acute herniation of the disk. More chronic spinal cord and nerve root symptoms are usually due to disk degeneration and/or herniation with associated osteophytes and degenerative changes in the joints, ligaments, and adjacent vertebral bodies. The levels most frequently affected by both disk herniation and cervical spondylosis are C5-6 and C6-7.

Cervical disk herniations typically cause pain and stiffness in the neck and intrascapular region but may differ with respect to the affected nerve root. The cervical nerves exit through neural foramina above the body of the same number. Thus a disk herniation or spurs at C5-6 will impact on the C6 nerve root.

Compression of the C4 nerve root can produce pain along one side of the neck radiating to the shoulder whereas compression of C5, 6, 7, and 8 and T1 can produce almost identical pain in the base of the neck, posterior scapular region, and shoulder. The involvement of muscle groups and reflex deficits are more accurate indicators of nerve root level.

Cervical disk herniation, especially when central or large, is well appreciated on routine sagittal and axial MR images (Figs. 3-46 and 3-47). Again, thin slices (3 mm or less) are critical for accurate diagnosis (Figs. 3-48 and 3-49). This may necessitate the use of three-dimensional volume sequences with partitions of 2 mm or less and/or reconstructions in other planes (Fig. 3-50). The T_2 signal intensity of intervertebral disks in the cervical region is not as helpful as in the lumbar region for identifying the presence or absence of degeneration. Cervical disk herniation is usually identified on sagittal images as an anterior or anterior-lateral extradural defect that may indent or compress the cervical cord. In a prospective study to compare the accuracy of surface coil MR with metrizamide myelography (MM) and computed tomography with metrizamide (CTM),[55] there was surgical agreement in 74% of patients with surface coil MR, 85% with CTM, and 67% with MM. When surface coil MR and CTM were used jointly, 90% agreement with surgical findings was seen, and when CTM and MM were used jointly, 92% agreement occurred. In general, surface coil MR was as sensitive as CTM for identifying disease level but not as specific for type of disease. Metrizamide myelography was least specific for disease type. (The major advantage of CTM was its ability to distinguish bone from soft tissue, for which contrast material would be unnecessary.) A follow-up study utiliz-

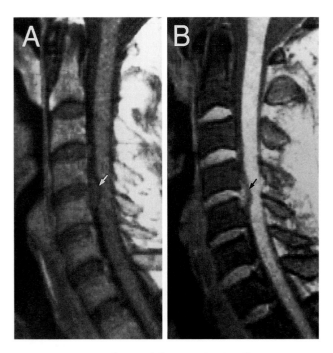

Fig. 3-46. Herniated C4-5 disk. **A,** Sagittal midline T_1-weighted (500/17) spin-echo image through the cervical spine. A moderately large soft tissue mass extends posteriorly from the disk space, indenting the anterior aspect of the cervical cord *(arrow)*. **B,** Sagittal midline FLASH (200/13/60 degrees) image. Note that the herniated disk is well demarcated from the cervical cord and surrounding CSF *(arrow)*.

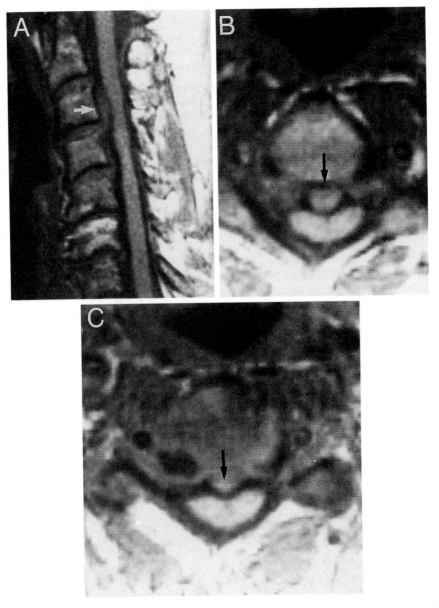

Fig. 3-47. Cervical free disk fragment. **A,** Sagittal midline T$_1$-weighted (500/17) spin-echo image through the cervical spine. Note the soft tissue mass posterior to C3 with its inferior extent at the C3-4 disk level *(arrow)*. The anterior aspect of the cervical cord is indented. A smaller disk herniation is evident at the C4-5 level, again with indentation of the cervical cord. High signal intensity in C6 is thought to represent type II degenerative change. **B** and **C,** Axial T$_1$-weighted (500/17) spin-echo images through C3 and the C3-4 disk. Note the ovoid soft tissue mass anterior to the cord at C3 *(arrow)*, which represents a free disk fragment that has migrated superiorly behind the posterior longitudinal ligament.

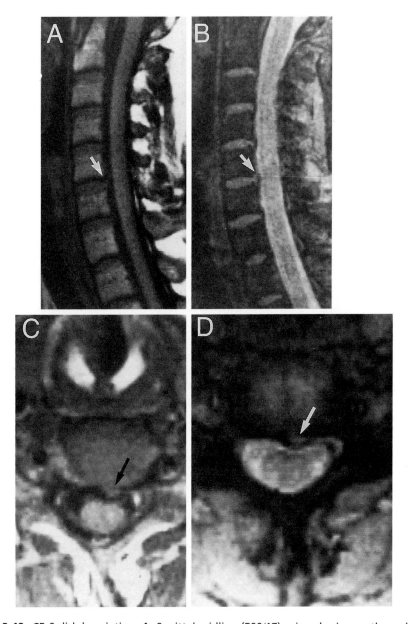

Fig. 3-48. C5-6 disk herniation. **A,** Sagittal midline (500/17) spin-echo image through the cervical spine. A small anterior extradural defect is evident at the C5-6 level *(white arrow).* **B,** Sagittal midline FLASH (200/13/10 degrees) through the cervical spine. The small anterior extradural defect *(white arrow)* is outlined by the high signal intensity of the adjacent CSF. **C,** T_1-weighted (500/17) spin-echo axial image through the C5-6 disk. The central left disk herniation is demarcated by the *black arrow.* **D,** Axial FLASH (200/13/10 degrees) through the C5-6 disk. The *white arrow* points to high signal intensity in the herniated disk at this level. Note the high signal intensity of the CSF relative to the cord. This contrast is characteristic of low–flip angle gradient echo scans and produces the so-called CSF myelogram effect.

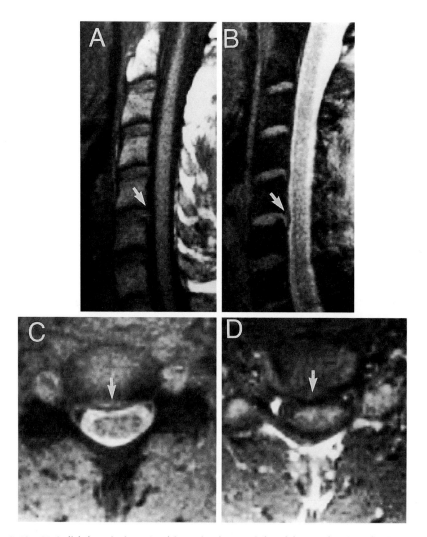

Fig. 3-49. C5-6 disk herniation. **A,** This sagittal T₁-weighted (500/17) spin-echo image through the cervical spine demonstrates an anterior extradural defect at the C5-6 level *(arrow).* **B,** A sagittal FLASH (200/13/10 degrees) through the cervical spine also shows the defect. **C** and **D** are a T₁-weighted (500/17) spin-echo and an axial FLASH (200/13/10 degrees) through the C5-6 disk. Note the soft tissue mass, which is of similar signal intensity to the adjacent intervertebral disk and evident in both sequences, projecting posteriorly *(arrow).* The conspicuousness of this extradural defect is better appreciated in **D,** however, because of the high signal of adjacent CSF.

ing oblique MR images of the lateral neural canal and foramen[56] improved the accuracy of MR by providing an additional orthogonal view of the foramen (Fig. 3-51). Because the routine parasagittal images fail to depict adequately the ventral, inferior, and lateral anatomic courses of the neural foramina in the cervical region, an additional view is often required. Thus, if routine sagittal and axial images fail to identify a definite extradural defect in the presence of well-defined radiculopathy, oblique images may be indicated; again, this is facilitated by three-dimensional imaging with reformatted images in planes orthogonal to the region of interest.

In another study comparing MRI to CT, plain film myelography, and CT-myelography in 35 patients operated on for cervical radiculopathy and myelopathy,[133] MRI correctly predicted 88% of the surgically proved lesions. The corresponding rates were 81% for CT myelography, 58% for plain myelography, and 50% for CT. The authors concluded that MRI, in combination with plain films, provided the best test for preoperative evaluations for cervical radiculopathy and myelopathy.

The major advantages of surface coil MR imaging are that it (1) displays the foramen magnum and cervical region in their entirety, (2) depicts the contour of the cord

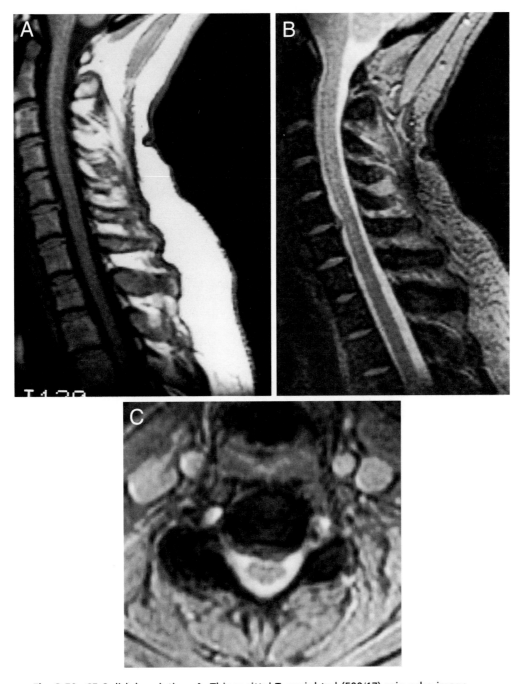

Fig. 3-50. C5-6 disk herniation. **A,** This sagittal T_1-weighted (500/17) spin-echo image through the cervical spine shows an anterior extradural defect at the C5-6 level. **B,** A sagittal FLASH (200/13/10 degrees) through the cervical spine also shows the defect. **C,** The 2 mm axial partition from a three-dimensional dataset with a low flip angle through C5-6 demonstrates the soft tissue mass, which is slightly more prominent on the left.

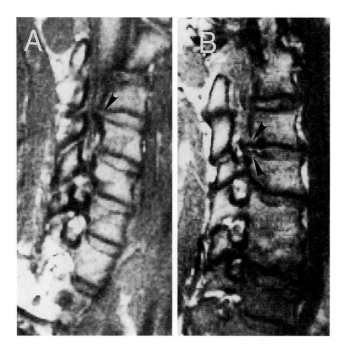

Fig. 3-51. Oblique 45-degree T$_1$-weighted (500/17) spin-echo images through the cervical neural foramina. In **A** the *arrow* points to a lateral disk herniation at the C3-4 disk level. **B** shows hypertrophic degenerative changes of the inferior-posterior aspect of C3 and the uncinate process of C4 producing bony foraminal stenosis. This additional orthogonal plane oriented in the true course of the neural foramina can be useful for better characterizing bone versus soft tissue abnormalities.

and delineates signal alterations in the cord substance accurately, (3) provides high-quality views of regions proximal or distal to a severe stenosis or block, (4) provides multiple orthogonal planar views of the neural foramina, and (5) avoids the need for contrast material. Nevertheless, preliminary work with Gd-DTPA enhancement has shown that it may play a role in evaluating cervical extradural disease. As demonstrated by Russell et al.[134] with intravenous CT, enhancement of the epidural plexus and/or peridiskal scar can significantly increase the conspicuousness of extradural defects (Fig. 3-52).

The occasional difficulty encountered in distinguishing bone from soft tissue on surface coil MR imaging is probably due to variable signal intensities from the herniated disk, ligamentous hypertrophy, and osteophytes as well as to partial volume averaging of adjacent structures. The reason for the variable signal from osteophytes is, we presume, related to the variable presence and composition of bone marrow within them. Relative to the disk or adjacent vertebral body, osteophytes can have markedly decreased signal intensity (when the bone is dense) or iso- or hyperintense signal (when fatty marrow is more abundant). Hypertrophic bony changes that produce no discernible signal on surface coil MR imaging may be indiscernible from adjacent cerebral spinal

fluid without careful T$_2$-weighted images or fast gradient echo scans with a small flip angle (Fig. 3-53).

Although we would maintain that most evaluations of the cervical spine for extradural disease can be done in an adequate fashion using spin-echo T$_1$-weighted sagittal and axial images, the introduction of fast gradient echo images with small flip angles (less than 15 degrees) has improved the accuracy of the examination by increasing the conspicuousness of extradural defects; and recent work[135-137] has confirmed its value (Figs. 3-46 to 3-49 and 3-53). Gradient echo scans with low flip angles provide a high signal intensity of CSF relative to the extradural structures, providing the so-called CSF-myelogram effect in a shorter period than can usually be accomplished with T$_2$-weighted spin-echo images. The major advantages are most apparent in the axial plane — sharp delineation of bone and disk margins, excellent contrast between the spinal cord and surrounding subarachnoid space, clear visualization of the neural foramina and exiting nerve roots. Degenerative bony ridging tends to be of a lower signal intensity than herniated disk material (Fig. 3-53).

This capability, coupled with the potential of utilizing very short TRs (50 msec or less), has provided the stimulus for using volume imaging in the evaluation of extradural disease, in hopes of shortening the examina-

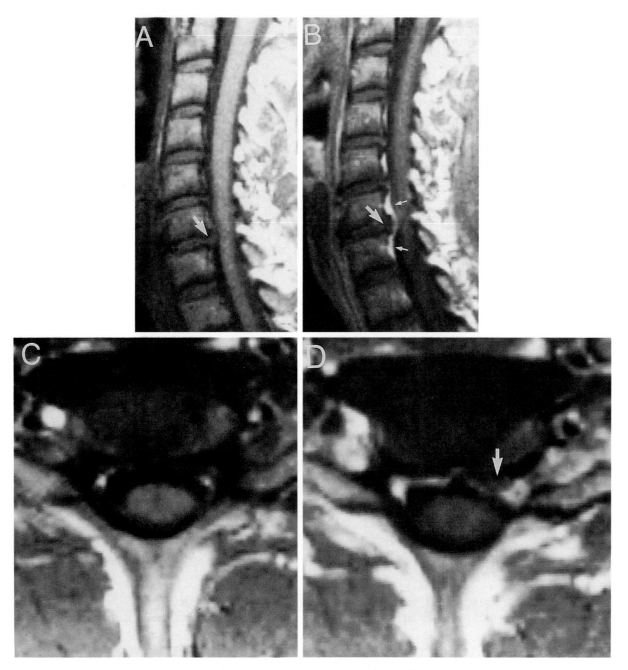

Fig. 3-52. C6-7 disk herniation with and without gadolinium-DTPA. **A** and **B** are T₁-weighted (500/17) spin-echo images through the cervical spine before and after the administration of 0.1 mmole/kg of contrast. The anterior extradural defect **(A)** is denoted by the *arrow.* After Gd-DTPA **(B)** the enhanced epidural venous plexus lateral to midline more clearly outlines the defect caused by the herniation *(arrows).* **C** and **D** are axial T₁-weighted (500/17) spin-echos through the C6-7 disk before and after gadolinium. The lateral herniation is not so well appreciated in the precontrast **(C)** as in the postcontrast **(D)** study because of adjacent enhancement of the epidural veins in the latter. This increases the conspicuousness of the extradural defect. Enhancement of the peripheral disk margin may represent some granulation tissue in addition to the epidural venous plexus.

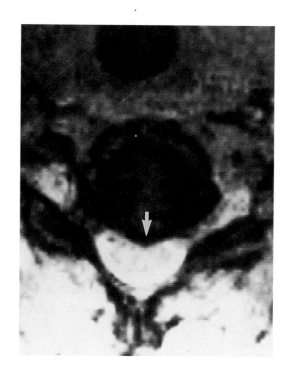

Fig. 3-53. Cervical osteophyte. An axial FLASH (200/13/10 degrees) through C5 shows the posterior osteophyte, which has indented both the thecal sac and the anterior aspect of the cord *(arrow)*. The high signal intensity of CSF on this gradient echo sequence with a low flip angle outlines the decreased signal of the osteophyte.

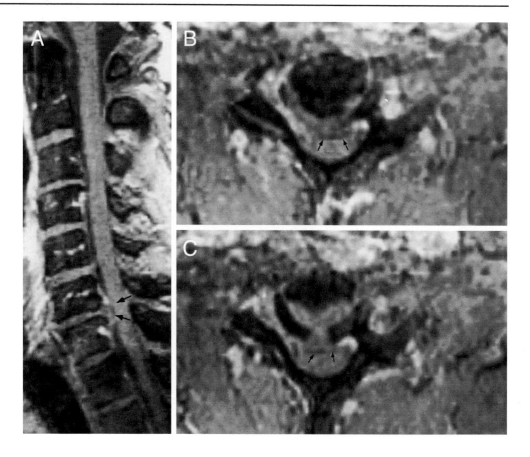

Fig. 3-54. For legend see opposite page.

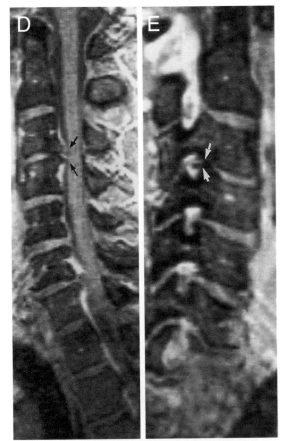

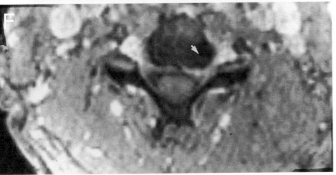

Fig. 3-54. C3-4 osteophyte and C6-7 disk herniation, MPRAGE* 3D dataset with contrast. **A** is a 1.5 mm sagittal midline partition from the dataset. *Arrows* point to the herniation. **B** and **C** are contiguous 1 mm multiplanar reformatted images in an axial plane from the original sagittal dataset. *Arrows* denote the herniation seen on these contiguous images. **D,** A 1.5 mm parasagittal partition to the left of midline demonstrates the extradural defect at C3-4. **E** and **F,** Oblique and axial multiplanar reformatted images highlighting the left C3-4 neural foramen. *Arrows* point to the osteophyte, which is narrowing the neural foramen

*Magnetization-prepared rapid-acquisition gradient echo.

tion time and decreasing slice thickness. Typically, an anisotropic volume acquired in the sagittal plane with a slab thickness of 10 cm or less can be obtained in less than 10 minutes with partitions producing a contiguous slice thickness of 3 mm or less. When the sagittal plane is used for acquisition, subsequent reconstructions in any plane can be obtained that will produce contiguous 2 mm or less slices through the entire field of view. Thus the entire length of the cervical or lumbar spine can be imaged in a multiplanar fashion with one acquisition (Fig. 3-54).

The disadvantages of gradient echo imaging relate to problems with field inhomogeneity and contrast detectability of pathologic processes within the cord itself. Thus, if patients present with radiculopathy and myelopathy or intrinsic cord symptoms alone, additional sagittal multislice multiecho refocused long TR/TE images (with or without gating) are needed.[135,138]

An adjunct to conventional MR in evaluating degenerative disk disease is the utilization of Gd-DTPA. Gadolinium diethylenetriamine pentaacetate is a paramagnetic contrast agent that shows variable degrees of transit from the intravascular space depending on tissue type. Studies with virgin disks and postoperative disk herniation[49] indicate that it is the most accurate means of separating epidural fibrosis and disk tissue. There is consistent enhancement of peridiskal fibrosis early (less than 15 minutes after injection), and variable enhancement occurs in herniated or degenerated parent disks late (30 minutes after injection). Enhancement of intervertebral disks does not appear to occur in the normal state and is likely a sequela of the degenerative process[49,125] (Fig. 3-55).

The degenerative changes in the anulus fibrosus of both cadavers and experimental models include several types of radial tear or rupture. These tears have several stages, including one in which abundant capillaries, precapillaries, and connective tissue enter the tear.[17] Similarly, other studies[27,126] have noted reactive granulation tissue surrounding herniated disks from nonoperated spines that was similar to that seen postoperatively and appeared to reflect scar tissue without evidence of an inflammatory exudate. It makes sense that degenerative disk disease with or without herniation involving the anulus, posterior longitudinal ligaments, and other associated support structures would result in an attempted reparative process that enhanced. Why some but not all degenerated and/or herniated disks exhibit this response and its relationship to the patients' clinical symptomatology remain unclear.

Thus it seems likely that Gd-DTPA may play a role in identifying the sequelae of degenerative disk disease by enhancing the reactive granulation tissue that forms secondary to disruption of the disk and associated structures. This enhancement increases the conspicuousness of extradural defects on T_1-weighted images (Figs. 3-56 and 3-57), as confirmed in part by the observation that even herniated virgin disks are usually outlined by enhancement on MR.

Gadolinium-DTPA may be useful in degenerative disk disease for a second reason. Following its intravenous injection, there is consistent and persistent enhancement of the epidural venous plexus for up to 30 or 40 minutes. This, again, produces increased contrast in the epidural venous structure surrounding the disk space and can heighten the conspicuousness of extradural disease when it impacts on the adjacent venous structures. Future applications of Gd-DTPA will include its utilization with fast gradient echo volume scans to produce contrast that may not be inherently apparent.

In addition to changes within the disk, including herniation, secondary changes are noted both in animal models and in humans following disk degeneration. The stability of a motion segment depends on the integrity of all its components. Diseases occurring in this area are circumferential, that in one joint affecting another, and degeneration of one disk leads to a loss of disk height and forces the facet joints into malalignment, so-called "rostrocaudal subluxation." This leads to increased biomechanical forces at the facet joint with increasing joint relaxation and instability, secondary facet and arthritic changes, and potential fractures. Similarly, abnormal movements allowed by disk degeneration and facet changes add stress to the posterior ligaments and can result in hypertrophy. A vicious degenerative cycle is established that includes degenerative disk disease, facet arthrosis, ligamentous and capsular hypertrophy, spinal instability, and lumbar stenosis.[139]

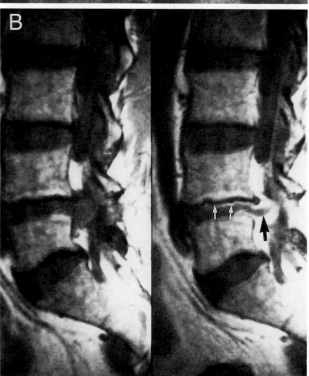

Fig. 3-55. Enhancement of degenerative disks. **A,** T_1-weighted (500/17) midline sections before and 30 minutes after the injection of gadolinium-DTPA. Type I vertebral body changes are evident in the inferior aspect of L5 and the contiguous portion of S1. Following injection there is enhancement of these regions *(tailed black arrows)* as well as the entire L5-S1 disk *(straight black arrow)*. The enhancement of the disk itself is presumably secondary to diffusion of contrast via fibrovascular granulation tissue within both the vertebral body and the endplate of the central disk. **B,** Epidural fibrosis and linear enhancement. These are T_1-weighted (500/17) and parasagittal sections before and 8 minutes after gadolinium. The preinjection scan demonstrates a soft tissue mass extending posteriorly and laterally from the L4-5 disk. Following injection there is enhancement of soft tissue surrounding this herniation *(black arrow)*. Pathology revealed granulation tissue. A thin line of enhancement just beneath the inferior cortical margin of L4 on the postinjection study was thought to represent granulation tissue within a disrupted endplate and/or peripheral disk margin *(small white arrows)*.

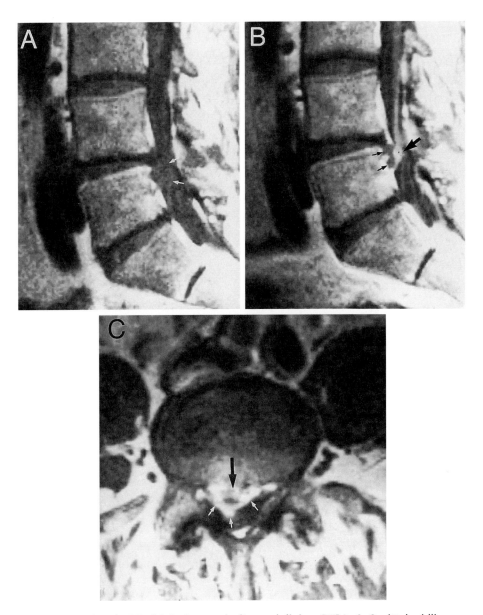

Fig. 3-56. Herniated L4-5 disk before and after gadolinium-DTPA. **A,** Sagittal midline T$_1$-weighted (500/17) spin-echo sequence through the lumbar spine. *Small white arrows* point to a poorly defined soft tissue mass posterior to the superior aspect of L5. **B,** Following the administration of contrast there is enhancement surrounding this soft tissue mass. **C,** An axial T$_1$-weighted (500/17) spin-echo through the inferior aspect of the L4-5 disk and superior L5 shows an enhancing mass with a central area of decreased signal *(arrows).* There is posterior displacement with compression of the thecal sac. At surgery the central portion of this mass was found to represent herniated disk surrounded by a peripheral portion (which enhanced on MR) that proved to be granulation tissue. This case demonstrates that in addition to enhancement of the epidural venous plexus by Gd-DTPA for increased conspicuousness of extradural defects, there may be enhancement of granulation tissue that is associated with virgin disks as well as the postoperative state.

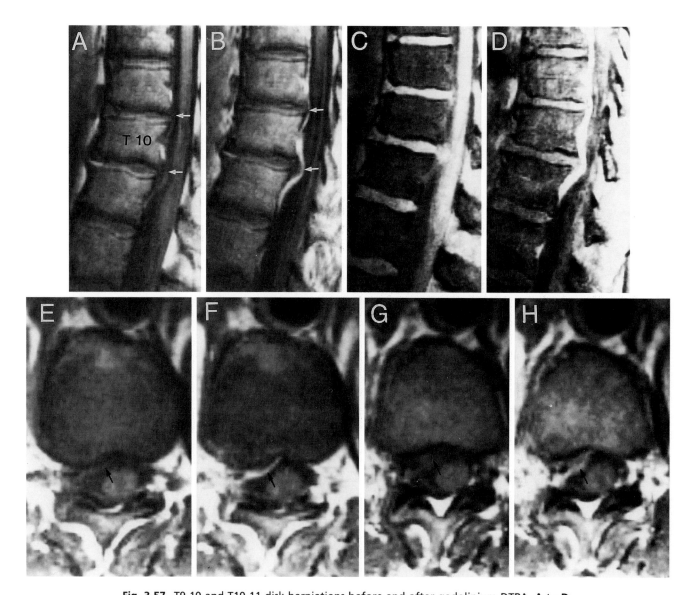

Fig. 3-57. T9-10 and T10-11 disk herniations before and after gadolinium-DTPA. **A** to **D** represent sagittal T$_1$-weighted (500/17) spin-echo pre- and postgadolinium and FLASH (200/13/60 degrees) pre- and postgadolinium. Note the anterior extradural defects at T9-10 and T10-11, which are more clearly outlined following contrast by linear areas of enhancement. **E** to **H,** Axial T$_1$-weighted (500/17) spin-echo images before and after Gd-DTPA at the T9-10 and 10-11 levels. Soft tissue–signal intensity herniations to the right of midline (larger at T10-11) are peripherally enhanced at T9-10 and both peripherally and diffusely enhanced at T10-11. Surgery showed them to be lateral thoracic disk herniations with peridiskal granulation tissue. In such cases the enhancement is a combination of venous plexus and peridiskal granulation tissue.

SPINAL STENOSIS

Spinal stenosis results from an overall diminution of the spinal canal, lateral recesses, or neural foramina. It occurs more commonly in the lumbar and cervical regions. The symptoms are usually a reflection of the compressive pathology. In the cervical region the most frequently observed manifestations are multiple unilateral or bilateral radiculopathy and/or myelopathy. Neck or shoulder pain is a frequent complaint but is not specific and may only reflect general myotomal innervation. Myelopathic syndromes usually present with some degree of spasticity and weakness secondary to involvement of the cortical spinal tracks, spinal thalamic tracks, and/or posterior columns below the level(s) of involvement.[140] In the lumbar region canal stenosis can cause compression of the cauda equina and/or individual nerve roots. The classic description of neurogenic claudication from spinal stenosis is bilateral radicular pain, disorders of sensory function, and motor deficits that develop when the patient is standing or walking, and are absent when the patient is recumbent. Interestingly, this claudication, unlike vascular claudication, may actually be more severe when standing still. More frequently arthritic symptoms such as back pain and the subjective symptoms of coldness, tingling, burning, and sciatica are noted. As a rule the symptoms and signs of spinal stenosis do not appear until the fifth or sixth decade but can occur much earlier for acquired disease superimposed on a developmental form.

Etiologically stenosis can be divided into two main types. The first is developmental or *congenital* stenosis, which is idiopathic and includes achondroplasia, Morquio's disease, and various bony dysplasias. It may be associated with thick pedicles and a reduced interpedicular distance and is often further complicated by the second type, *acquired* stenosis, which may be seen after trauma and with degenerative disease, spondylolisthesis, postoperative changes, and various miscellaneous disorders including ankylosing spondylitis, ossification of the posterior longitudinal ligament or ligamentum flavum, Paget's disease, acromegaly, and fluorosis.

Three factors, either alone or in combination, are thought to be responsible for the development of symptoms in most cases[140]: The first is some degree of developmental narrowing of the neural canal. The second is tethering of the involved nerve roots secondary to hypertrophic vertebral body or facet joint disease that may interfere with the normal vascular supply. The third is rotary or lateral instability following disk and facet degeneration. Regardless of the etiology, the common denominator of spinal stenosis is narrowing of the canal, which may be central, peripheral, or both.

From a therapeutic standpoint it seems more practical to describe the changes of spinal stenosis in relation to the regions and anatomic structures involved. *Central* changes encompass the bony spinal canal bounded by the pedicles laterally, the facet joints, laminae, and spinous processes posteriorly, and the disks anteriorly. *Subarticular* involvement refers to the subarticular segments of the nerve root canals, including the lateral recesses. *Intervertebral canal* (foraminal) involvement includes the infrapedicular segments of the nerve root canals and the intervertebral foramina. When these last two regions are involved, the condition is often referred to as peripheral stenosis. Central and peripheral stenosis may coexist.

Lumbar Spine

Central stenosis tends to occur at multiple levels but is most frequent and usually most severe at the L4-5 level, where it may occur alone (Figs. 3-58 to 3-61). Central stenosis tends to produce complicated radicular signs and symptoms with or without claudication. This region is particularly susceptible to impingement by osteophytes from the vertebral bodies or facet joints, thickening of the ligaments, and bulging of the intervertebral disks. Ligamentous stenosis can occur even when the dimensions of the central bony canal are normal and includes reduction of the overall dimensions by hypertrophy of the ligamentum flavum as well as calcification of the posterior longitudinal ligament. Although this reduction is more common in the cervical region, it can also occur in the thoracic or lumbar region and is seen in up to 25% of patients with diffuse idiopathic skeletal hyperostosis. Paget's disease may also cause spinal canal narrowing secondary to diffuse bony overgrowth. Following surgery, secondary stenosis of the spinal canal may occur with hypertrophy of bone grafts, overgrowth of bone, or spondylolisthesis.

The transverse and sagittal dimensions of the central neural canal are best depicted by integrating orthogonal (e.g., axial and sagittal) planes. Gradient echo images with low flip angles or more T_2-weighted spin-echo sequences provide the best views of thecal sac dimensions by furnishing a gray-scale inversion of the CSF and extradural elements.[135,136] Besides an overall reduction in size of the neural canal, several ancillary signs may be noted that often are a cause for confusion. First, especially in the lumbar regions, central canal stenosis can cause central consolidation of the nerve roots, resulting in an intermediate signal intensity within the thecal sac on T_1-weighted images. This may be confused with clumping secondary to arachnoiditis or an intradural mass. Second, canal stenosis can damp the CSF pulsations, resulting in a diffuse or focal higher signal intensity distally on both sagittal and axial images, again not to be confused with arachnoiditis or an intradural mass. There is often a reduction of ghosting, and the signal intensity of the CSF is well preserved on T_2-weighted sequences for similar reasons.

Text continued on p. 138.

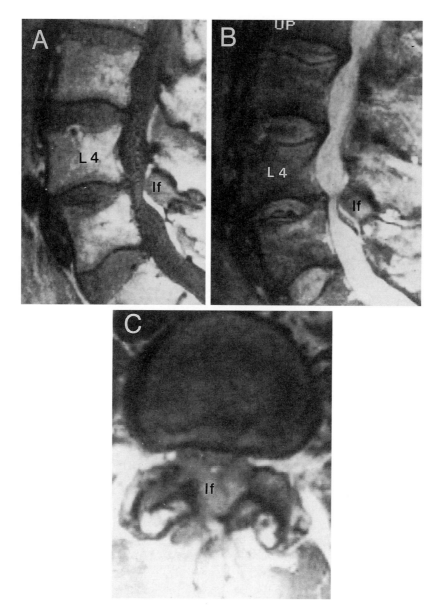

Fig. 3-58. Central lumbar canal stenosis at L4-5. **A,** Sagittal midline T$_1$-weighted (500/17) spin-echo image. There is marked narrowing of the canal at the L4-5 interspace caused primarily by enlargement of the ligamentum flavum *(lf)*. **B,** Sagittal T$_2$-weighted (2000/90) spin-echo through the same level. Again, marked canal stenosis is evident at the L4-5 interspace. **C,** An axial T$_1$-weighted (500/17) spin-echo through the L4-5 disk shows the enlarged ligamentum *(lf)*. The thecal sac is of reduced size. Also the facet joints are enlarged and show evidence of hypertrophic degenerative change.

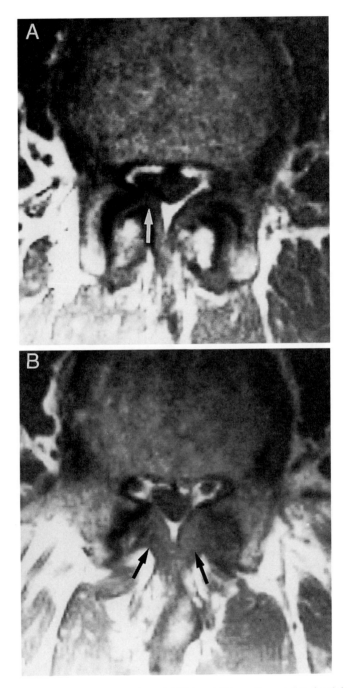

Fig. 3-59. Central canal stenosis at the mid-L3 level. These T_1-weighted axial (500/17) spin-echo images show the stenosis produced by hypertrophic changes in the facets *(white arrow)* as well as posterolateral indentation of the thecal sac from the enlarged facet-capsule complex. Note the thickened and enlarged ligamentum flavum posteriorly *(black arrows)*.

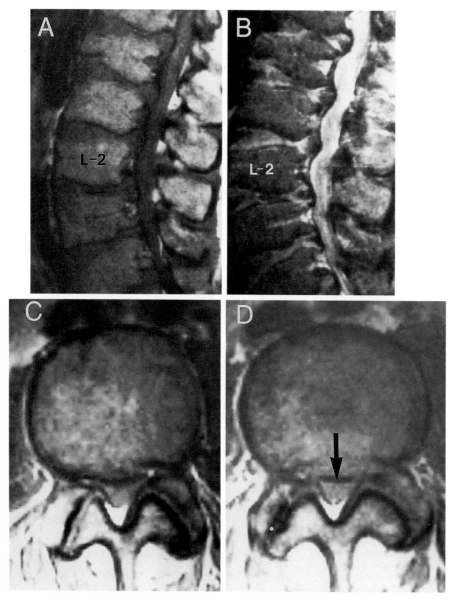

Fig. 3-60. Lumbar canal stenosis. **A,** Sagittal midline T_1-weighted (500/17) spin-echo, **B,** sagittal midline T_2-weighted (2000/90) spin-echo, and, **C** and **D,** axial T_1-weighted (500/17) spin-echo images through the L4 neural foramina demonstrate diffuse central and peripheral stenosis in this 36-year-old woman. There is complete obliteration of the normal neural foramina caused by hypertrophic degenerative changes of the facet joints and vertebral bodies at all levels. The signal intensity of the CSF is higher than one would anticipate on the T_1-weighted images and is due to both the decreased pulsations of thoracic CSF and the central clumping of nerve roots in the cauda equina (*arrow* in **D**).

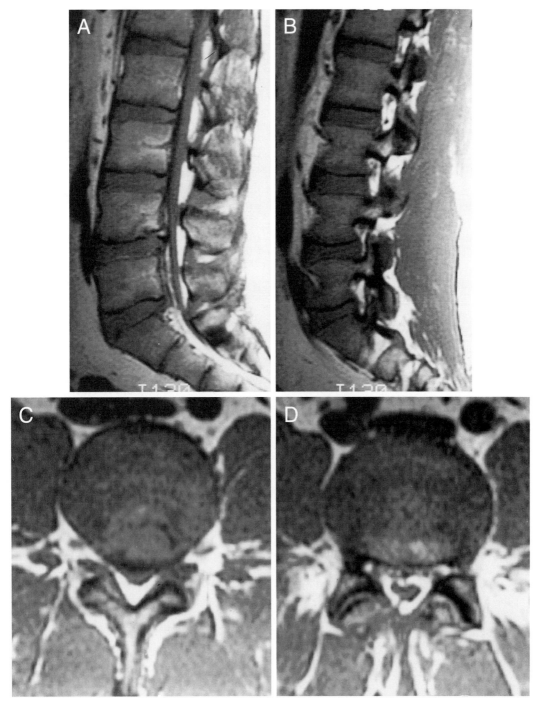

Fig. 3-61. Developmental lumbar canal stenosis. **A** and **B,** Midline and parasagittal
T_1-weighted spin-echo images and, **C** and **D,** axial T_1-weighted spin-echos through the
L4-5 disk. There is diffuse central canal stenosis presumably of developmental origin. The
neural foramina show some narrowing at the L4-5 level but otherwise remain widely
patent. The stenosis is complicated by superimposed degenerative disk disease, as
evidenced at the L4-5 and S-1 levels.

Peripheral stenosis may occur alone or in combination with central stenosis (Fig. 3-62). The height of the lateral recess is defined as the distance between the most anterior portion of the superior articular facet and the posterior portion of the vertebral body in the same plane. A height of 4 mm or less is usually associated with symptoms. More laterally a neural foraminal stenosis can occur from bony overgrowth, spondylolisthesis, and/or degenerative bulging or herniation of the intervertebral disk. Postoperative fibrosis can also cause symptoms identical to those of bony stenosis. It must be remembered, however, that severe morphologic changes can occur without symptomatology because the nerve root occupies only a small portion of the superior neural foramen. Narrowing of the inferior portion is a relatively common finding in the aging population and is less likely to cause symptoms.

Peripheral stenosis is best appreciated on T_1-weighted images, which maintain the separation between neural structures and epidural fat quite well. The signal intensity between neural elements and fat is less well seen on more T_2-weighted and gradient echo images, although bony overgrowth can be identified. In the lumbar region the parasagittal and axial images together allow accurate identification of the lateral recesses and neural foramina and their relationship to the vertebral body, disk, and facets. In this fashion an accurate description of the various anatomic zones where stenosis may occur can be obtained. It should be noted that lateral disk bulging into the inferior aspect of a foramen is commonly noted in the aging population. This by itself, however, is rarely a cause of symptoms since the neural elements pass laterally in a more superior plane beneath the pedicle. In the cervical region oblique images are more useful than parasagittal images because they provide a more accurate second orthogonal plane in conjunction with the axial images.

The malalignment concomitant with spondylolisthesis produces anatomic derangement of the neural foramina that causes stenosis. Associated true disk herniation is uncommon at the level of a pars defect but may be seen at the interspace above. Compression of the nerve roots in spondylolisthesis may be due to a buildup of fibrocartilage rather than to the pars defect (and malalignment) itself. The height of the neural foramina becomes reduced at the level of the segment involved by the pedicles, which forms the roof as it is positioned more inferiorly. Encroachment of the central spinal canal also occurs secondary to forward displacement.

Thoracic Spine

Symptomatic spinal stenosis in the thoracic region is much less common than in the cervical and lumbar regions, unless it is associated with metabolic disease or spinal trauma. This is, to a large degree, due to the relatively large size of the thoracic canal relative to the cord. Thus there must be a marked decrease in the overall dimensions of the thoracic canal to produce compressive symptomatology. The symptoms of thoracic spinal stenosis are varied and may consist of myelopathy, sensory changes, radiculopathy, and a syndrome of claudication with low back pain similar to that seen with lumbar disease but without leg pain. The pathology noted is usually hypertrophy of the posterior spinal bony and/or ligamentous elements.[141] Thoracic radiculomyelopathy from cord compression by the posterior spinal elements has been reported[142] under categories such as thoracic spinal stenosis, developmental stenosis of thoracic vertebrae, hypertrophic ligamentum flavum with ossification, ossified ligamentum flavum, thoracic spondylosis, osteophyte of the articular process, and narrowing of the spinal canal by thickened laminae. Reports to date with MR demonstrate decreased signal intensity from ossified lesions.[142]

A less common form of cord compression secondary to spinal stenosis is that induced by epidural lipomatosis. Asymptomatic epidural lipomatosis is not uncommon in classic pituitary-dependent Cushing disease and is even more common in the ectopic adrenocorticotropic hormone syndrome. It is part of the central or truncal lipomatosis associated with both exogenous and endogenous hypercortisolemia. Symptomatic epidural lipomatosis, however, is rarely encountered in endogenous cases, being more often seen in exogenous hypercortisolism. It has been speculated[143] that this is related to the shorter duration and the lesser severity of hypercortisolism seen with endogenous cases. Most of the lesions are located in the thoracic region, but there can be extensive involvement of the lumbosacral junction as well. Characteristic thoracic locations are likely accounted for by the fact that the thoracic region generally has a large amount of normal spinal canal fat, which is usually posteriorly or posterolaterally located in the canal.[144] Recently it has been suggested[145] that patients with spinal epidural lipomatosis may be at greater risk for cord compression from osteopenic compression fracture.

Cervical Spine

In the cervical spine degenerative changes affect all major spinal articulations, including the intervertebral disks, apophyseal joints, ligamentous connections between vertebral bodies, and the vertebral bodies themselves. The term *spondylosis* is used to refer to changes involving the intervertebral disk and vertebral bodies, in contrast to degenerative changes of the apophyseal joints, which are more often classified as osteoarthritis. A common factor in both spondylosis and osteoarthritis is concomitant degenerative disease of the intervertebral disk that results in the loss of elasticity of the disk and surrounding ligaments. Bulging of the disk margin tends

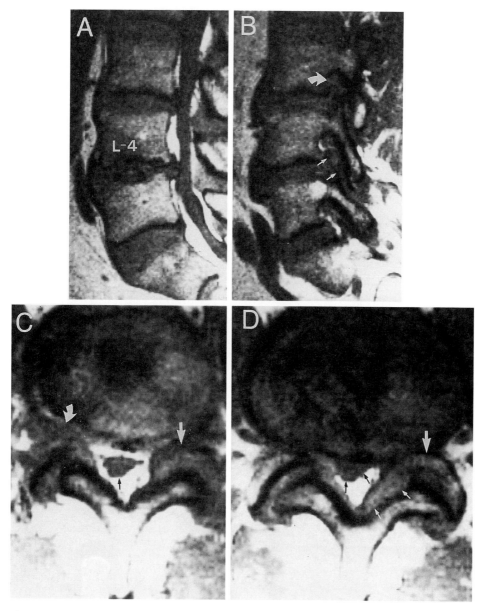

Fig. 3-62. Lumbar canal stenosis. **A** and **B,** Midline and parasagittal T_1-weighted spin-echo (500/17) and, **C** and **D,** axial T_1-weighted spin-echo (500/17) images through the neural foramina at L4 show diffuse central and peripheral stenosis. The normal epidural fat signal is obliterated, and it is impossible to discern the dorsal root ganglia beneath the pedicles in **B** *(curved arrow* and *small arrows).* The axial images demonstrate marked hypertrophy of the ligamentum flavum, facet joints, and capsule, totally obliterating the neural foramina *(white arrows).* The thecal sac is small, and despite the severe stenosis *(black arrows)* there is abundant epidural fat centrally. The L4-5 disk is diffusely herniated both centrally and laterally.

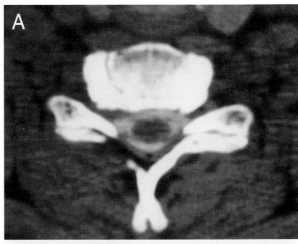

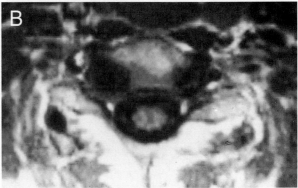

Fig. 3-63. Lateral cervical stenosis. **A,** This high-resolution CT obtained after myelography demonstrates marked hypertrophic degenerative changes of the uncinate process of C7 bilaterally. **B,** Axial T_1-weighted (500/17) spin-echo image through the same level. Note the marked decrease in signal of the hypertrophic degenerative changes within the uncinate process, causing bilateral foraminal stenosis.

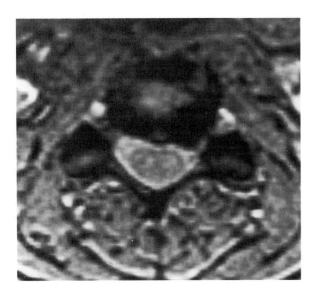

Fig. 3-64. Cervical foraminal stenosis. Axial FLASH (200/13/60 degrees) through the C5-6 neural foramina. Hypertrophic degenerative changes of the left uncinate process have resulted in bony stenosis on the left.

to exert traction on the longitudinal ligaments of the vertebral bodies, producing an irritative reaction that results in the formation of osteophytes. Ironically, the formation of osteophytes may have a stabilizing effect on the spine. This mechanism is important in the formation more of anterior than of posterior or posterolateral osteophytes, which are usually the most important clinically.

With degenerative collapse of the intervertebral disk space and/or posterior intervertebral joints, there is narrowing of the intervertebral foramina that tends to compress the individual nerve roots. The development of uncovertebral spurs that lie medially and laterally in the spinal canal usually occurs concomitantly (Figs. 3-63 and 3-64). Thus the major cause of cervical spinal stenosis is osteophytic overgrowth at the posterolateral margins of the body, posterior protrusion of the disk material, hypertrophy of the ligamentum flavum, and dorsal intrusions into the canal by osteophytes secondary to apophyseal arthritic changes (Figs. 3-65 and 3-66). Not all individuals with evidence of cervical spondylosis and osteoarthritis have cord compression, and those who do tend to have small spinal canals irrespective of the secondary changes. This is exacerbated in extension, since maximal canal size is achieved in slight flexion. Relaxation or bulging of the ligamentum flavum into the canal and hyperextension may also be a cause of stenosis. (One of the reasons that stenosis may appear more severe at myelography than at MR is the difference in positions, i.e., hyperextensional with myelography and neutral with MR.) Degenerative changes of the posterior articulations can allow mild retrolisthesis of the superior vertebra on the inferior, which also tends to decrease the sagittal diameter.

A less common cause of cervical spinal stenosis is ossification of the posterior longitudinal ligament (OPLL) (Fig. 3-67). Until recently this was considered endemic in Japan. A large comprehensive epidemiologic study of elderly Japanese[146] determined the prevalence to be 2.4%. Recently a number of reports of OPLL in non-Orientals have appeared. OPLL seems to be more frequent in diffuse idiopathic skeletal hyperostosis; and a variant, ossification of the yellow ligament (OYL), can be responsible for compression of the thoracic spinal cord. The basic pathophysiologic process of OPLL is similar to that of heterotopic bone formation elsewhere secondary to mechanical stress. With time the OPLL mass progressively enlarges (thickness, width, and length). Again, OPLL is more likely to produce symptomatic cord compression in a canal already compromised by congenital stenosis, spondylosis, or hypertrophy of the ligamentum flavum than in a canal with normal dimensions.[147] Cervical OPLL can be divided into segmental and continuous types. Calcification is usually identified on MR as an area of hypointensity, but

bands of intermediate or high signal intensity may be observed within the areas of ossification; these most likely represent marrow formation with lipid elements. The degree of cord compression is usually more severe in segmental OPLL, which is characteristically more hypointense than the continuous variety.

Whereas asymptomatic cervical cord compression is often seen, it has only recently been directly implicated in the etiology of cervical myelopathy. As mentioned previously, it is often secondary to a combination of spondylitic ridges, disk disease, hypertrophy of the ligamentum flavum, and congenital narrowing of the spinal canal. The suggestion has been made[148] that myelopathy or stenosis is associated with an average canal diameter less than 12 mm. Care must be taken, however, when using gradient echo images since the degree of spinal narrowing can be overestimated because of susceptibility effects. The degree of spinal narrowing may not be the only factor in the development of myelopathy. Increasing cervical motion may also contribute to neurologic deterioration; for, despite the canal's being slightly wider in mild flexion, repeated flexion might actually traumatize the cord by forcing it against the anterior osteophytes. In extension there is some narrowing of the canal, and buckling of the posterior longitudinal ligament can narrow the canal even further.[148] Another method suggested for determining cervical spinal stenosis[149] is the vertebral body–canal ratio, which has been suggested to correct for body size. A spinal canal–vertebra body ratio of less 0.82 would indicate significant cervical spinal stenosis.

The mechanism for ischemia of the cord in compressive states is unclear, but experimental data suggest that lateral compression and masses have less effect on central cord perfusion than anterior-posterior compression does. These disproportionate ischemic effects of anterior as compared to lateral compression have been attributed to the cord's limited capacity for posterior displacement as contrasted with freer side-to-side mobility.[150]

MR and myelographic CT studies appear to be equivalent in measuring the degree of cord compression. There may be a correlation between compression and the amount of neurologic dysfunction.[151]

It has been suggested[152] that high signal intensity on T_2-weighted images within the spinal cord indicates parenchymal damage (Fig. 3-68). In a study of 668 patients with lesions chronically compressing the cervical canal,[152] high signal was observed within the cord of 99 patients (14.8%). The frequency of this finding was directly proportionate to the severity of clinical myelopathy and the degree of cord compression seen on MR images. Patients with this high signal intensity responded less favorably than those without it when treated either surgically or medically.[152] In another study[153] the incidence of this finding was highest in herniated disk dis-

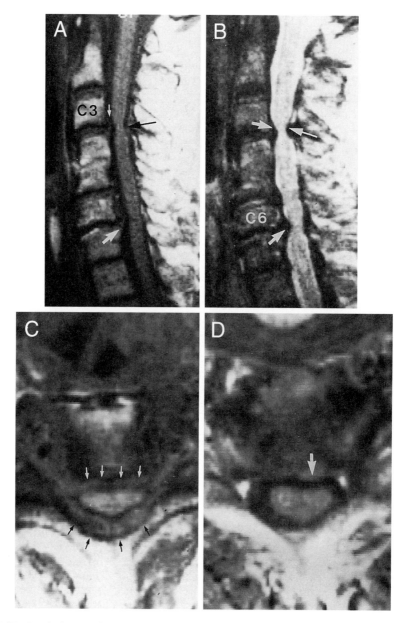

Fig. 3-65. Cervical stenosis. **A** and **B,** Sagittal T_1-weighted (500/17) and T_2-weighted (2000/90) spin-echo images show stenosis at the C3-4 level both anteriorly and posteriorly *(small white arrow, large black arrow)* as well as hypertrophic degenerative changes and canal narrowing at the C6-7 level anteriorly. **C** and **D,** Axial T_1-weighted (500/17) spin-echo images through the C3-4 and C6-7 levels. At C3-4 the *small white* and *black arrows* point to marked ligamentous and soft tissue stenosis with compression of the cord. The intermediate signal in **D** arising from hypertrophic degenerative bone on the superior aspect of C7 *(white arrow)* has caused an anterior extradural defect with the stenosis.

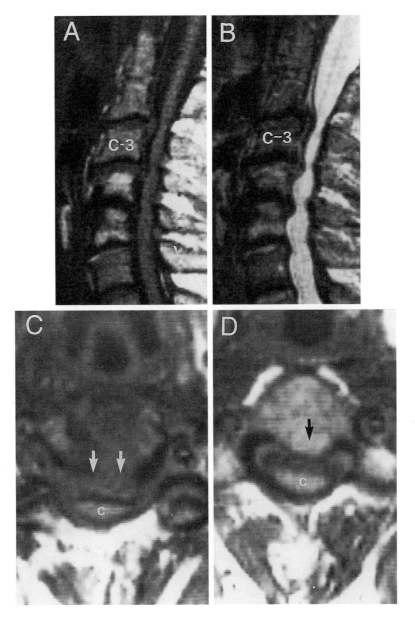

Fig. 3-66. Cervical stenosis. **A** and **B** are sagittal T$_1$-weighted (2000/90) spin-echo images through the cervical spine showing severe stenosis from C2-3 through C4-5. **C,** An axial T$_1$-weighted (500/17) spin-echo through C2-3 demonstrates herniation of the disk *(white arrows)* with marked compression of the cord. **D,** Another axial T$_1$-weighted (500/17) spin-echo through C5 reveals a large osteophyte anteriorly *(black arrow)* along with the compression.

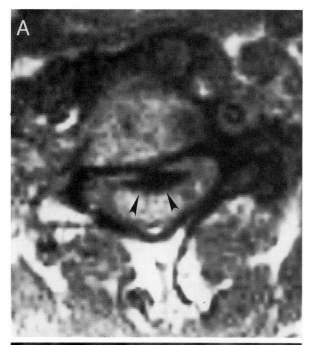

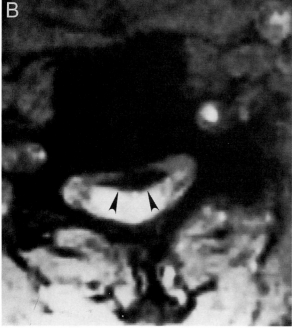

Fig. 3-67. Ossification of the posterior longitudinal ligament. **A,** An axial T$_1$-weighted (500/17) spin-echo and, **B,** a FLASH (200/13/60 degrees) show decreased signal anterior to the cord at C6 *(arrowheads)*. Although both acquisitions depict the ossification, the gradient echo tends to show it better, presumably because of the susceptibility effect of heterotopic bone formation within the ligament.

ease (32.4%), atlantoaxial dislocation (28.6%), and OPLL (22.7%) whereas it was only sporadic in cervical spondylosis and vertebral body tumors. Local spinal cord constriction seemed to be the most important predisposing factor in producing the high signal intensity change. The authors speculated that the pathophysiologic basis of this change was myelomalacia or cord gliosis secondary to a long-standing compressive effect on the cord.[153] Others[154] have suggested that the high signal intensity on proton density and T$_2$-weighted images is related to shear stress rather than vascular occlusion or direct mechanical trauma.

Although there are no good studies to indicate that MR has led to improved therapeutic choices, there is at present sufficient evidence to suggest that MR is adequate for most therapeutic planning to allow physicians to stop further testing, obviating the need for a myelogram or CT.[155,156]

On MR the following features are important for analysis: facet joint size and contour, osteophyte formation of the facet joints or vertebral bodies, hypertrophy and/or calcification of ligamentous structures, and transverse and sagittal dimensions of the neural canal, lateral recess, and neural foramina.

Bony osteophytes can be of decreased, intermediate, or high signal intensity relative to the adjacent vertebral body and facet joints.[55] Signal differences presumably reflect variable amounts of yellow marrow. Despite usually being well appreciated on T$_1$-weighted images, they are reportedly easier to see and distinguish from soft tissue on long TR/short TE images. On T$_1$-weighted images, osteophytes with a higher lipid marrow content are easier to identify than sclerotic osteophytes (which usually have a low signal intensity that may blend with adjacent ligamentous structures or CSF). Gradient echo images, especially with low flip angles, depict hypertrophic changes as decreased signal, in contrast to the CSF or adjacent paraspinal fat.

Thickening of the ligamentum flavum can be identified in both the axial and the sagittal plane.[157] In the axial plane of normal persons the mean thickness is 5.5 ± 1.3 mm. Hypertrophy can be unilateral or asymmetric (Fig. 3-58). In the cervical region it measures 1 to 3 mm, and in the thoracic region approximately 2 mm. Thickening—identified with degeneration, aging, or buckling—is usually seen concomitantly with degenerative disease of the facets and disks. The high signal intensity of the ligamentum flavum relative to the PLLs, especially on T$_1$-weighted or gradient echo images, has been reported[157] to be related to its high elastin (80%) and low type I collagen (20%) content. Calcification of the ligamentous structures may be difficult to appreciate on T$_1$-weighted spin-echo images because the decreased signal intensity from adjacent CSF may blend with that

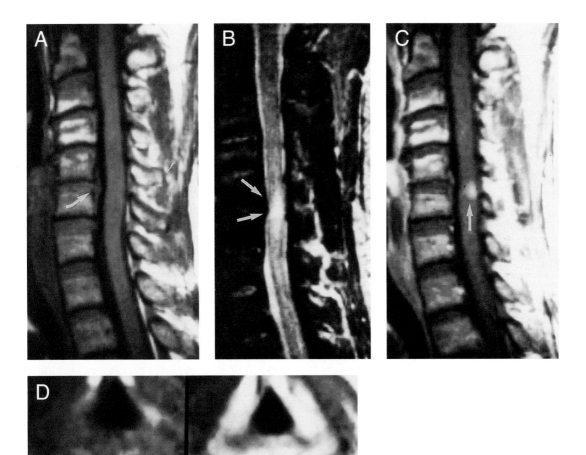

Fig. 3-68. Cervical myelopathy. **A** and **B,** T_1- and T_2-weighted sagittal spin-echo images through the cervical cord reveal a disk that is indenting the cord anteriorly (*arrow* in **A**). On the T_2-weighted image there is high signal in the cord immediately contiguous with the herniated disk *(arrows)*. After the administration of gadolinium, **C,** high signal intensity can be seen posteriorly within the cord. **D,** Pre- and postcontrast axial images through the area of enhancement demonstrate the posterior-lateral margins of the cord *(arrows).*

of the thecal sac. This is particularly true in OPLL, where the decreased signal sharply contrasts with that of the CSF on more T_2-weighted images. Alternatively, gradient echo scans appear to be more sensitive to calcification, because of a susceptibility effect, thus allowing their identification with greater accuracy than on T_1-weighted spin-echo sequences (Fig. 3-67).

Facet Joints

Although facet arthrosis constitutes an important cause of acquired lumbar stenosis, degenerative change can occur independently of it and may be a cause of low back pain and radiculopathy.[139,158] Like any diarthrodial synovium-lined joint, the facets are predisposed to arthropathies. These may result in alterations of the articular cartilage leading to osteochondral fragments, which can act like joint mice. With advancing disease and progressive evolution of the articular cartilage, subchondral bony sclerosis and degenerative cysts develop. Synovial villi can become entrapped, and joint effusions may be produced. Osteophytes often develop in areas of bone stress, which may, in addition, lead to hypertrophy of the entire facet joints or parts thereof, usually the superior articular facet. Herniation of synovium through the facet joint capsule can then result in a synovial cyst that will act as a mass lesion.

Back pain may be caused by two mechanisms of facet joint disease. The first is direct compression of nerve roots secondary to facet hypertrophies, osteophytes, or rostrocaudal subluxation and expansion of the facet joint capsule secondary to joint effusions. Second, and perhaps more importantly, because the synovial linings and joint capsule of the facet joint are richly innervated,[137] pain may be produced by local internal derangements, resulting in direct irritation of pain fibers that can lead to muscular spasm, focal or diffuse back pain, and sciatica.

As mentioned, degenerative changes of the facet joints most commonly involve the superior articular facet, which can with hypertrophy and focal osteophyte formation produce both central and lateral stenosis. Enlargement of the superior articular facet can cause stenosis in the region of the lateral recess and with rostrocaudal subluxation can lead to narrowing in the upper portion of the neural canal. Posterolateral protrusion of the facet joint into the central canal can also occur. It must be emphasized that undiagnosed facet disease has been implicated as one of the causes of the failed back surgery syndrome and thus must be looked for carefully in all preoperative evaluations. Postoperative changes may also be seen with the development of contralateral facet joint disease following a foraminotomy and diskectomy. This procedure can lead to additional stress on the facet joints, which most often is manifested on the con-

tralateral side since the ipsilateral side is usually sufficiently decompressed.[137]

On MR the facet joints are best evaluated by visually integrating sagittal and axial images. Again, osteophytes are easier to identify on gradient echo or spin-echo images with long TRs. Those that contain marrow are also better demarcated than those that are sclerotic, which can be confused with the adjacent capsular ligamentous structures (particularly at the posterior-inferior aspect of the joint, where the capsule always demonstrates low signal intensity). Altered signal intensity in bone marrow consistent with fatty replacement has also been reported to be commonly associated.[157] Although both facet joints may be involved, the superior is more common. The articular cartilage can be directly visualized on both T_1- and T_2-weighted spin-echo images, but thinning is difficult to measure accurately because of variable axial obliquity and chemical shift artifact from the adjacent facet. Nevertheless, notable changes appear to correlate well with those identified on CT. More recently gradient echo examinations have demonstrated that they provide better conspicuousness of the articular cartilage itself as distinct from adjacent osseous structures. Preliminary data suggest that they are better appraised with this technique, which potentially could allow direct visualization of thinning and irregularities of the cartilage itself not possible with other modalities. Changes in the underlying bone such as facet erosions or cyst formation might also be noted.

REFERENCES

1. Kelsey JL, White AA III, Pastides H, et al: The impact of musculoskeletal disorders in the population of the United States. *J Bone Joint Surg [Am]* 1979;61:959-964.
2. Dillane JB, Frye J, Colton G: Acute back syndrome: a study from general practice. *Br Med J* 1966;2:82-84.
3. Rowe ML: Low back pain in industry: a position paper. *J Occup Med* 1969;11:161-169.
4. Frymoyer JW: Back pain and sciatica. *N Engl J Med* 1988;318:291-300.
5. Frymoyer JW: Are we performing too much spinal surgery? *Iowa Orthop J* 1989;9:32-36.
6. Cypress BK: Characteristics of physician visits for back symptoms: a national perspective. *Am J Public Health* 1983;73:389-395.
7. Deyo RA: Early diagnostic evaluation of low back pain. *J Gen Intern Med* 1986;1:328-338.
8. Resnick D: Degenerative diseases of the vertebral column. *Radiology* 1985;156:3-14.
9. Mooney V: The syndromes of low back disease. *Orthop Clin North Am* 1983;14:505-515.
10. Waddell G: A new clinical model for the treatment of low back pain. *Spine* 1987;12:632-644.
11. Parke WW: The innervation of connective tissues of the spinal motion segment. Presented at the International Symposium on Percutaneous Lumbar Discectomy, 1987.

12. Pedowitz RA, Rydevik BL, Hargens AR, et al: Morot and sensory nerve root conduction deficit induced by acute graded compression of the pig cauda equina. Presented at the 34th annual meeting of the Orthopaedic Research Society, 1988.

13. Smyth MJ, Wright V: Sciatica and the intervertebral disc. *J Bone Joint Surg [Am]* 1958;40:1401-1418.

14. Howe JF, Loeser JD, Calvin WH: Mechanosensitivity of dorsal root ganglia and chronically injured axons: a physiological basis for the radicular pain of nerve root compression. *Pain* 1977;3:25-41.

15. Rydevik B, Brown MD, Lundborg G: Pathoanatomy and pathophysiology of nerve root compression. *Spine* 1984;9:11-15.

16. Weinstein JN, Rydevik BL: The pain of spondylolisthesis. *Semin Spine Surg* 1989;1:100-105.

17. Haughton VM: MR imaging of the spine. *Radiology* 1988;166:297-301.

18. Penning L, Wilmink JT, Woerden HH, et al: CT myelographic findings in degenerative disorders of the cervical spine: clinical significance. *AJNR* 1986;7:119-127.

19. Teresi LM, Lufkin RB, Reicher MA, et al: Asymptomatic degenerative disk disease and spondylosis of the cervical spine: MR imaging. *Radiology* 1987;164:83-88.

20. Rothman SL, Glenn WV: Spondylosis and spondylolisthesis. In Newton TH, Potts DG (eds): *Computed tomography of the spine and spinal cord*. San Anselmo Calif, Clavadel, 1983, pp 267-280.

21. Johnson DW, Farnum GN, Latchaw RE, Erba SM: MR imaging of the pars interarticularis. *AJNR* 1988;9:1215-1220.

22. Pritzker KP: Aging and degeneration in the lumbar intervertebral disc. *Orthop Clin North Am* 1977;8(1):66-77.

23. White AA, Gordon SL: Synopsis: Workshop on idiopathic low-back pain. *Spine* 1982;7(2):141-149.

24. Tertti MO, Salminen JJ, Paganen HEK, et al: Low back pain and disk degeneration in children: a case-control MR imaging study. *Radiology* 1991;180:503-507.

25. Paajanen H, Alanen A, Erkintalo M, et al: Disc degeneration in Scheuermann disease. *Skeletal Radiol* 1989;18(7):523-526.

26. Quinet RJ, Hadler NM: Diagnosis and treatment of backache. *Semin Arthritis Rheum* 1979;8(4):261-287.

27. Coventry MB: Anatomy of the intervertebral disk. *Clin Orthop* 1969;67:9-15.

28. Adams P, Eyre DR, Muir H: Biochemical aspects of development and ageing of human lumbar intervertebral discs. *Rheumatol Rehabil* 1977;16:22-29.

29. Brown MD: The pathophysiology of disc disease. Symposium on disease of the intervertebral disc. *Orthop Clin North Am* 1971;2(2):359-370.

30. Lipson SJ, Muir H: Experimental intervertebral disc degeneration: morphological and proteoglycan changes over time. *Arthritis Rheum* 1981;24(1):12-21.

31. Lipson SJ, Muir H: Proteoglycans in experimental intervertebral disc degeneration. *Spine* 1984;6(3):194-210.

32. Naylor A: Intervertebral disc prolapse and degeneration: the biochemical and biophysical approach. *Spine* 1976;1(1):108-114.

33. Bisla RS, Marchisello PJ, Lockshin MD, et al: Autoimmunological basis of disk degeneration. *Clin Orthop Rel Res* 1976(Nov/Dec);121:205-211.

34. Bobechko WP, Hirsch C: Auto-immune response to nucleus pulposus in the rabbit. *J Bone Joint Surg [Br]* 1965;47(3):574-580.

35. Battie MC, Videman T, Gill K, et al: Smoking and lumbar intervertebral disc degeneration: an MRI study of identical twins. 1991 Volvo Award in Clinical Sciences. *Spine* 1991;16(9):1015-1021.

36. Moskowitz RW, Adler JH: Spondylosis in sand rats: a model of intervertebral disk degeneration. [Abstract.] *Arthritis Rheum* 1986;29:S17.

37. Yu S, Haughton VM, Sether LA, et al: Criteria for classifying normal and degenerated lumbar intervertebral disks. *Radiology* 1989;170:523-526.

38. Yu S, Haughton VM, Ho PSP, et al: Progressive and regressive changes in the nucleus pulposus. II. The adult. *Radiology* 1988;169:93-97.

39. Hirsch C, Schajowikz F: Studies on structural changes in the lumbar annulus fibrosus. *Acta Orthop Scand* 1952;22:185-231.

40. Brown T, Hansen RJ, Yorra AJ: Some mechanical tests on the lumbosacral spine with particular reference to the intervertebral discs: a preliminary report. *J Bone Joint Surg [Am]* 1957;39:1135-1164.

41. Evans FG, Lissner HR: Strength of intervertebral discs. [Abstract.] *J Bone Joint Surg [Am]* 1954;36:185.

42. Nachemson A: The load on lumbar disks in different positions of the body. *Clin Orthop* 1966;45:107-122.

43. Roaf R: A study of the mechanics of spinal injuries. *J Bone Joint Surg [Br]* 1960;42:810-823.

44. Eyre D: Intervertebral disk. B. Basic science perspectives. In Frymoyer JW, Gordon SL (eds): *New perspectives on low back pain*. Chicago, American Academy of Orthopaedic Surgeons, 1989, pp 187-188.

45. Donohue PJ, Jahnke MR, Blaha JD, et al: Characterization of link protein(s) from human intervertebral-disc tissues. *Biochem J* 1988;251:739-747.

46. Axel LL: Surface coil magnetic resonance imaging. *J Comput Assist Tomogr* 1984;8:381-384.

47. Enzmann DR, Rubin JB, Wright A: Use of cerebral spinal fluid gating to improve T2 weighted images. I. The spinal cord. *Radiology* 1987;162:763-767.

48. Haacke EM, Lenz G: Improving MR image quality in the presence of motion by using rephasing gradients. *AJR* 1987;148:1251-1258.

49. Hueftle M, Modic MT, Ross JS, et al: Lumbar spine: postoperative MR imaging with Gd-DTPA. *Radiology* 1988;167:817-824.

50. Edelman RR, Atkinson DJ, Silver MS, et al: FRODO pulse sequences: a new means of eliminating motion, flow and wrap around artifacts. *Radiology* 1986;166:231-236.

51. Chafetz NI, Genant HK, Moon KL, et al: Recognition of lumbar disk herniation with NMR. *AJR* 1983;141:1153-1156.

52. Edelman RR, Shoukimas GM, Stark ED, et al: High resolution surface coil imaging in lumbar disk disease. *AJR* 1985;144:1123-1229.

53. Maravilla KR, Lash HP, Weinreb JC, et al: Magnetic resonance imaging of the lumbar spine with CT correlation. *AJNR* 1985;6:237-245.

54. Modic MT, Masaryk TJ, Boumphrey F, et al: Lumbar herniated disc disease and canal stenosis: Prospective evaluation by surface coil MR, CT and myelography. *AJNR* 1986;7:709-717.

55. Modic MT, Masaryk TJ, Mulopulos GP, et al: Cervical radiculopathy: prospective evaluations with surface coil MR imaging, CT with metrizamide and metrizamide myelography. *Radiology* 1986;161:753-759.

56. Modic MT, Masaryk TJ, Ross JS, et al: Cervical radiculopathy: value of oblique MR imaging. *Radiology* 1987;163:227-231.

57. Ross JS, Perez-Reyes N, Masaryk TJ, et al: Thoracic disk herniation: MR imaging. *Radiology* 1987;165:511-515.

58. Modic MT, Pavlicek W, Weinstein MA, et al: Magnetic resonance imaging of intervertebral disk disease: clinical and pulse sequence considerations. *Radiology* 1984;152:103-111.

59. deRoos A, Kressel H, Spritzer C, et al: MR imaging of marrow changes adjacent to end plates in degenerative lumbar disk disease. *AJR* 1987;149:531-534.

60. Modic MT, Steinberg PM, Ross JS, et al: Degenerative disk disease: assessment of changes in vertebral body marrow with MR imaging. *Radiology* 1988;166:193-199.

61. Aoki J, Yamamoto I, Kitamura N, et al: End plate of the discovertebral joint: degenerative change in the elderly adult. *Radiology* 1987;164:411-414.

62. Masaryk TJ, Boumphrey F, Modic MT, et al: Effects of chemonucleolysis demonstrated by MR imaging. *J Comput Assist Tomogr* 1986;10:917-923.

63. Modic MT, Feiglin DH, Piraino DW, et al: Vertebral osteomyelitis: assessment using MR. *Radiology* 1985;157:157-166.

64. Kenney JB, Hughes PL, Whitehouse GH: Discovertebral destruction in ankylosing spondylitis: the role of computed tomography and magnetic resonance imaging. *Br J Radiol* 1990;63:448-455.

65. Rafto SE, Dalinka MK, Schiebler ML, et al: Spondyloarthropathy of the cervical spine in long-term hemodialysis. *Radiology* 1988;166:201-204.

66. Yu S, Ho PS, Sether LM, et al: Nucleus pulposus degeneration: MR imaging. Presented at the RSNA, 1987.

67. Sether LA, Yu S, Haughton VM, Fischer ME: Intervertebral disk: normal age-related changes in MR signal intensity. *Radiology* 1990;177:385-388.

68. Friberg R, Hirsch C: Anatomical and clinical studies on lumbar disc degeneration. *Acta Orthop Scand* 1949;19:222-242.

69. Hirsch C: Studies on the pathology of low back pain. *J Bone Joint Surg [Br]* 1959;41:237-243.

69a. Coventry MB: Anatomy of the intervertebral disk. *Clin Orthop* 1969;67:9-15.

70. Grenier N, Grossman RI, Schiebler ML, et al: Degenerative lumbar disk disease: pitfalls and usefulness of MR imaging in detection of vacuum phenomenon. *Radiology* 1987;164:861-865.

71. Berns DH, Ross JS, Kormos D, Modic MT: The spinal vacuum phenomenon: Evaluation by gradient echo MR imaging. *J Comput Assist Tomogr* 1991;15(2):233-236.

72. Bielecki DK, Sartoris D, Resnick D, et al: Intraosseous and intradiscal gas in association with spinal infection: report of three cases. *AJR* 1986;147:83-86.

73. Kumpan W, Salomonowitz E, Seidl G, Wittich GR: The intravertebral vacuum phenomenon. *Skeletal Radiol* 1986;15:444-447.

74. Resnick D, Niwayama G, Guerra J, et al: Spinal vacuum phenomena: anatomical study and review. *Radiology* 1981;139:341-348.

75. Naul LG, Peet GJ, Maupin WB: Avascular necrosis of the vertebral body: MR imaging. *Radiology* 1989;172:219-222.

76. Maldague BE, Noel HM, Malghem JJ: The intravertebral vacuum cleft: a sign of ischemic vertebral collapse. *Radiology* 1978;129:23-29.

77. Gagnerie F, Taillan B, Euller-Ziegler L, Ziegler G: Intravertebral vacuum phenomenon in multiple myeloma. *Clin Rheumatol* 1987;6(4):597-599.

78. Castillo M, Malko JA, Hoffman JC: The bright intervertebral disk: an indirect sign of abnormal spinal bone marrow on T1-weighted MR images. *AJNR* 1990;11:23-26.

79. Ho PS, Yu S, Sether L, Wagner M, et al: Calcification of the nucleus pulposus with pathologic confirmation in a premature infant: abbreviated report. *AJNR* 1989;10:201-202.

80. Lester JW, Miller WA, Carter MP, Hemphill JM: MR of childhood calcified herniated cervical disk with spontaneous resorption. *AJNR (Suppl)* 1989;10:S48-S50.

81. Brown TR, Quinn SF, D'Agostino AN: Deposition of calcium pyrophosphate dihydrate crystals in the ligamentum flavum: evaluation with MR imaging with CT. *Radiology* 1991;178:871-873.

82. Otake S, Matsuo M, Nishizawa S, et al: Ossification of the posterior longitudinal ligament: MR evaluation. *AJNR* 1992;13:1059-1067.

83. Gomori JM, Grossman RI, Goldbert HI, et al: Intracranial hematomas: imaging by high-field MR. *Radiology* 1985;157:87-93.

84. Gomori JM, Grossman RI, Hackney DB, et al: Variable appearances of subacute intracranial hematomas on high-field spin-echo MR. *AJNR* 1987;8:1019-1026.

85. Nabatame H, Fujimoto N, Nakamura K, et al: High intensity areas on noncontrast T1-weighted MR images in cerebral infarction. *J Comput Assist Tomogr* 1990;14(4):521-526.

86. Mirowitz SA, Sartor K, Gado M: High-intensity basal ganglia lesions on T1-weighted MR images in neurofibromatosis. *AJNR* 1989;10:1159-1163.

87. Mirowitz SA, Westrich TJ, Hirsch JD: Hyperintense basal ganglia on T1 weighted MR images in patients receiving parenteral nutrition. *Radiology* 1991;181:117-120.

88. Mirowitz SA, Westrich TJ: Basal ganglial signal intensity alterations: reversal after discontinuation of parenteral manganese administration. *Radiology* 1992;185:535-536.

89. Maeder PP, Holtas SL, Basibuyuk LN, et al: Colloid cyst of the third ventricle: correlation of MR and CT findings with histology and chemical analysis. *AJNR* 1990;11:575-581.

90. Som PM, Dillon WP, Fullerton GD, et al: Chronically obstructed sinonasal secretion: observations on T1 and T2 shortening. *Radiology* 1989;172:515-520.

91. Abe K, Hasegawa H, Kobayashi Y, et al: A gemistocytic astrocytoma demonstrated high intensity on MR images: protein hydration layer. *Neuroradiology* 1990;32:166-167.

92. Boyko OB, Burger PC, Shelburne JD, Ingram P: Non-heme mechanisms for T1 shortening: pathologic, CT, and MR elucidation. *AJNR* 1992;13:1439-1445.

93. Henkelman RM, Watts JF, Kucharczyk W: High signal intensity in MR images of calcified brain tissue. *Radiology* 1991;179:199-206.

94. Dell LA, Brown MS, Orrison WW, et al: Physiologic intracranial calcification with hyperintensity on MR imaging: case report and experimental model. *AJNR* 1988;9:1145-1148.

95. Tien RD, Hesselink JR, Duberg A: Rare subependymal giant-cell astrocytoma in a neonate with tuberous sclerosis. *AJNR* 1990;11:1251-1252.

96. Araki Y, Furukawa T, Tsuda K, et al: High field MR imaging of the brain in pseudohypoparathyroidism. *Neuroradiology* 1990;32:325-327.

97. Bangert BA, Modic MT, Ross JS, et al: Hyperintense signal of the intervertebral discs on T1WSE imaging. RSNA, 1992.

98. Jackson RP, Cain JE, Jacobs RR, et al: The neuroradiographic diagnosis of lumbar herniated nucleus pulposus. II. A comparison of computed tomography (CT), myelography, CT-myelography, and magnetic resonance imaging. *Spine* 1989;14(12):1362-1367.

99. Ross JS, Modic MT, Masaryk TJ, et al: Assessment of extradural degenerative disease with Gd-DTPA-enhanced MR imaging: correlation with surgical and pathologic findings. *AJNR* 1989;10:1243-1249.

100. Boden SD, Davis DO, Dina TS, et al: Abnormal magnetic resonance scans of the lumbarspine in asymptomatic subjects. *J Bone Joint Surg [Am]* 1990;72:403–408.

101. Jensen MC, Brant-Zawadzki MN, Obuchowski N, et al: Lumbar back studies in asymptomatic subjects. ASNR, 1993.

102. Fardon D, Pinkerton S, Balderston R, et al: Terms used for diagnosis by English speaking spine surgeons. *Spine* 1993;18:274-277.

103. Masaryk TJ, Ross JS, Modic MT, et al: High-resolution MR imaging of sequestered lumbar intervertebral disks. *AJNR* 1988;150:1155-1162.

104. Yu S, Haughton VM, Sether LA, Wagner M: Anulus fibrosus in bulging intervertebral disks. *Radiology* 1988;169:761-763.

105. Yu S, Sether LA, Ho PSP, et al: Tears of the anulus fibrosus: correlation between MR and pathologic findings in cadavers. *AJNR* 1988;9:367-370.

106. Schellinger D, Manz HJ, Vidic B, et al: Disk fragment migration. *Radiology* 1990;175:831-836.

107. Holtas S, Nordstrom CH, Larsson EM, Pettersson H: MR imaging of intradural disk herniation: case report. *J Comput Assist Tomogr* 1987;11(2):353-356.

108. Castillo M: Neural foramen remodeling caused by a sequestered disk fragment: case report. *AJNR* 1991;12:566.

109. Glickstein MF, Burke L, Kressel HY: Magnetic resonance demonstration of hyperintense herniated discs and extruded disk fragments. *Skeletal Radiol* 1989;18:527-530.

110. Pech P, Haughton VM: Lumbar intervertebral disk: correlative MR and anatomic study. *Radiology* 1985;156:699-701.

111. Jinkins JR. MR of enhancing nerve roots in the unoperated lumbosacral spine. *AJNR* 1993;14:193-202.

112. Kobayashi S, Yoshizawa H, Hachiya Y: Blood nerve barrier and spinal nerve root. 18th annual meeting of the International Society for the Study of the Lumbar Spine, 1991.

113. Jackson RP, Cain JE, Jacobs RR, et al: The neuroradiographic diagnosis of lumbar herniated nucleus pulposus. II. A comparison of computed tomography (CT), myelography, CT-myelography, and magnetic resonance imaging. *Spine* 1989;14(12):1362-1367.

114. Thornbury JR, Fryback DG, Turski PA, et al: Disk-caused nerve compression in patients with acute low back pain: diagnosis by MR, CT myelography, and plain CT. *Radiology* 1993;186:731-738.

115. Bozzao A, Gallucci M, Masiocchi C, et al: Lumbar disk herniation: MR imaging assessment of natural history in patients treated without surgery. *Radiology* 1992;185:135-141.

116. Saal JA, Saal JS, Herzog RJ: The natural history of lumbar intervertebral disc extrusions treated nonoperatively. *Spine* 1990;15(7):683-686.

117. Bush K, Cowan N, Katz DE, Gishen P: The natural history of sciatica associated with disc pathology. *Spine* 1992;17(10):1205-1212.

118. Maigne JY, Rime B, Delignet B: Computed tomographic follow-up study of forty-eight cases of nonoperatively treated lumbar intervertebral disc herniation. *Spine* 1992;17(9):1071-1074.

119. Fagerlund MKJ, Thelander U, Friberg S: Size of lumbar disc hernias measured using computed tomography and related to sciatic symptoms. *Acta Radiol* 1990;31:555-558.

120. Modic MT, Ross JS, Obuchowski N, et al: Contrast enhanced MR in acute lumbar radiculopathy. ASNR, 1993.

121. Ross JS, Delamarter R, Masaryk TJ, et al: Gadolinium-DTPA enhanced postoperative lumbar spine MRI: biodistribution and mechanism. RSNA, 1987.

122. Lindblom K, Hultqvist G: Absorption of protruded disk tissue. *J Bone Joint Surg [Am]* 1950;22(3):557-560.

123. Liu SS, Williams KD, Drayer BP, et al: Synovial cysts of the lumbosacral spine: diagnosis by MR imaging. *AJNR* 1989;10:1239-1242.

124. Nijensohn E, Russel EJ, Milan M, Brown T: Calcified synovial cyst of the cervical spine: CT and MR evaluation. *J Comput Assist Tomogr* 1990;14(3):473-476, 1990.

125. Awwad EE, Martin DS, Smith KR, Bucholz RD: MR imaging of lumbar juxtaarticular cysts. *J Comput Assist Tomogr* 1990;14(3):415-417.

126. Silbergleit R, Gebarski SS, Brunberg JA, et al: Lumbar synovial cysts: correlation of myelographic CT, MR and pathologic findings. *AJNR* 1990;11:777-779.

127. Williams MP, Cherryman GR, Husband JE: Significance of thoracic disc herniation demonstrated by MR imaging. *J Comput Assist Tomogr* 1989;13(2):211-214.

128. Blumenkopf B: Thoracic intervertebral disc herniations: diagnostic value of magnetic resonance imaging. *Neurosurgery* 23:36-40, 1988.

129. Parizel PM, Rodesch G, Baleriaux D, et al: Gd-DTPA-enhanced MR in thoracic disc herniations. *Neuroradiology* 1989;31(1):75-79.

130. Horst M, Brinckmann P: Measurement of the distribution of axial stress on the end-plate of the vertebral body. *Spine* 1981;6:217-232.

131. Enzmann DR, Griffin L, Rubin J: Potential false-negative MR images of the thoracic spine in disk disease with switching of phase and frequency-encoding gradients. *Radiology* 1987;165:635-637.

132. Boden SD, McCowin PR, Davis DO, et al: Abnormal magnetic resonance scans of the cervical spine in asymptomatic subjects: a prospective investigation. *J Bone Joint Surg [Am]* 1990;72:8;1178-1184.

133. Brown BM, Schwartz RH, Frank E, et al: Preoperative evaluation of cervical radiculopathy and myelopathy by surface-coil MR imaging. *AJNR* 1988;9:859-866.

134. Russell EJ, D'Angelo CM, Zimmerman RD, et al: Cervical disk herniation: CT demonstration after contrast enhancement. *Radiology* 1984;152:703-712.

135. Hedberg MC, Drayer BP, Flom RA, et al: Gradient echo (GRASS) MR imaging and cervical radiculopathy. *AJNR* 1988;9:145-151.

136. Enzmann DR, Rubin JB: Cervical spine: MR imaging with a partial flip angle, gradient refocussed pulse sequence. I. General considerations and disk disease. *Radiology* 1988;166:467-472.

137. Yousem DM, Atlas SW, Goldberg HI, Grossman RI: Degenerative narrowing of the cervical spine neural foramina: evaluation with high-resolution 3DFT gradient-echo MR imaging. *AJNR* 1991;12:229-236.

138. Enzmann DR, Rubin JB: Cervical spine: MR imaging with a partial flip angle, gradient refocussed pulse sequence. II. Spinal cord disease. *Radiology* 1988;166:473-478.

139. Schellinger D, Wener L, Ragsdale BD: Facet joint disorders and their role in the production of back pain and sciatica. *RadioGraphics* 1987;7(5):923-944.

140. Dorwart RH, Vogler JB III, Helms CA: Spinal stenosis: Symposium on CT of the lumbar spine. *Radiol Clin North Am* 1983;21(2):301-323.

141. Yamamoto I, Matsumae M, Ikeda A, et al: Thoracic spinal stenosis: experience with 7 cases. *J Neurosurg* 1988;68(1):37-40.

142. Hanakita J, Suwa H, Ohta F, et al: Neuroradiological examination of thoracic radiculomyelopathy due to ossification of the ligamentum flavum. *Neuroradiology* 1990;32:38-42.

143. Doppman JL: Epidural lipomatosis. Letters to the Editor. *Radiology* 1989;171:581-582.

144. Quint DJ, Boulos RS, Sanders WP, et al: Epidural lipomatosis. *Radiology* 1988;169:485-490.

145. Jungreis CA, Cohen WA: Spinal cord compression induced by steroid therapy: CT findings. *J Comput Assist Tomogr* 1987;11(2):245-247.

146. Yamashita Y, Takahashi M, Matsuno Y, et al: Spinal cord compression due to ossification of ligaments: MR imaging. *Radiology* 1990;175:843-848.

147. Harsh GR III, Sypert GW, Weinstein PR, et al: Cervical spine stenosis secondary to ossification of the posterior longitudinal ligament. *J Neurosurg* 1987;67:349-357.

148. Freeman TB, Martinez CR: Radiological evaluation of cervical spondylotic disease: limitations of magnetic resonance imaging for diagnosis and preoperative assessment. *Perspect Neurol Surg* 1992;3(1):34-54.

149. Pavlov H, Torg JS, Robie B, Jahre C: Cervical spine stenosis: determination with vertebral body ratio method. *Radiology* 1987;164:771-775.

150. Doppman JL: The mechanism of ischemia in anteroposterior compression of the spinal cord. *Invest Radiol* 1990;25:543-550.

151. Fukushima T, Ikata T, Taoka Y, Takata S: Magnetic resonance imaging study on spinal cord plasticity in patients with cervical compression myelopathy. *Spine (Suppl)* 1991;16(10):S534-S538.

152. Takahashi M, Yamashita Y, Sakamoto Y, Kojima R: Chronic cervical cord compression: Clinical significance of increased signal intensity on MR images. *Radiology* 1989;173:219-224.

153. Takahashi M, Sakamoto Y, Miyawaki M, Bussaka H: Increased MR signal intensity secondary to chronic cervical cord compression. *Neuroradiology* 1987;29:550-556.

154. Haupts M, Hahn J: Further aspects of MR signal enhancements in stenosis of the cervical spinal canal: MRI investigations in correlation to clinical and cerebrospinal fluid (CSF) findings. *Neuroradiology* 1988;30:545-546.

155. Statham PF, Hadley DM, MacPherson P, et al: MRI in the management of suspected cervical spondylotic myelopathy. *J Neurol Neurosurg Psychiatry* 1991;54(6):484-489.

156. Brown BM, Schwartz RH, Frank E, Blank NK: Preoperative evaluation of cervical radiculopathy and myelopathy by surface coil MR imaging. *AJR* 1988;15:1205-1212.

157. Grenier N, Kressel HY, Schiebler ML, et al: Normal and degenerative posterior spinal structures: MR imaging. *Radiology* 1987;165:517-525.

158. Harris RI, McNab I: Structural changes in the lumbar intervertebral disks: their relationship to low back pain and sciatica. *J Bone Joint Surg (Br)* 1954;36:304-322.

4

Postoperative Spine

JEFFREY S. ROSS

LUMBAR SPINE

A difficult diagnostic problem from the clinical and radiographic viewpoints is the evaluation of patients with symptoms following spinal surgery. This failed back surgery syndrome is a spectrum of diseases characterized by pain and functional incapacitation. From 10% to 40% of patients may fall into this category following spinal surgery. The causative factors accounting for the failed back surgery syndrome include recurrent disk herniation (12% to 16%), lateral (58%) or central (7% to 14%) spinal stenosis, arachnoiditis (6% to 16%), and epidural fibrosis (6% to 8%).[1] Less frequent causes are meningocele formation, mechanical instability (including facet subluxations and pseudoarthroses), nerve injury, and wrong-level surgery. In evaluating the postoperative patient, plain radiographs are generally unrewarding since they reveal only the usual postoperative bone changes such as laminectomy site, fusion masses, and degenerative disk-space narrowing. Myelography may show arachnoiditis or a focal extradural defect at the surgical site. However, the myelographic distinction between scar and herniated disk is considered by many to be impossible.[2-4] High-resolution computed tomographic (CT) scanning of the lumbar spine was a major advance in understanding the causes of failed back surgery syndrome, and the CT findings in postoperative spines have been described.[5] Magnetic resonance (MR) has become a mainstay in the evaluation of postoperative spines, with excellent results in the diagnosis of a wide variety of disease entities reported.[6]

Pulse Sequences

T_1-weighted spin-echo sagittal and axial images are the mainstay of postoperative spine imaging. The use of surface coils is mandatory for achieving optimum signal-to-noise. T_2-weighted images are not an absolute necessity but will occasionally better define the extradural tissues, extradural interface, and nerve roots than is possible with only a T_1-weighted sequence. Gradient echo images with variable flip angles (usually 40 to 60 degrees for the lumbar spine) may also contribute to better definition of the extradural interface. Gradient echo or T_2-weighted spin-echo images are also necessary if there is any clinical concern regarding postoperative hematoma, which will be more apparent because of the T_2 dephasing that the paramagnetic hemoglobin breakdown products induce. Four-millimeter slice thickness is adequate for lumbar spine imaging, usually with a 40% to 50% interslice gap. In the cervical spine 3 to 4 mm slice thicknesses are the maximum that should be used, because of the smaller anatomy that needs to be imaged (particularly the foramina). If contrast is employed to diagnose epidural scar from residual or recurrent disk herniation, then the sequences are simply a sagittal and an axial T_1-weighted spin echo before and after contrast administration. We prefer not to separate the image slices into groups related to each disk level, but rather to lengthen the TR slightly to accommodate contiguous slices throughout the area of interest. Fat-suppressed T_1-weighted images may also be useful, and have the potential to eliminate precontrast images, since enhancement and fat are readily separated on these sequences. The disadvantage of fat-suppressed sequences is their decreased signal-to-noise.

Unenhanced Magnetic Resonance Imaging

Before images of abnormalities in postoperative patients can be interpreted, knowledge of the normal postoperative sequence of events that is demonstrable by MR is a necessity. The following findings are based on 15 patients who underwent MR imaging before, 1 to 10 days after, and 2 to 6 months after a variety of lumbar spinal surgeries. The majority of surgeries were laminectomy and diskectomies (Fig. 4-1): Laminectomy sites

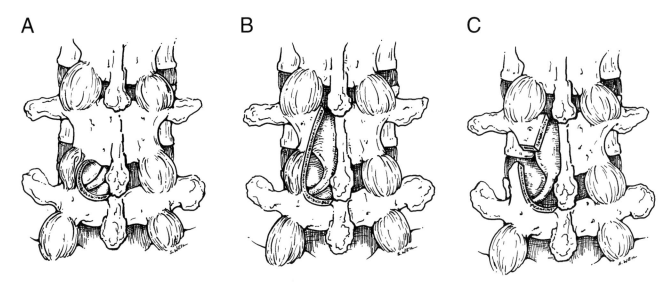

Fig. 4-1. A, Laminotomy. Only a small amount of bone is removed from the inferior and superior laminae above and below the herniated nucleus pulposus *(HNP)* level. **B,** Laminectomy. The length of the lamina is removed to improve exposure of the HNP. **C,** Laminectomy and facetectomy. The exposure is widened by removal of a variable amount of facet, not only to better visualize the HNP but also to relieve stenosis of the lateral recess or foramen.

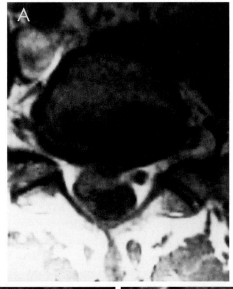

Fig. 4-2. Normal sequence of events following laminectomy and diskectomy. **A,** Preoperative axial T$_1$-weighted MR. Note the large central disk herniation at L5-S1 compressing the thecal sac. **B,** An immediately postoperative axial T$_1$-weighted shows disruption of the epidural soft tissues and an indistinct thecal sac margin. **C,** Late postoperative (6 months) axial T$_1$-weighted MR. The thecal sac margin is restored and now surrounded by epidural fibrosis.

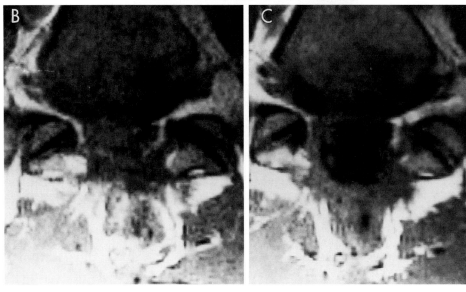

were quite apparent because of the bone removal involved (Figs. 4-2, *B*, and 4-3, *B*). The regions of missing lamina were identified on T_1-weighted axial and sagittal images as a loss of the normal low-signal cortical bone and high-signal marrow. In the immediate postoperative period this was replaced by a variable amount of postoperative soft tissue edema, exhibiting slightly heterogeneous intermediate signal on T_1-weighted images and hyperintense signal on T_2-weighted images (Figs. 4-2 and 4-3).

This soft tissue signal obliterates the normal muscle-fat planes of the paraspinal musculature along the operative tract. Mass effect is not usually present on the dural tube from such posterior edema. Midline sagittal images also well define the portions of the spinous processes remaining because of their high-signal fatty marrow. The minimal soft tissue disruption caused by microsurgical techniques may be difficult or impossible to

localize. With a laminotomy, only the absence of the ligamentum flavum will denote the site of previous surgical intervention. Studies obtained 2 to 6 months postoperatively show persistence of these posterior soft tissue changes (i.e., scar), which have become more homogeneous in appearance. The disruption of the normal muscle-fat planes continues. Following laminectomy, the thecal sac will maintain a smooth rounded contour, although it may be slightly posteriorly displaced or may protrude into the soft tissues. Expansion of the thecal sac to normal contour will occur quite rapidly in the immediate postoperative period, even if there has been severe canal stenosis preoperatively (Fig. 4-4).

Diskectomy produces unique changes on MR. Sagittal and axial T_1-weighted images immediately following diskectomy will show intermediate soft tissue signal anterior to the thecal sac at the original site of disk herniation and operation, which will blend smoothly with the

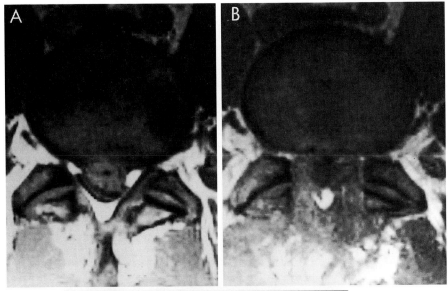

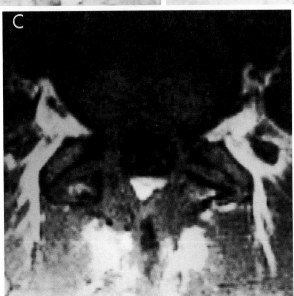

Fig. 4-3. Normal sequence of events following laminectomy and diskectomy. **A,** An axial T_1-weighted image shows the enormous central disk herniation. **B,** An immediately postoperative T_1-weighted axial shows disruption of the epidural tissues and an indistinct thecal sac. The herniation appears to have been removed. **C,** Late postoperative axial T_1-weighted. Note the normal thecal sac contour but extensive epidural fibrosis.

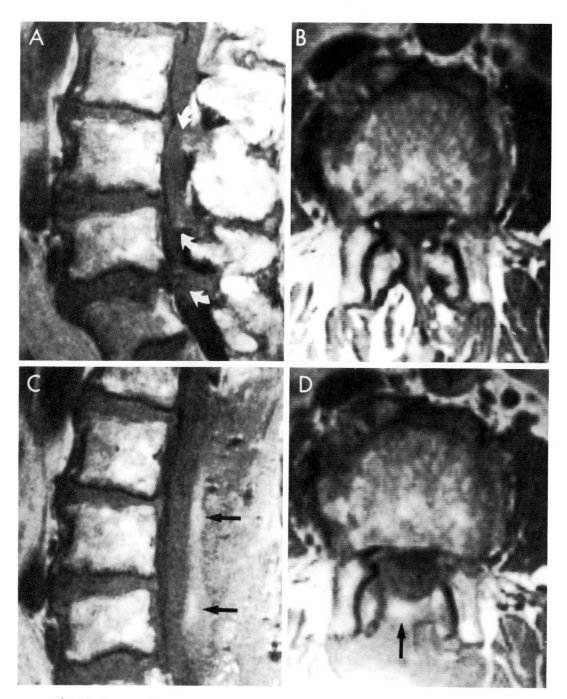

Fig. 4-4. Preoperative sagittal, **A,** and axial, **B,** T$_1$-weighted images demonstrate severe canal stenosis at several levels. The hypertrophied ligaments are seen as indistinct masses encroaching on the thecal sac in the sagittal view *(arrows).* Increased signal is present from CSF in the lumbar spine because of dampened CSF pulsation secondary to the stenosis. Postoperative sagittal, **C** and **D,** T$_1$-weighted images show a more normal contour to the thecal sac following an extensive laminectomy. High signal intensity posterior to the sac *(arrows)* is presumed to be blood (methemoglobin). (From Ross JS, Masaryk TJ, Modic MT, et al: *Radiology* 1987;164:851-860.)

posterior portion of the disk, especially at the site of diskectomy on T_1-weighted images, and show increased signal on T_2-weighted images. This soft tissue can be as large as the original disk herniation and may produce mass effect on the anterior dural tube (Fig. 4-2, *B*). Of the 13 patients we studied who underwent diskectomy, mass effect mimicking preoperative findings was present in 9. The amount of this anterior extradural soft tissue usually decreased by 2 to 6 months postoperatively. Spe-

cifically, these anterior extradural changes were seen to improve in appearance by the late postoperative study in 8 of 9 cases in which an initial mass effect was present (Figs. 4-2 and 4-3, *C*). Anular disruption can also be identified in patients who are post–percutaneous diskectomy (Fig. 4-5).

Sagittal T_2-weighted images are excellent for showing the distribution of the normally low signal of outer fibers of the posterior anulus fibrosus–posterior longitu-

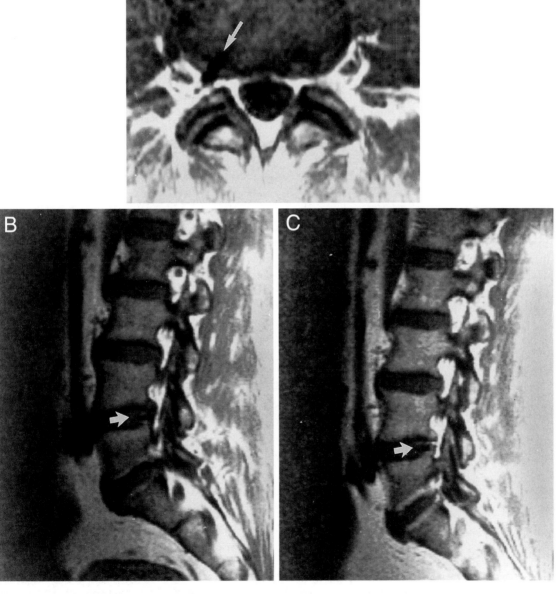

Fig. 4-5. Percutaneous diskectomy. Unenhanced axial, **A,** and sagittal, **B,** images following percutaneous diskectomy demonstrate the well-defined low-signal tract in the posterolateral aspect of the disk *(arrow)* from the nucleotome. A small amount of enhancement can be seen at the tract site in **C.**

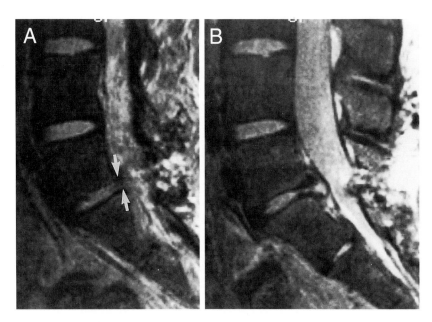

Fig. 4-6. A, An immediately postoperative T$_2$-weighted image following laminectomy and diskectomy shows the site of disruption of the posterior anulus fibrosus–posterior longitudinal ligament due to disk curettage *(arrows)*. **B,** Another image, lateral to **A,** shows the apparently continued disk herniation. These generally decrease in size with time. (From Ross JS, Masaryk TJ, Modic MT, et al: *Radiology* 1987;164:851-860.)

dinal ligament at the site of diskectomy. The high signal of the nucleus pulposus also may be seen on T$_2$-weighted images extending posteriorly to where the anulus has been disrupted by surgery (Fig. 4-6). This area will merge with the high cerebrospinal fluid (CSF) signal in the region. Axial T$_2$-weighted images can show similar findings, with a tract of increased signal extending laterally from the diskectomy site into the central portion of the nucleus pulposus where curettage has been done. This disruption of the posterior aspect of the anulus fibrosus ("anular rent") is generally not visible on T$_1$-weighted images, although it was seen on T$_2$-weighted images in 11 of 13 cases in the immediate postoperative period. It is important to realize that the anulus lateral to the site of diskectomy can retain its preoperative appearance (whether normal in configuration, bulging, or even protruded) if imaged soon enough after surgery.

Late follow-up studies 2 to 6 months postoperatively will show that the rent in the anulus at the diskectomy site is less, or no longer, apparent. In the 10 patients in whom a comparison could be made on last postoperative studies, the anular rent resolved in 8 out of 10. With "healing," the original high signal on T$_2$-weighted images from the rent is replaced by linear vertically decreasing signal on T$_2$-weighted sagittal images, similar to the appearance of the preoperative anulus fibrosus. Whereas the configuration of the anulus away from this site of diskectomy may remain unchanged, more com-

monly the disk bulge or protrusion will become less apparent with a concomitant decrease in disk-space height as further degeneration occurs. This lack of change in the appearance of the disk herniation, combined with the epidural surgical disruption, makes an unenhanced MR examination within the first 8 weeks following surgery nearly useless in defining residual disk material.

Changes in the adjacent lumbar vertebral bodies are uncommon with simple diskectomy. Only 1 of our 15 patients showed a rectangular area of hypodensity in the posterior-superior endplate of the L5 vertebral body following L5-S1 diskectomy (Fig. 4-7). This was presumably due to curettage of the endplate during diskectomy. In an additional three patients, type I vertebral body marrow changes occurred adjacent to the site of diskectomy on the late postoperative study.[7]

In the immediate postoperative period, soft tissue changes following foraminotomy are confined to the level where foraminal exploration and operation have been performed. These are seen on T$_1$-weighted images as an increased amount of soft tissue signal surrounding the nerve roots that obliterates the usual foraminal fat. This soft tissue commonly will show increased signal on T$_2$-weighted images.

Increased soft tissue signal lateral to the dural tube can be seen immediately after a variety of surgeries and is not limited to foraminotomy or fasciotomy. Lateral epidural soft tissue signal changes are present in virtu-

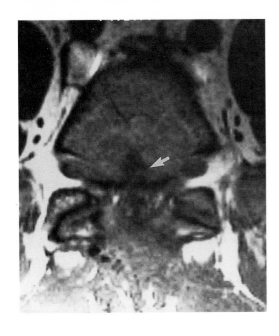

Fig. 4-7. Area of decreased signal within the superior S1 endplate *(arrow)* due to inadvertent curettage during surgery. (From Ross JS, Masaryk TJ, Modic MT, et al: *Radiology* 1987;164:851-860.)

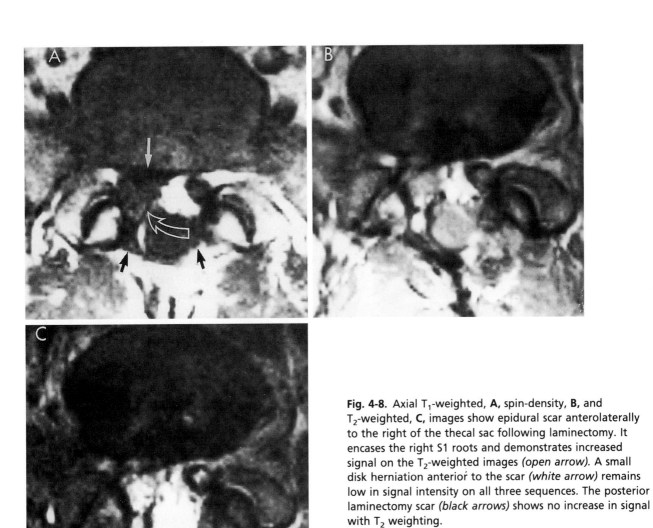

Fig. 4-8. Axial T$_1$-weighted, **A,** spin-density, **B,** and T$_2$-weighted, **C,** images show epidural scar anterolaterally to the right of the thecal sac following laminectomy. It encases the right S1 roots and demonstrates increased signal on the T$_2$-weighted images *(open arrow)*. A small disk herniation anterior to the scar *(white arrow)* remains low in signal intensity on all three sequences. The posterior laminectomy scar *(black arrows)* shows no increase in signal with T$_2$ weighting.

ally all patients following laminectomy and diskectomy, usually merging with the soft tissue edema anterior and posterior to the thecal sac in a circumferential pattern. Increased signal on T_2-weighted images is also seen with lateral epidural edema. Initially, mass effect can displace the dural tube away from the operative site, but 2 to 3 months postoperatively the changes become smaller and more homogeneous, with a loss of the initial mass effect. However, these areas of epidural fibrosis continue to show increased signal on T_2-weighted images (Fig. 4-8).

In the immediate postoperative period, posterior and posterolateral fusions appear as large areas of soft tissue signal intensity on T_1-weighted images containing scattered pieces of graft bone in the region of the transverse processes and facet joints. The involved regions show a loss of the normal fat signal and muscle-fat planes. The appearance of the bone grafts is quite variable and depends on their type. Allografts tend to show decreased signal on T_1- and T_2-weighted images. Autografts tend to show higher signal on T_1-weighted image due to the presence of marrow. However, decreased signal on T_1-weighted images and increased signal on T_2-weighted images may also be seen with autografts. The thecal sac contour is not disrupted by the posterior soft tissue signal. This soft tissue signal will merge imperceptibly with that of the posterior and lateral epidural scar from the operation.

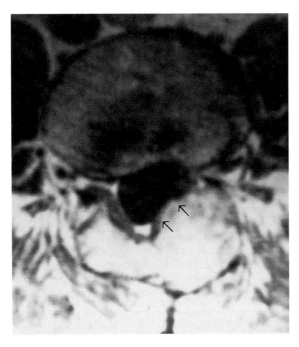

Fig. 4-9. Bony stenosis. A posterior fusion mass compresses the left posterolateral aspect of the thecal sac *(arrows).* (From Ross JS, Modic MT, Masaryk TJ, Hueftle MG: *Semin Roentgenol* 1988;13:125-136.)

Solid bony fusion masses are outlined by the low signal intensity of cortical bone on T_1- and T_2-weighted images. They show increased signal on T_1-weighted images because of the marrow content (Fig. 4-9). Fibrous portions of the fusions generally show decreased signal on T_1- and T_2-weighted images, but low signal-intensity areas may be either fibrous or bony if fatty marrow is not present. The continuity of fusion masses is generally quite difficult to determine by MR, due to the variable signal of graft marrow. CT or tomography is generally more helpful in defining areas of nonunion or pseudarthrosis.

Acute and subacute soft tissue hemorrhage has a fairly characteristic MR appearance, showing increased signal on T_1-weighted images (Fig. 4-4). In several patients we have observed moderately well-defined homogeneous areas of increased signal on T_1- and T_2-weighted images around the dural tube. Although pathologic confirmation was not available in these asymptomatic patients, we felt the areas to be compatible with postoperative hematomas.[8-10] Small postoperative hematomas may also demonstrate decreased signal intensity on T_2-weighted sequences. A significant mass effect on the thecal sac was not observed in our cases. One patient who was imaged 2 months postoperatively showed complete resolution of these areas of increased signal on T_1- and T_2-weighted images, the areas having been replaced by homogeneous scar formation. Patients imaged within 24 hours following surgery also may show a different hematoma appearance, isointense on T_1-weighted images with strikingly decreased signal on T_2-weighted images because of deoxyhemoglobin (Fig. 4-10).

We have been unable to predict the clinical course of patients by the appearance of their initial postoperative MR studies. Patients who were pain free may show significant anterior and lateral epidural scar tissue on late postoperative studies. Because of the tremendous changes in epidural soft tissues and intervertebral disks following surgery, caution must be used in MR interpretation during the first 6 weeks following surgery. There may be a large amount of tissue disruption and edema, producing mass effect on the anterior thecal sac. MR may be used during the immediate postoperative period for a more gross view of the thecal sac and epidural space—to exclude significant postoperative hemorrhage at the laminectomy site, pseudomeningocele, or disk space infection. Small fluid collections are not uncommonly seen in the posterior tissues following laminectomy. The signal intensities can vary somewhat depending on whether the collections are serous (following CSF signal intensity) or serosanguineous (increased on T_1-weighted images because of hemoglobin breakdown products). The distinction between small benign postoperative fluid collections and infected collections cannot be made by MR morphology or signal intensity.

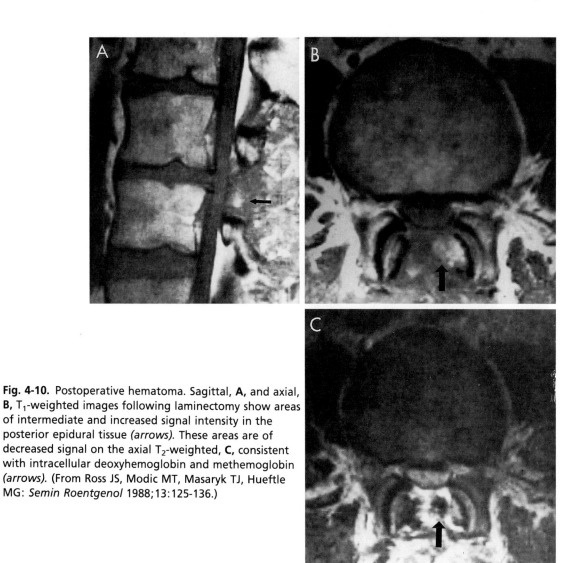

Fig. 4-10. Postoperative hematoma. Sagittal, **A,** and axial, **B,** T_1-weighted images following laminectomy show areas of intermediate and increased signal intensity in the posterior epidural tissue *(arrows)*. These areas are of decreased signal on the axial T_2-weighted, **C,** consistent with intracellular deoxyhemoglobin and methemoglobin *(arrows)*. (From Ross JS, Modic MT, Masaryk TJ, Hueftle MG: *Semin Roentgenol* 1988;13:125-136.)

Scar versus disk

The distinction between epidural fibrosis and recurrent disk herniation is of considerable importance since removal of extradural scar often leads to further scar formation whereas removal of disk herniation is generally beneficial. Intravenous contrast–enhanced CT is felt by some investigators[11,12] to be a reliable means of separating scar from disk but has not gained widespread usage in the routine workup of postoperative patients. A prospective study on 27 patients to evaluate MR and secondarily intravenous contrast–enhanced CT in the differentiation of epidural scar from herniated disk material[13] showed that MR correctly foretold surgical findings in 83%. Epidural fibrosis exhibited increased signal intensity relative to protruded disks on T_2-weighted sequences. Free fragments demonstrated slightly increased signal relative to epidural fibrosis on T_1-weighted images but a hyperintense signal intensity on T_2-weighted images similar to scar.

The intensity characteristics of epidural scar differed according to their location.[13] Anterior epidural scars ranged between hypointense and isointense relative to the adjacent disk material on T_1-weighted images but were hyperintense on both spin-density and T_2-weighted sequences (Fig. 4-8). Lateral scars, in general, exhibited similar characteristics but not so consistently. As one moved posteriorly toward the site of laminectomy, the signal intensity of the scar became more variable although increased intensity was generally seen in the paraspinal musculature at the operative site on T_2-weighted sequences. This study showed that, when the criteria of morphology, epidural location, and mass effect are used, scar and disk may be differentiated on unenhanced MRI with an accuracy comparable to that of intravenous contrast–enhanced CT. Except for free fragments, herniated disks will show continuity with the intervertebral disk space and mass effect. Scarring will generally show increased signal on T_2-weighted images

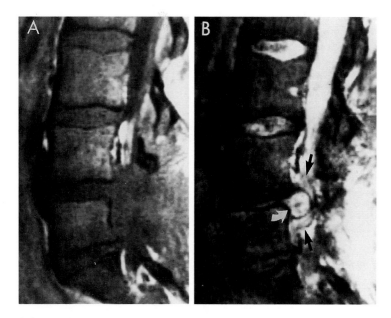

Fig. 4-11. Postoperative recurrent disk herniation. **A,** Sagittal T_1-weighted image. Note the large area of intermediate signal at the L4-5 level extending inferiorly over the L5 body *(arrows).* **B,** Sagittal T_2-weighted image. A large high-signal mass, representing recurrent disk material *(curved arrow),* extends into the canal from the L4-5 interspace. Epidural scar surrounds the disk herniation and is also of increased intensity *(black arrows).* No abnormal increased signal is seen in the central portion of the L4-5 disk or of the adjacent vertebral endplates to suggest disk space infection despite the rather ominous-appearing T_1-weighted images.

without mass effect. Large protruded or extruded disks may show decreased signal along their periphery on T_2-weighted images while the central portion shows increased signal (similar to nucleus pulposus) (Fig. 4-11).

The signal intensity of a severe extrusion or free fragment can be increased relative to that of the apparent disk or adjacent vertebral bodies on T_2-weighted sequences. Similar signal intensity changes are observed with epidural scar. In this small study,[13] half the surgically proved free disk fragments showed hyperintensity relative to epidural fibrosis on T_1-weighted sequences. No surgically demonstrated free fragments appeared hypointense relative to the desiccated postoperative disk or adjacent bone. However, scar was slightly hypointense or isointense on T_1-weighted images where it could be easily separated from fat. Both epidural scar and fat conform to the available space whereas herniated disk compresses and distorts it. Mass effect may be the only finding that aids in discriminating free fragments from anterior or lateral recess scar.

Sotiropoulos et al.[14] compared enhanced CT to nonenhanced MR in 25 patients and found that MR had a 79% accuracy and CT a 71% accuracy relative to surgery. Hochhauser et al.[15] suggested that configuration and margination were also important determinants for scar versus disk. In their study, preoperative MR find-

ings agreed with surgery in 13 of 17 patients—recurrent herniations having a smooth polypoid configuration, and scar an irregular unsharp margination. They also noted a hypointense rim outlining the high–signal intensity herniations, which would agree with our findings on T_2-weighted images, that helped to separate the herniated material from the adjacent CSF. This hypointense rim may represent the combination of posterior longitudinal ligament and outer anular fibers surrounding the herniated disk material. However, unenhanced MR suffers from the necessity of using T_2-weighted images (with their inherent poor signal-to-noise and long acquisition times). Additionally, the signal intensity changes associated with epidural scar as distinct from disk may be subtle on T_2-weighted images. In contradistinction, scar enhancement with Gd-DTPA is intense and generally unmistakable.

Besides differentiating scar from disk, which is usually the primary concern in these postoperative patients, MR is also capable of defining a wide variety of additional postoperative findings.

Fluid collections

A pseudomeningocele results from a dural tear during surgery.[17] The fluid collection may be formed as arachnoid herniates through the tear and proliferates into

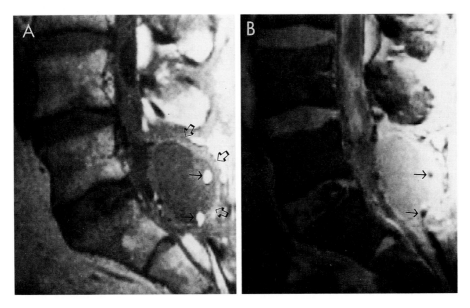

Fig. 4-12. Pseudomeningocele. Sagittal T$_1$-weighted image, **A,** showing a posterior CSF collection *(open arrows)* with well-defined capsule. Small droplets of iophendylate (Pantopaque) lie in the dependent portion of the pseudomeningocele. Note the clumped nerve roots at the L4 level, indicating arachnoiditis. **B,** Gradient echo FISP image (angle, 60 degrees). Findings are similar to those in **A** except that the Pantopaque is now low in signal.

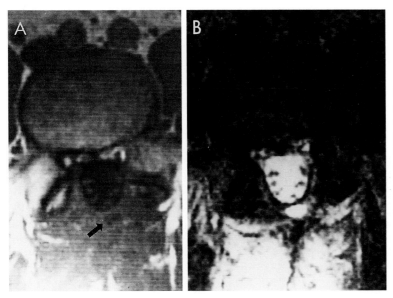

Fig. 4-13. The small round area of decreased signal *(arrow)* on this axial T$_1$-weighted, **A,** and the increased signal on a T$_2$-weighted, **B,** in the posterior epidural tissue are consistent with small serous fluid collections. Note the abnormal high signal intensity from the paraspinal muscles along the operative tract. (From Ross JS, Masaryk JJ, Modic MT, et al: *Radiology* 1987;164:851-860.)

an arachnoid pouch, or the CSF may extravasate into soft tissues that develop a fibrous capsule. Magnetic resonance will show a rounded area of CSF intensity immediately posterior to the thecal sac at the site of previous laminectomy (Fig. 4-12). If the fluid contains blood products, then the T$_1$-weighted images may show slightly increased signal. This was present in one patient who had a large fluid collection of the right and posterior to the thecal sac following resection of an extradu-

ral component of a dumbbell-shaped neurofibroma. This collection demonstrated increased signal on the T$_1$- and T$_2$-weighted images. At reoperation the presence of a pseudomeningocele containing xanthochromic fluid was verified.

Not uncommonly, well-defined areas of decreased signal on T$_1$-weighted and of increased signal on T$_2$-weighted images will be seen in the midline posteriorly along the incision site (Fig. 4-13). Out of five patients we have examined with these small collections, no clinical symptoms were referable to the areas. The collections are presumed to be small postoperative serous fluid accumulations. A similar-appearing fluid collection that may also lie posteriorly along the incision site is a wound abscess. This, likewise, shows low signal on T_1-weighted and increased signal on T_2-weighted images. The MR changes are nonspecific for these fluid collections, and MR is unable to differentiate by signal characteristics or morphology a benign postoperative fluid collection, pseudomeningocele, or wound abscess. A pseudomeningocele should not be mistaken for the normal posteriorly placed thecal sac that occurs with simple laminectomy.

Stenosis

In a recent series of 73 postoperative patients,[1] recurrent disk herniation was present in only 67% of cases. On the other hand, lateral bony stenosis was implicated as a cause of failed back surgery syndrome in up to 60% of the cases. An additional cause of stenosis is the upward migration of a superior facet (with concomitant narrowing of the foramen) secondary to disk degeneration and loss of height after diskectomy. Bony stenosis may have a wide variety of appearances on MR. This is due to the variability of the marrow content of the vertebral body and bony fusion masses as well as to various degrees of bony sclerosis. Osteophytes of compact or sclerotic bone will have low signal intensity on T_1- and T_2-weighted images (Fig. 4-14). These may be apparent only by the displacement of the epidural fat or mass effect on the thecal sac and nerve roots. At the other extreme, spurs containing fatty marrow are easily recognized by their high signal intensity on T_1-weighted images (Fig. 4-9). We have seen postoperative bony stenosis in 10 of 62 patients in our series. In 5 of these, the narrowing was generalized secondary to disk degeneration. In our series with MR, as well as in the series of Teplick and Haskins[5] using CT, epidural fibrosis has been a much more common finding than severe bony stenosis.

One method used in an attempt to decrease epidural fibrosis is the placement of free fat or pedicle fat grafts over the laminectomy site.[18] Posterior fat grafts are easily recognized as globular collections of increased signal on T_1-weighted images posterior to the dural tube (Fig. 4-15). The fat grafts may be associated with minimal epidural scarring or be included in extensive scarring that appears to stop just where the graft is present. A small amount of posterior epidural scar is often interposed between the dural tube and the graft.

Arachnoiditis is covered more fully in Chapter 6. Magnetic resonance is capable of demonstrating central adhesions of nerve roots as increased soft tissue signal within the central portion of the thecal sac on T_1- and T_2-weighted images. Peripheral adhesions of roots to the meninges may also occur, giving rise to an apparently "empty thecal sac," seen as homogeneous CSF signal within the dural tube on both T_1- and T_2-weighted images (Fig. 4-16). With more severe arachnoiditis, in-

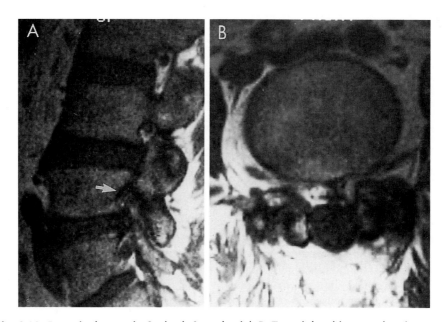

Fig. 4-14. Foraminal stenosis. Sagittal, **A,** and axial, **B,** T_1-weighted images showing severe bilateral foraminal stenosis in a patient who is status postlaminectomy. The superior articular facets compress the exiting nerve roots *(arrow).* (From Ross JS, Modic MT, Masaryk TJ, Hueftle MG: *Semin Roentgenol* 1988;13:125-136.)

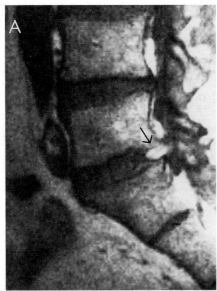

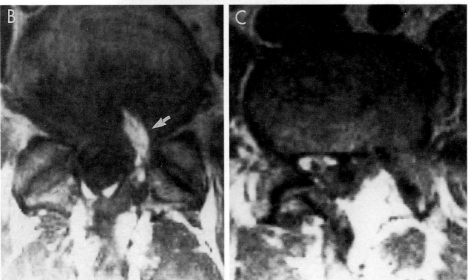

Fig. 4-15. Fat grafts. Sagittal, **A,** and axial, **B,** T$_1$-weighted images show a fat graft extending from the left epidural space into the disk at the site of previous curettage *(arrow).* **C,** A more typical-appearing fat graft fills in the left hemilaminectomy site, precluding significant epidural fibrosis.

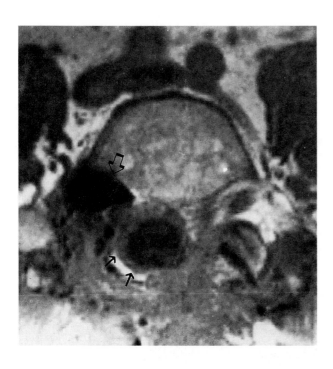

Fig. 4-16. Metal artifact. The oval area of decreased signal overlying the right foramen *(large arrow)* is secondary to minute metal fragments sheared off instruments during surgery. A CT scan showed no metallic density. Additionally, the nerve roots adhere to the meninges, giving an "empty thecal sac" appearance of arachnoiditis. The small posterior protrusion of the thecal sac *(arrows)* is normal following laminectomy.

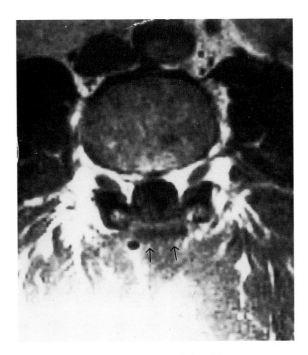

Fig. 4-17. Gelfoam. An axial T_1-weighted image demonstrates a linear band of decreased signal posterior to the thecal sac immediately following laminectomy *(arrows)*. This most likely represents Gelfoam placed at surgery. The small dot of decreased signal posterolateral to the Gelfoam is a gas bubble.

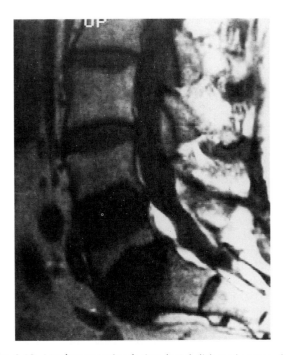

Fig. 4-18. Lumbar anterior fusion (total disk replacement). Disk replacements performed at L4-5 and L5-S1 are seen as well-defined areas of decreased signal on this sagittal T_1-weighted image.

creased soft tissue signal may be seen in the thecal sac obliterating the normal CSF signal. This finding correlates with marked irregularity of the thecal sac or a myelographic block.[19]

Field distortion from changes in magnetic susceptibility is frequently observed in postoperative spine patients because of minute metallic particles from surgical instruments. During surgery, small metallic fragments that are not visible on plain x-ray or CT can be sheared off the instruments either by contact with other metal instruments or when dense sclerotic bone is drilled (Fig. 4-16). In the lumbar spine these artifacts are commonly seen in the regions of the foramina and lateral recesses. They consist of field distortion, a loss of signal, or a halo of increased signal. Occasionally they are great enough to impede diagnosis.[20]

Gelfoam (an absorbable gelatin sponge used primarily for hemostasis during surgery) can act as a matrix for thrombus formation.[21] It appears to have a characteristic appearance by MR (i.e., decreased signal on T_1- and T_2-weighted images). In two patients we have seen linear well-defined areas of decreased signal on both T_1- and T_2-weighted images posterior to the dural tube where Gelfoam had been placed at surgery (Fig. 4-17). Follow-up study 60 days later in one patient showed apparent reabsorption of the Gelfoam, with loss of the areas of decreased signal intensity.

Methyl methacrylate is commonly used in orthopedic procedures to distribute the mechanical forces imposed by metal hardware on endosteal or cancellous bony surfaces. It shows decreased signal on T_1- and T_2-weighted images.[20] Occasionally the appearance of the methacrylate will be rather unusual, depending on its area of placement. One patient from whom fusion hardware that had been placed through the pedicles and into the vertebral bodies was removed showed linear areas of low signal intensity representing residual methyl methacrylate within the pedicles. These appeared as "ghost shadows" of the spiral configuration of the screws. Areas of previous pedicle fixation (which may also be seen as ghost shadows of high signal intensity on T_1-weighted images) are presumably related to fatty marrow.

Lumbar interbody fusions often utilize bank bone grafts. These demonstrate a uniformly decreased signal intensity on T_1- and T_2-weighted images within the graft. The margins of the graft are well defined and linear. Axial images show the graft as a square-shaped area of low signal intensity on T_1-weighted images at the level of the intervertebral disk (Fig. 4-18). We have not observed adjacent vertebral body marrow signal changes with these grafts.

Fibular grafts may be utilized for posterior interbody fusions of the lumbar spine in severe spondylolisthesis. The fibular grafts demonstrate a rim of decreased signal on T_1- and T_2-weighted images, representing cortical

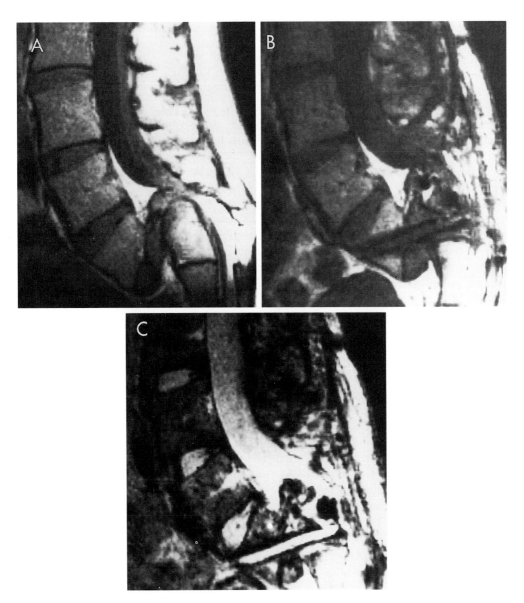

Fig. 4-19. Interbody fusion. The preoperative sagittal T_1-weighted image, **A,** demonstrates a grade IV spondylolisthesis of L5 on S1. Postoperative sagittal T_1-weighted, **B,** and T_2-weighted, **C,** images show a fibular strut through L5 and S1 to stabilize the spine. The strut is outlined by low-signal cortical bone. The marrow signal is increased on the T_2-weighted image, which could reflect edema due to the operative procedure. (From Ross JS, Masaryk TJ, Modic MT, et al: *Radiology* 1987;164:851-860.)

bone, with the marrow spaces showing more variable appearance (Fig. 4-19). Commonly the graft marrow space will show decreased signal on T_1-weighted and increased signal on T_2-weighted images compared to the normal fibular marrow. This change in the central marrow signal, which can be seen in the immediate postoperative period, may persist over at least a 6-month period. Other grafts will show only the high signal on T_1-weighted images from normal-appearing marrow. Whether these signal changes on MR relate to graft revascularization is presently unknown.

Gd-DTPA–Enhanced Magnetic Resonance Imaging

Gadolinium diethylenetriamine pentaacetic acid (Gd-DTPA), the paramagnetic contrast agent used in MR imaging, has been shown to enhance the MR intensity of various tissues following its intravenous administration in humans and animal models.[22-26] It has a biodistribution compatible with the extracellular fluid compartment and is rapidly excreted by the kidneys. With a high degree of paramagnetism, it exhibits strong complex formation and appears to be well tolerated.[27-28] It is useful as a contrast agent for evaluating inflammatory or tumorous lesions, as well as for denoting any disruption within the blood-brain barrier. It has a short half-life in blood (approximately 20 minutes) and a relatively high LD_{50} in rats (18 mmole/kg).[24]

The normal spectrum of enhanced MR findings following diskectomy, foraminotomy, and laminectomy has been described by Boden et al.[29] They evaluated 15 patients who had relief of symptoms following surgery and found enhancement of the nerve roots in 62% at 3 weeks following surgery, which was gone by 6 months postsurgery. Areas of peripheral enhancement with mass effect at the site of the original disk herniation were common. This study parallels the MR findings in the early postoperative patient studied without contrast—that is, a residual mass effect can simulate residual disease or disk fragment despite complete relief of leg pain.

As previously indicated in this chapter, the differentiation of epidural fibrosis from recurrent or persistent disk herniation is of prime importance in imaging patients with the failed back surgery syndrome. A large amount of time and effort has been expended in trying to identify an imaging modality and/or diagnostic criteria that would allow this distinction. Myelography has not proved useful.[3,4] In the series of Firooznia et al.,[30] unenhanced CT scanning was diagnostic in 60% of cases. The accuracy of intravenously enhanced computed tomography (IVCT) has been variously reported in the literature[31-35] as ranging between 67% and 100%.

Unenhanced MR was recently addressed by Bundschuh et al.,[13] who found a similar accuracy to that of IVCT. More recently, Gd-DTPA–enhanced MR has been used to evaluate scar and disk herniations. Based on our experience,[16] we feel that Gd-DTPA–enhanced MR is very accurate at differentiating scar from residural or recurrent disk herniation.

The use of Gd-DTPA–enhanced MR in the evaluation of scar versus disk has been examined by Hueftle et al.[16] Thirty patients were evaluated with MR before and after administration of 0.1 mmol/kg Gd-DTPA, with reoperation correlation in 17 patients. Enhanced MR correctly predicted the surgical findings in all 17 patients. These findings could be divided into three categories: (1) scar only, (2) disk only, and (3) scar plus disk.

Scar tissue was consistently seen to enhance immediately following injection. This occurred regardless of the time since surgery (Figs. 4-20 and 4-21). Epidural scar was also seen to enhance in patients whose surgery had been over 20 years earlier. Scar tissue showed mass effect only occasionally, and this criterion thus should not be used as the major discriminator of disk versus scar. Because of its avascularity disk material did not enhance on the early postinjection images (Figs. 4-22 to 4-28). However, if delayed images were obtained (greater than 20 to 30 minutes following injection), disk material did

enhance because contrast diffused into it from the adjacent vascularized scar tissue. In cases with a mixture of scar and disk material, scar was seen to enhance and the disk material not to enhance on early postinjection images. Nevertheless, disk material consistently enhanced if enough time was given for diffusion of contrast into it from the surrounding vascular scar. Similar findings have been noted using iodinated contrast material with CT.[36]

A couple of points need to be stressed about the technique: It is important to obtain both sagittal and axial T_1-weighted images before and after contrast. Ideally, to assure precise comparison between the same regions of interest, the patient should not be moved between the pre- and postcontrast scans. It is also important to complete the postinjection images within the first 20 minutes following contrast administration. We routinely place a heparin lock in patients with a history of previous lumbar spine surgery before any imaging. Once the precontrast images have been obtained, the patient is removed from the bore of the magnet, injected, and returned to the same position. This technique minimizes patient motion associated with the contrast administration.

Although time constraints are always a consideration, nevertheless, it is important to obtain as much diagnostic information in this population as possible. Toward that end, we continue to obtain both sagittal and axial T_1-weighted images before and after contrast administration. We do not get T_2-weighted spin-echo images in the postoperative population unless there is a question of disk space infection or epidural abscess. Preliminary data in a postoperative dog model[37] suggest that 0.3 mmol/kg of contrast improves the visualization of scar tissue.

More recently,[38] we have increased the patient numbers in our series by adding 27 patients who underwent reoperation following contrast-enhanced MR. These data, when combined with those of Hueftle et al.,[16] give pre- and postcontrast MR a 96% accuracy in differentiating scar from disk in 44 patients and at 50 reoperated levels. The missed MR diagnoses occurred in one patient in whom scar and disk were called on MR but scar and osteophyte were present at surgery and in another in whom scar only was called on MR but scar and disk were present at surgery.

Problems can occur in two situations: when the volume of nonenhancing herniated disk is small relative to the volume of enhancing scar tissue, partial volume averaging may obscure the disk (Fig 4-27); additionally, when scar tissue invades the herniated disk material as part of the body's reparative process, the disk material may show enhancement. Overall, in patients 6 weeks or more postsurgery, sagittal and axial T_1-weighted MR before and after Gd-DTPA remains the single most effective method of evaluating the postoperative lumbar spine.

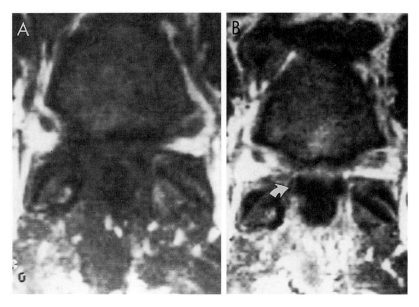

Fig. 4-20. Gd-DTPA enhancement of epidural fibrosis. A precontrast axial T_1-weighted image, **A,** shows circumferential soft tissue signal about the thecal sac. The differentiation of a recurrent disk from scar is not possible. Following Gd-DTPA (0.1 mmole/kg) the epidural scar is enhanced, **B,** allowing definition of the thecal sac and nerve roots *(arrow)*. No disk herniation is seen. (From Ross JS, Modic MT, Masaryk TJ, Hueftle MG: *Semin Roentgenol* 1988;13:125-136.)

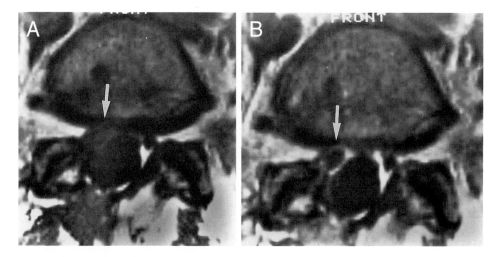

Fig. 4-21. Gd-DTPA enhancement of epidural fibrosis. **A,** A precontrast axial T_1-weighted image shows increased tissue surrounding the right lateral aspect of the thecal sac, and around the right L5 nerve root, with an indistinct thecal sac margin *(arrow)*. **B,** Postcontrast image. The thecal sac margin and right L5 root sleeve can be seen, with no evidence of recurrent herniation. Root sleeves surrounded by scar may show increased size compared to the contralateral normal side *(arrow)*, as in this case.

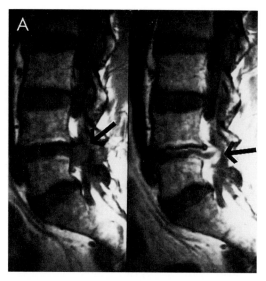

Fig. 4-22. Scar and disk herniation. **A,** Precontrast T$_1$-weighted sagittal MR. The image on the left shows a large mass of aberrant soft tissue anterior to the thecal sac at the L4-5 level *(arrow)* in this patient with a previous L4-5 diskectomy. The postcontrast sagittal image *(right)* shows marked enhancement of the peridiskal fibrosis *(arrow)* with nonenhancing disk present centrally. **B,** The precontrast axial image *(top)* shows aberrant tissue anterior and to the left of the dural tube. The immediate postcontrast axial image *(middle)* shows enhancement of peripheral scar *(arrow)* but no enhancement of the disk herniation. The late postcontrast axial image *(bottom)* (more than 30 minutes after injection) shows enhancement of the herniation and scar *(arrow).* (From Hueftle MG, Modic MT, Ross JS, et al: *Radiology* 1988;1167:817-824.)

Fig. 4-23. Scar and recurrent disk herniation. **A,** Axial precontrast image showing aberrant soft tissue anterior and to the left of the dural tube. **B,** Axial postcontrast image showing enhancement of the median scar *(white arrow),* with good definition of the lateral disk herniation *(black arrow).* (From Hueftle MG, Modic MT, Ross JS, et al: *Radiology* 1988;167:817-824.)

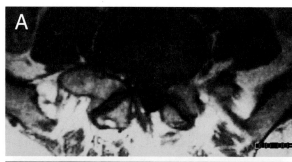

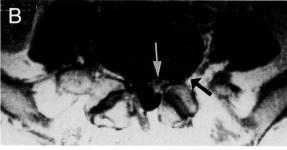

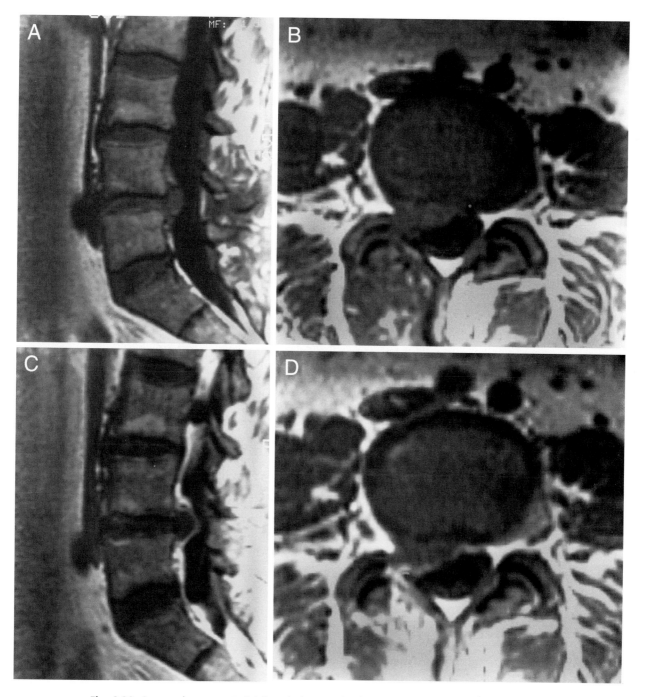

Fig. 4-24. Scar and recurrent disk herniation. Sagittal, **A,** and axial, **B,** T_1-weighted images before contrast show a fairly well-defined anterior epidural mass posterior to the L4-5 disk space, extending toward the right neural foramina. T_1-weighted sagittal, **C,** and axial, **D,** images following contrast show a thin rind of enhancing scar tissue outlining the large nonenhancing recurrent herniation.

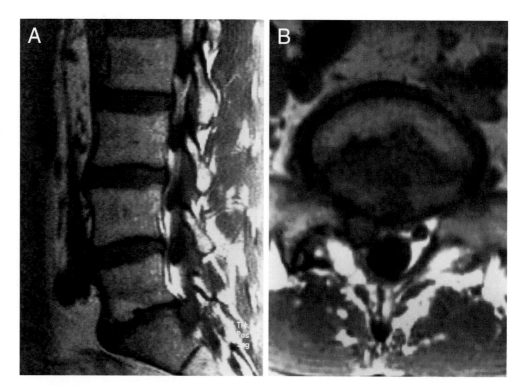

Fig. 4-25. Scar and recurrent disk herniation. Sagittal, **A,** and axial, **B,** T_1-weighted images before contrast show a fairly well-defined anterior epidural mass posterior to the L5-S1 disk space, extending toward the right neural foramina and obliterating the right S1 root. T_1-weighted, **C,** fat-suppressed, **D,** and axial T_1-weighted, **E,** images following contrast show a thin rim of enhancing scar tissue outlining the large nonenhancing recurrent herniation.

There are not enough data in the literature to allow one to comment on the use of contrast in the more immediate postoperative period, other than to say that enhancement within the epidural space can be seen quite early following surgery (i.e., within 2 or 3 days). The problem in this immediate postoperative group is not enhancement but differentiating pathology from the usual changes that occur surrounding the thecal sac after even successful surgery.

The important criteria for evaluation of scar versus disk in the postoperative patient can be summarized as follows:

1. Scar tissue enhances immediately after injection, irrespective of the time since surgery.
2. Disk material does not enhance immediately following injection.
3. A smoothly marginated, polypoid anterior epidural mass is disk.
4. Scar can have mass effect and be contiguous with the disk space.

In our experience anterior epidural scar consistently enhances regardless of the time since surgery. In general, three things are necessary for contrast enhancement

of any tissue: a vascular supply, a route for contrast material to exit the vasculature, and some amount of interstitial space to sequester the contrast. Epidural scar has all these attributes.[39] Light microscopy and electron microscopy have shown a considerable vascular supply within scar tissue. The potential pathways out of the vasculature and into the large interstitial space of scar consist of two major routes: one through the junctional complexes between adjacent scar capillary endothelial cells (which have various degrees of "leakiness" and in scar appear wide enough to allow the egress of low–molecular weight contrast material) and one through areas of endothelial discontinuity (where contrast can go directly from the lumen to the capillary basement membrane).

There are a couple of possibilities as to why enhancement occurs in scar even years following surgery. It may not mean that scar tissue that enhances in a patient 30 years postdiskectomy is, in fact, 30 years old. We have frequently observed a mixture of fibrous tissue ages in these patients, ranging from highly vascularized granulation tissue to cicatrized poorly vascularized "mature" scar. It could be that the ongoing degenerative disease

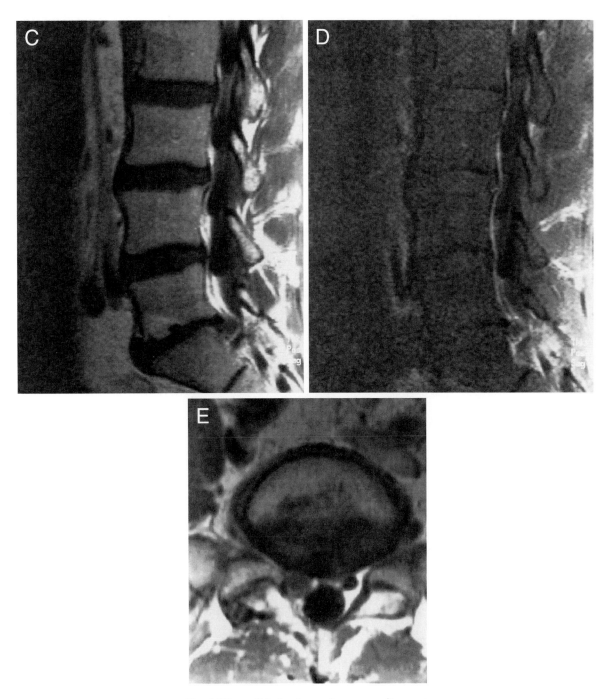

Fig. 4-25, cont'd. For legend see opposite page.

process that caused these individuals to again seek treatment and subsequent imaging has instigated new scar tissue formation and this is what is seen to enhance. Scar tissue may be intimately associated with and surround disk herniations in the previously unoperated patient and will enhance in much the same manner as scar tissue does in the postoperative patient.[40] Clearly, the scar tissue present in these postoperative patients is not solely due to the operative trauma but is also in some measure generated as the body's "reparative" response to the her-

niated material, if present. One other factor to be considered regarding epidural scar enhancement is whether anterior epidural scar can be treated in an equivalent fashion (from an imaging or physiologic standpoint) to other areas of epidural scar formation, such as posterior to the thecal sac. We have shown[41] that a simple lumbar laminectomy in dogs will produce abundant posterior epidural scar tissue but this does not follow the same time course of enhancement as anterior epidural scar. Posterior epidural scar tends to show a rapid decline in

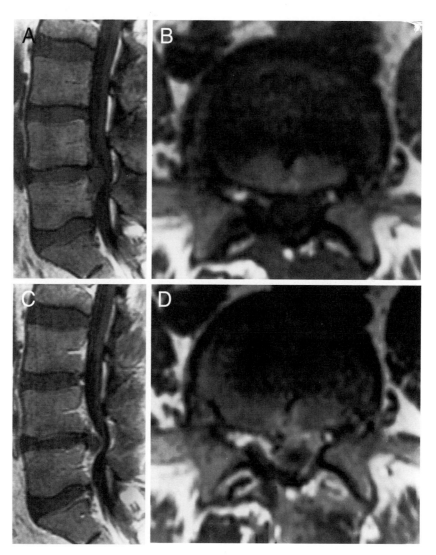

Fig. 4-26. Scar and recurrent disk herniation. Sagittal, **A,** and axial, **B,** T_1-weighted images before contrast show a large soft tissue mass in the anterior epidural space at L4-5, with mass effect on the left lateral thecal sac. Postcontrast sagittal, **C,** and axial, **D,** images show peripheral enhancement of epidural scar and a large central nonenhancing disk herniation.

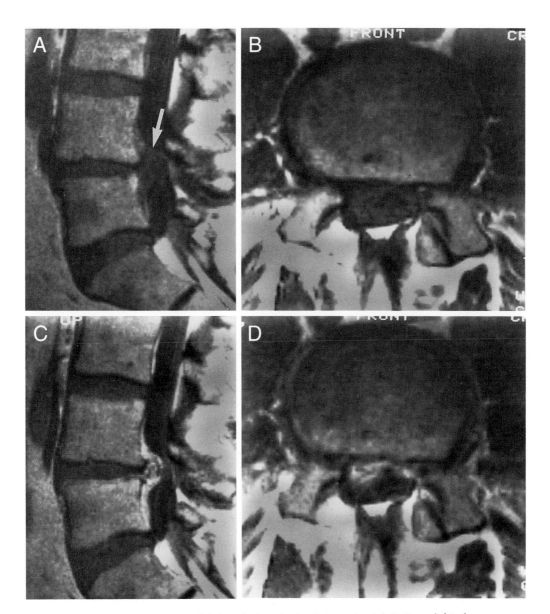

Fig. 4-27. Scar and recurrent disk herniation. Sagittal, **A,** and axial, **B,** T$_1$-weighted images before contrast show an indistinct soft tissue mass in the anterior epidural space at L4-5 *(arrow).* Differentiation of disk and scar is not possible. Postcontrast sagittal, **C,** and axial, **D,** images show a pattern of heterogeneous enhancement of epidural scar, admixed with fragments of nonenhancing disk material.

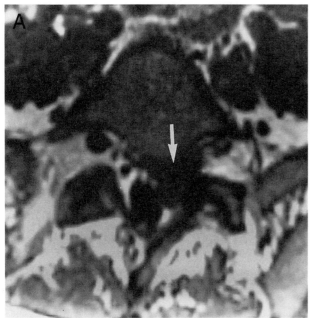

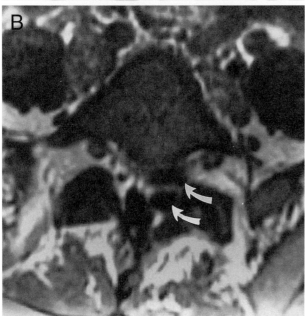

Fig. 4-28. Scar and recurrent disk herniation. The axial, **A,** T₁-weighted image before contrast shows a soft tissue mass in the anterior epidural space at L5-S1 *(arrow),* with mass effect on the anterior and left lateral thecal sac. Differentiation of disk and scar is not possible. The postcontrast sagittal axial, **B,** image shows predominately peripheral enhancement of epidural scar, with bilobular-appearing nonenhancing disk material *(arrows).*

the amount of enhancement present over a period of 4 months, unlike the consistent enhancement seen in anterior epidural scar.[16] The reason for the difference is unknown, but it could relate to the close physical relationship of anterior epidural scar to the intervertebral disk and the process of disk degeneration.

Epidural scar, and not just disk material, is capable of showing mass effect on the thecal sac. The enhancement characteristics, in our experience, are more useful diagnostically than the presence of mass effect from an ill-defined anterior epidural soft tissue lesion in distinguishing scar from disk material. Retraction of the thecal sac toward aberrant epidural soft tissue can be a helpful sign of scar when present. Obviously, no morphologic sign should be ignored; but the presence or absence of mass effect should be a secondary consideration compared to the presence or absence of enhancement.

Venous plexus and basivertebral vein

Enhancement of the venous plexus and basivertebral vein is a consistent finding following the instillation of contrast. It may help to outline nonenhancing disk herniations when there is dilation of the plexus above and below the lesion, similar to the enhancement of cervical herniations with iodinated contrast for CT.[42] The enhancement in type I vertebral endplate changes is associated with degenerative disease (decreased signal on T₁-weighted, increased signal on T₂-weighted, images)[43,44] and is due to the replacement of normal cellular marrow by vascularized fibrous marrow with acute disk degeneration. It should not be misinterpreted as metastatic disease. Type I enhancement parallels the endplates, is linear, and always accompanies evidence of disk degeneration on T₂-weighted images (e.g., loss of disk space height or a decrease in signal). Enhancement is also commonly seen within the intervertebral disk itself—spotty, linear, or diffuse—and is probably related to disk degeneration with ingrowth of granulation tissue into the disk material. Likewise, enhancement may be seen within the anulus and posterior nucleus pulposus at the site of previous diskectomy and surgical curettage (Fig. 4-29). In this case it may be triangular or rectangular and, again, is presumably scar tissue filling in the surgical site.

Disk space infection and vertebral osteomyelitis

The MR appearance of disk space infection and vertebral osteomyelitis is more fully covered in Chapter 6. Briefly, with disk space infection, T₁-weighted images show confluent decreased signal intensity from the intervertebral disk space and contiguous vertebral bodies relative to the normal vertebral body marrow signal. On T₂-weighted images there is increased signal intensity of these tissues. The intervertebral disk shows abnormal increased signal intensity in a nonanatomic morphology—that is, the intranuclear cleft, a normal anatomic finding in disks of adults over 30 years of age, is absent. The abnormal signal from the endplates may precede the signal changes from the disk itself. MR provides more anatomic detail regarding the adjacent soft tissues and neural elements than radionuclide scanning.[45]

A real advantage of MR is its ability to image directly in the sagittal plane, in contrast to CT. This point is especially important in evaluating enhancement and in preventing partial volume averaging. The continuity of abnormal soft tissue extending from the parent disk space can be evaluated exquisitely with sagittal MR in a manner unobtainable with other imaging modalities. In addition, the multislice capabilities of MR allow numerous levels to be studied at one time. Gd-DTPA–enhanced MR is the most accurate means for identifying and characterizing aberrant soft tissue in the postoperative lumbar spine. If there is a discrepancy in the diagnosis, ability to be enhanced should supersede any other diagnostic criterion. In other words, if it is enhanced on the early T_1-weighted studies, it is epidural fibrosis. Sagittal and axial scans are needed to prevent partial volume averaging and to evaluate the enhancement optimally.

Conclusion

Early postoperative changes demonstrated by MR are dramatic and affect every portion of the neural canal. In the immediate postoperative period following diskectomy, the anular rent where diskectomy and curettage have taken place is easily demonstrated. Increased soft tissue signal (edema) that obliterates the normal epidural fat signal is commonly seen anterior and lateral to the dural tube. These changes also greatly distort the dural tube contour. The intervertebral disk may continue to show a herniation in the immediate postoperative period. This lack of disk change, coupled with extensive epidural disruption, precludes the usefulness of an unenhanced MR study in the immediate postoperative period for continuing symptomatology except to exclude postoperative hemorrhage. The high signal intensity of hemorrhage on T_1- and T_2-weighted images allows tissue contrast with the intermediate intensity of epidural edema.

Immediately postoperative T_2-weighted sagittal images appear to be more helpful than T_1-weighted images in discerning the site of anulus disruption and the morphology of the remaining disk. T_1-weighted images generally show ill-defined increased soft tissue signal involving the anulus, nucleus, and anterior and lateral epidural tissues. Later in the postoperative course the anular rent will heal and become inapparent, with concomitant disk degeneration and resolution of any remaining disk protrusion away from the diskectomy site. Epidural

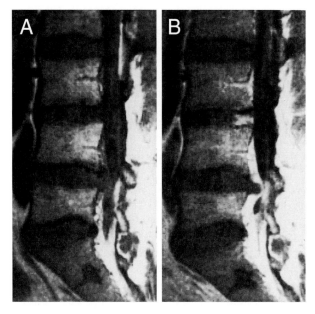

Fig. 4-29. Anular rent enhancement following laminectomy and diskectomy at L3-4. The precontrast sagittal T_1-weighted image, **A,** shows a large anterior extradural defect at L4-5. The postcontrast sagittal T_1-weighted image, **B,** shows a rectangular area of enhancement involving the L3-4 disk that abuts on the anterior thecal sac. This likely represents scar tissue within the disk at the site of previous curettage. The dura may adhere to it. The disk herniation is outlined by an enhancing epidural plexus at L4-5. (From Hueftle MG, Modic MT, Ross JS, et al: *Radiology* 1988;167:817-824.)

changes will improve in appearance and become more homogeneous as any initial mass effect is lost. Scar formation tends to be ubiquitous in lumbar surgery, except for a simple laminectomy or laminectomy and fusion. Epidural fibrosis conforms to the dural tube outline and usually does not demonstrate mass effect. Scarring anterior and lateral to the dural tube will generally show increased signal on T_2-weighted images. The changes present in the immediate postoperative period are a consequence of the surgical intervention and should not be confused with pathology. They reflect instead the dynamic course of the normal repair process.

CERVICAL SPINE

A multiplicity of surgical procedures has been developed for cervical disk disease and spondylosis. The initial surgical approach for treating spondylosis was posterior. The problem with this approach is the difficulty in removing anteriorly compressive structures.

Most surgeons today agree that the anterior approach has the best clinical response for radicular pain at one or two levels. This approach was initially developed by

Robinson and Smith,[48] Cloward,[47] and Baley and Badgley. In general, this surgical approach involves a dissecting plane lateral to the esophagus and trachea and medial to the carotid sheath. Once the correct disk space is determined, the disk material is removed. The disk space is then distracted, and disk remnants are removed back to the posterior longitudinal ligament. DePalma et al.[49] reported 63% good to excellent results, and 29% fair results, in 229 patients treated for intractable radicular pain by the anterior approach. Anterior diskectomies are performed with graft placement for fusion. Some surgeons have advocated diskectomy without fusion, although long-term follow-up is limited. Graft material may be autografts (generally iliac crest) or allografts (banked iliac crest, tibia, fibula, and femoral head). With longer segments of disease, partial corpectomies or more radical decompressions may occur, with placement of larger iliac grafts or fibular strut grafts.

Anterior cervical spine fusion may be roughly grouped into three types: Smith-Robinson, Cloward, and the strut graft. These fusions involve removing the offending intervertebral disk and a portion of the vertebral bodies, including osteophytes, and inserting a bone graft (Fig. 4-30). The bone graft functions for fusion as well as for maintaining the proper disk space height and alignment. Anterior fusion can be applied to a variety of cervical spine disorders, including disk disease with radiculopathy, spondylosis, instability, dislocations and fractures, tumors, and infections.

The Smith-Robinson technique[48] involves removing the disk material and cartilaginous endplates from an anterior approach. The bony osteophytes are generally not removed. A rectangular iliac bone graft is then cut to fit the curetted disk space. Traction is applied to widen the space, and the graft is inserted and countersunk.

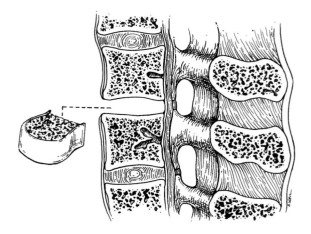

Fig. 4-30. Appearance of iliac crest bone graft and positioning for a Smith-Robinson anterior diskectomy and fusion.

The Cloward technique[47] involves drilling a round hole in the disk space and adjacent endplates with a specialized tool. Into this drilled space is inserted a prefit dowel of bone. Before graft insertion, the posterior and posterolateral osteophytes are removed. The graft material may be iliac, autograft, or allograft.

Strut grafts are larger segments of bone used to obtain stabilization following multilevel diskectomy or corpectomy. The graft material may be iliac, rib, tibial, or fibular bone. The anterior aspects of the uppermost and lowermost receptor vertebral bodies must be carefully preserved so the graft ends will lock in place and not become dislodged.

As in the anterior approach, the posterior approach may be used for unilateral radiculopathy at one or more levels. In this instance the procedure is a posterior foraminotomy. Up to 96% excellent results have been reported[50] for the posterior decompression of cervical disk disease. Cervical myelopathy with spinal cord compression at multiple levels may be treated with a posterior laminectomy. Degenerative subluxation may necessitate facet joint fusion in addition to the laminectomy. A more recent variant on laminectomy is the open-door laminoplasty, which is thought to limit the instability associated with long segment laminectomies. In this procedure a thin trough is drilled in the lamina on one side, and completely through the lamina on the other side. The spinous process and lamina are then lifted posteriorly, with the trough acting as a hinge. Often the spinous processes are sutured to the facet capsule to keep the laminoplasty "open."

Some immediate surgical complications of the anterior approach include pneumothorax, perforation of the esophagus, permanent cord damage, infection, graft extrusion, and damage to the recurrent laryngeal nerve.[51] Late complications that will be considered include bony stenosis, degenerative disease (including disk herniations above and below the fusion site), bony deformity, and intrinsic cord abnormalities.

Anterior Diskectomy and Fusion

Patients imaged within the first few days following anterior diskectomy and fusion (ADF) will demonstrate a fairly characteristic appearance[52] (Fig. 4-31). The bone grafts are visible as discrete rectangular areas of altered signal intensity within the central portion of the disk space. The signal intensities of the grafts themselves may be quite variable. Hyperintense, hypointense, and isointense signals from cervical graft material have been seen when compared with adjacent normal marrow signal (Fig. 4-32). These signal changes most likely reflect the state of the graft marrow, whether cellular or fatty. The adjacent vertebral body endplates and subchondral bone may be normal or, just as commonly, may show de-

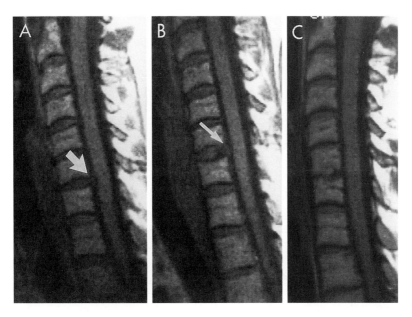

Fig. 4-31. Normal postoperative changes following anterior diskectomy and fusion. **A,** Preoperative T_1-weighted image demonstrating a large disk herniation *(arrow)* at C6-7. **B,** The immediately postoperative study shows a graft as intermediate signal within the disk space causing an apparent anterior extradural defect. **C,** A T_1-weighted image 9 months following surgery shows incorporation of the graft, which now has indistinct margins. The anterior extradural defect is no longer apparent. (From Ross JS, Masaryk TJ, Modic MT: *J Comput Assist Tomogr* 1987;11:955-962.)

creased signal on T_1-weighted images. If decreased signal on a T_1-weighted image is present within the bony endplates, these areas will show increased signal on a T_2-weighted images. Such changes are presumed to represent marrow edema from the operative trauma.

Patients imaged months to 1 or 2 years following ADF will show a wide variety of graft and adjacent vertebral body signal changes. In general, the grafts continue to be visible as horizontal linear areas of decreased signal on T_1- and T_2-weighted images. The adjacent vertebral body signal changes will vary from isointense or hypointense on T_1-weighted to isointense or hyperintense on T_2-weighted images. The etiology of these varied grafts and vertebral body signal changes in the postoperative spine is unknown. They probably represent a combination of (1) the initial status of the vertebral body and graft marrow, (2) the amount of trauma received by the endplate vertebral body and graft during the operative procedure, (3) the postoperative stress placed on the fusion mass, and (4) the amount of revascularization that is present (Fig. 4-33). In addition, a series of vertebral body signal changes occurs in the spine associated with acute and chronic disk degeneration. Acute disk degeneration as seen with chymopapain injection in the lumbar spine shows decreased signal on T_1-weighted and increased signal on T_2-weighted images from the vertebral endplates.[53] Changes within the vertebral endplates associ-

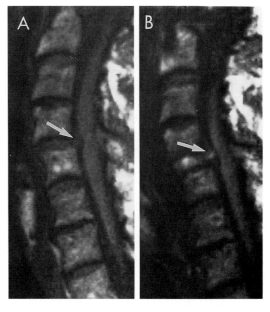

Fig. 4-32. Complication of anterior diskectomy. **A,** Preoperative T_1-weighted image showing a large disk herniation at C4-5 compressing the cord *(arrow)*. **B,** The immediately postoperative T_1-weighted image shows extension of the graft posteriorly to continue compressing the cord *(arrow)*. The high signal within the graft is presumably due to yellow marrow. (From Ross JS, Masaryk TJ, Modic MT: *J Comput Assist Tomogr* 1987;11:955-962.)

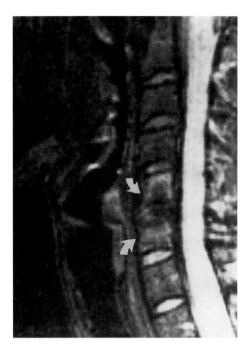

Fig. 4-33. Postoperative vertebral body changes. An immediately postoperative T$_1$-weighted image following anterior diskectomy and fusion at C5-6 shows increased signal from the adjacent vertebral body *(arrows)* thought to represent marrow edema. (From Ross JS, Masaryk TJ, Modic MT: *J Comput Assist Tomogr* 1987;11:955-962.)

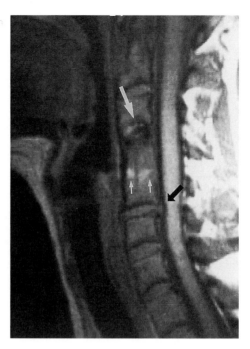

Fig. 4-34. Late appearance of cervical fusions. A sagittal T$_1$-weighted image shows the typical appearance of a solid fusion at C4-5 9 years following surgery. The linear area of high signal *(small arrows)* presumably represents focal increased yellow marrow. A mixed-intensity graft is present at C3-4 9 months following surgery *(white arrow).* Note the new disk herniation below the fusion mass *(black arrow).* (From Ross JS, Masaryk TJ, Modic MT: *J Comput Assist Tomogr* 1987;11:955-962.)

ated with chronic disk degeneration typically show increased signal on T$_1$-weighted and isointense to slightly increased signal on T$_2$-weighted images. This is secondary to fatty marrow conversion.[44] Similar changes have been seen within the cervical spine. Trauma effects on the vertebral body and graft marrow reflect marrow edema, showing decreased signal on T$_1$-weighted and increased signal on T$_2$-weighted images or perhaps even the varied signal intensities of hemorrhage.

Solid bony fusions are more consistent in their appearance. They are seen as continuous marrow signal without evidence of an original intervertebral disk space or definable bone graft. The marrow of the fusion mass may be isointense to the adjacent normal marrow (approximately 50% of the time) or can demonstrate a more patchy or spotty increased signal on T$_1$-weighted images (Fig. 4-34).

Vertebral Body Resection

Vertebral body resections appear as homogeneous areas of decreased signal with respect to the normal mar-

row signal on T$_1$-weighted images. These areas may be isointense or, more commonly, may show increased signal on T$_2$-weighted images. Disk material is not visible within the midportion of the disk spaces, where corpectomy has been performed. However, away from the corpectomy site at the lateral aspects of the vertebral bodies, the intervertebral disk space again will become well defined and retain its normal signal intensity.

The outlines of the strut graft material itself are well defined by the low-signal cortical bone (Fig. 4-35). Strut graft marrow may be isointense or may demonstrate increased signal on T$_1$-weighted images when compared to the adjacent normal vertebral body. The precise positioning of the ends of the strut grafts is visible as very low signal graft cortical bone, in contrast to the variable signal intensity (slightly hypointense or isointense) of the corpectomy site. Portions of strut graft marrow commonly show increased signal on T$_2$-weighted images, corresponding to the areas of decreased signal on T$_1$-weighted images, and most likely reflect graft marrow edema or revascularization.

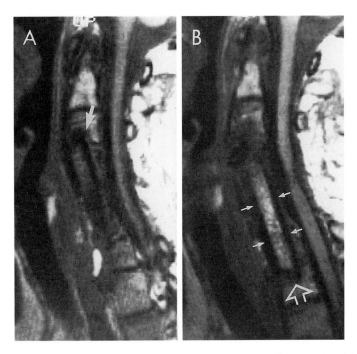

Fig. 4-35. Cervical strut graft. Immediately postoperative sagittal T_1-weighted images show a fibular strut graft placed from C3 to C7. The sequential 4 mm slices allow good definition of the superior (*arrow,* **A**) and inferior (*open arrow,* **B**) extent of the graft. The anterior-posterior dimensions of the graft are also visualized due to the cortical bone (*small arrows,* **B**). A focal area of cord atrophy is present at the C5 level. This patient had previously undergone a C3-5 laminectomy. (From Ross JS, Masaryk TJ, Modic MT: *J Comput Assist Tomogr* 1987;11:955-967.)

Bony Stenosis

The most significant postoperative changes that we have identified by MR in the postoperative cervical spine are bony stenosis and new disk herniations. We have identified bony stenosis at the fusion sites in up to 26% of our patients. This stenosis was most often secondary to hypertrophic bone from the anterior fusion mass that encroached on the cord or neural foramen (Figs. 4-36 and 4-37). The hypertrophic bone can be visualized as an anterior extradural defect that is isointense with the vertebral body on T_1-weighted images, showing increased signal or very low signal. The osteophytes may be visible only by the mass effect they exert on the cord. In these cases, when the osteophytes are very low signal, T_2-weighted or gradient echo low flip-angle images are necessary to confirm their presence. The sensitivity of MR for extradural disease, but its lack of specificity regarding the differentiation of disk versus bone, has been previously noted.[54] However, at least in the cervical spine, this nonspecific appearance may be of less importance since recurrent disk herniations (which can be totally removed under direct vision) are uncommon.

An additional type of bony stenosis seen immediately following ADF is anterior or posterior graft extrusion.

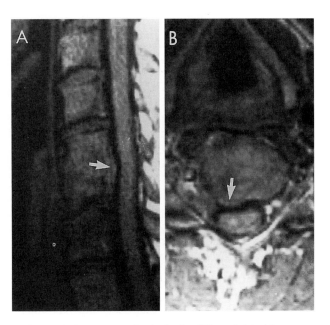

Fig. 4-36. Bony stenosis. **A,** Sagittal T_1-weighted image showing a solid fusion mass at C5-6. An area of bony hypertrophy compresses the cord *(arrow).* **B,** An axial T_1-weighted confirms the bony compression of the cord *(arrow).*

180

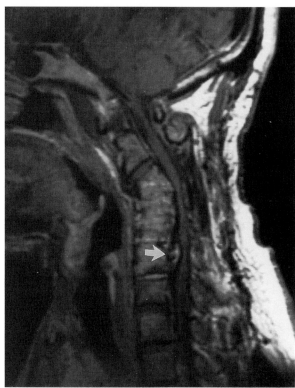

Fig. 4-37. Bony stenosis. A sagittal T₁-weighted image shows that the patient is post–multilevel laminectomy and anterior diskectomy at C3-5. The cord is small and draped over the kyposis at C3-4. Additionally, there is a large osteophyte arising from the posterior aspect of C5 *(arrow)* that causes severe canal stenosis and cord compression.

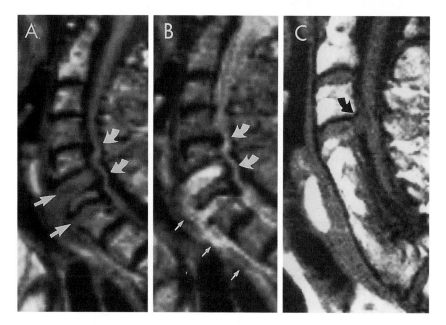

Fig. 4-38. A, Initial sagittal T₁-weighted image in a 79-year-old woman who underwent anterior diskectomy and fusion at C5-6 levels with postoperative quadriparesis. Homogeneous low signal arises from the diskectomy sites *(straight arrows)*. There continue to be large extradural defects at C4-5 and C5-6 with marked cord compression *(curved arrows).* **B,** The sagittal T₂-weighted also shows large anterior extradural defects at C4-5 and C5-6 *(curved arrows)* with a smaller defect at C3-4. The grafts and prevertebral space *(small arrows)* show high signal intensity. **C,** Follow-up T₁-weighted sagittal image 2 years after fibular graft placement from C4 through C7. The graft appears well incorporated into the bodies. There is now a very large disk herniation at the C3-4 level *(arrow).* (From Ross JS, Masaryk TJ, Modic MT: *J Comput Assist Tomogr* 1987;11:955-962.)

We have seen two cases of graft extrusion in which MR defined the extruded graft when patients were imaged within the first few days following ADF. In one case no new symptomatology was present following a Smith-Robinson ADF at C4-5. The postoperative images showed the graft in close approximation to the cord, which mimicked the preoperative appearance of the disk herniation (Fig. 4-32). One other patient underwent a C5-6, C6-7 ADF with postoperative quadriparesis. The MR examination performed 5 days postoperatively showed a large anterior extradural defect at C4-5 that compressed the cervical cord. Additional cord compression was produced by a large anterior extradural defect at C5-6, at the site of the bone graft (Fig. 4-38). All these findings were confirmed at reoperation.

Disk Herniation and Degeneration

Following anterior diskectomy with fusion, instability and disk degeneration or herniation can develop above or below the fusion site due to excess stress placed on these joints. This is especially true when multiple levels have been fused. Disk degeneration at levels adjacent to the fusion may occur in as many as 81% of cases.[55] We have observed disk herniations in up to 29% of our cases, fairly evenly distributed above and below the fusion site. These herniations have the typical appearance of intermediate soft tissue signal on T_1-weighted images and low signal anterior extradural defects on gradient echo images (Figs. 4-34 and 4-38, *C*). The vast majority were seen in patients following ADF. Occasionally, multiple herniations were seen in patients who had undergone wide cervical laminectomies since they were the cause for the initial operation.

Disk herniations, for all practical purposes, do not recur at the operated levels in the cervical spine as they do in the lumbar spine. This is due to the different surgical techniques: in the cervical spine the intervertebral disk material is removed under direct vision back to the posterior longitudinal ligament, the disk space is then widened by traction, and the graft is sunk into the space. This technique removes the vast bulk of the disk material at the time of surgery, in contrast to a lumbar diskectomy, wherein the bulk of the disk material remains behind.

Soft Tissues

Areas of high signal intensity may be present within the prevertebral region on T_2-weighted images immediately following anterior diskectomy and fusion. These regions are isointense with muscle on T_1-weighted images and most likely represent edema along the operative tract (Fig. 4-38, *B*). With time, the size and signal intensity of the prevertebral space will return to normal. Any high signal intensity within the prevertebral space

on T_1-weighted images should be considered suspicious for a hematoma.

Bony Deformity with Instability

Midline sagittal images allow excellent definition of bony deformities such as kyphosis and subluxation. We observed cervical kyphosis in 6 of 73 postoperative patients, all of whom had undergone anterior diskectomy and fusions. Of significance, every patient had evidence of bony encroachment on the canal and cervical cord from the fusion sites.

Cervical laminectomy has been previously used in the treatment of tumors, trauma, and spondylosis. The problem with it, however, is the development of a kyphotic or swan-neck deformity months or years following surgery. This is more likely to occur with multilevel laminectomy. Johnson et al.[56] showed that laminectomy by itself decreased spinal stability by only 20%, but with associated disruption of the facet joints, spinal stability decreased by 60%. Patient groups who appear most susceptible to postoperative deformity include those under 25 years of age, those having undergone laminectomy coupled with foraminotomy, and those having undergone laminectomy following trauma, in whom spinal stability was already compromised.[57,58] Simple T_1-weighted spin-echo sagittal images are generally all that are necessary in cases of severe deformity. Depending upon angulation, the axial plane may need to be rotated to achieve a true transverse image. With more severe kyphosis, signal dropoff may be excessive with use of a surface coil. In these cases body coil images may be the only way to achieve a diagnostically useful scan (with the inherent decreased resolution).

Metal Artifacts and Posterior Approaches

Cervical laminectomies are easily recognized by the absence of bony posterior elements. Axial images commonly show loss of the normal muscle-fat interfaces at the surgical site, which can be replaced by relatively homogeneous intermediate signal on T_1-weighted images (representing scar) or high signal (representing fat).

Posterior cervical fusions involving sublaminar or intraspinous process wiring are defined by the local metal artifacts they produce. The metal artifacts are usually confined to the posterior soft tissues or perhaps to the posterior margin of the subarachnoid space when spin-echo images are used (Fig. 4-39). Gradient echo images are more susceptible to metal artifacts, which commonly extend to involve the cervical canal. Occasional patients will have metal artifacts anteriorly at the side of anterior diskectomy and fusion produced by a shearing off of small metal drill particles during the diskectomy or corpectomy. The artifacts vary in size from small (mimicking a small anterior extradural defect) to large (obscuring the fusion mass and cervical cord)[59] (Fig. 4-40).

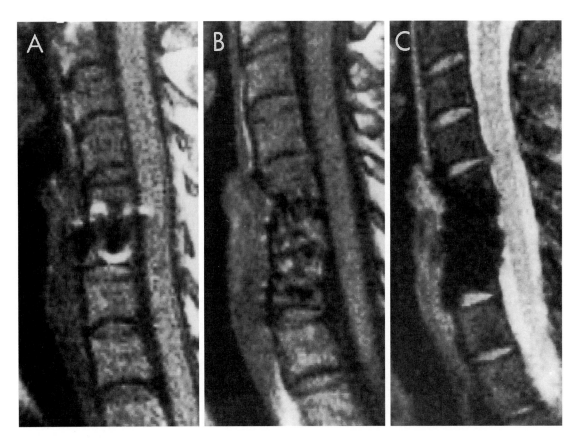

Fig. 4-39. Metal artifacts. **A,** Spin-echo T_1-weighted image. Decreased signal with a halo of increased signal is seen at the site of anterior fusion. **B,** Spin-echo T_1-weighted image in a different patient. Note the mottled, diffuse low signal from the C5-6—C6-7 fusions. **C,** Gradient echo 10-degree flip-angle image in the same patient showing an extensive area of low signal due to minute metal fragments within the fusions.

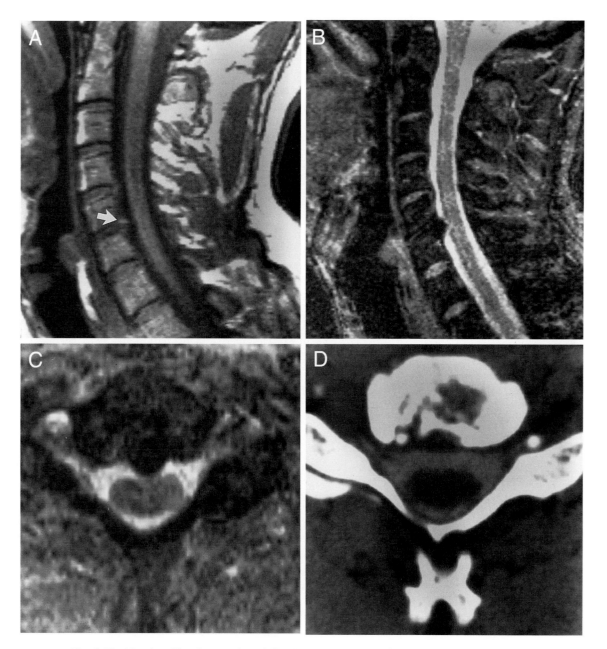

Fig. 4-40. Metal artifact in a patient following C5-6 anterior diskectomy. The sagittal T$_1$-weighted image, **A,** shows a slightly hyperintense anterior extradural defect at C5-6. Note that it is low in signal on the sagittal, **B,** and axial, **C,** gradient echo images. Also the extradural defects are considerably larger on the gradient echo sequences. An axial postmyelogram CT image, **D,** demonstrates no anterior extradural defect and no visible metal particles.

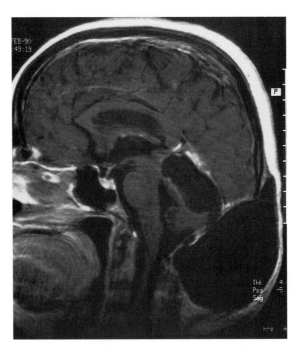

Fig. 4-41. Pseudomeningocele. Sagittal T₁-weighted images in a patient after suboccipital craniectomy and upper cervical laminectomy shows a large CSF signal collection over the operative site.

Pseudomeningocele

Pseudomeningoceles are defined as sharply marginated areas of decreased signal on T_1-weighted and increased signal on T_2-weighted images, similar to CSF. They are most commonly seen posterior to the upper cervical thecal sac following suboccipital craniotomy and decompression. Sagittal and axial images are usually necessary to define the full extent of a pseudomeningocele and the site of its connection with the subarachnoid space (Fig. 4-41).

Intrinsic Cord Abnormalities

A variety of abnormalities involving the cervical cord can be defined by MR in the postoperative patient. Diffuse cord atrophy may occur from cervical spondylosis, trauma, or tumor surgery.

Severe cervical spondylosis can allow repetitive trauma to take place with limited amounts of flexion and extension, causing cord cavitation (Fig. 4-42). This is usually seen as well-defined areas of decreased signal intensity on T_1-weighted images within the central portion of the cord[60-62] (Fig. 4-43). If the patient is imaged within a few days following trauma and posterior stabilization, evidence of cord hematoma may be seen, appearing as an ill-defined area of high signal intensity on T_1-weighted images within the cord secondary to the methemoglobin content.

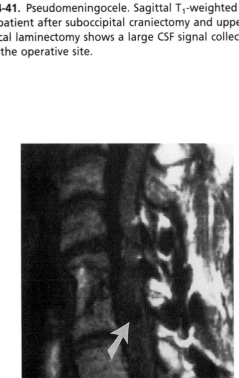

Fig. 4-42. Posttraumatic cord cavitation. Sagittal T₁-weighted MR following a fracture-subluxation of C5 and C6, with subsequent fusions anteriorly and posteriorly. The cord is enlarged and contains a small cyst (arrow). Posterior fusion wires give moderate artifact.

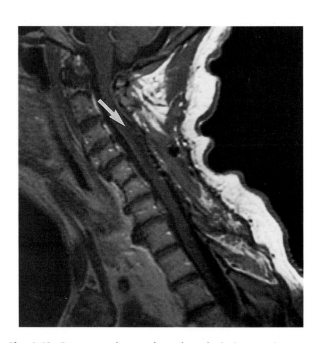

Fig. 4-43. Postoperative cord myelomalacia in a patient after multilevel laminectomy for cervical spondylosis. The cord, tethered at the operative site, demonstrates linear low signal intensity at the C4 and C5 levels (arrow) consistent with myelomalacia. Note the multilevel herniations and osteophytes.

Conclusion

A variety of signal changes are present with postoperative graft healing in the cervical spine. These would appear to represent, in and of themselves, not a pathologic process but rather a complex series of graft–vertebral body interactions in the course of healing. Magnetic resonance can define numerous postoperative abnormalities, the most common being disk herniation above or below the fusion level and bony stenosis from the fusion mass.

THORACIC SPINE

The initial surgical assaults on thoracic disk disease and vertebral body fractures with cord compromise were by means of laminectomy, the intention being to decompress the spinal cord. From this experience, it became quite clear that laminectomy resulted in an unacceptably high incidence of neurologic deterioration and instability. These complications occurred without any attempts to remove the offending anterior bone or disk fragments responsible for cord compression.[63]

Since the first reports of transthoracic (1958)[64] and anterolateral (1960)[65] procedures for thoracic disk disease, it is now agreed that a lateral or anterior approach gives the best neurologic results, without compromising spine stability.

There are three general types of anterior or lateral approaches[66]: (1) posterior-lateral (costotransversectomy), (2) extrapleural anterior-lateral (modified costotransversectomy), and (3) transthoracic, transpleural (Fig. 4-44).

These procedures allow removal of the pedicle on the side of approach, as well as a variable amount of vertebral body above and below the disk space, and the intervertebral disk. The amount of vertebral body removed will depend on the cause for surgery. A thoracic diskectomy may require only removal of a small amount of the posterior-inferior and posterior-superior endplates above and below the herniation, respectively. Correction of kyphosis, burst fracture, or tumor may necessitate radical corpectomy. The surgical procedures requiring that larger amounts of vertebral body be removed call for graft placement. Bone graft material may be either iliac or rib. The superior and inferior ends of the graft are carefully incorporated into the central recesses of the upper and lower receptor vertebral bodies. Cancellous bone chips may be placed anterior to the graft itself.[67]

Pulse Sequences

The usual postoperative evaluation of the thoracic spine includes sagittal and axial T$_1$-weighted images as well as sagittal T$_2$-weighted images. The T$_1$-weighted images allow assessment of both the vertebral body marrow condition at the operative site and the amount and

A

B

C

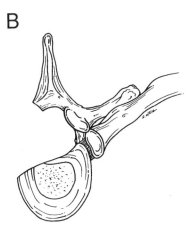

Fig. 4-44. Approaches for thoracic cord decompression. **A,** The posterolateral or lateral gutter approach allows more of an anterior decompression than is possible with a conventional posterior exposure. **B,** The lateral approach or costotransversectomy allows access to the entire posterior margin of the vertebral body. **C,** The anterolateral or transthoracic-transpleural approach allows wide resection of the offending vertebral body.

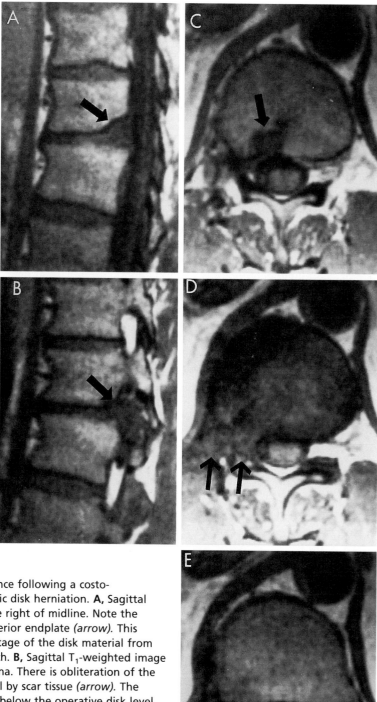

Fig. 4-45. Normal appearance following a costo-transversectomy for thoracic disk herniation. **A,** Sagittal T$_1$-weighted MR just to the right of midline. Note the operative defect in the inferior endplate *(arrow)*. This allows room for safe curettage of the disk material from an anterior-lateral approach. **B,** Sagittal T$_1$-weighted image through the neural foramina. There is obliteration of the normal foraminal fat signal by scar tissue *(arrow)*. The pedicle has been removed below the operative disk level. **C,** An axial T$_1$-weighted image shows the defect in the inferior endplate *(arrow)* comparable to that in **A. D,** The axial T$_1$-weighted just inferior to **C** shows scar within the right neural foramen *(arrows)*. The posterior disk margin is slightly convex, but otherwise normal. **E,** Axial T$_1$-weighted image just inferior to **D.** The pedicle is absent on the right.

location of scar. T_1-weighted images are usually adequate for evaluating the presence or absence of extradural mass effect on the cord. However, with more extensive corpectomies, occasionally the interface between the surrounding postoperative soft tissue edema and scar cannot be discerned from the dural tube itself. In these situations, a gradient echo image with higher flip angles (approximately 40 to 60 degrees) is useful. With this degree of flip angle, CSF has a lower signal intensity than does the cord, which usually allows better definition of the cord than may be possible with a standard spin-echo T_2-weighted image. The disadvantage of using the gradient echo is its increased susceptibility to local magnetic field inhomogeneity. This is often present due to the surgical clips used to ligate vessels in these surgeries.

The appearance of the postoperative thoracic spine might be expected to parallel that of the cervical spine since the approaches, types of surgeries, and grafts are similar. This is indeed the case, up to a certain point.

Posterior lateral approaches for thoracic disk disease show absence of the pedicle below the operated disk level, as well as a portion of the posterior vertebral body adjacent to the dural tube. These areas are replaced by intermediate soft tissue signal material (scar) on T_1-weighted images (Fig. 4-45). The scar can be fairly homogeneous and extend medially to conform to the smooth outer border of the dural tube. Its anterior extent is to the region of the costotransverse articulation, which may also be removed during the operation. Laterally, the scar will be seen to encompass the neural foramen, with obliteration of the normal foraminal fat signal. With a posterolateral approach, the dural tube should continue to be well defined and oval in shape. The epidural and paravertebral scarring shows a more variable appearance on T_2-weighted images, being either isointense or hyperintense with respect to normal marrow signal. The margins of the dural tube are graphically defined by the high-signal CSF.

We have not as yet observed changes in signal intensity within the vertebral body marrow adjacent to the intervertebral disk space in the thoracic spine following anterior graft placement. This is more common in the cervical and lumbar regions. The thoracic vertebral bodies adjacent to the disk continue to show normal marrow signal on T_1- and T_2-weighted images. A small amount of metal artifact is commonly seen along the lateral aspect of the vertebral body due to clipping of the segmental vessels.

Regions of more extensive corpectomy also show replacement with intermediate soft tissue signal scar on T_1-weighted images. The interface of the scar with the remaining normal vertebral bodies is well defined. Areas of scar can show very high signal on T_2-weighted images, similar to CSF. Of considerable importance is the

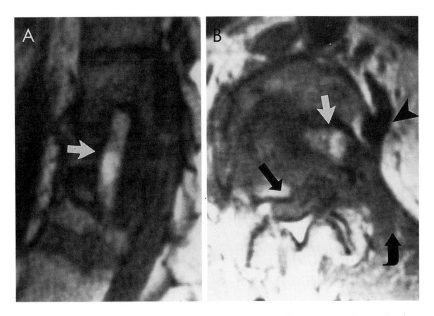

Fig. 4-46. Corpectomy and iliac grafting following a burst fracture. **A,** The sagittal T_1-weighted image shows a rectangular high-signal graft *(arrow)* spanning the corpectomy site that is hypointense. **B,** An axial T_1-weighted image shows the graft to the left *(white arrow)*. The circular hypointensity with a hyperintense halo *(arrowhead)* is a metal artifact. There continues to be compression of the cord by a retropulsed bone fragment with hyperintense signal *(straight black arrow)*. Note the low signal intensity following the extraperitoneal approach on the left *(tailed arrow)*.

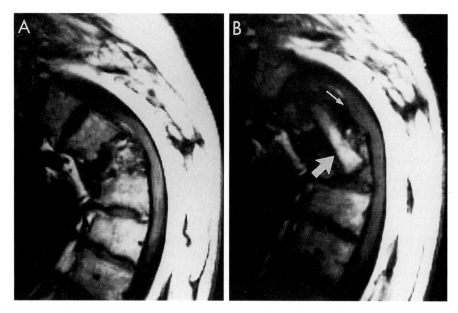

Fig. 4-47. Thoracic osteonecrosis. **A,** A preoperative sagittal T_1-weighted image shows heterogeneous signal from a collapsed vertebral body. There is mild compression of the cord at this level with severe kyphosis. **B,** Sagittal T_1-weighted image following corpectomy and iliac grafting. Note the well-defined graft traversing the corpectomy site *(large arrow).* The caudal portion of the graft is well defined and seated within the inferior vertebral body. The cord now follows the concavity of the corpectomy site *(small arrow).*

fact that normal postoperative soft tissue changes can obscure the dural tube on sagittal and axial images. This soft tissue precludes adequate evaluation of the potential mass effect on the thecal sac postoperatively.

Graft material may have a wide variety of signal intensities, as it has within the cervical spine (Figs. 4-46 and 4-47). On T_1-weighted images, graft marrow signal may be isointense, slightly hyperintense, or quite hyperintense with respect to the normal vertebral body marrow. The edges of the grafts are well defined due to the decreased signal of the cortical bone. With more extensive corpectomies, metal artifact may be a more significant impediment to interpretation, especially when gradient echo images are used.

Laminectomies

Thoracic laminectomies are performed for a variety of reasons, including resection of tumors and syringes and exploration of the cord. The site of a thoracic laminectomy, as in other areas of the spine, is defined by the lack of posterior elements. A variable amount of scar tissue may be present in the posterior epidural region. This has intermediate signal intensity on T_1-weighted sequences and is usually isointense to slightly hyperintense on T_2-weighted sequences.

Conclusion

The effectiveness of MR in evaluating the postoperative thoracic spine remains undocumented. However, the success of MR imaging in evaluating the lumbar and cervical spine postoperatively, combined with the ease of examination, makes MR the first choice for evaluating postoperative thoracic spines.

REFERENCES

1. Burton CV, Kirkaldy-Willis WH, Young-Hing K, et al: Causes of failure of surgery on the lumbar spine. *Clin Orthop* 1981;157:191-199.
2. Cronqvist S: The postoperative myelogram. *Acta Radiol [Stockh]* 1959;52:45-51.
3. Quencer RM, Tenner M, Rothman L: The postoperative myelogram. *Radiology* 1977;123:667-679.
4. Shapiro R: *Myelography,* ed 3, Chicago, Year Book, 1975, p 203.
5. Teplick JG, Haskin ME: Computed tomography of the postoperative lumbar spine. *AJR* 1983;141:865-884.
6. Ross JS, Masaryk TJ, Modic MT, et al: Lumbar spine: postoperative assessment with surface-coil MR imaging. *Radiology* 1987;164:851-860.
7. Modic MT, Steinberg PM, Ross JS, et al: Degenerative disk disease: assessment of changes in vertebral body marrow with MRI. *Radiology* 1988;166:193-199.

8. Ehrman RL, Berquist TH: Magnetic resonance imaging of musculoskeletal trauma. *Radiol Clin North Am* 1986;2:291-319.

9. Unger EC, Glazer HS, Lee JKT, et al: MRI of extracranial hematomas: preliminary observations. *AJR* 1986;146:403-407.

10. Dooms GC, Fisher MR, Hricak H, et al: MR imaging of intramuscular hemorrhage. *J Comput Assist Tomogr* 1985;9:908-913.

11. Teplick JG, Haskin ME: Intravenous contrast enhanced CT of the postoperative lumbar spine. *AJR* 1984;143:845-855.

12. Braun IF, Hoffman JC, Davis PC, et al: Contrast enhancement in CT differentiation between recurrent disk herniation and postoperative scar: prospective study. *AJR* 1985;145:785-790.

13. Bundschuh CV, Modic MT, Ross JS, et al: Epidural fibrosis and recurrent disk herniation in the lumbar spine: assessment with MR. *AJNR* 1988;9:169-178.

14. Sotiropoulos S, Chafetz NI, Lang P, et al: Differentiation between postoperative scar and recurrent disk herniation: prospective comparison of MR, CT, and contrast-enhanced CT. *AJNR* 1989;10:639-643.

15. Hochhauser L, Kieffer SA, Cacayorin ED, et al: Recurrent postdiskectomy low back pain: MR-surgical correlation. *AJNR* 1988;9:769-774.

16. Hueftle M, Modic MT, Ross JS, et al: Lumbar spine: postoperative MR imaging with Gd-DTPA. *Radiology* 1988;167:817-824.

17. Teplick JG, Peyster RG, Teplick S, et al: CT identification of post laminectomy pseudomeningocele. *AJNR* 1983;4:179-182.

18. Gill GG, Scheck M, Kelley ET, et al: Pedicle fat grafts for the prevention of scar in low-back surgery. *Spine* 1985;10:662-667.

19. Ross JS, Masaryk TJ, Modic MT, et al: Magnetic resonance of lumbar arachnoiditis. *AJNR* 1987;8:885-892 and *AJR* 1987;149:1025-1032.

20. Heindel W, Friedman G, Burke J, et al: Artifacts in MR imaging after surgical intervention. *J Comput Assist Tomogr* 1986;10:596-599.

21. Harrington DP: Particulate embolization materials. In Abrams HL (ed): *Abrams angiography: vascular and interventional radiology,* ed 3, Boston, Little Brown, 1983, pp 2138-2139.

22. Brasch RC, Weinmann HJ, Wesley GE: Contrast enhanced MR imaging: animal studies using gadolinium-DTPA complex. *AJR* 1984;142:625-630.

23. Runge VM, Clanton JA, Herzer WA, et al: Intravascular contrast agents suitable for magnetic resonance imaging. *Radiology* 1984;153:171-176.

24. Weinmann HJ, Brasch RC, Press WR, et al: Characteristics of gadolinium-DTPA complex: a potential NMR contrast agent. *AJR* 1984;142:619-624.

25. Carr DH, Brown J, Bidder GM, et al: Gadolinium-DTPA as a contrast agent in MRI: Initial clinical experience in 20 patients. *AJR* 1984;143:215-224.

26. Felix R, Schoerner W, Laniado M, et al: Brain tumors: MR imaging with gadolinium-DTPA. *Radiology* 1985;156:681-688.

27. Gadian DG, Payne JA, Bryant DJ, et al: Gadolinium-DTPA as a contrast agent in MR imaging—theoretical projections. *J Comput Assist Tomogr* 1985;9:242-248.

28. Wolf GL, Fobben ES: The tissue proton T1 and T2 response to gadolinium-DTPA injection in rabbits: a potential renal contrast agent for NMR imaging. *Invest Radiol* 1984;19:324-328.

29. Boden SD, Davis DO, Dina TS, et al: Contrast-enhanced MR imaging performed after successful lumbar disk surgery: prospective study. *Radiology* 1992;182:59-64.

30. Firooznia H, Kricheff II, Rafii M, Golimbu C: Lumbar spine after surgery; examination with intravenous contrast enhanced CT. *Radiology* 1987;163:221-226.

31. Yang PJ, Seeger JF, Dzioba RB, et al: High dose IV contrast in CT scanning of the postoperative lumbar spine. *AJNR* 1986;7:703-707.

32. Teplick GJ, Haskin ME: Intravenous contrast enhanced CT of the postoperative lumbar spine: improved identification of recurrent disc herniation, scar, arachnoiditis and diskitis. *AJNR* 1984;5:373-383.

33. Braun IF, Hoffman JC Jr, Davis PC, et al: Contrast enhancement in CT differentiation between recurrent disc herniation and postoperative scar: prospective study. *AJNR* 1985;6:607-612.

34. Schubiger O, Valavanis A: CT differentiation between recurrent disc herniation and postoperative scar formation: the value of contrast enhancement. *Neuroradiology* 1982;22:251-254.

35. Weiss T, Treisch J, Kazner E, et al: CT of the postoperative lumbar spine: The value of intravenous contrast. *Neuroradiology* 1986;28:241-245.

36. DeSantis M, Crisi G, Folch I, et al: Late contrast enhancement in the CT diagnosis of herniated disc. *Neuroradiology* 1984;26:303-307.

37. Nguyun CM, Haughton V, et al: Dose effectiveness of intravenous contrast medium in MR imaging of postlaminectomy scar tissue. (Abstract.) RSNA, 1991.

38. Ross JS, Masaryk TJ, Modic MT: MRI of the postoperative spine: further assessment. *AJNR* 1990;11:771-776.

39. Ross JS, Delamarter R, Hueftle MG, et al: Gadolinium-DTPA-enhanced MR imaging of the postoperative lumbar spine: time course and mechanism of enhancement. *AJNR* 1989;10:37-46.

40. Ross JS, Modic MT, Masaryk TJ, et al: Assessment of extradural degenerative disease with Gd-DTPA-enhanced MR imaging: correlation with surgical and pathologic findings. *AJNR* 1989;10:1243-1249.

41. Ross JS, Blaser S, Masaryk TJ, et al: Gd-DTPA enhancement of posterior epidural scar: an experimental model. *AJNR* 1989;10:1083-1088.

42. Russell EJ, D'Angelo CM, Zimmerman RD, et al: Cervical disk herniation: CT demonstration after contrast enhancement. *Radiology* 1984;152:703-712.

43. Modic MT, Masaryk TJ, Ross JS, Carter JR: Imaging of degenerative disk disease. *Radiology* 1988;168:177-186.

44. Modic MT, Steinberg PM, Ross JS, et al: Degenerative disk disease: assessment of changes in vertebral body marrow with MR imaging. *Radiology* 1988;166:193-199.

45. Modic MT, Feiglin DH, Piraino DW, et al: Vertebral osteomyelitis: assessment using MR. *Radiology* 1987;157:157-166.

46. Jacobs B: Anterior cervical spine fusion. *Surg Annu* 1976;8:413-446.

47. Cloward RB: The anterior approach for removal of ruptured cervical discs. *Neurosurgery* 1958;15:602-614.

48. Robinson RA, Smith GW: Anterolateral cervical disc removal and interbody fusion for cervical disc syndrome. *Bull Hopkins Hosp* 1955;96:223.

49. DePalma A, Rothman R, Lewinnek G, et al: Anterior interbody fusion for severe cervical degeneration. *Surg Gynecol Obstet* 1972;134:755-758.

50. Henderson CM, Hennessy RG, Shirey HM Jr, et al: Posterior-lateral foraminotomy as an exclusive operative technique for cervical radiculopathy: a review of 846 consecutively operated cases. *Neurosurgery* 1983;13:504.

51. Whitecloud TS: Management of radiculopathy and myelopathy by the anterior approach. In Cervical Spine Research Society: *The cervical spine,* Philadelphia, Lippincott, 1983, pp 411-424.

52. Ross JS, Masaryk TJ, Modic MT: Postoperative cervical spine: MR assessment. *J Comput Assist Tomogr* 1987;11:955-962.

53. Masaryk TJ, Boumphrey F, Modic MT, et al: Effects of chemonucleolysis demonstrated by MR imaging. *J Comput Assist Tomogr* 1986;10:917-923.

54. Modic MT, Masaryk TJ, Mulopulous GP, et al: Cervical radiculopathy: prospective evaluation with surface coil MR imaging, CT with metrizamide and metrizamide myelography. *Radiology* 1986;161:753-759.

55. Simone FA, Rothman RH: Cervical disc disease. In Rothman RH, Simone FA (eds): *The spine,* Philadelphia, Saunders, 1982, p 491.

56. Johnson RM, Owen JR, Panjobi MM, et al: Biomechanical stability of the cervical spine using a human cadaver model. *Orthop Trans* 1980;4:46.

57. Callahan RA, Johnson RM, Margolis RN, et al: Cervical facet fusion for central instability following laminectomy. *J Bone Joint Surg [Am]* 1977;59:991-1002.

58. Fielding JW, Tolli TC: Surgical management of post-laminectomy kyphosis. *Semin Spine Surg* 1989;1(4):271-275.

59. Heindel W, Friedmann G, Burke J, et al: Artifacts in MR imaging after surgical intervention. *J Comput Assist Tomogr* 1986;10:596-599.

60. Regenbogen VS, Rogers LF, Atlas SW, et al: Cervical spinal cord injuries in patients with cervical spondylosis. *AJR* 1986;146:277-284.

61. Jinkins JR, Baskir R, Al-Mefty O, et al: Cystic necrosis of the spinal cord in compressive cervical myelopathy: demonstration by Iopamidol CT-myelography. *AJR* 1986;147:767-775.

62. Sherman JL, Barkovich AJ, Citrin CM: The MR appearance of syringomyelia: new observations. *AJR* 1987;148:381-391.

63. Benjamin V: Diagnosis and management of thoracic disk disease. *Clin Neurosurg* 1983;30:577-605.

64. Crafoord C, Hiertonn T, Lindblom K, et al: Spinal cord compression caused by a protruded thoracic disc: report of a case treated with antero-lateral fenestration of the disc. *Acta Orthop Scand* 1958;28:103-107.

65. Hulme A: The surgical approach to thoracic intervertebral disc protrusion. *J Neurol Neurosurg Psychiatry* 1960;23:133-137.

66. Dohn DF: Thoracic spinal cord decompression: alternative surgical approaches and basis of choice. *Clin Neurosurg* 1980;27:611-623.

67. Bohlman HH, Eismont FJ: Surgical techniques of anterior decompression and fusion for spinal cord injuries. *Clin Orthop Rel Res* 1981;154:57-67.

5

Cervicomedullary and Craniovertebral Junctions

JEFFREY S. ROSS

Magnetic resonance imaging has opened vistas in diagnosing disorders of the brain stem, medulla, upper cervical cord, cervicomedullary junction (CMJ), and encompassing bony and ligamentous structures of the craniovertebral junction (CVJ). The neurologic symptoms produced from the diverse disorders of this region relate to compression or distortion of the neurovascular structures of the CMJ from either intrinsic diseases or alterations (acquired and congenital) of the CVJ. These abnormalities may be congenital, osseous, neoplastic, inflammatory, or traumatic.

MRI has proved extremely useful in evaluating this region because of its ability to image directly in the sagittal and coronal planes.[1] Although the lack of signal from cortical bone may cause some initial trepidation in the examiner trying to determine bony outlines, this is not so large a problem as was once feared. The lack of signal on MRI from cortical bone is, in fact, a diagnostic asset when compared to computed tomography of the posterior fossae. The role of conventional evaluation of the complex anatomy in this region is undergoing revision, with the result that MR has assumed the place of a primary imaging modality.

SEQUENCES AND TECHNIQUES

Sagittal images provide the best views of the brain stem, fourth ventricle, and upper cervical spine. Short echo time (TE) – repetition time (TR) spin-echo (SE) sequences are optimal for defining the gross anatomy of the cervicomedullary junction while keeping the CSF signal intensity low. The precise imaging planes, however, are determined by the need to image particular anatomic structures; for instance, the cerebellar tonsils can be evaluated best by a combination of coronal and sagittal planes. The key to diagnosing a large part of CVJ pathology lies in precise definition of the anatomy, which is best done with high signal-to-noise T_1-weighted images. Parenchymal lesions (tumors, multiple sclerosis) may be better identified with long TR/TE sequences. In particular, refocused and/or gated T_2-weighted images allow high signal from CSF and pathology while minimizing CSF pulsation artifact. Additional rephasing gradients may also be added to improve spatial misregistration and dephasing from CSF flow. Gradient echo techniques with low flip angles (10 degrees) are also capable of giving a CSF-myelogram–like effect, with the advantage of short imaging times. The gradient echo examination appears excellent for extradural disease but fairly unreliable for intramedullary disease. A potentially useful technique for the CMJ is to obtain sagittal T_1-weighted images of the patient in neutral, flexed, and extended positions so the atlantodental interval (ADI), basion-dental interval (BDI), and effects of the dens and ligaments on it can be assessed. Our routine examination consists of sagittal and axial T_1-weighted images (3 mm slice thickness, 50% gap, 256 matrix) with a sagittal low flip-angle (10 degrees) gradient echo or sagittal fast spin echo (TR 4000 msec, TE 90). If there is a question of instability, then flexion and extension sagittal T_1-weighted images may be obtained.

NORMAL ANATOMY

Figures 5-1 through 5-4 show normal anatomy of the CMJ and CVJ at various planes. The occipitoatlantoaxial joint consists of two atlantooccipital articulations and three atlantoaxial articulations. Each of the atlantooccipital joints involves the superior facet of the lateral mass

Text continued on p. 199.

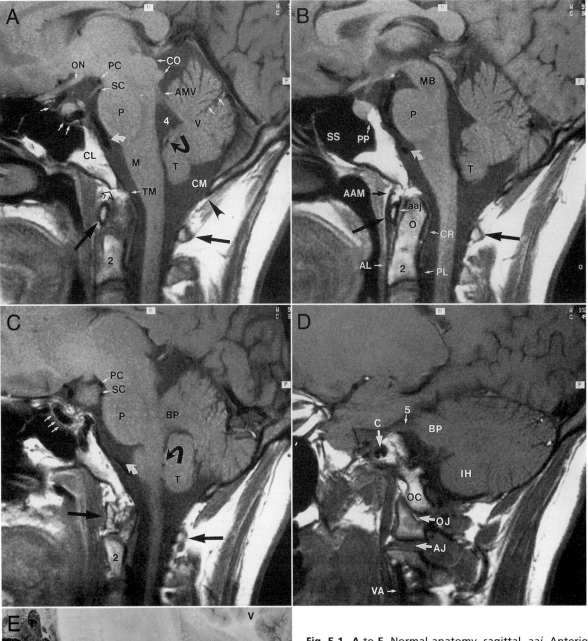

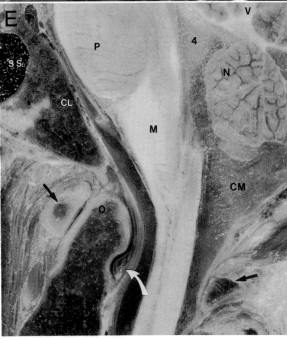

Fig. 5-1. A to **E,** Normal anatomy, sagittal. *aaj,* Anterior atlantoaxial joint; *AAM,* anterior atlantooccipital membrane; *AJ,* lateral atlantoaxial joint; *AL,* anterior longitudinal ligament; *AMV,* anterior medullary velum; *BP,* brachium pontis; *C,* carotid artery; *CL,* clivus, *CM,* cisterna magna; *CO,* colliculi; *IH,* inferior hemisphere of cerebellum; *M,* medulla; *MB,* midbrain; *N,* nodulus; *O,* odontoid; *OC,* occipital condyle; *OJ,* occipitoatlantal joint; *ON,* optic nerve; *P,* pons; *PC,* posterior cerebral artery; *PP,* posterior pituitary; *SC,* superior cerebellar artery; *SS,* sphenoidal sinus; *T,* cerebellar tonsil; *TM,* tectorial membrane; *V,* vermis; *VA,* vertebral artery; *2,* C2 body; *4,* fourth ventricle; *5,* fifth nerve. *Black arrow,* C1; *arrowhead,* opisthion; *small open arrow,* basion; *three white arrows,* carotid siphon; *two white arrows,* primary cerebellar fissure; *small curved white arrow,* basilar artery; *large curved white arrow,* transverse ligament; *curved black arrow,* PICA. (**E** courtesy Shiwei Yu, M.D., Syracuse NY.)

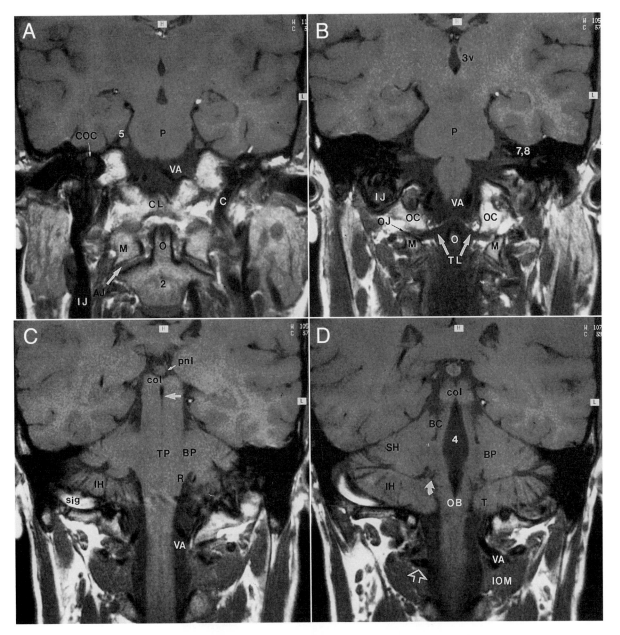

Fig. 5-2. A to **G,** Normal anatomy, coronal. *AJ,* Atlantoaxial joint; *AL,* alar ligament; *BC,* brachium conjunctivum (superior cerebellar peduncle); *BP,* brachium pontis (middle cerebellar peduncle); *C,* carotid artery; *CL,* clivus; *CM,* cisterna magna; *COC,* cochlea; *col,* colliculi; *IH,* inferior hemisphere of cerebellum; *IJ,* internal jugular vein; *IOM,* inferior oblique muscle; *M,* lateral mass at C2; *N,* nodulus; *OB,* obex; *O,* odontoid; *OC,* occipital condyle; *OJ,* occipitoatlantal joint; *P,* pons; *pnl,* pineal; *R,* restiform body (inferior cerebellar peduncle); *SH,* superior hemisphere of cerebellum; *sig,* sigmoid sinus; *som,* superior oblique muscle; *svr,* superior vermis; *TP,* tegmentum of pons; *T,* tonsil; *TL,* transverse ligament; *VA,* vertebral arteries; *VR,* vermis; *2,* body of C2; *3v,* third ventricle; *7,8,* cranial nerves VII and VIII within internal auditory canal; *5,* cranial nerve V; *4,* fourth ventricle. *White arrow,* Aqueduct of Sylvius; *curved white arrow,* lateral recess of fourth ventricle; *vertical black arrows,* foramen magnum margin; *open white arrow,* posterior arch of C1. (**G** courtesy Shiwei Yu, M.D., Syracuse NY.)   *Continued.*

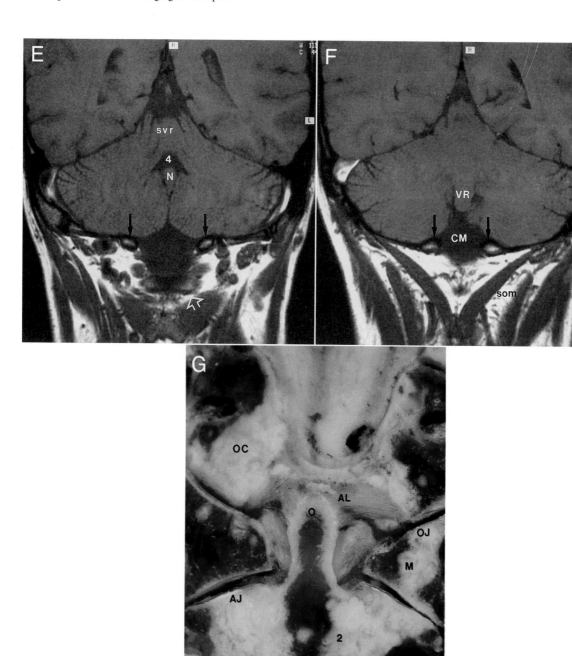

Fig. 5-2. cont'd. A to **G,** Normal anatomy, coronal. *AJ,* Atlantoaxial joint; *AL,* alar ligament; *BC,* brachium conjunctivum (superior cerebellar peduncle); *BP,* brachium pontis (middle cerebellar peduncle); *C,* carotid artery; *CL,* clivus; *CM,* cisterna magna; *COC,* cochlea; *col,* colliculi; *IH,* inferior hemisphere of cerebellum; *IJ,* internal jugular vein; *IOM,* inferior oblique muscle; *M,* lateral mass at C2; *N,* nodulus; *OB,* obex; *O,* odontoid; *OC,* occipital condyle; *OJ,* occipitoatlantal joint; *P,* pons; *pnl,* pineal; *R,* restiform body (inferior cerebellar peduncle); *SH,* superior hemisphere of cerebellum; *sig,* sigmoid sinus; *som,* superior oblique muscle; *svr,* superior vermis; *TP,* tegmentum of pons; *T,* tonsil; *TL,* transverse ligament; *VA,* vertebral arteries; *VR,* vermis; *2,* body of C2; *3v,* third ventricle; *7,8,* cranial nerves VII and VIII within internal auditory canal; *5,* cranial nerve V; *4,* fourth ventricle. *White arrow,* Aqueduct of Sylvius; *curved white arrow,* lateral recess of fourth ventricle; *vertical black arrows,* foramen magnum margin; *open white arrow,* posterior arch of C1. (**G** courtesy Shiwei Yu, M.D., Syracuse NY.)

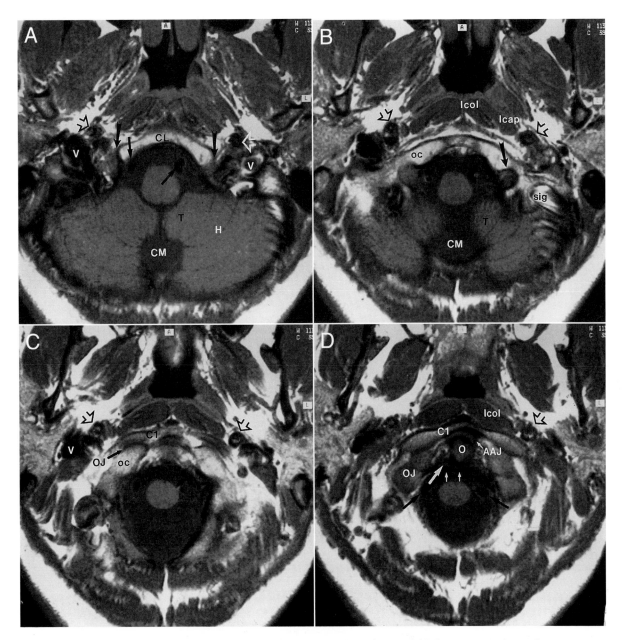

Fig. 5-3. A to **J,** Normal anatomy, axial. *AAJ,* Anterior atlantoaxial joint; *C1,* anterior arch of C1; *CL,* clivus; *CM,* cisterna magna; *C2,* body of C2; *H,* cerebellar hemisphere; *LAJ,* lateral atlantoaxial joint; *lcap,* longus capitus muscle; *lcol,* longus colli muscle; *M,* lateral mass at C1; *O,* odontoid; *oc,* occipital condyle; *OJ,* atlantooccipital joint; *PC1,* posterior arch of C1; *C2,* body of C2; *sig,* sigmoid sinus; *T,* tonsil; *TL(tl),* transverse ligament; *V(v),* jugular vein. *Straight black arrows,* Vertebral arteries; *tailed arrows,* hypoglossal canal; *open arrows,* carotid arteries; *small white arrows,* tectorial membrane; *large white arrow,* alar ligament. (**I** and **J** courtesy Shiwei Yu, M.D., Syracuse NY.)   *Continued.*

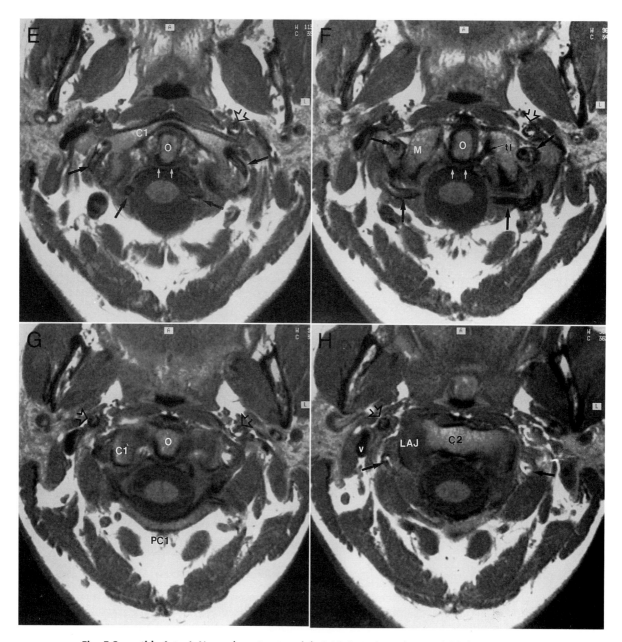

Fig. 5-3 cont'd. A to **J,** Normal anatomy, axial. *AAJ,* Anterior atlantoaxial joint; *C1,* anterior arch of C1; *CL,* clivus; *CM,* cisterna magna; *C2,* body of C2; *LAJ,* lateral atlantoaxial joint; *lcap,* longus capitus muscle; *lcol,* longus colli muscle; *M,* lateral mass at C1; *O,* odontoid; *oc,* occipital condyle; *OJ,* atlantooccipital joint; *PC1,* posterior arch of C1; *C2,* body of C2; *sig,* sigmoid sinus; *T,* tonsil; *TL(tl),* transverse ligament; *V(v),* jugular vein. *Straight black arrows,* Vertebral arteries; *tailed arrows,* hypoglossal canal; *open arrows,* carotid arteries; *small white arrows,* tectorial membrane; *large white arrow,* alar ligament. (**I** and **J** courtesy Shiwei Yu, M.D., Syracuse NY.)

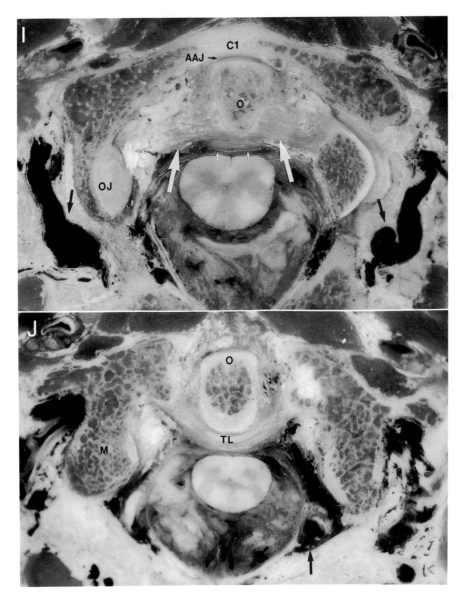

Fig. 5-3 cont'd. A to **J,** Normal anatomy, axial. *AAJ,* Anterior atlantoaxial joint; *C1,* anterior arch of C1; *CL,* clivus; *CM,* cisterna magna; *C2,* body of C2; *LAJ,* lateral atlantoaxial joint; *lcap,* longus capitus muscle; *lcol,* longus colli muscle; *M,* lateral mass at C1; *O,* odontoid; *oc,* occipital condyle; *OJ,* atlantooccipital joint; *PC1,* posterior arch of C1; *C2,* body of C2; *sig,* sigmoid sinus; *T,* tonsil; *TL(tl),* transverse ligament; *V(v),* jugular vein. *Straight black arrows,* Vertebral arteries; *tailed arrows,* hypoglossal canal; *open arrows,* carotid arteries; *small white arrows,* tectorial membrane; *large white arrow,* alar ligament. (**I** and **J** courtesy Shiwei Yu, M.D., Syracuse NY.)

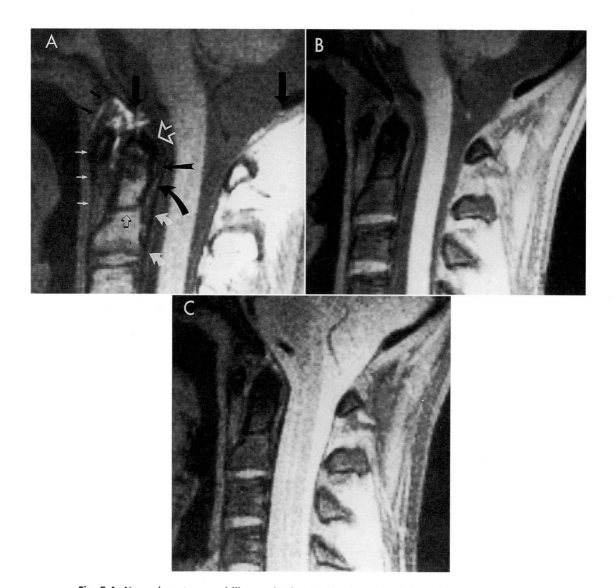

Fig. 5-4. Normal anatomy, midline sagittal. **A,** Spin-echo; T$_1$-weighted image; **B,** gradient echo scan (a = 60 degrees); **C,** gradient echo scan (a = 10 degrees). *Small white arrows,* Anterior longitudinal ligament; *curved white arrows,* posterior longitudinal ligament; *small open arrow,* subdental synchrondosis; *small black arrows,* atlantooccipital membrane; *curved black arrow,* inferior fascicle of cruciate ligament; *open white arrow,* tectorial membrane and superior fascicle cruciate ligament; *tailed black arrow,* transverse ligament; *vertical black arrows,* foramen magnum margin.

of the atlas and an occipital condyle. The atlantal facets are concave and tilt medially, articulating with the ellipsoidal surface of the occipital condyle. There is intercommunication of the synovial joints of the lateral masses of C1 and C2, as well as the joints between the dens and atlas arch anteriorly and the transverse ligament posteriorly. The unique combination of stability and complex motion of the CVJ is provided by the complex ligaments of the region. The anterior ligaments consist of (1) the anterior atlantooccipital membrane, which is the superior extension of the anterior longitudinal ligament and connects the anterior margin of the foramen magnum to the anterior arch of the atlas; (2) the transverse ligament, which consists of a broad band that crosses the ring of the atlas and secures the dens in contact with the anterior arch of C1 (a small upper band connects the basilar part of the occipital bone and a lower band attaches to the posterior surface of the body of the axis, the whole ligament thus forming a cross and referred to as the cruciform ligament); (3) the alar ligaments, which are strong bands that connect the dens to the medial aspect of the occipital condyles; (4) the apical ligament, which connects the tip of the odontoid to the anterior margin of the foramen magnum; and (5) the tectorial membrane, which is a cephalad extension of the posterior longitudinal ligament and attaches to the upper surface of the basilar occipital bone in front of the foramen magnum (Fig. 5-4).

The posterior structures that are responsible for stability are the ligamentum nuchae, interspinous ligament, posterior atlantooccipital membrane, ligamentum flavum, and cervical musculature.

Since cortical bone does not produce signal on MR, care must be taken when the bony margins are identified, as with the foramen magnum. Nevertheless, the low signal from the cortical bone of the foramen magnum's anterior margin (basion) and posterior margin (opisthion) usually provides enough contrast against the surrounding soft tissue and CSF to allow fairly precise measurements. The high-signal yellow marrow in the skull base is quite variable and should not be used as an indicator of bony margins. The signal intensity of the dens is also quite variable depending on the marrow content (e.g., red or yellow) and pathologic alterations (edema, erosions, bony sclerosis). The odontoid often has decreased signal on parasagittal images due to partial volume averaging of the cortical bone and periodontoid soft tissue. A variable amount of fat is routinely seen between the tip of the dens and the basion. Absence of fat should signify CVJ pathology.

Certain measurements of the CVJ relationships, first applied to plain films, are identifiable and applicable with MR. Some of the more classic ones will be described briefly:

1. Platybasia: An increase in the basal angle of the skull. This may be defined by the angle between lines drawn along the plane of the sphenoid bone and along the clivus. Platybasia exists if this angle is greater than 143 degrees (normal range, 125 to 143 degrees).[2]

2. Basilar impression
   a. Chamberlain's line: Drawn between the hard palate and the opisthion. Projection of up to one third of the top of the dens above this line has been considered normal.[2]
   b. McGregor's line: Drawn between the hard palate to the caudal point of the occipital curve.[3] It has the same significance as Chamberlain's line.
   c. Fischgold's digastric line: Drawn tangent to the digastric grooves. This line in the article by Fischgold et al.[4] relates to the location of the skull base; that is, if the skull base is above the line, basilar invagination is present. Other publications[5] have related this line to the location of the odontoid tip.
   d. Wachenheim's line: Drawn along the posterior surface of the clivus. The dens should lie inferior to this line, and any intersection is considered abnormal.[6]

3. Foramen magnum margin
   a. McRae's line: Drawn between the basion and opisthion. This is normal if it measures approximately 35 mm in diameter.[7]

4. Vertical setting
   a. Redlund-Johnell method: Assesses the distance between the base of C2 and McGregor's line on the lateral view. Normal value is 34 mm or greater in men, and 28 mm or greater in women[8] (Fig. 5-5).

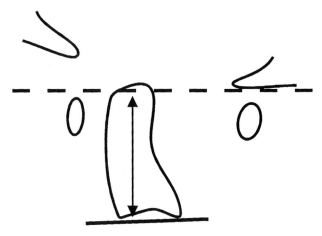

Fig. 5-5. Redlund-Johnell measurement. The *row of dashes* denotes McGregor's line.

b. Ranawat method: Assesses collapse of the C1-2 articulation by measuring from the center of the C2 pedicle to a line connecting the anterior arch and the spinous process of C1. Normal value is 14 mm or greater in men, and 13 mm or greater for women[9] (Fig. 5-6).

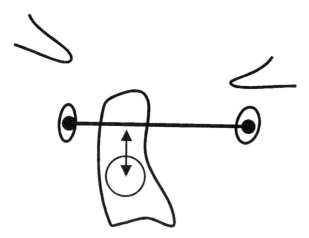

Fig. 5-6. Ranawat measurement.

CONGENITAL ANOMALIES
Chiari I Malformation

The Chiari I malformation consists of tonsillar displacement through the foramen magnum into the cervical spinal canal. The fourth ventricle retains its normal position. Commonly reported associations are syringo-hydromyelia and bony CVJ anomalies. Symptomatic populations tend to be older children and adults. A variety of symptoms can be present, including brain stem and cranial nerve findings such as facial pain, deafness, and vertigo. Cerebellar signs and paresthesias also occur. Multiple sclerosis is a common mimicking diagnosis.

Magnetic resonance findings

Minor downward displacement of the tonsils ("tonsillar ectopia") and the Chiari I malformation tend to form a spectrum of abnormalities. In tonsillar ectopia the cerebellar tonsils project slightly below the foramen magnum but retain their normal globular configuration. The brain stem and fourth ventricle are usually normal, and there is no syrinx. Various minor degrees of caudal displacement have been described. A reasonable upper limit of normal by sagittal MR is that the tonsils may project 2 mm below a line drawn from the inferior margin of the basion to the opisthion[10] (Fig. 5-7).

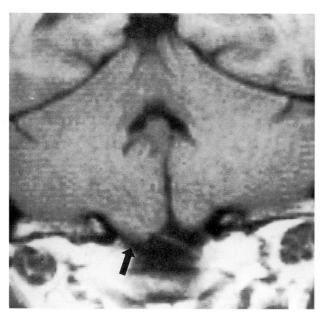

Fig. 5-7. Tonsillar ectopia. A coronal T$_1$-weighted image shows slight inferior displacement of the right cerebellar tonsil *(arrow)*. Note that it maintains its normal globular configuration.

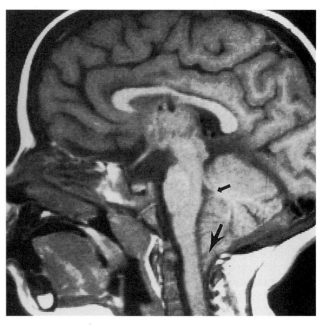

Fig. 5-8. Chiari I malformation. There is downward displacement of the cerebellar tonsils, which have an abnormal peglike configuration *(large arrow)*. The fourth ventricle maintains its normal position *(small arrow)*.

More recent evaluation of tonsillar position[11] has shown a striking variation with age, the tonsils ascending in older patients. The criteria of Mikulis et al.[11] for the lower limits of normal (2 standard deviations out of normal range) are as follows: first decade of life, 6 mm; second and third decades, 5 mm; fourth to eighth decades, 4 mm; ninth decade, 3 mm. The tonsils should have a smooth rounded configuration in both the coronal and the sagittal plane.

In the classic Chiari I malformation the tonsils assume an abnormal "peglike" configuration. Arachnoiditis can mat the tonsils, medulla, and cord together. Occasionally the tonsils may be so adherent that they are difficult to separate from the dorsal cord surface (Fig. 5-8). An additional clue to the diagnosis would be the presence of a syrinx cavity. Basilar invagination has been reported in up to 50% of Chiari I patients. The cisterna magna is usually small, and the incidence of hydrocephalus varies greatly from 0% to 44%.[12-14]

Chiari II Malformation

The Chiari II (Arnold-Chiari) malformation is defined by downward displacement of the brain stem and inferior cerebellum into the cervical spinal canal (Fig. 5-9). The fourth ventricle is a long sagittally flattened cavity with no obvious lateral recesses. The fourth ventricle also extends into the cervical spinal canal. The medulla may characteristically buckle in on itself (the cervicomedullary kink or spur) as it descends behind and below the upper cervical cord. This kink usually occurs between C2 and C4. The bony posterior fossa is quite small, and the foramen magnum symmetrically enlarged. The sagittal diameter of the C1 ring is less than that of the foramen magnum, so C1 may be displaced upward into the foramen. The lower vertebral column invariably demonstrates a myelocele or myelomeningocele. A syrinx is present to 40% to 90% of cases. Approximately 6% of cases will demonstrate diastematomyelia below C3.[15-19] McLone and Nadich[20] have put forth a unified theory as to the cause of Chiari II. The anomaly starts with a dorsal myeloschisis and subsequent failure to occlude the spinal neurocele. The primitive ventricular system thus fails to distend, which leads to a series of defects described as Chiari II.

Depending on the source consulted, basilar impression and/or assimilation of C1 to the occiput may or may not be associated with Chiari I and Chiari II malformations. With the superb anatomic fidelity of MR, determining this association becomes a matter of simply defining the parenchymal pathology and any bony CVJ anomalies present.

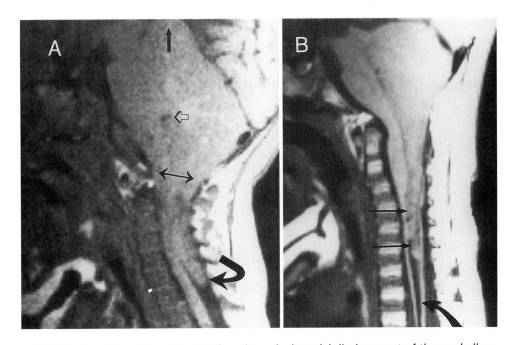

Fig. 5-9. Chiari II malformation. **A,** There is marked caudal displacement of the cerebellar tonsils *(curved arrow)* below the foramen magnum margin *(double arrow)*. The fourth ventricle is attenuated and barely visible *(open arrow)*. Note the superior projection of the vermis *(arrow)*, also called the cerebellar "pseudomass." **B,** Chiari II malformation wherein the choroid plexus *(arrows)* lies entirely within the cystic prolongation of the fourth ventricle, contiguous with the cervical syrinx cavity *(curved arrow)*.

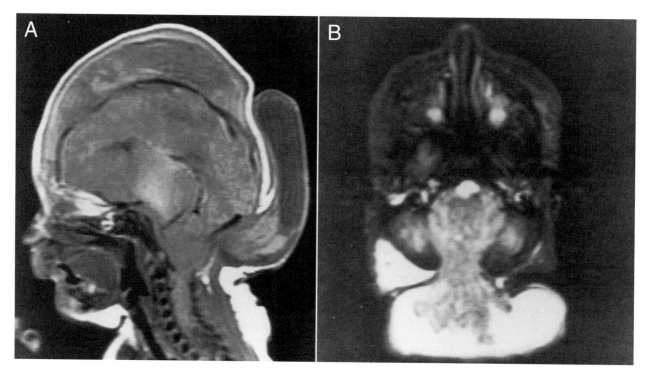

Fig. 5-10. Chiari III malformation. A sagittal T$_1$-weighted, **A**, and an axial T$_2$-weighted, **B**, demonstrate the large occipital high cervical myelomenigocele with herniation of cerebellar tissue. (Courtesy M. Shah, M.D., Cleveland.)

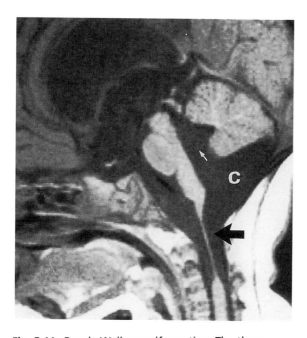

Fig. 5-11. Dandy-Walker malformation. The three components of this malformation are demonstrated: (1) hydrocephalus, (2) inferior vermian dysplasia, and (3) a retrovermian cyst *(C)* that communicates with the fourth ventricle *(white arrow)*. There is marked atrophy of the cervicomedullary junction *(black arrow)* due to birth trauma.

Chiari III Malformation

The Chiari III malformation is a rare abnormality that includes downward displacement of the medulla with herniation of the cerebellum through a high cervical spina bifida (Fig. 5-10).

Dandy-Walker Malformation

The Dandy-Walker malformation is a well-defined entity consisting of three features (Fig. 5-11):

1. Hydrocephalus
2. Incomplete fusion of the cerebellar vermis
3. Retrovermian cyst contiguous with the fourth ventricle[21,22]

The size of the cyst and whether it communicates with the subarachnoid space have no bearing on the diagnosis. The term *Dandy-Walker variant* (which has been applied to cases with a narrow slit between the cerebellar hemisphere) may be inappropriate since these cases do have the three necessary conditions to be simply Dandy-Walker. Other associated congenital anomalies include agenesis of the corpus callosum, holoprosencephaly, heterotopic gray matter, and occipital encephalocele (Fig. 5-12). Sagittal and axial T$_1$-weighted images are usually all that is required for identification of the malformation. Sagittal images are especially useful in defining the dysplastic vermis and connection of the cyst to the fourth ventricle. Look-alikes include a large cisterna magna and posterior fossa arachnoid cyst. However, neither of these shows the dysplasia and connection to the fourth ventricle of a true Dandy-Walker malformation.

Basilar Invagination

Basilar impression (or invagination) is a common congenital anomaly in the atlantooccipital region. It involves upward migration of the skull base around the foramen magnum and may be associated with intracranial extension of the dens. A primary congenital cause is occipitalization of the atlas. There are several secondary causes related to abnormal bone conditions—such as osteogenesis imperfecta (Fig. 5-13), Paget disease, rickets, osteomalacia, and hyperparathyroidism. Midline T_1-weighted images are ideal for defining the position of the odontoid process with respect to the foramen magnum and, more important, its effect in neutral, flexion, and extension on the cervicomedullary junction.

Achondroplasia

Achondroplasia is a congenital abnormality transmitted as an autosomal dominant. In the lumbar spine its features, such as a small spinal canal with progressively narrowing interpediculate spaces, are well known. More of a problem in the pediatric population is a small foramen magnum, or coarctation of the foramen (Fig. 5-14), which can cause respiratory problems, quadriparesis, and communicating hydrocephalus.[23] The hydrocephalus is sometimes secondary to obstruction of the small foramen magnum, or perhaps to venous outflow obstruction.[24] The foramen may be extremely small and narrowed in the transverse plane, with coronal imaging necessary to reveal the precise degree of cord impingement laterally. Basilar impression is seen in up to 50% of cases.[25]

Morquio Syndrome

The Morquio syndrome is a lysosomal storage disease thought to be secondary to an enzyme defect (galactosamine-6-sulfate-sulfatase β-galactosidase) and is transmitted as an autosomal recessive. Atlantoaxial subluxation secondary to ligamentous laxity is a regular feature. The foramen magnum may also be transversely small and narrow, similar to that seen in achondroplasia.[23] Patients with mucopolysaccharidosis can have leptomeningeal thickening and dural involvement as well as spinal stenosis and subluxation. Cord compression may be caused by atlantoaxial subluxation or by deposits of mucopolysaccharide in the anterior soft tissues. Water-soluble contrast myelography has been recommended for evaluating the cervical spine in these patients to define the spinal soft tissues precisely. MRI may also define CVJ abnormalities, including the deposits of mucopolysaccharide.[26,27]

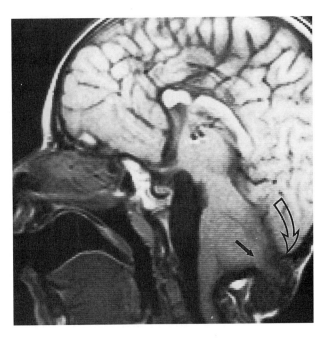

Fig. 5-12. Occipital encephalocele. The brain stem is tethered posteriorly when the cerebellum *(arrow)* herniates through the occipital-bone defect *(curved arrow).* (Courtesy Alison S. Smith, M.D., Cleveland.)

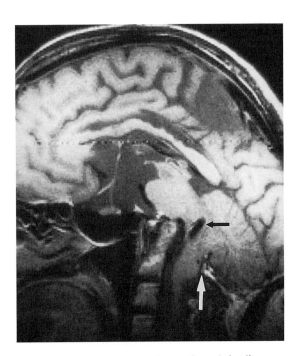

Fig. 5-13. Osteogenesis imperfecta. There is basilar invagination, with the odontoid compressing the pontomedullary junction. The opisthion is also superiorly displaced, with mass effect on the posterior medulla *(white arrow).* Note the extreme platybasia *(arrow* points to a tortuous vertebral artery).

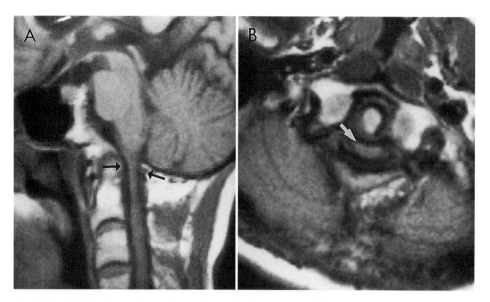

Fig. 5-14. Achrondroplasia. **A,** There is marked narrowing of the foramen magnum with compression of the cervicomedullary junction *(arrows).* **B,** An axial image confirms the anterior compression of the cord *(arrow).*

Down Syndrome

A variety of cervical spinal abnormalities have been reported in the Down syndrome. Atlantoaxial subluxation occurs, with a prevalence of between 10% and 22%, and several cases of atlantoaxial dislocation with cord compression have been reported.[28-32] Various other CVJ abnormalities are known, including odontoid hypoplasia, an os odontoideum, and hypoplasia of the posterior arch of C1.[33-35]

Martich et al.[34] evaluated the C1 posterior arch in 38 Down syndrome patients and found isolated hypoplasia in 26%. This has direct clinical relevance, since a small posterior arch causes more dramatic canal narrowing, which would be exacerbated with any atlantoaxial subluxation.

Osseous Abnormalities

The CVJ osseous abnormalities may consist of a variety of segmentation errors and subluxations. Polytomography or CT scanning with bone algorithms may be necessary to define the bony anatomy precisely. MR is capable of roughly defining the bony anatomy using a combination of signal void produced by cortical bone and high signal from yellow marrow (e.g., clivus, anterior and posterior arches of C1, and dens). MR excels at defining any distortion of the brain stem or cervical cord by its portrayal of the osseous abnormalities on T_1-weighted sagittal images. Flexion and extension views add the element of motion and can disclose C1-2 subluxations and basilar invagination as well as whether they are reducible (Fig. 5-15).

Atlantoaxial Subluxations

In children the ADI should be no larger than 4 mm whereas in adults the upper limit of normal is 2.5 to 3 mm. It must be kept in mind that these measurements are based on ossified portions of the C1 anterior arch as shown by plain radiographs. Care is needed in applying any measurements to MR images in children, in whom cartilage and synovial joints may be readily visualized. Congenital causes of atlantoaxial instability include the Down syndrome, spondyloepiphyseal dysplasia, osteogenesis imperfecta, and neurofibromatosis. However, with these congenital causes the presence of an increased ADI in flexion may not signal the need for stabilization nor are the patients necessarily symptomatic. Of more physiologic importance is the space available for the cord (SAC), measured from the dens to the nearest posterior bony structure (e.g., the opisthion or the posterior arch of C1). Cord impression always occurs if the SAC is 14 mm or less.[36]

Klippel-Feil Syndrome

The Klippel-Feil syndrome is a condition in patients with congenital fusion of the cervical vertebrae (Figs. 5-16 and 5-17). The classic triad consists of a low posterior hairline, limited range of motion, and a short neck. Although occipitalization of the atlas, hemivertebrae, and basilar impression occur more frequently in this syndrome, as isolated entities they are not designated Klippel-Feil.[37] Sagittal T_1-weighted sequences define the levels of congenital fusion by the thinner, "wasp-waist" appearance of the fused segments. The segments dem-

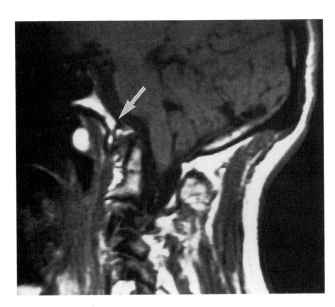

Fig. 5-15. Assimilation of C1 with the basiocciput. The high signal of the marrow of the lower clivus merges with that of the anterior arch of C1 *(arrow)*. The anterior arch is abnormally positioned with respect to both the clivus and the dens. There is an increased atlantodental interval.

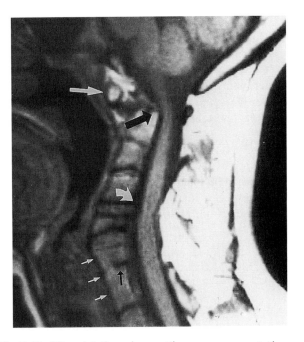

Fig. 5-16. Klippel-Feil syndrome. There are segmentation anomalies involving C2-3 and C6-7. Level C6-7 has no "wasp-waist" configuration *(small white arrows),* with only a small remnant of the disk space *(small black arrow).* Note the reverse atlantoaxial subluxation with compression of the cervicomedullary junction *(black arrow).* Additionally, the C4-5 disk is herniated *(curved arrow). White arrow,* Anterior arch of C1.

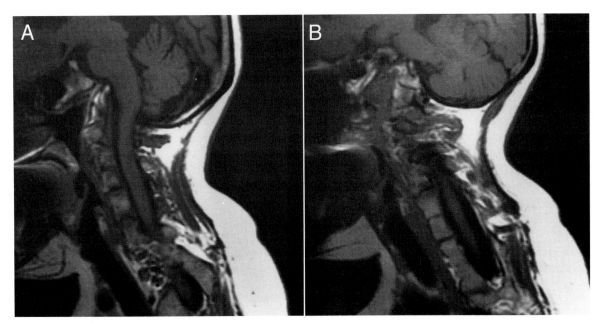

Fig. 5-17. Klippel-Feil syndrome. There are multiple segmentation abnormalities involving the entire cervical spine. Note the upward translocation of the dens and the multiple fusions of lower cervical and upper thoracic bodies in the typical "wasp-waist" configuration.

onstrate normal marrow signal. Frequently a thin horizontal line of decreased signal intensity is present in a central portion of the fusion, representing the rudimentary disk space. Flexion and extension views are useful for determining any atlantoaxial instability. Changes in stress on the spine secondary to fusion can cause disk herniations above and below the fusion levels.

Os Odontoideum

A true os odontoideum is relatively rare—manifesting as a separate bone between the basion and the normal odontoid tip. Many cases described as os odontoideum are the result of an unrecognized fracture through the base of the odontoid, which subsequently becomes distracted by the alar ligaments toward the basion[38] (Figs. 5-18 and 5-19). When there is complete resorption of the fractured dens, the mistake is to consider this a congenital absence of the dens.

Sherman and Kopits[39] reported the MR findings in 80 patients with a variety of skeletal dysplasias. An os odontoideum was present in eight of the patients, with evidence of C1-2 instability in all eight and signs of myelopathy in five. The types of dysplasias included mucopolysaccharidosis, spondylometaphyseal dysplasia, metatropic dysplasia, and Conradi disease. The authors stated that patients with skeletal dysplasia are more likely

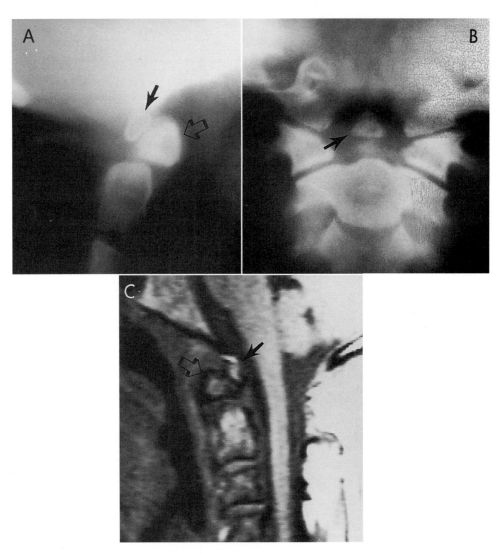

Fig. 5-18. Old odontoid fracture. **A,** Sagittal tomogram. Note the hyperplastic anterior arch of C1 *(open arrow)* and the small remnant of odontoid *(arrow)*. **B,** A coronal tomogram demonstrates the smoothly corticated odontoid fragment *(arrow)*. **C,** A sagittal MR also demonstrates the fragment *(arrow)* relative to the anterior C1 arch *(open arrow)*. The odontoid fracture occurred after posterior fusion.

to have an os odontoideum and are at increased risk of subluxation with acute or chronic myelopathy. This is particularly important because of the high incidence of associated bony disorders in these patients leading to orthopedic procedures and the risks of anesthesia with the CVJ abnormality.[39]

Infection

Pyogenic osteomyelitis of the occiput, atlas, and axis is a rare entity, with less than 10 cases reported in the literature. Diabetes mellitus appears to be a predisposing factor. Nevertheless, it is important to consider since it can be fatal due to cervical instability and cord compression from lysis of the transverse ligament. The clinical diagnosis may be difficult, with vague symptoms and no severe pain. *Staphylococcus aureus* is the organism most commonly involved. MR findings in more advances cases include the typical loss of endplate definition, with prevertebral soft tissue, and epidural extension with cord compression[40] (Figs. 5-20 and 5-21).

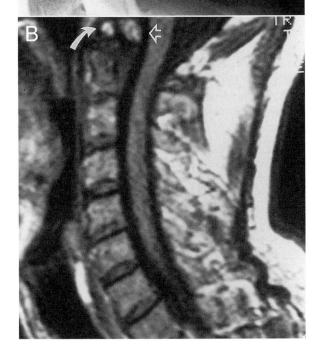

Fig. 5-19. Os odontoideum. The lateral view of a myleogram, **A,** and a sagittal T₁-weighted MR, **B,** both demonstrate the large odontoid tip remnant *(open arrow)* and the posteriorly displaced hyperplasic anterior arch of C1 *(curved arrow).*

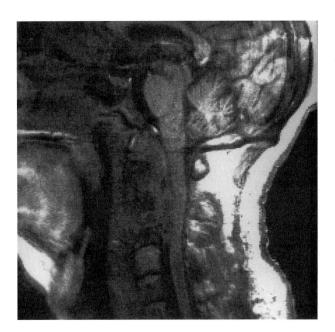

Fig. 5-20. Pyogenic infection of the upper cervical spine. Note the diffuse low signal intensity involving C2 through C4, with obliterated disk spaces, and the large posterior epidural abcess that displaces the cord. (From Smith AS, Blaser SI: *Radiol Clin North Am* 1991;29[4]:809-827.)

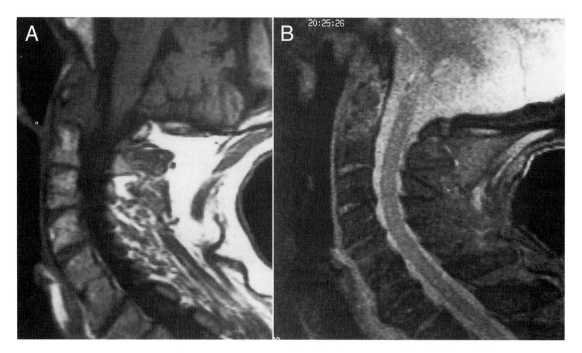

Fig. 5-21. Pyogenic infection of C2. *Staphylococcus aureus*–caused osteomyelitis with low signal intensity involving the upper portion of C2 on this T_1-weighted spin-echo sequence and obscuration of the periodontoid fat planes, **A.** The sagittal gradient echo shows destruction of the odontoid (with increased signal), **B.**

TUMORS

Brain stem gliomas are a fairly common tumor, representing 10% to 15% of childhood neoplasms or 20% of infratentorial childhood tumors. Histologic evidence of malignancy is common. Sagittal and axial T_1- and T_2-weighted images are best for defining areas of pathology as well as compression of adjacent structures (e.g., the fourth ventricle or midbrain) (Fig. 5-22). Brain stem gliomas usually show marked expansion of the brain stem, which will appear hypointense on T_1-weighted and hyperintense on T_2-weighted images. The exophytic components and their relationship to the basilar artery (seen well because of the flow void) are also easily defined. A large expansile mass in the brain stem with these signal characteristics is pathognomonic for brain stem glioma in a child.[41] In adults metastatic disease must be a prime consideration (Fig. 5-23). Other intraparenchymal lesions of the posterior fossae that must be included in the differential are cerebellar hemispheric or tonsillar gliomas, infection, and infarction. Tumors and infection distort the architecture and produce mass effect. Infarcts generally preserve the gross morphology of gray and white matter (albeit abnormal in signal intensity) and produce less mass effect for the overall lesion size.

The most common extraaxial lesions occurring at the CVJ are meningiomas and neurinomas (Figs. 5-24 to 5-26). The posterior fossa accounts for approximately 10% of intracranial meningiomas. These are usually smooth well-defined tumors that displace the CMJ, caus-

ing symptoms by pressure or vascular compromise rather than by parenchymal destruction. On T_1- and T_2-weighted images meningiomas are commonly isointense to brain parenchyma, so the gross anatomic picture must be carefully evaluated. Neurinomas, being well-defined extramedullary lesions, closely resemble meningiomas; they are usually isointense on T_1-weighted sequences but may be isointense to hyperintense on T_2-weighted images. Both neurinomas and meningiomas show marked enhancement with paramagnetic contrast agents on T_1-weighted images. However, not all extramedullary tumoral masses of the CVJ are neurofibromas or meningiomas. We have seen one case of a posterior inferior cerebellar arterial (PICA) aneurysm that was initially interpreted as a meningioma because of its low signal on T_1- and T_2-weighted images that, in retrospect, was secondary to organized thrombus within the aneurysm (Fig. 5-27). Other extraaxial prepontine tumors that must be considered include chordoma, nasopharyngeal carcinoma, metastasis, multiple myeloma, chondroma, osteochondroma, and osteoma (Figs. 5-28 and 5-29). All these may present as a soft tissue mass destroying the clivus.

Chordomas are uncommon tumors derived from notochordal remnants. They tend to be locally aggressive and infrequently metastasize. Plain films and CT will show calcification (20% to 70%) and bone destruction. Because they arise from notochordal remnants, they may be found throughout the spinal column, with a prepon-

Text continued on p. 213.

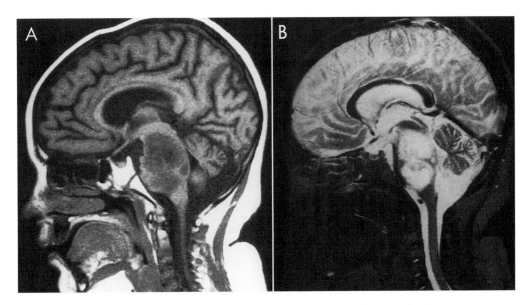

Fig. 5-22. Brain stem glioma. T_1-weighted, **A,** and cardiac-gated T_2-weighted, **B,** images show a large exophytic brain stem mass with prolonged T_1 and T_2 relaxation times. The caudal and cephalic edges of the tumor are well defined.

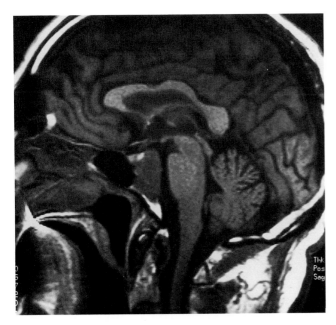

Fig. 5-23. Metastatic adenocarcinoma. A sagittal T_1-weighted image demonstrates a low–signal intensity mass replacing the basisphenoid marrow signal.

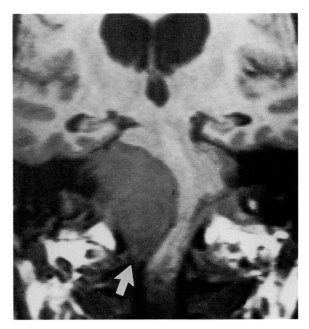

Fig. 5-24. Meningioma. The large extraaxial mass compresses the brain stem and has caused hydrocephalus. Note its extension below the level of the foramen magnum *(arrow).*

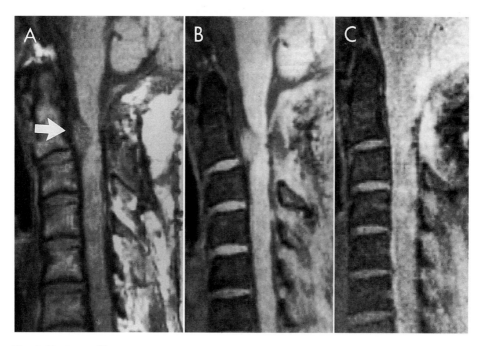

Fig. 5-25. Neurofibroma. **A,** A sagittal T_1-weighted spin-echo image shows the extramedullary mass arising anteriorly at the C2 level *(arrow).* **B,** The gradient echo fast low-angle shot (FLASH) with a 60-degree flip angle demonstrates an extramedullary lesion. **C,** A gradient echo FLASH with a 10-degree flip angle causes the CSF to increase in signal relative to the parenchyma, thus obscuring the tumor.

Fig. 5-26. Neurofibroma. A sagittal T_1-weighted image shows the large soft tissue mass at C1 displacing the cord out of the midline *(arrow).*

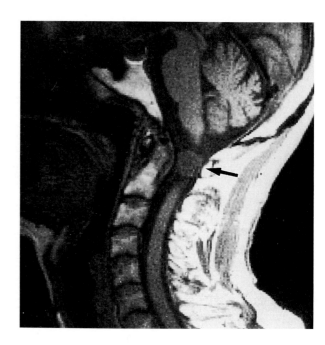

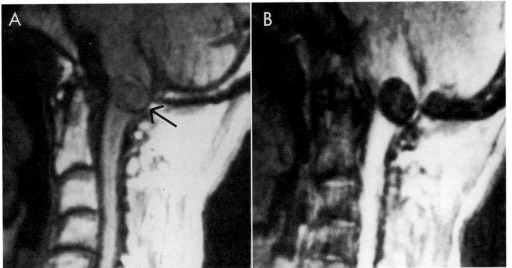

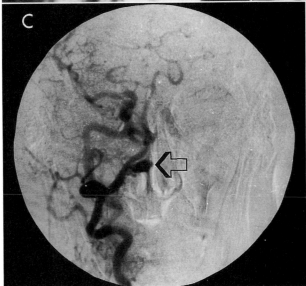

Fig. 5-27. Partially thrombosed posterior inferior cerebellar arterial (PICA) aneurysm. **A,** The sagittal T$_1$-weighted image shows a well-defined circular mass *(arrow)* of peripheral low signal intensity at the foramen magnum level. **B,** A T$_2$-weighted image shows markedly decreased signal from the aneurysm due to preferential T$_2$ relaxation from the thrombus. **C,** An anteroposterior digital subtraction angiogram (DSA) shows the aneurysm rising off the origin of the right PICA *(arrow).*

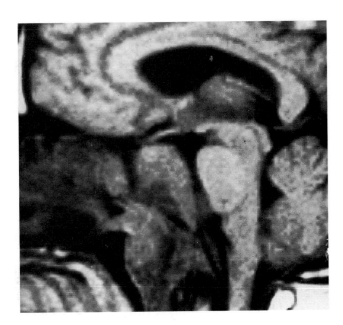

Fig. 5-28. Nasopharyngeal carcinoma. A sagittal T$_1$-weighted image shows soft tissue replacing the nasopharynx, clivus, and prevertebral space. The pituitary is not distinctly seen. (Courtesy Frederick Dengel, M.D., Cleveland.)

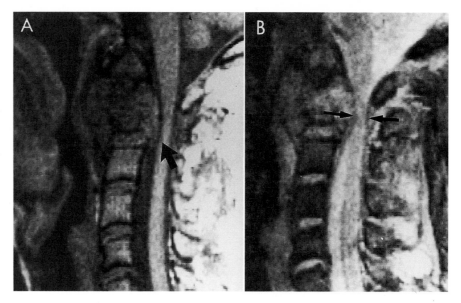

Fig. 5-29. Metastatic paraganglioma. **A,** Sagittal T$_2$-weighted image. A large soft tissue mass has destroyed the C2 body and is compressing the cervical cord *(arrow)*. **B,** Gradient echo (FLASH) with 10-degree flip angle. The destruction of C2 and the cord compression *(arrows)* are well visualized.

Fig. 5-30. Chordoma. Sagittal, **A,** and axial, **B,** T$_1$-weighted images show a homogeneous mass involving the right basisphenoid with extension into the prepontine cistern. The tumor surrounds the petrous carotid on three sides. An axial T$_2$-weighted image, **C,** shows heterogeneous signal from the mass and increased signal from the anterior pons (related to previous radiation therapy).

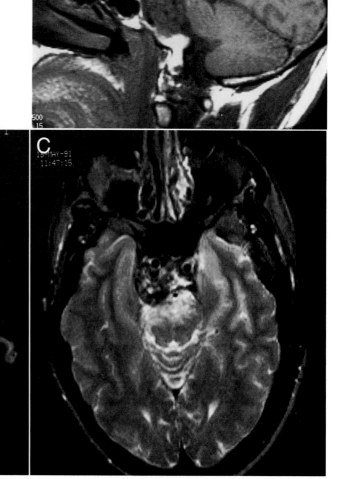

derance in the sacrococcygeal (50% to 70%) and clival (15% to 25%) regions. In the spine the cervical (especially C2) region is the most common location.

The MR findings with chordoma are nonspecific — intermediate signal on T_1-weighted images destroying or involving bone. Like other tumors, they will show increased signal on T_2-weighted images (Fig. 5-30).

DOLICHOECTASIA OF THE BASILAR ARTERY AND VERTEBRAL ARTERIES

The most common correctable reason for trigeminal neuralgia and hemifacial spasm is vascular compression of the fifth and seventh cranial nerves. This may be caused by a tortuous or dolichoectatic vertebral basilar system. A loop of the superior cerebellar artery usually is responsible for fifth-nerve symptoms whereas a loop of the anterior inferior cerebellar artery (AICA) compresses the seventh nerve exit zone.[42]

The course of the vascular system is usually well defined on T_1-weighted sagittal and axial images, as is the mass effect on the brain stem (Figs. 5-31 and 5-32).

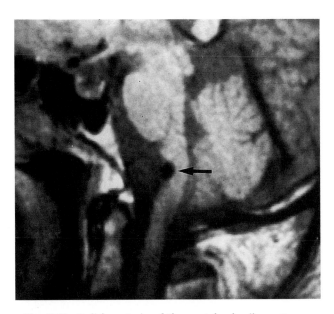

Fig. 5-31. Dolichoectasia of the vertebrobasilar system. A tortuous vertebral artery *(arrow)* indents the anterior medulla.

Fig. 5-32. Left hemifacial spasm. The axial T_2-weighted image, **A,** shows a flow void adjacent to the root exit zone of cranial nerves VII and VIII *(arrow)*. The anterior view of an MR angiogram maximum intensity projection, **B,** demonstrates a tortuous left vertebral artery extending to the left of midline *(arrow)*. Note on an individual slice from the MR angiogram, **C,** the proximity of the left vertebral artery to the exiting VII and VIII nerve complex *(arrow)*.

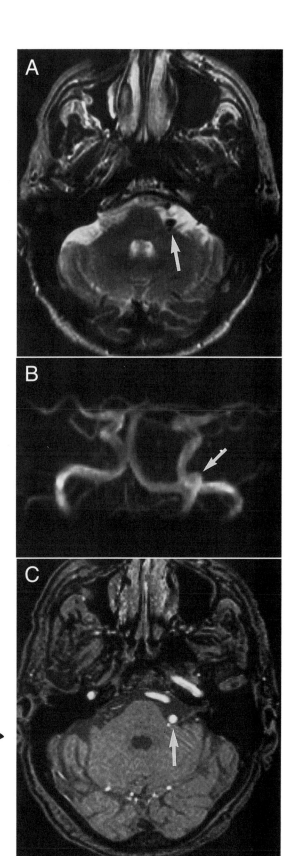

Long TR/TE odd-echo images provide excellent contrast between the increased-signal CSF and the flow void within the vessels. Even-echo T_2-weighted images may rephase enough flow to decrease the conspicuousness of the vessels. Slow flow can demonstrate increased signal on T_1-weighted images. MR angiography defines with high detail the vascular loops implicated in nerve compression. Both the maximum intensity projections and the individual slices need to be evaluated for subtle mass effect and vessel position. However, a significant degree of compression by MR may or may not correlate with a patient's symptomatology.

REFERENCES

1. Lee, BC, Kneeland JB, Deck MDF, et al: Posterior fossae lesions: magnetic resonance imaging. *Radiology* 1984;153:137-143.
2. Taveras JM, Wood EH: *Diagnostic neuroradiology.* Baltimore, Williams & Wilkins, 1976, pp 51-60.
3. McGregor M: The significance of certain measurements of the skull in diagnosis of basilar impression. *Br J Radial* 1948;21:171-181.
4. Fischgold H, David M, Bregeat P: *La tomographie de la base du crâne en neurochirurgie et neuro-ophtalmologie.* Paris, Masson, 1952.
5. Hinck VC, Hopkins CE: Measurement of the atlanto-dental interval in the adult. *AJR* 1960;84:945-951.
6. VanGilder JC, Meneges AH: Craniovertebral junction abnormalities. *Clin Neurosurg* 1983;30:514-530.
7. McRae DL, Barnum AS: Occipitalization of the atlas. *AJR* 1953;70:23-46.
8. Redlund-Johnell I, Petterson H: Radiographic measurements of the cranio-vertebral region. *Acta Radiol Diagn* 1984;25:23-28.
9. Ranawat CS, O'Leary P, Pellicci P, et al: Cervical spine fusion in rheumatoid arthritis. *J Bone Joint Surg [Am]* 1979;61:1003-1010.
10. Barkovich AJ, Wippold FJ, Sherman JL, et al: Significance of cerebellar tonsillar position on MR. *AJR* 1986;97:795-799.
11. Mikulis DJ, Diaz O, Egglin TK, Sanchez R: Variance of the position of the cerebellar tonsils with age: preliminary report. *Radiology* 1992;183:725-728.
12. DuBoulay G, Shah SH, Currie JC, et al: The mechanism of hydromyelia in Chiari type I malformations. *Br J Radiol* 1974;47:579-587.
13. Rhoton AL: Microsurgery of Arnold-Chiari malformations in adults with and without hydromyelia. *J Neurosurg* 1976;45:473-487.
14. Forbes WS, Isherwood I: Computed tomography in syringomyelia and the associated Arnold-Chiari type I malformation. *Neuroradiology* 1978;15:73-78.
15. Naidich TP, Pudlowski RM, Naidich JB, et al: Computed tomographic signs of the Chiari II malformation. I. Skull and dural partitions. *Radiology* 1980;134:65-71.
16. Naidich TP, Pudlowski RM, Naidich JB: Computed tomographic signs of Chiari II malformation. II. Midbrain and cerebellum. *Radiology* 1980;134:391-398.
17. Naidich TP, Pudlowski RM, Naidich JB: Computed tomographic signs of the Chiari II malformation. III. Ventricles and cisterns. *Radiology* 1980;134:657-663.
18. Naidich TP, McLane DG, Fulling KH: The Chiari II malformation. IV. The midbrain deformity. *Neuroradiology* 1983;25:179-197.
19. Wolpert SM, Anderson M, Scott RM, et al: Chiari II malformation: MR imaging evaluation. *AJNR* 1987;8:783-792.
20. McLone DG, Naidich TP: Developmental morphology of the subarachnoid space, brain vasculature, and contiguous structures, and the cause of the Chiari II malformation. *AJNR* 1992;13:463-482.
21. Harwood-Nash DC, Fitz CR: Congenital malformations of the brain. In Harwood-Nash DC, Fitz CR (eds): *Neuroradiology in infants and children.* St Louis, Mosby, 1976; vol 3, pp 998-1053.
22. Masdeu JC, Dobben GD, Azar-Kia B: Dandy-Walker syndrome studied by computed tomography and pneumoencephalography. *Radiology* 1983;147:109-114.
23. Naidich TP, McLane DG, Harwood-Nash DC: Systemic malformations. In Newton TH, Potts DG (eds): *Computed tomography of the spine and spinal cord.* San Anselmo Calif, Clavadel, 1983.
24. Yamada H, Nakamura S, Tajima M, et al: Neurological manifestations of pediatric achondroplasia. *J Neurosurg* 1981;54:49-57.
25. Luyendijk W: Proceedings of the Society of British Neurological Surgeons. (Abstract.) *J Neurol Neurosurg Psychiatry* 1978;41:1053.
26. Edwards MK, Harwood-Nash DC, Fitz CR, et al: CT metrizamide myelography of the cervical spine in Morquio syndrome. *AJNR* 1982;3:666-669.
27. Kulkarni MV, Williams JC, Yeakley JW, et al: Magnetic resonance imaging in the diagnosis of the cranio-cervical manifestations of the mucopolysaccharidoses. *Magn Reson Imaging* 1987;5:317-323.
28. Martel W, Tishler JM: Observations on the spine in mongoloidism. *AJR* 1966;97:630-638.
29. Pueschel SM, Scola FH: Atlantoaxial instability in individuals with Down syndrome: epidemiologic, radiographic, and clinical studies. *Pediatrics* 1987;80:555-560.
30. Burke SW, French HG, Roberts JM, et al: Chronic atlantoaxial instability in Down syndrome. *J Bone Joint Surg [Am]* 1985;67:1356-1360.
31. Hreidarsson S, Magram G, Singer H: Symptomatic atlantoaxial dislocation in Down syndrome. *Pediatrics* 1982;69:568-571.
32. Martel W, Uyham R, Stimson CW: Subluxation of the atlas causing spinal cord compression in a case of Down's syndrome with a "manifestation of an occipital vertebra." *Radiology* 1969;93:839-840.
33. Coria F, Quintana F, Villalba A, et al: Craniocervical abnormalities in Down's syndrome. *Develop Med Child Neurol* 1983;25:252-254.
34. Elliott S: The odontoid process in children; is it hypoplastic? *Clin Radiol* 1988;39:391-393.
35. Martich V, Ben-Ami T, Yousefzadeh DK, et al: Hypoplastic posterior arch of C-1 in children with Down syndrome: a double jeopardy. *Radiology* 1992;183:125-128.

36. Greenberg AD: Atlanto-axial dislocations. *Brain* 1968;91:655.

37. Pizzutillo PD: Klippel-Feil. In Cervical Spine Research Society: *The cervical spine*. Philadelphia, Lippincott, 1983, pp 174-188.

38. Fielding JW, Hensinger RN, Hawkins RJ: Os odontoideum. *J Bone Joint Surg [Am]* 1980;62:376.

39. Sherman JL, Kopits SE. MR imaging appearance of os odontoidium in skeletal dysplasia. Presented at the SMRI, 1992.

40. Zigler JE, Bohlman HH, Robinson RR, et al: Pyogenic osteomyelitis of the occiput, the atlas, and the axis. *J Bone Joint Surg [Am]* 1987;69:1069-1073.

41. Hueftle MG, Han JS, Kaufman B, et al: MR imaging of brainstem gliomas. *J Comput Assist Tomogr* 1985;9:263-267.

42. Sobel D, Norman D, Yorke CH, et al: Radiography of trigeminal neuralgia and hemifacial spasm. *AJNR* 1980;1:251-253.

6

Inflammatory Disease

JEFFREY S. ROSS

Inflammatory disorders of the spine that will be covered in this chapter include arachnoiditis, disk space infection (DSI), epidural abscess, tuberculous and brucellar spondylitis, hemodialysis spondyloarthropathy, ankylosing spondylitis, and rheumatoid arthritis. These diverse processes have sarcoidosis, presenting symptomatologies that are often nonspecific. Imaging plays a key role in defining the abnormalities and guiding the clinician toward proper management. Magnetic resonance imaging has replaced the more conventional imaging modalities (myelography for arachnoiditis, scintigraphy for DSI) and can help in early and specific diagnosis.

ARACHNOIDITIS

It has been stated[1] that in 6% to 16% of patients who have undergone spinal surgery, spinal arachnoiditis is the cause of persistent symptoms. However, to date no rigorous scientific study has been published that would substantiate this figure. Furthermore, there is no established correlation of morphologic features with patient symptomatology. The clinical diagnosis of arachnoiditis is often difficult since the disease has no distinct symptom complex. The pathogenesis of spinal arachnoiditis is similar to the repair process in serous membranes, such as the peritoneum, which demonstrate little inflammatory cellular or fibrinous exudate. The fibrin-covered roots stick to themselves and to the thecal sac. With time, dense collagenous adhesions are formed by the proliferating fibrocytes during the repair phase.[2]

Previously the diagnosis of arachnoiditis was confirmed by myelography and, less commonly, by computed tomography and surgery. Myelography in spinal arachnoiditis may show a variety of patterns—including prominent cauda equina nerve roots, a homogeneous contrast pattern without nerve root shadows, and subarachnoid filling defects with concomitant narrowing and

shortening of the thecal sac. Jorgensen et al.[3] divided the myelographic patterns into a *type I* group, which is due to adhesions of the roots inside the meninges, giving a root "sleeveless" appearance, and a *type II* group, which demonstrates filling defects, narrowing, shortening, and occlusion of the thecal sac. Type I is seen with mild disease whereas type II is the picture accompanying more extensive adhesions.[4] By CT myelography the early adhesions are seen in the distal thecal sac as a loss of nerve root sleeve filling. Roots become adherent to each other and to the meninges, which leads to the appearance of an "empty sac."[5] As this transmeningeal fibrosis continues, clumping becomes more prominent until the thecal sac and roots are one confluent soft tissue mass. This produces a myelographic block and has been considered the end stage of arachnoiditis.[6] Surface coil MR utilizing slice thicknesses less than 5 mm can also define abnormal patterns of nerve roots within the thecal sac.

Sequences

Both T_1- and T_2-weighted sequences are useful for the optimum definition of arachnoiditis. The single most efficient sequence is probably the axial T_1-weighted, for it allows a moderate degree of confidence in defining all types of arachnoiditis. A recent report[7] has stated that the heavily T_2-weighted sequence cannot distinguish inflammatory tissue (e.g., arachnoiditis) within the thecal sac by using body coil MR. In our experience with surface coil MR, however, the T_2-weighted axial study is helpful for defining the distribution of roots within the thecal sac and provides greater contrast sensitivity than is possible with T_1-weighted images, at least in the less severely affected groups. Nevertheless, the pathology in the type II group of Jorgensen et al.[3] (large soft tissue mass within the thecal sac) could be masked by the high signal from fibrosis and adhesions, which mimics normal cerebrospinal fluid signal on the T_2-weighted study.

Normal Variations

Since the pattern and positioning of new roots within the thecal sac are critical for defining arachnoiditis, the normal variations must first be considered. We examined 20 patients with no previous history of myelography or spinal surgery referred for an MR study for low back pain, to be used as a control group for nerve root distribution. Ten of these patients had had plain film myelograms or CT myelograms within a week of the MR study. We examined a total of 54 vertebral body levels.

At the L2 level the roots are seen as a mass of intermediate soft tissue signal on T_1-weighted images in the dependent portion of the thecal sac, forming a smooth crescent that follows the curvature of the sac. At the L3 level they are often amassed posteriorly (the dependent position) and may be globular and irregular or crescentic and smooth in appearance. The roots about to exit the dural tube are placed anterolaterally in a symmetric pattern. At the L4 level they have dispersed and are seen as separate delicate entities arranged in a symmetric pattern within the CSF. By the L5 level the few roots present are equally spaced within the thecal sac. Central conglomeration is conspicuously lacking at the L5 level. Midline sagittal images show the roots as a single band of intermediate signal intensity on T_1-weighted images, following the curvature of the posterior thecal sac. This band gradually tapers from the conus to the L4 level. Parasagittal images nicely demonstrate the roots fanning out from the conus as they travel from the posterior-superior position of the conus to the anterior-inferior L5 level.

Pathology

The MR morphologic changes of arachnoiditis can be divided into three groups[8]:

In group I large conglomerations of nerve roots reside centrally within the thecal sac (Fig. 6-1) and are seen on T_1-weighted images as well-defined rounded areas of intermediate soft tissue signal. Some improvement in definition occurs with the high contrast provided by the CSF signal on T_2-weighted images. The CT-myelographic appearance in this group is similar to that of T_2-weighted MR images, showing a central thickening of the roots. Myelograms may vary in appearance, from loss of definition of the root sleeves with thickened roots present intrathecally to moderate narrowing and irregularity of the contrast column.

In group II clumped nerve roots are attached peripherally to the meninges (Figs. 6-2 to 6-4) and appear as areas of focal thickening of the meninges, with few or no nerve roots visible in the subarachnoid space. T_2-weighted images provide the best definition of peripheral nerve roots and the central homogeneous CSF signal. The appearance is essentially one of an "empty thecal sac." CT-myelograms also show the focal thickening of soft tissue–attenuation nerve roots peripherally along the meninges. The central portion of the subarachnoid space shows homogeneous intrathecal contrast, with no appreciable nerve roots. Myelograms in this group will disclose a capacious thecal sac with a smooth outer border, amputation of the root sleeves, and no nerve roots in the caudal thecal sac.

In group III increased soft tissue signal within the thecal sac below the conus obliterates most of the subarachnoid space on T_1-weighted images (Fig. 6-5). T_2-weighted images show increased signal diffusely from the thecal sac without definition of individual nerve roots. CT-myelography shows increased–soft tissue attenuation material within the subarachnoid space. Small loculated areas of contrast may be seen peripherally. Myelography commonly demonstrates a block of distally visualized subarachnoid space, with an irregular "candle dripping" appearance.

Of course, variations and combinations of these groups may be seen. One fairly frequently observed combination is group I with group II (Fig. 6-6). Often at the L3 or L4 level the roots are seen to clump centrally. As they progress caudally, they fan out and attach peripherally to the meninges, giving an empty thecal sac appearance by the L5 level.

These abnormalities of nerve roots are uniformly seen at the L3 level or below. In more than 25 patients we have studied with lumbar arachnoiditis the abnormal configuration of nerve roots was seen over at least two vertebral body levels.

In one series[8] we identified the changes of arachnoiditis by MR in 11 of 12 cases that had been demonstrated by CT-myelography and plain film myelography. This represented a sensitivity of 92%, a specificity of 100%, and an accuracy of 99%. Our group I and group II patients appeared to fall within the type I category of Jorgensen et al.,[3] the main difference being the distinction between central and peripheral clumping of nerve roots. More severe disease, categorized as Jorgensen type II, was reflected in our group III, with soft tissue replacing the subarachnoid space on CT and MR (giving rise to the myelographic block).

False-negative and false-positive MR studies are inevitable. Both may be caused by suboptimal MR scans, in which patient motion or poor signal-to-noise can give the appearance of no nerve roots within the thecal sac as well as central clumping.

It is possible for the normal appearance of nerve roots at the L2 or L3 level to be mistaken for arachnoiditis. In routine practice, however, this is not a problem since arachnoiditis involves the L3 level and below and also extends over at least two lumbar body levels. Arachnoid-

Text continued on p. 222.

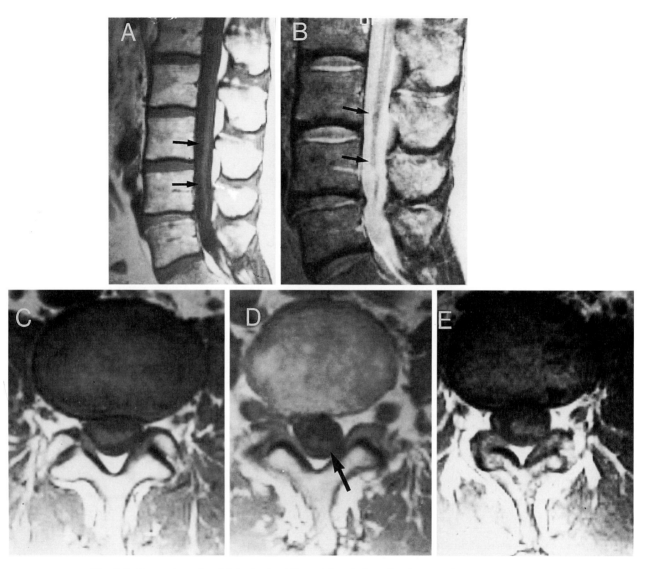

Fig. 6-1. Group I arachnoiditis. Sagittal T$_1$-weighted, **A** and **B,** images show nerve roots conglomerating centrally into a linear mass of soft tissue signal *(arrows)*. An axial T$_1$-weighted image, **C,** at the L3-4 level also demonstrates the abnormally clumped roots. At the L5 body level, **D,** the roots continue to be centrally clumped *(arrow)*. An axial T$_1$-weighted image, **E,** in a different patient shows the typical appearance of centrally clumped nerve roots. (From Ross JS, Masaryk TJ, Modic MT, et al: *AJNR* 1987;8:885-892.)

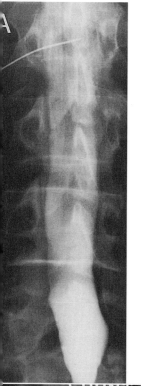

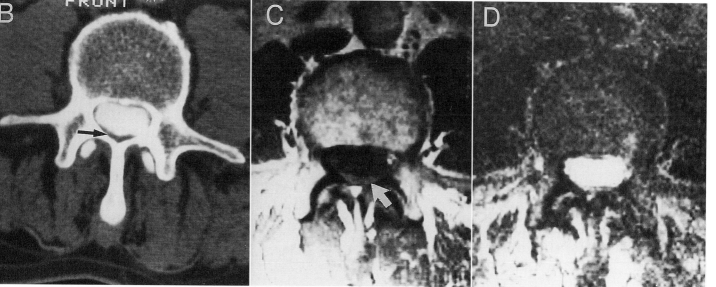

Fig. 6-2. Group II arachnoiditis. A water-soluble contrast myelogram, **A,** shows an amorphous collection of contrast in the caudal thecal sac, with no visible nerve roots or root sleeves. CT following the myelogram, **B,** confirms that the roots are adhering peripherally to the meninges *(arrow).* An axial T_1-weighted MR, **C,** also shows the "empty thecal sac" and the peripherally clumped roots *(arrow).* **D,** The axial T_2-weighted image confirms that no roots are visible within the sac. (From Ross JS, Masaryk TJ, Modic MT, et al: *AJNR* 1987;8:885-892.)

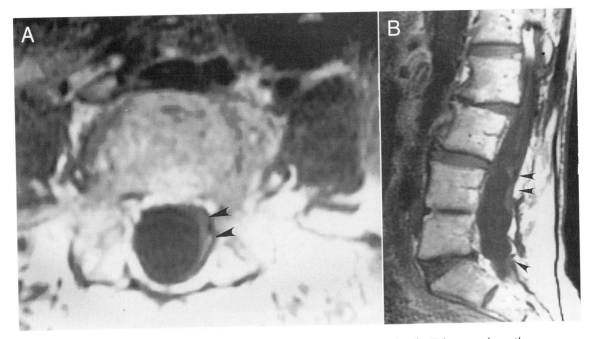

Fig. 6-3. Group II arachnoiditis. **A,** Axial and, **B,** sagittal T_1-weighted MR images show the distal "empty thecal sac" and peripherally clumped roots *(arrowheads)*.

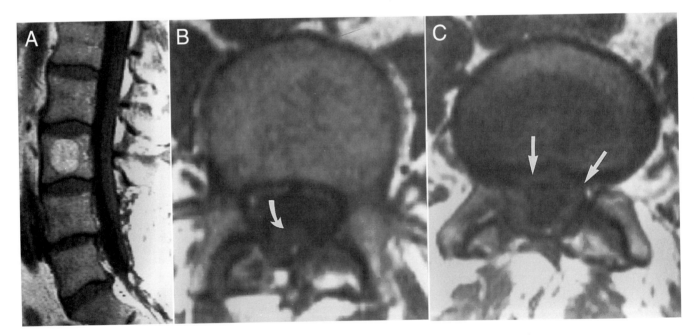

Fig. 6-4. Combination group I and group II arachnoiditis. A sagittal T_1-weighted, **A,** demonstrates the nerve roots posteriorly displaced at the L4 and L5 levels. An axial MR at the superior aspect of L4, **B,** shows the central clumping of group I arachnoiditis *(curved arrow)* whereas the inferior slice at the L4-5 disk level, **C,** shows peripheral clumping of group II *(arrows)*.

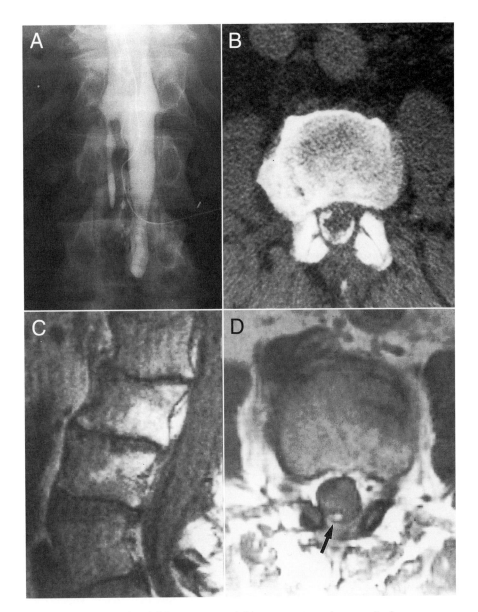

Fig. 6-5. Group III arachnoiditis. A water-soluble contrast myelogram, **A,** shows an irregular block at the L2-3 level with a "candle-dripping" appearance. (The thin wire along the midline is a dorsal column simulator for pain control.) A CT scan following the myelogram, **B,** shows abnormal soft tissue attenuation material within the thecal sac. The sagittal T_1-weighted MR, **C,** shows a large mass of inflammatory tissue filling the thecal sac. Note the extensive laminectomy. **D,** Axial T_1-weighted MR also showing the intrathecal soft tissue mass with a small amount of Pantopaque posteriorly *(arrow).* (From Ross JS, Masaryk TJ, Modic MT, et al: *AJNR* 1987;8:885-892.)

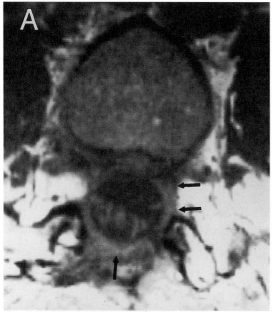

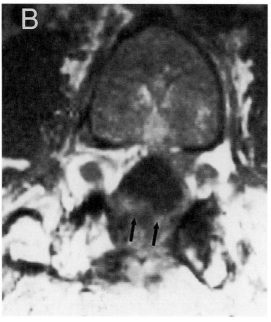

Fig. 6-6. Group I and II arachnoiditis. An axial T$_1$-weighted MR at the L4 level, **A,** shows central clumping of the nerve roots. Peripherally there is a rind of soft tissue consisting of thickened meninges and/or epidural fibrosis *(arrows).* At the L5 level, **B,** the roots have become peripherally adherent to the meninges *(arrows).* (From Ross JS, Modic MT, Masaryk TJ, et al: *Semin Roentgenol* 1988;23:125-136.)

itis is difficult to diagnose on a single axial image. A much more confident diagnosis can be made by visually integrating the appearance of the roots over several levels. Clumping of lumbar nerve roots is commonly seen with lumbar canal stenosis and may mimic a group III arachnoiditis. However, the associated findings in bone and ligament allow a correct diagnosis to be made. The distinction between group III arachnoiditis and an intrathecal tumor may be impossible by MR, except for any secondary findings of previous surgery and/or iophendylate (Pantopaque) myelography. If the tumor has been present long enough, ancillary findings such as scalloping of the posterior margins of the vertebral bodies may be an additional clue. Although neoplastic CSF seeding can produce soft tissue masses within the thecal sac indistinguishable from group I changes, more commonly the roots seen with group I arachnoiditis are smooth and tapered, in contradistinction to the focal and irregular tumor masses seen with CSF seeding.

Thoracic arachnoiditis may appear as thickening of the leptomeninges, which is best imaged using axial T$_1$-weighted spin-echo (SE) sequences. The cord may or may not be involved in the inflammation, with subsequent adhesion to the dura. If the cord is adherent, it will lie eccentrically within the canal. Thoracic arachnoiditis appears to predispose it to syringomyelia. The syringes have relatively indistinct margins when compared to the archetype syrinx associated with a Chiari I malformation. They form presumably because of the markedly altered CSF dynamics secondary to the adhesions. Arachnoid cysts are also commonly formed in association with thoracic arachnoiditis.[9]

Causes of spinal arachnoiditis are varied and include infection, intrathecal steroids or anesthetic agents, surgery, trauma, and intrathecal hemorrhage.[10] Although surgery is probably the most common cause, retained Pantopaque is an additional source of fairly characteristic signals on MR. The T$_1$ value of Pantopaque is approximately 134 msec, slightly less than that of subcutaneous fat, and thus it has high signal intensity on T$_1$ images.[11-12] Its signal intensity, however, decreases more rapidly than that of subcutaneous fat as images become progressively more T$_2$ weighted.

The literature concerning the appearance of arachnoiditis by MR is at present quite scarce and deals mainly with moderate to severe degrees of inflammation. Nevertheless, for the diagnosis of arachnoiditis MR has excellent correlation with CT-myelographic and plain film myelographic findings.

Gd-DTPA appears not to play a significant role in the evaluation of arachnoiditis. Johnson and Sze[13] used it in evaluating 13 patients with lumbar arachnoiditis. Three patients had no abnormal enhancement, and the remainder showed variable amounts. The noncontrast images depicted abnormal morphology of the nerve roots in all patients. The authors noted that the enhancement of arachnoiditis was quite inconsistent: there were patients with severe arachnoiditis but no enhancement.

DISK SPACE INFECTION

Before the advent of antibiotic therapy, spinal osteomyelitis was often an acute virulent disease that caused death from septic complications. Patients who survived long enough to develop abscesses were generally treated by abscess drainage and immobilization. Since antibiotic therapy has become all pervasive, the disease has changed to an insidious disorder of the geriatric population. Dilemmas may arise because clinical and laboratory findings mimic a neoplastic, traumatic, or inflammatory condition. Reliance on conventional radiographs can allow extensive bony destruction to take place before therapy is instituted.[14]

The sources for bacteremia that seed vertebral osteomyelitis are generally genitourinary, dermal, and respiratory. The bacteria find their way to the vascularized disk in children where the destruction causes loss of disk space height. As the infection spreads to the adjacent endplates, plain films show the characteristic irregularity. Hematogeneous spread also occurs in adults, even though the disk has lost a great deal of its vascularity. The seeding is to the vascularized endplates, with the disk and opposite endplates becoming infected secondarily.

Infection may not be considered in the differential for back pain since it remains an uncommon disorder (less than 1% of all cases of osteomyelitis). Once infection is considered, accurate imaging is necessary to provide invasive tests for a microbiologic diagnosis or surgical drainage. Since abnormalities that appear on plain radiographs usually take days to weeks to become manifest, radionuclide studies have been the primary imaging modality for vertebral osteomyelitis.

Radionuclides most commonly used for detecting inflammatory changes of the spine are technetium 99m (^{99m}Tc) phosphate complexes, gallium (^{67}Ga) citrate, and indium-111–labeled white blood cells. Although scintigraphy with ^{99m}Tc and ^{67}Ga compounds is sensitive to infection, it is also nonspecific. Healing fractures, sterile inflammatory reactions, tumors, and loosened prosthetic devices can show increased uptake.[15-18] Indium-111 has several advantages compared to other radionuclides, including higher target-to-background ratios, better image quality (compared to gallium), and more intense uptake by abscesses. Its main disadvantage is its accumulation within any inflammatory lesion, whether infectious or not.[19] The radionuclide study also takes time to perform—hours to days. Computed tomog-

raphy has played a minor role in cases with bony or soft tissue components and is not considered a mainstay for the diagnosis of disk space infection.[20,21] Literature comparing MR with the more conventional modalities in diagnosing inflammatory processes continues to grow. In appropriate situations MR appears to have a sensitivity for detecting vertebral osteomyelitis that exceeds that of plain films and CT and approaches or equals that of radionuclide studies.[22,23]

Pulse Sequences and Technical Considerations

For the evaluation of inflammatory changes in the spine, sagittal images are usually obtained first. They are optimal for outlining a relationship of the involved area with the thecal sac and neural structures and for determining the presence or absence of cord compromise. Also the relationship and visibility of the disk space and endplates (quite important for the proper diagnosis of disk space infection) are best appreciated in the sagittal plane. It is imperative to obtain both T_1-weighted and T_2-weighted images in at least the sagittal plane for optimum sensitivity to disease. The T_1-weighted SE image allows detection of the increased water content or marrow fluid seen with inflammatory exudate or edema. Like most pathologic processes, disk space infection or vertebral osteomyelitis results in an increased signal intensity on T_2-weighted images secondary to an increased proton density or prolonged T_2 relaxation time. The diagnostic specificity of MR is provided by the signal intensity changes on T_1- and T_2-weighted images, as well as by the anatomic pattern of disease involvement and the appropriate clinical situation. Short time-to-inversion recovery (STIR) scans have been advocated for use in osteomyelitis and epidural abscess because of improved tissue contrast. These sequences suppress fat signal (with a T_1 of 150 msec and a TR of 1400 msec) and may allow clearer separation of infection from normal structures. Motion and pulsation artifacts are reduced by keeping the TR fairly short to decrease the CSF signal.[24]

Magnetic Resonance Findings: Pyogenic

Knowledge of the normal MR appearance of intervertebral disks on T_2-weighted images is critical for the correct interpretation of disk space infections. On T_2-weighted images the normal intervertebral disk usually shows an increased signal intensity within its central portion that is bisected by a thin horizontal line of decreased signal. Although the precise histologic correlation of this intranuclear cleft has not been conclusively proved, it appears to represent fibrous tissue secondary to fissuring (Fig. 6-7). After the age of 30 years the cleft is almost a constant feature of normal intervertebral disks.[25]

Certain characteristic changes are seen by MR with disk space infections:

On T_1-weighted images a confluently decreased signal intensity of the adjacent vertebral bodies and the involved intervertebral disk space is noted as compared to the normal vertebral body marrow. A margin between the disk and adjacent vertebral bodies cannot be defined (Figs. 6-7 to 6-10).

On T_2-weighted images there is increased signal intensity at the vertebral bodies adjacent to the involved disk. Also an abnormal configuration, with increased signal intensity from the disk itself, is usually noted that may take the form of a streaky linear appearance of the absence of the intranuclear cleft.

These MR findings are much more typical of pyogenic than of tuberculous spondylitis.[26] In a comparative study of patients with suspected vertebral osteomyelitis[25] MR had a sensitivity of 96%, a specificity of 92%, and an accuracy of 94%. Gallium-67 and technetium-99m bone scintigraphy had a sensitivity of 90%, specificity of 100%, and accuracy of 94% when combined. In this study MR was as accurate and sensitive as radionuclide scanning for the detection of osteomyelitis.[25]

The decreased signal intensity seen on T_1-weighted images most likely results from increased water content of the exudative polymorphonuclear leukocyte response and local ischemia, which together overwhelm and/or replace the normal marrow signal. As the inflammatory process becomes more established, it progresses to involve the intervertebral disk and adjacent vertebral body and results in the confluent decreased signal intensity that was noted in the majority of our cases.[27,28]

The increased signal intensity on T_2-weighted images is a nonspecific response, in and of itself, and is probably secondary to the prolonged T_2 relaxation time of the inflammatory exudate or areas of ischemia.

The typical disk space infection presents no problem in diagnosis, provided both T_1-weighted and T_2-weighted images are obtained. However, atypical-appearing disk space infections do exist and complicate a usually unequivocal diagnosis. One atypical form may be seen if DSI complicates a degenerated disk with an associated type II marrow change (i.e., increased signal from the endplates on T_1-weighted images). In these cases the T_1-weighted images may continue to show increased signal, in effect masking the usual characteristically confluent decreased intensity (Fig. 6-11). The key in these cases is the abnormal disk signal intensity on T_2-weighted images, something that does not occur in uncomplicated type II marrow change. Very early on in vertebral osteomyelitis, there may be decreased signal involving the endplates without an appreciable increase in signal from the bodies or disk on T_2-weighted images.

The differentiation of degenerative disease and tumor from vertebral osteomyelitis is easier on MR than on radionuclide studies or plain radiographs. Degenerated disks show decreased signal intensity within their cen-

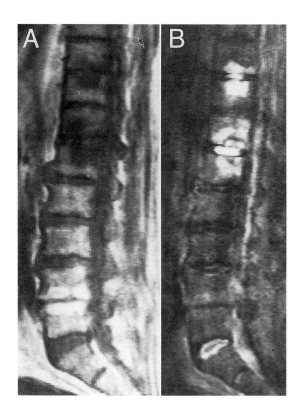

Fig. 6-7. Lumbar vertebral osteomyelitis. A sagittal T_1-weighted image, **A,** shows decreased signal intensity from the T10-11 and T12-L1 disks and adjacent vertebral body endplates involved with osteomyelitis. The disk margins are indistinct. The high signal from the endplates adjacent to the L4 disk denotes chronic degenerative change (type II marrow). A T_2-weighted image, **B,** shows the characteristic findings of disk space infections at T10 and T12: (1) abnormal high signal intensity of the adjacent endplates and (2) high signal intensity from the intervertebral disk without the intranuclear cleft. Compare T10 and T12 to the normal L5 disk with an intranuclear cleft. Disks L1 through L4 are degenerated, as evidenced by the low signal on T_2-weighted images.

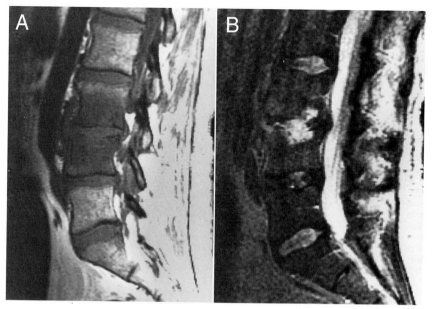

Fig. 6-8. Lumbar vertebral osteomyelitis. A sagittal T_1-weighted image, **A,** shows decreased signal intensity from the L3-4 intervertebral disk and adjacent vertebral body endplates involved with osteomyelitis. The disk margins are indistinct, and there is disruption of the usual low signal intensity from the cortical endplates. Note the anterior prevertebral soft tissue. The T_2-weighted image, **B,** shows characteristic findings of disk space infections, with abnormal high signal intensity of the adjacent endplates and abnormally shaped high signal from the intervertebral disk.

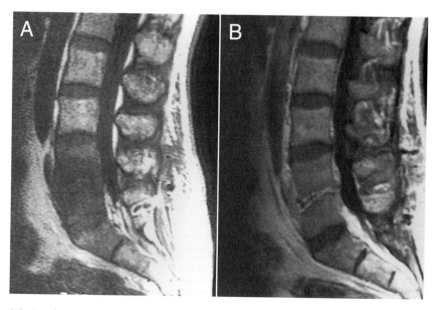

Fig. 6-9. Lumbar vertebral osteomyelitis with contrast. A sagittal T_1-weighted image before contrast, **A,** shows decreased signal intensity from the L4-5 intervertebral disk and adjacent vertebral body endplates. There is a question of posterior epidural extension that is difficult to define. The sagittal image after contrast, **B,** shows enhancement of the vertebral bodies now isointense with normal marrow obscuring the pathology. However, there is better definition of the posterior epidural extension. The markedly abnormal enhancement of the disk proper may persist for months following successful treatment.

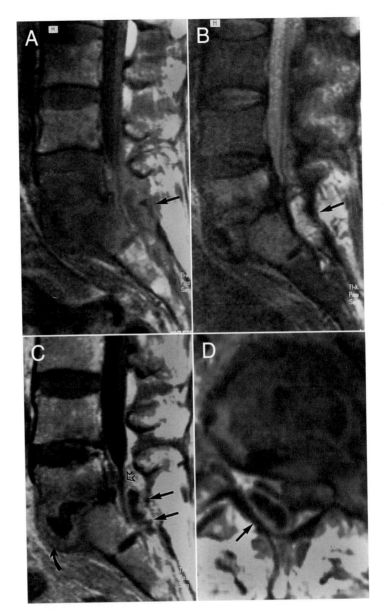

Fig. 6-10. Lumbar vertebral osteomyelitis and epidural abscess with contrast. A sagittal T_1-weighted image before contrast, **A,** shows decreased signal from the L5-S1 intervertebral disk and adjacent vertebral body endplates. There is heterogeneous obscuration of the distal thecal sac because of the abscess. Anterior prevertebral extension is also present. The sagittal T_2-weighted, **B,** shows abnormal increased signal from the L5 and S1 bodies and abnormally shaped increased signal from the disk space. The posterior abscess shows increased signal *(arrow).* Sagittal, **C,** and axial, **D,** postcontrast images show the vertebral bodies now nearly isointense with normal marrow. There is excellent definition of the abscess *(straight arrows),* with peripheral enhancement surrounding the nonenhancing liquid abscess. Note the marked compression of the distal thecal sac *(open arrow)* and the abnormal enhancement outlining the intradiskal abscess in the anterior portion of the disk space *(curved arrow).*

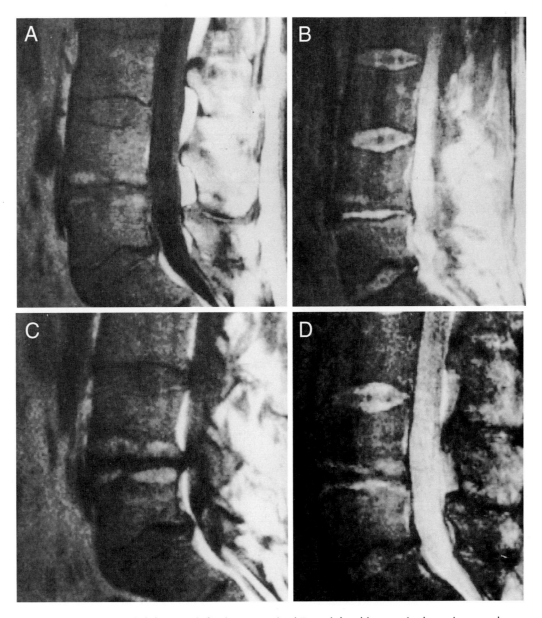

Fig. 6-11. Atypical disk space infection. A sagittal T_1-weighted image, **A,** shows increased signal from the L4-5 endplates consistent with type II marrow change. The sagittal T_2-weighted image, **B,** shows abnormal increased signal from the L4-5 disk without an intranuclear cleft in the biopsy-proved disk space infection. There is little increased signal from the adjacent endplates. A posttreatment T_1-weighted image, **C,** shows more extensive type II marrow change. The sagittal T_2-weighted after treatment, **D,** shows resolution of the increased signal from the disk space and more prominent marrow changes. This type II endplate change likely masked the usual confluent low signal seen from marrow with pyogenic disk space infections.

tral portion on T_2-weighted images that can be distinguished from the high signal of active inflammation. It may be difficult to differentiate metastatic disease, postoperative changes, or degenerative changes from osteomyelitis by scintigraphic means. These entities can usually be differentiated from osteomyelitis on MR by the lack of confluent decreased signal of the vertebral body and disk on the T_1-weighted images. Likewise, metastatic disease can be distinguished from osteomyelitis by the lack of disk space involvement. Although rare instances of metastatic involvement of the disk have been reported,[29,30] this continues to be a reliable sign of benign disease in the overwhelming majority of cases. In the initial stages of vertebral osteomyelitis, when the disk space is not yet involved, it may be difficult to exclude neoplastic disease or compression fracture from the differential diagnosis using only MR. Follow-up studies are usually necessary to further define the nature of the lesion. A single report[31] exists of vertebral osteomyelitis from *Streptococcus* wherein the vertebral endplates were intact, although the adjacent bodies and disk were involved. It may be that MR can detect vertebral body infection before endplate destruction.[31]

On plain films and radionuclide studies severe degenerative changes can produce alterations that are similar to those seen in vertebral osteomyelitis. On MR degenerative disk disease occasionally shows decreased signal intensity within the adjacent vertebral bodies on T_1-weighted images and increased signal intensity on T_2-weighted images. The disk space itself, however, is always distinct from the adjacent vertebral body endplate on T_1-weighted images. Also the disk almost always shows decreased signal on T_2-weighted images in degenerative disease whereas inflammation shows high signal intensity.[32] Rarely a cystic type of degenerative change with fluid in the disk space will mimic disk space infection. Similar changes within the adjacent vertebral bodies can be seen following surgical instrumentation or chymopapain injection into the intervertebral disk.[33] As with the changes of degenerative disk disease, the signal intensity of the disk usually remains decreased on both T_1- and T_2-weighted images and the borders of the disk are maintained.

Radionuclide studies have several advantages over surface coil MR. They are not as sensitive to patient positioning, claustrophobia, or motion. They have a broader field of view, and involvement of the extravertebral osseous or soft tissue structures is better appreciated. Also images produced by ^{67}Ga scintigraphy may revert to normal following antibiotic therapy, and may thus be used as an indication of appropriate therapy, which does not appear possible with MR. The effects of antibiotics on MR signal intensity have not been described. Although the MR findings are altered, they apparently are not obscured in the early stages of treatment

as can occur with ^{67}Ga imaging. The findings in vertebral osteomyelitis with MR and ^{67}Ga appear approximately at the same time.

With treated osteomyelitis any abnormal signal-intensity changes revert to normal within 6 weeks to a year. Changes in signal intensity reflect the resolution of inflammatory exudate or ischemia, with fibrous tissue replacement and a small amount of new bone formation. MRI is highly sensitive to detection of inflammatory diseases of the spine; but, because of the characteristic pattern of involvement, it can also be highly specific.

EPIDURAL ABSCESS

The incidence of spinal epidural abscess ranges from 0.2 to 1.96 cases per 10,000, with the higher rates found in more recent literature.[34] This apparent increase may relate to the general aging of the population as well as to the increasing number of spinal procedures and incidents of IV drug abuse.

Risk factors for the development of epidural abscess include altered immune status (e.g., diabetes mellitus), renal failure requiring dialysis, alcoholism, and malignancy. Although intravenous drug abuse is a risk factor for epidural abscess, HIV infection does not appear to play a role in the overall increasing incidence of the disease.[34]

Staphylococcus aureus is the organism most commonly associated with epidural abscess, constituting approximately 60% of the cases. It is ubiquitous, tends to form abscesses, and can infect compromised as well as normal hosts. Other gram-positive cocci account for approximately 13% of cases, and gram-negative organisms for approximately 15%. Most patients are infected by a hematogenous route, with the skin and soft tissues a leading portal. The sites for abscess formation are mainly cervical (25%) and lumbosacral (38%), with half being anterior and a third circumferential in position. Clinical acute symptomatology classically includes back pain, fever, obtundation, and neurologic deficits. Chronic cases may have less pain and no elevated temperature. The classic course of epidural abscess was described by Rankin and Flothow[35] in four stages: spinal ache, root pain, weakness, paralysis. Acute deterioration from spinal epidural abscess, however, remains unpredictable. Patients may present with abrupt paraplegia and anesthesia. The cause for this precipitous course is unknown, but it is thought to be related to a vascular mechanism (epidural thrombosis and thrombophlebitis, venous infarction).[36-39]

The primary diagnostic modality in the evaluation of epidural abscess is MR (Figs. 6-12 to 6-19). MR is as sensitive as CT myelography for epidural infection, but it also allows the exclusion of other diagnostic choices such as herniation, syrinx, tumor, and cord infarc-

Text continued on p. 234.

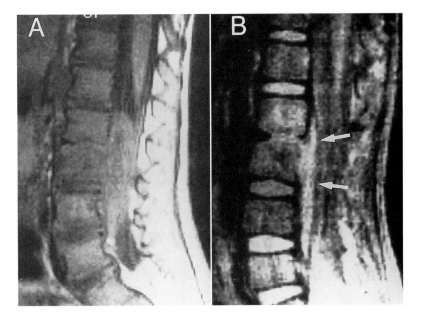

Fig. 6-12. Epidural abscess in a 10-year-old boy. The T$_1$-weighted image, **A,** shows confluent decreased signal from the vertebral bodies and disk space. Epidural spread of infection is seen as an intermediate-signal mass compressing the anterior thecal sac. The spin-density image, **B,** shows high signal from the involved vertebral bodies and epidural abscess *(arrows).*

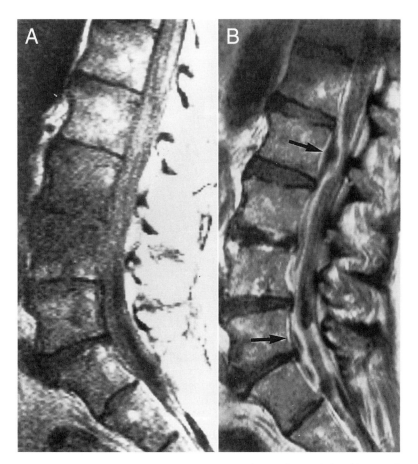

Fig. 6-13. Lumbar epidural abscess. A sagittal nonenhanced T$_1$-weighted image shows disk space infection at L3-4, with abnormal increased signal in the anterior epidural space from L2 to S1. The postcontrast image, **B,** shows extension of the abscess from L1 to S1, with nonenhancing pockets at L2 and L5 *(arrows).* Note the enhancement of the involved vertebral bodies and disk.

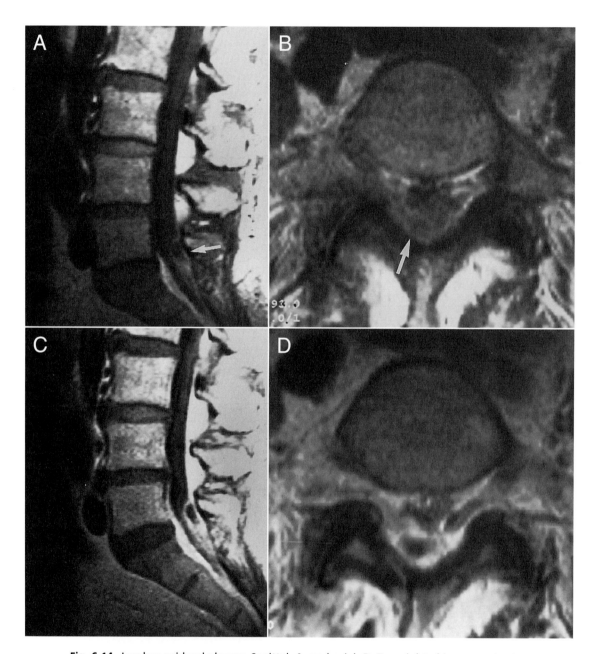

Fig. 6-14. Lumbar epidural abscess. Sagittal, **A**, and axial, **B**, T$_1$-weighted images prior to contrast show an ill-defined soft tissue signal mass posterior to the thecal sac at the L5-S1 level *(arrow)*. Sagittal, **C**, and axial, **D**, postcontrast images now show a well-defined peripherally enhancing mass confined to the posterior epidural space. There is no vertebral body or disk space involvement.

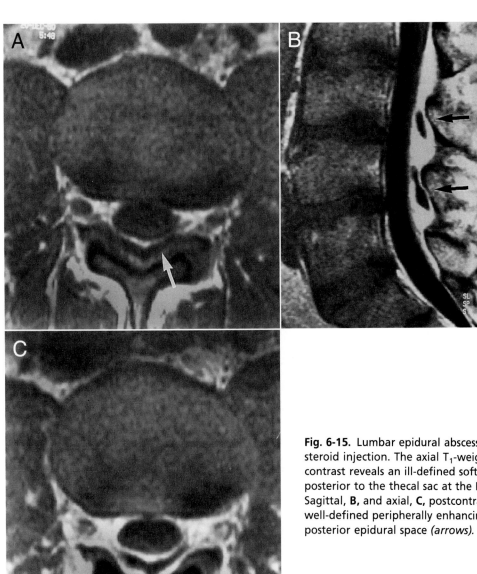

Fig. 6-15. Lumbar epidural abscess following epidural steroid injection. The axial T$_1$-weighted image, **A,** prior to contrast reveals an ill-defined soft tissue–signal mass posterior to the thecal sac at the L4-5 level *(arrow)*. Sagittal, **B,** and axial, **C,** postcontrast images show the well-defined peripherally enhancing masses confined to the posterior epidural space *(arrows)*.

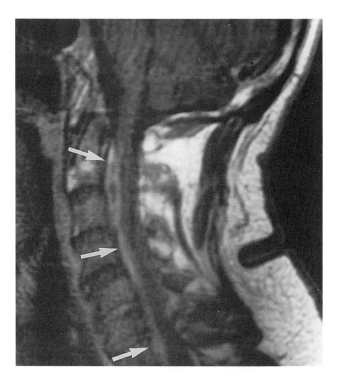

Fig. 6-16. Cervical epidural abscess. A sagittal postcontrast T$_1$-weighted shows the extensive enhancing abscess from C2 to C7 *(arrows)*, with mass effect and posterior displacement of the thecal sac. There is also abnormal enhancement of the C5-6 disk, the site of disk space infection.

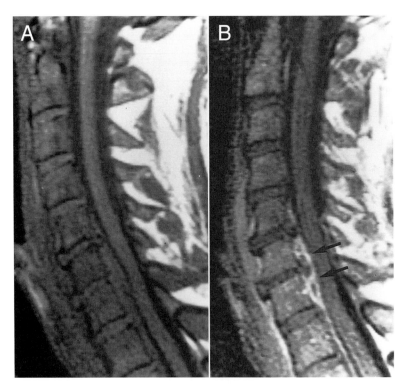

Fig. 6-17. Cervical epidural abscess. Sagittal precontrast, **A,** and postcontrast, **B,** T$_1$-weighted images show an enhancing anterior epidural abscess from C5 to C7 *(arrows),* with mass effect and posterior displacement of the thecal sac and cervical cord. In **A** note that the usual low signal intensity from the posterior anulus—posterior longitudinal ligament complex at C6-7 and C7-T1 is lost where there are disk space infections.

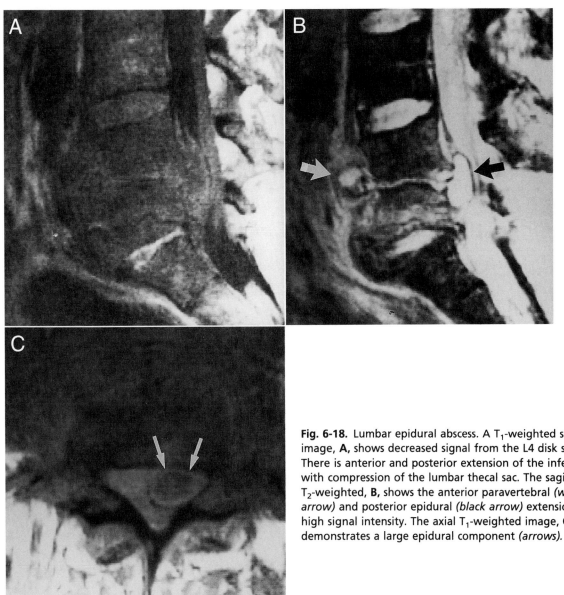

Fig. 6-18. Lumbar epidural abscess. A T$_1$-weighted sagittal image, **A,** shows decreased signal from the L4 disk space. There is anterior and posterior extension of the infection with compression of the lumbar thecal sac. The sagittal T$_2$-weighted, **B,** shows the anterior paravertebral *(white arrow)* and posterior epidural *(black arrow)* extensions as high signal intensity. The axial T$_1$-weighted image, **C,** also demonstrates a large epidural component *(arrows).*

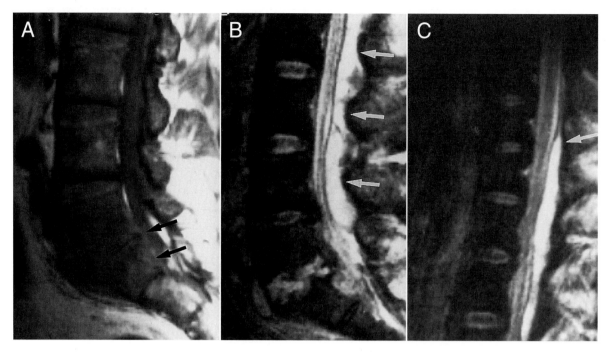

Fig. 6-19. Epidural abscess. A sagittal T_1-weighted image, **A**, shows confluent low signal intensity from the L5 and S1 vertebral bodies. There is an ill-defined anterior epidural mass *(arrows)*. A sagittal T_2-weighted image, **B**, discloses abnormal increased signal from the L5 disk as well as a large posterior epidural collection extending cephalad *(arrows)*. The sagittal T_2-weighted image of the upper lumbar spine, **C**, shows a high–signal intensity fluid collection extending to the thoracolumbar junction *(arrow)*.

tion.[34,40] MR imaging of epidural abscess demonstrates a soft tissue mass in the epidural space with tapered edges and an associated mass effect on the thecal sac and cord. The epidural masses are usually isointense to the cord on T_1-weighted images and of increased signal on T_2-weighted images.[41] Occasionally an epidural mass will be difficult to distinguish when there is associated meningitis (which increases the CSF signal intensity). Post et al.[41,42] recommended that in these ambiguous cases either CT myelography or perhaps Gd-DTPA* enhancement is necessary for full elucidation of the abscess (Figs. 6-13 to 6-17). The patterns of Gd-DTPA enhancement of epidural abscess include (1) diffuse and homogeneous, (2) heterogeneous, and (3) thin peripheral.[42] Post et al.[41,42] found that Gd-DTPA enhancement was a very useful adjunct for identifying the extent of a lesion when the plain MR scan was equivocal, for demonstrating activity of an infection, and for directing needle biopsy and follow-up treatment. Successful therapy should cause a progressive decrease in enhancement of the paraspinal soft tissues, disk, and vertebral bodies. The role of Gd-DTPA in attempts to distinguish between frank pus and granulation tissue is not clinically significant since both pus and granulation tissue can cause neurologic compromise.[34]

Treatment for epidural abscess remains immediate surgical drainage. There is a significant risk to medical management because of its unpredictable clinical course. Despite improvements in imaging and surgical techniques, the mortality rate remains high (23%).

TUBERCULOUS SPONDYLITIS

Tuberculous spondylitis has been noted[43] to demonstrate findings more typical of neoplasms than of pyogenic spondylitis. These findings include (1) sparing of the intervertebral disk space, with no abnormal increased signal on T_2-weighted images, (2) preferential involvement of the posterior elements and posterior portions of the vertebral bodies, (3) involvement of more than two vertebral bodies, and (4) large paraspinal soft tissue masses (Figs. 6-20 and 6-21).

Tuberculous spondylitis begins in the anterior-inferior portion of the vertebral body, with spread beneath the longitudinal ligaments.[44] The intervertebral disk is commonly not involved. The lack of proteolytic enzymes in mycobacteria has been touted[45] as the cause of intervertebral disk space preservation.

*Gadolinium–diethylenetriamine pentaacetate.

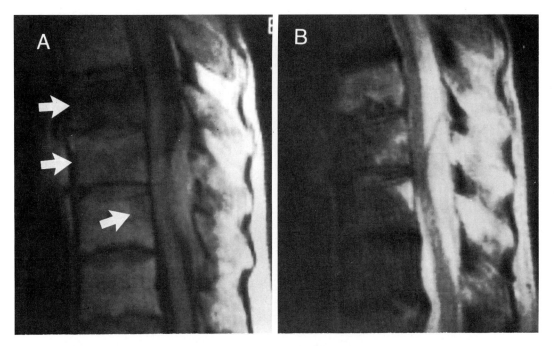

Fig. 6-20. Tuberculous spondylitis. A sagittal T$_1$-weighted image, **A,** reveals areas of decreased signal within T7 and T9 *(arrows),* with preservation of the T7-8 and T8-9 intervertebral disks. A large posterior soft tissue mass displaces the cord anteriorly. The sagittal T$_2$-weighted, **B,** shows abnormal increased signal from the involved vertebral bodies, without abnormal signal from the disks. The posterior mass also shows high signal intensity. (From Smith AS, Weinstein MA, Mizushima A, et al: *AJR* 1989;153:399-405.)

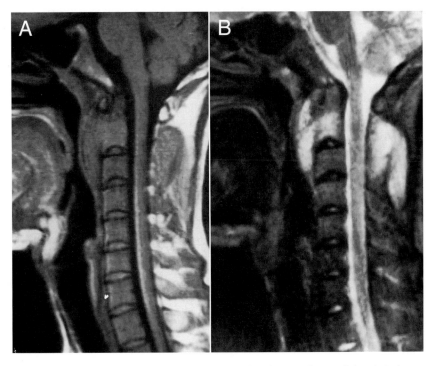

Fig. 6-21. Tuberculous spondylitis. Sagittal T$_1$-weighted, **A,** and T$_2$-weighted, **B,** images of the cervical spine show abnormal signal within the C2 body with anterior prevertebral extension down to C3. There is also prominent posterior element involvement at the C2 and C3 levels with extension into the posterior paraspinal muscles. Note the sparing of the intervertebral disk at the C2-3 level. (Courtesy H.S. Sharif, M.D., Riyadh Armed Forces Hospital.)

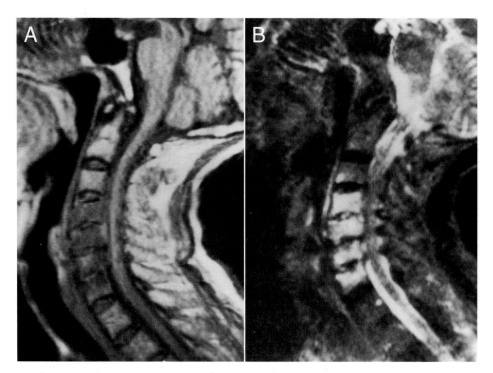

Fig. 6-22. Brucellar spondylitis. Sagittal T_1-weighted, **A,** and T_2-weighted, **B,** images demonstrate extensive involvement of the C4 to C7 vertebral bodies. The disk spaces also show abnormal increased signal on the T_2-weighted images at C4-6. Findings leading toward the diagnosis of brucellar spondylitis include the lack of posterior element involvement, reduced disk space size despite the evidence of involvement, and relative paucity of epidural involvement. (Courtesy H.S. Sharif, M.D., Riyadh Armed Forces Hospital.)

With the predilection for multiple vertebral body and posterior element involvement, the distinction from metastatic disease may be impossible, except when correlated with history. In North America, spinal tuberculosis is most common in young adults (30 to 45 years) and has an insidious onset (months to years).[43,44] Also to be included in the differential diagnosis are other unusual infections, such as actinomycosis (which can also spread by a subligamentous route) and hydatid disease (which can produce vertebral body destruction and a paraspinal mass). Type I vertebral body changes should, likewise, be considered since both type I changes and spinal tuberculosis can show increased signal on T_1-weighted images from adjacent vertebral bodies and a narrowed disk space without increased signal on T_2-weighted images.

BRUCELLAR SPONDYLITIS

Brucellosis is caused by a small gram-negative bacillus, which can affect the spine in either a focal or a diffuse fashion. The focal form is localized to the anterior aspect of an endplate, most typically the superior endplate of L4. The diffuse form initially involves an endplate and spreads to involve the entire vertebral body, with subsequent extension into the adjacent body and disk.

Early diagnosis allows for effective antibrucellar chemotherapy, and the need for surgical intervention is uncommon.[46,47] The differential diagnosis of brucellosis is against that of tuberculous infection.

The MR findings of brucellosis have been described by Sharif et al.[47,48] Brucellar spondylitis is more common in the lower lumbar spine, demonstrates intact vertebral body margins despite high signal intensity vertebral bodies on T2 weighted images, and does not show posterior element involvement or paraspinal abscesses or gibbus deformity as does TB[48] (Figs. 6-22 and 6-23). Sharif et al.[47,48] did not see the combination of vertebral body collapse, paraspinal abscess, and gibbus deformity in any of their 17 patients with brucellosis.

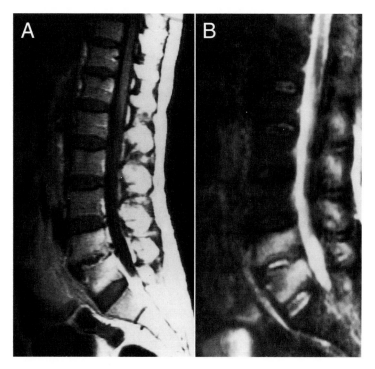

Fig. 6-23. Brucellar spondylitis. Sagittal enhanced T_1-weighted, **A,** and T_2-weighted, **B,** images demonstrate extensive involvement of the L4 and L5 vertebral bodies. The intervertebral disk space and anterior prevertebral tissues show abnormal increased signal on the T_2-weighted. There is also enhancement of the L4 disk in a peripheral fashion, which is a nonspecific finding that may be seen with brucellosis, tuberculosis, or pyogenic infection. (Courtesy H.S. Sharif, M.D., Riyadh Armed Forces Hospital.)

HEMODIALYSIS SPONDYLOARTHROPATHY

Spondyloarthropathy has been described[49-52] in patients undergoing long-term hemodialysis. The duration of dialysis was approximately 5 to 9 years.[49,50] The plain film changes included disk space narrowing and irregular endplate destruction (Figs. 6-24 and 6-25).

The cervical and thoracic vertebrae are typical locations of involvement and may be associated with pain. The major differential diagnostic feature for hemodialysis spondyloarthropathy is pyogenic disk space infection. As in ankylosing spondylitis, there is a lack of associated soft tissue disease on T_2-weighted images as well as, usually, a decrease in signal intensity from the intervertebral disk (although this latter is not pathognomonic).

The cause of this noninfectious spondyloarthropathy is unknown. Theories put forth include crystal induced (e.g., calcium pyrophosphate and hydroxyapatite deposition) and amyloid induced.[1] Long-term hemodialysis patients may experience carpal tunnel syndrome, shoulder pain, and erosive arthritis. Histology in these cases shows amyloid deposits, which stain with Congo red. The amyloid consists of β_2 microglobulin, which accumulates in dialysis patients.

ANKYLOSING SPONDYLITIS

Ankylosing spondylitis (Marie-Strümpell disease) is a spondyloarthropathy that affects mainly young men and has a specific association with the histocompatibility antigen (HLA) B27. It involves primarily the sacroiliac joints and spine, at the insertion of the ligaments and capsules in bone. Nonmusculoskeletal manifestations include uveitis, pulmonary fibrosis, cardiac valvular disease, and amyloidosis.

Spinal involvement includes ankylosis, atlantoaxial subluxation, traumatic fractures, and extradural hematoma[53] (Fig. 6-26). An unusual complication in longstanding cases is a cauda equina syndrome, first reported by Bowie and Glasgow.[54] Radiographic description exists for plain films, CT, and myelography.[55-57] A few

Fig. 6-24. Hemodialysis spondyloarthropathy. A lateral plain radiograph, **A,** shows near complete collapse of the C5 body *(arrow)* with irregularity of the inferior endplates of C4, C5, and C6, highly suggestive of disk space infection. A sagittal T$_1$-weighted image, **B,** shows similar findings but without evidence of epidural or prevertebral extension. A sagittal T$_2$-weighted, **C,** shows no abnormal increased signal from the disk spaces. This lack of paravertebral soft tissue extension plus a lack of increased signal from the disk space makes the possibility of pyogenic infection less likely. (From Smith AS, Blaser SI: *Crit Rev Diagnost Imaging* 1991;32[3]:165-189.)

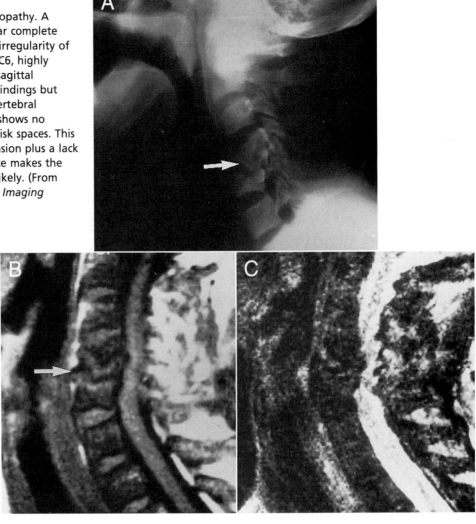

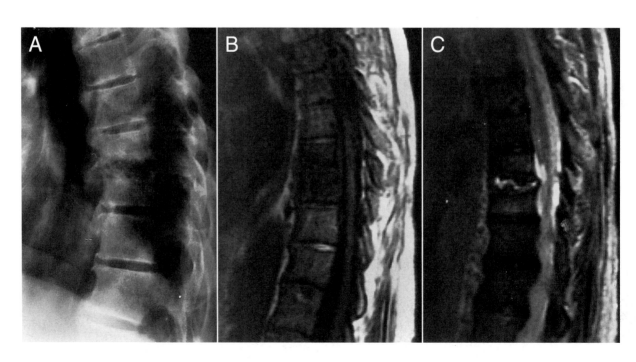

Fig. 6-25. For legend see opposite page.

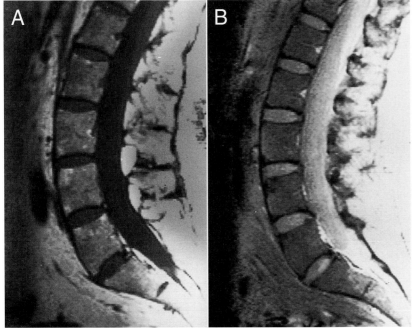

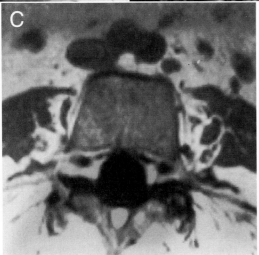

Fig. 6-26. Long-standing ankylosing spondylitis with multilevel fusion. Sagittal T₁-weighted and gradient echo, **A** and **B,** images show a prominent low-signal line involving the anterior cortex and anterior disk levels with squaring of the body shapes. Squaring is particularly evident on the axial image, **C.**

Fig. 6-25. Hemodialysis spondyloarthropathy. A lateral plain radiograph of the thoracic spine, **A,** shows destruction of the endplates of T9 and T10, highly suggestive of disk space infection. The sagittal T₁ weighted image, **B,** shows abnormal low signal from the T9 and T10 bodies with an indistinct disk space, also consistent with disk space infection. The sagittal T₂-weighted, **C,** shows abnormal increased signal from the disk space, with minimally increased signal from the adjacent vertebral bodies. This patient was receiving chronic dialysis, and multiple biopsies had been negative for infection.

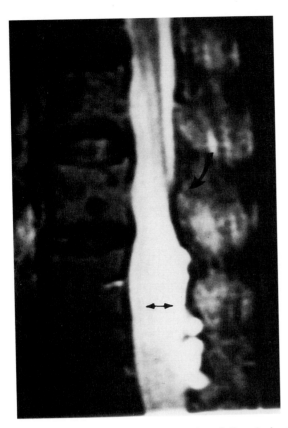

Fig. 6-27. Ankylosing spondylitis with dorsal diverticula. A sagittal T_2-weighted image shows dorsal thecal sac diverticula within areas of erosion of the L3 and L4 posterior elements with expansion of the bony canal *(double arrow)*. There is posterior clumping of the nerve roots *(curved arrow)*. (From Tullous MW, Skerhut HEI, Story JL, et al: *J Neurosurg* 1990;73:441-447.)

reports describe MR images.[58-60] MR findings include a large lumbosacral thecal sac, with multiple dorsal diverticula lying within the lamina, and spinous process bone erosions[58] (Fig. 6-27). Multiple root sleeves may be enlarged, and nerve roots may adhere posteriorly to the dura.

The cause of the cauda equina syndrome in ankylosing spondylitis is not known. Tullous et al.[58] concluded that most likely a primary ligamentous inflammation leads to inflammation of the local meninges and posterior elements. This could produce dorsal dural inflammation and arachnoid adhesions with lamina erosion. Nerve injury thus may relate to the arachnoiditis, with subsequent vasculitis and adhesion formation.

In 3% to 28% of cases frank diskovertebral destruction may be seen in ankylosing spondylitis without infection.[61] Andersson[62] first described this condition, which most frequently affects the thoracolumbar region and consists of disk space narrowing, bone destruction, surrounding sclerosis, and kyphosis. These features (of "Andersson lesions") may mimic those of disk space infection, particularly with tuberculosis. However, the spondylitic destruction does not have soft tissue swelling or a soft tissue prevertebral mass, as would be seen in most cases of tuberculosis. MR distinguishes Andersson lesions from infective spondylitis by usually showing decreased signal intensity on T_2-weighted images within the intervertebral disk space itself. This signal decrease corresponds to fibrous replacement of the disk and has been demonstrated histologically.[61]

SARCOIDOSIS

Sarcoidosis is a multisystem granulomatous disease of unknown cause. It is diagnosed by noncaseating granulomas, with supportive laboratory and imaging findings. These include primarily chest radiographs and angiotensin converting enzyme (ACE) levels. The true positive yield from ACE is 75%. Areas of involvement are most commonly the lung and hila, with eye and skin involvement next most common. The CNS is affected in up to 5% of cases. Areas of CNS involvement include the cranial nerves (cranial polyneuritis), basal cisterns (meningitis with hydrocephalus), and hypothalamus (diabetes insipidus). Other clinical syndromes include a peripheral neuropathy and myopathy. Spinal cord involvement is less common than brain involvement, with approximately 69 cases reported in the literature.[63-65] Pathologic changes include sarcoid tissue in the meninges and parenchyma, with areas of infarction resulting from occlusion of small vessels by the granulomas.

MR shows direct cord involvement (increased cord size) and increased signal on T_2-weighted images, combined with evidence of leptomeningeal enhancement. Patchy multifocal enhancement of the cord (which is broad based) and adjacent to the cord surface is fairly typical.

RHEUMATOID ARTHRITIS

Garrod[66] first reported involvement of the cervical spine by rheumatoid arthritis in 1890, in which he found 36% of rheumatoid arthritis patients to have cervical spinal involvement. Involvement of the upper cervical spine occurs in 36% to 88% of patient affected with rheumatoid arthritis.[67,68] Conditions such as atlantoaxial subluxation can lead to cervical myelopathy, progressive disability, and even sudden death. The instabilities are caused by ligamentous laxity of the transverse, alar, apical, and capsular ligaments, in addition to bone erosion.

There are several types of subluxation, which are defined first by plain films:

Anterior atlantoaxial
Vertical of the odontoid
Posterior atlantoaxial (associated with an eroded
   odontoid)
Lateral of the lateral masses of C1
Subaxial

Anterior atlantoaxial subluxation

The diagnosis of anterior C1-C2 subluxation is based on the atlantodental interval (ADI) measured in flexion on lateral views. In adults a distance greater than 2.5 to 3 mm indicates anterior atlantoaxial subluxation. Anterior subluxations are primarily caused by laxity of the transverse ligament. Erosions occur around the odontoid and at the atlantoaxial joint margins. As disease progresses, frank ligamentous rupture can occur, increasing instability. Clinical manifestations include occipital, temporal, and retroorbital pain. Cord myelopathy results from cord compression between the odontoid and the anteriorly displaced posterior arch of C1. Vertebral basilar insufficiency may be due to vascular kinking around the anteriorly displaced C1. Cervical cord compression can be estimated by measuring the space available for the cord (SAC).

Vertical subluxation

Vertical subluxation of the odontoid into the foramen magnum has various terms in the literature: atlantoaxial impaction, cranial settling, vertical settling, vertical subluxation, and upward translocation. It occurs with progressive collapse of the occipital condylar articulations as well as the lateral masses and facet joints of C1 and C2, and it may compress the cervicomedullary junction, leading to myelopathy or death. The diagnosis is made on a lateral view using the Redlund-Johnell method, which evaluates the distance between the base of C2 and McGregor's line.[69] Normal values are 34 mm or greater in men and 28 mm or greater in women.[67] The method of Ranawat et al.[70] assesses collapse of the C1-2 articulation by measuring from the center of the C2 pedicle to a line connecting the anterior arch and the spinous process of C1. Normal Ranawat values are considered to be 14 mm or greater in men and 13 mm or greater in women.[67] Kawaida et al.[71] evaluated plain films and MRI in 55 rheumatoid arthritis patients and found that all who had an abnormal Redlund-Johnell value and a Ranawat value of 7 mm or less showed medullary compression. The upper cervical cord was compressed in all patients with an SAC of 13 or less.

Posterior atlantoaxial subluxation

This unusual form of subluxation results from either extensive erosion or a pathologic fracture of the odontoid.[72] The anterior arch of C1 can slip posteriorly to impinge on the cervical cord.

Lateral subluxation

Collapse and asymmetric erosions with joint capsule weakening that involve the lateral masses of C1 and C2 can lead to lateral subluxation and/or rotation. More than 2 mm of offset of the C1-C2 lateral masses is abnormal.[73] A nonreducible rotational head tilt with lateral mass collapse was seen in 10% of patients with advanced rheumatoid arthritis in the series by Halla et al.[74]

Subaxial subluxation

Subluxation below the C1-C2 level occurs in up to 40% of rheumatoid arthritis patients, the incidence increasing with long-standing disease.[75] A "stepladder" or "staircase" appearance of the vertebral bodies is characteristic and due to the multilevel involvement. Involvement of the facet joints, with laxity of the anterior and posterior longitudinal ligaments, is a prime cause.

Severe subaxial subluxation may cause cord compression and myelopathy. Vertebral artery compromise with cortical blindness has also been described.[76] Pannus arising from the uncovertebral joints may cause cord compression. The diskovertebral joints may demonstrate subchondral erosions and loss of disk space height without osteophytes, termed *spondylodiskitis*.[77] Lushka joint synovitis can lead to erosions of the disk and adjacent bone, or the cervical instability can lead to trauma of the diskovertebral complex.[78,79]

MRI Technique

Sagittal unenhanced T_1-weighted spin-echo sequences are a mainstay of the MR evaluation of rheumatoid arthritis patients (Figs. 6-28 to 6-33). They allow good evaluation of anatomic relationships of the cervicovertebral junction and any mass effect on the cervical cord. Although the CVJ proper is best evaluated by imaging the patient in a head coil, the field of view of the lower cervical spine is limited by such placement and a surface coil examination is necessary for complete cervical spine coverage. Occasionally a severe subluxation or kyphosis will necessitate use of the body coil. T_2-weighted spin-echo images are useful for evaluating the cord proper and for identifying any–signal intensity bony or ligamentous pathology that may not be easily visualized on T_1-weighted spin-echo images alone.

The use of "dynamic" or "functional" MRI (wherein neutral, flexion, and extension T_1-weighted sagittal images are acquired) is controversial. Bell and Stearns,[80] reporting on the use of flexion-extension MRI in seven rheumatoid arthritis patients, found that dynamic MRI clearly delineated the odontoid, foramen magnum, and cervical cord relationships, which aided in operative candidate selection in four cases, and concluded that flexion-extension MRI was the diagnostic study of choice for dynamically evaluating the cervical spine. Similarly, Dvorak et al.,[81] studying 34 patients with dy-

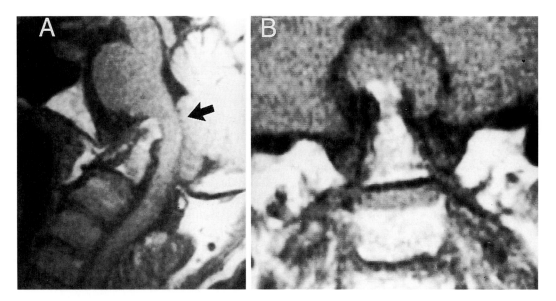

Fig. 6-28. Rheumatoid arthritis. **A,** There is severe upward translocation of a severely eroded dens, which compresses and kinks the pontomedullary junction *(arrow).* **B,** A coronal T$_1$-weighted image shows the severely eroded dens outlined by the pons superiorly.

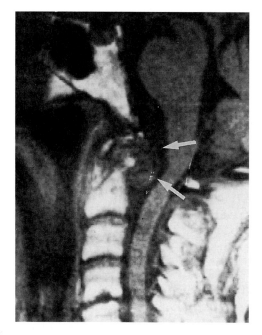

Fig. 6-29. Rheumatoid arthritis. A large mass of pannus *(arrows)* has eroded the odontoid and extends posteriorly to encroach on the cervicomedullary junction.

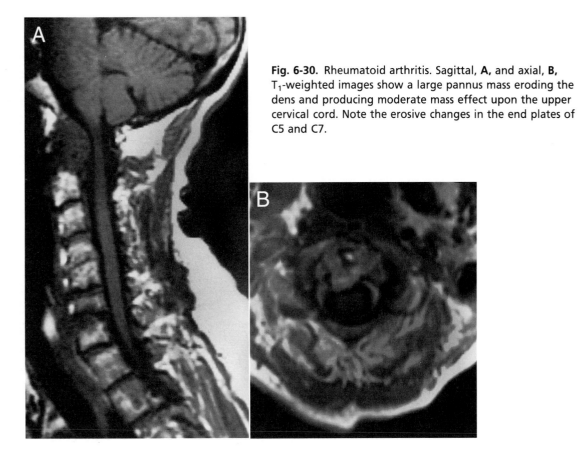

Fig. 6-30. Rheumatoid arthritis. Sagittal, **A,** and axial, **B,** T$_1$-weighted images show a large pannus mass eroding the dens and producing moderate mass effect upon the upper cervical cord. Note the erosive changes in the end plates of C5 and C7.

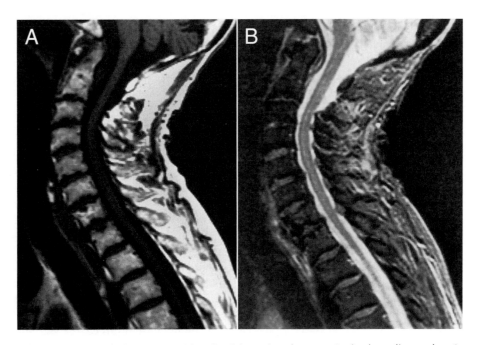

Fig. 6-31. Rheumatoid arthritis with subaxial erosive changes. Sagittal gradient echo, **A,** and T$_1$-weighted, **B,** images reveal extensive endplate erosions at multiple levels, without subluxation. A small amount of pannus is present at C2.

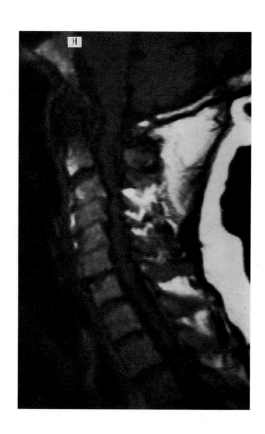

Fig. 6-32. Rheumatoid arthritis with fusion. A large amount of pannus engulfs the odontoid and anterior arch of C1, with moderate mass effect on the cervicomedullary junction. The is also fusion of C3, C4, C5, and C6, with fixed subaxial subluxations and severe canal stenosis.

namic MRI, found that most with myelopathy showed cord diameters less than 6 mm only in the flexion MRI images. They recommended functional MR in patients with atlantoaxial instability. Krodel et al.,[82] studying 11 patients with either rheumatoid arthritis or ankylosing spondylosis, concluded that flexion-extension MRI was an "absolute necessity" for the planning of stabilizing operations. In particular, they found that it was important to define any remaining cord compression following a trial reduction since this would alter the surgical approach. If functional MRIs showed cord compression in the reduced position, then they would resect the posterior arch of the atlas, with subsequent cervical occipital-C2 fusion, to allow more decompression of the cord.

However, the practical need for flexion-extension imaging has been challenged by Petterson et al.[83] They studied 23 patients with rheumatoid arthritis and found that neutral position sagittal MR, combined with lateral flexion-extension plain films, provided all the information necessary for clinical management. They also found that in most patients with neurologic disturbances cord compression was obvious by neutral position MR. Provocative positioning for MR is theoretically hazardous, for it increases the amount of cord compression. Nonetheless, Dvorak et al.[81] had no worsening of symptoms in their 34 patients during the dynamic examinations. These authors took care to have the patients move their

head only as far as tolerable without suffering additional pain or symptoms.

MR Findings

Bundschuh et al.[84] studied 15 patients with rheumatoid arthritis and compared MR images to plain films and tomography for defining subluxations and erosions (Figs. 6-12 and 6-13). All patients with MR-identifiable cervicomedullary angles of less than 135 degrees had brain stem compression, myelopathy, or C2 root pain. Surface coil T_1-weighted MR was as accurate as tomography in evaluating the atlantodental interval (ADI), dens erosion, osteophytes, and the various C1-C2 subluxations and subaxial subluxations. Magnetic resonance was not as efficient in evaluating the basion-dental interval (BDI), apophyseal disease, and cystic changes of the C1 and C2 facets. In 70% of the cases the dental opacity correlated well with the MR appearance; for example, the sclerotic regions of the dens appeared dark and the osteopenic regions bright on T_1-weighted images. Pannus was most commonly found in a retrodental location as an increased amount of intermediate soft tissue signal. Loss of the normal supradental fat pad implies the presence of thickened ligaments or pannus.

When brain stem symptoms are present, MR will consistently show marked craniovertebral junction (CVJ) abnormalities.[85] Facet erosive changes can be difficult to detect with MR because of their small size and the diffi-

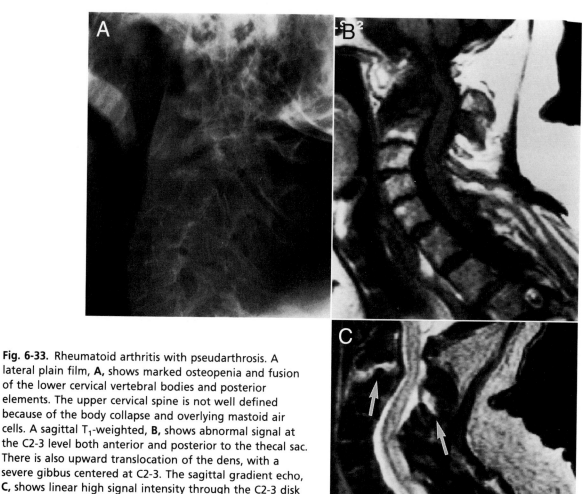

Fig. 6-33. Rheumatoid arthritis with pseudarthrosis. A lateral plain film, **A,** shows marked osteopenia and fusion of the lower cervical vertebral bodies and posterior elements. The upper cervical spine is not well defined because of the body collapse and overlying mastoid air cells. A sagittal T_1-weighted, **B,** shows abnormal signal at the C2-3 level both anterior and posterior to the thecal sac. There is also upward translocation of the dens, with a severe gibbus centered at C2-3. The sagittal gradient echo, **C,** shows linear high signal intensity through the C2-3 disk level extending to the posterior elements and representing the pseudarthrosis *(arrows)*. The relationship of the dens to the foramen magnum and anterior arch of C1 is better appreciated in **C.**

culty of orienting imaging slices. Erosions of the odontoid can be overestimated, especially when the cortex is thin and there is osteoporosis.[83] Measuring bony margins can be difficult with MR because, if the direction of the frequency encoding gradient is anterior-posterior, chemical shift may distort the apparent AP bony margins.

Postoperative Changes

Larsson et al.[86] described pre- and postoperative MR findings in 10 patients with chronic rheumatoid arthritis. The size of preoperative periodontoid pannus in patients with atlantoaxial subluxation decreased following stabilization surgery in all cases (average 6 months' follow-up). They assumed that the pannus reduction was the result of atlantoaxial immobility from surgery and con-

cluded that routine postoperative MR was not necessary but should be reserved for cases with residual or new symptomatology. Posterior fixation artifacts interfered with their evaluation of the periodontal region using T_1-weighted spin-echo sequences in two of five patients.[83] The use of biocompatible titanium wires allows undistorted imaging of the cervical spine, however.[87] Zygmunt et al also found a reduction or disappearance of pannus following posterior fixation.[88,89] They concluded that posterior fixation, by itself, may lead to sufficient decompression by resolving the periodontal pannus. This is to be contrasted with the other treatment option, the combined trans oral anterior decompression followed by posterior occipital cervical fusion.[90]

REFERENCES

1. Burton CV, Kirkaldy-Willis WH, Yong-Hing K, et al: Causes of failure of surgery on the lumbar spine, *Clin Orthop* 1981;157:191-199.
2. Smolik E, Nash F: Lumbar spinal arachnoiditis: a complication of the intervertebral disc operation, *Ann Surg* 1951;133:490-495.
3. Jorgensen J, Hansen PH, Steenskrov V, et al: A clinical and radiological study of chronic lower spinal arachnoiditis, *Neuroradiology* 1975;9:139-144.
4. Smith RW, Loesser JD: A myelographic variant in lumbar arachnoiditis, *J Neurosurg* 1972;36:441-446.
5. Simmons JD, Newton TH: Arachnoiditis. In Newton TH, Potts DG (eds): *Computed tomography of the spine and spinal cord,* San Anselmo Calif, Clavadel, 1983, p 224.
6. Quencer RM, Tenner M, Rothman L: The postoperative myelogram, *Radiology* 1977;123:667-679.
7. Reicher MA, Gold RH, Halboch VV, et al: MR imaging of the lumbar spine: Anatomic correlations and the effects of technical variations, *AJR* 1986;147:891-898.
8. Ross JS, Masaryk TJ, Modic MT, et al: MR imaging of lumbar arachnoiditis. *AJNR* 1987;8:885-892.
9. Mark AS, Andrew B, Sanches J, et al: MR imaging of syringomyelia secondary to arachnoid adhesions. Presented at the 73rd annual meeting of the RSNA, 1987.
10. Quiles M, Marchisello PJ, Tsairis P: Lumbar adhesive arachnoiditis, etiologic and pathologic aspects, *Spine* 1978;3:45-50.
11. Braun IF, Malko JA, Davis PC, et al: The behavior of Pantopaque on MR: in vivo and in vitro analyses, *AJNR* 1986;7:997-1001.
12. Marnourian AC, Briggs RW: Appearance of Pantopaque on MR images, *Radiology* 1986;158:457-460.
13. Johnson CE, Sze G: Benign lumbar arachnoiditis: MR imaging with gadopentetate dimeglumine. *AJNR* 1990;11(4):763-770.
14. McHenry MC, Weinstein AJ: Lumbar vertebral osteomyelitis. In Hardy RW (ed): *Lumbar disc disease,* New York, Raven, 1982, pp 229-254.
15. Lisbona R, Rosenthal L: Observations on the sequential use of Tc-99m phosphate complex and Ga-67 imaging in osteomyelitis, cellulitis, and septic arthritis, *Radiology* 1977;123:123-129.
16. Gelman MI, Coleman RE, Stevens PM, et al: Radiography radionuclide imaging and arthrography in the evaluation of total hip and knee replacement, *Radiology* 1978;128:677-682.
17. Weiss PPE, Mall JC, Hoffer PB, et al: Tc-99m methylene diphosphonate bone imaging in the evaluation of total hip prosthesis. *Radiology* 1979;133:727-729.
18. Rosenthal L, Lisbona R, Hernandez M, et al: Tc-99m PP and Ga-67 imaging following insertion of orthopedic devices. *Radiology* 1979;133:717-721.
19. McAfee JG, Samin A: In-111 labeled leukocytes: a review of problems in image interpretation. *Radiology* 1985;155:221-229.
20. Golimbu C, Firooznia H, Rafii M: CT of osteomyelitis of the spine. *AJR* 1984;142:159-163.
21. Jeffrey RB, Callen PW, Federle MP: Computed tomography of psoas abscesses. *J Comput Assist Tomogr* 1980;4:639-641.
22. Modic MT, Feiglin DH, Piraino DW, et al: Vertebral osteomyelitis: assessment using MR. *Radiology* 1985;157-166.
23. Modic MT, Weinstein MA, Pavlicek W, et al: Nuclear magnetic resonance imaging of the spine. *Radiology* 1983;148:757-762.
24. Bertino RE, Porter BA, Stimac G, Tepper S: Imaging spinal osteomyelitis and epidural abscess with short TI inversion recovery. *AJNR* 1988;9:563-564.
25. Aguila LA, Piraino DW, Modic MT: Magnetic resonance imaging of the intranuclear cleft. *Radiology* 1985;155:155-158.
26. deRoos A, Van Meerten EL, Bloem JL, et al: MRI of tuberculosis spondylitis. *AJR* 1986;146:79-82.
27. Fletcher BD, Scoles PV, Nelson AD: Osteomyelitis in children: detection by magnetic resonance. *Radiology* 1984;150:57-60.
28. Kahn DS, Pritzker KPH: The pathophysiology of bone infection. *Clin Orthop* 1973;961:12-20.
29. Norman A, Kambolis CP: Tumors of the spine and their relationship to the intervertebral disc. *AJR* 1964;92:1270-1274.
30. Resnick D, Niwayama G: Intervertebral disc abnormalities associated with vertebral metastases: observation in patients and cadavers with prostatic cancer. *Invest Radiol* 1978;13(3):182-190.
31. Michael AS, Mikhael MA: Spinal osteomyelitis: unusual findings on MR imaging. *Comput Med Imaging Graph* 1988;12:329-331.
32. Modic MT, Steinberg PM, Ross JS, et al: Degenerative disk disease: Assessment of changes in vertebral body marrow with MR imaging. *Radiology* 1987;166:193-199.
33. Masaryk TJ, Modic MT, Boumphrey F, et al: The effects of chemonucleolysis demonstrated by magnetic resonance imaging. *J Comp Assist Tomog* 1986;10:917-923.
34. Hlavin ML, Kaminski HJ, Ross JS, Ganz E: Spinal epidural abscess: a ten-year perspective. *Neurosurgery* 1990;27(2):177-184.
35. Rankin RM, Flothow PG: Pyogenic infection of the spinal epidural space. *West J Surg Obstet Gynecol* 1946;54:320-323.
36. Baker AS, Ojemann RG, Swartz MN, Richardson EP: Spinal epidural abscess. *N Engl J Med* 1975;293:463-468.
37. Browder J, Meyers R: Pyogenic infections of the spinal epidural space. *Surgery* 1941;10:296-308.
38. Heusner AP: Nontuberculous spinal epidural infections. *N Engl J Med* 1948;239:845-854.
39. Lasker BR, Harter DH: Cervical epidural abscess. *Neurology* 1987;37:1747-1753.
40. Angtuaco EJC, McConnell JR, Chadduck WM, et al: MR imaging of spinal epidural sepsis. *AJNR* 1987;8:879-883.
41. Post MJD, Quencer RM, Montalvo BM, et al: Spinal infection: evaluation with MR imaging and intraoperative US. *Radiology* 1988;169:765-771.
42. Post MJD, Sze G, Quencer RM, et al: Gadolinium-enhanced MR in spinal infection. *J Comput Assist Tomogr* 1990;14(5):721-729.
43. Smith AS, Weinstein MA, Mizushima A, et al: MR imaging characteristics of tuberculous spondylitis vs vertebral osteomyelitis. *AJR* 1989;153:399-405.
44. Weaver P, Lifeso RM: The radiological diagnosis of tuberculosis of the adult spine. *Skeletal Radiol* 1984;12:178-186.
45. Chapman M, Murray RO, Stoker DJ: Tuberculosis of the bones and joints. *Semin Roentgenol* 1979;14:266-282.

46. Young EJ: Human brucellosis. *Rev Infect Dis* 1983;5:821-842.

47. Sharif HS, Osarugue AA, Clark DC, et al: Brucellar and tuberculous spondylitis: comparative imaging features. *Radiology* 1989;171:419-425.

48. Sharif HS, Clark DC, Aabed M, et al: Granulomatous spinal infections: MR imaging. *Radiology* 1990;177:101-107.

49. Naidich JB, Mossey RT, McHeffey-Atkinson B, et al: Spondyloarthropathy from long-term hemodialysis. *Radiology* 1988;167:761-764.

50. Rafto SE, Dalinka MK, Schiebler ML, et al: Spondyloarthropathy of the cervical spine in long-term hemodialysis, *Radiology* 1988;166:201-204.

51. Kaplan P, Resnick D, Murphey M, et al: Destructive noninfectious spondyloarthropathy in hemodialysis patients: a report of four cases, *Radiology* 1987;162:241-244.

52. Maruyama H, Gejyo F, Arakawa M: A magnetic resonance imaging study of destructive spondyloarthropathy in long-term hemodialysis patients, *Nephron* 1991;59:71-74.

53. Garza-Mercado R: Traumatic extradural hematoma of the cervical spine, *J Neurosurg* 1989;24(3):410-414.

54. Bowie EA, Glasgow GL: Cauda equina lesions associated with ankylosing spondylitis: report of three cases, *Br Med J* 1916;2:24-27.

55. Calin A: Ankylosing spondylitis, *Clin Rheum Dis* 1985;11:41-60.

56. Grosman H, Gray R, St Louis EL: CT of long-standing ankylosing spondylitis with cauda equina syndrome, *AJNR* 1983;4:1077-1080.

57. Weinstein PR, Karpman RR, Gall EP, et al: Spinal cord injury, spinal fracture, and spinal stenosis in ankylosing spondylitis, *J Neurosurg* 1982;57:609-616.

58. Tullous MW, Skerhut HEI, Story JL, et al: Cauda equina syndrome of long-standing ankylosing spondylitis: case report and review of the literature, *J Neurosurg* 1990;73:441-447.

59. Rubenstein DJ, Alvarez O, Ghelman B, Marchisello P: Cauda equina syndrome complicating ankylosing spondylitis: MR features (case report), *J Comput Assist Tomogr* 1989;13(3):511-513.

60. Abello R, Rovira M, Sanz MP, et al: MRI and CT of ankylosing spondylitis with vertebral scalloping, *Neuroradiology* 1988;30:272-275.

61. Kenny JB, Hughes PL, Whitehouse GH: Discovertebral destruction in ankylosing spondylitis: the role of computed tomography and magnetic resonance imaging, *Br J Radiol* 1990;63:448-455.

62. Andersson O: Röntgenbiden vid spondylarthritis ankylopoetica, *Nord Med Tidskr* 1937;14:200.

63. Nesbit GM, Miller GM, Baker HL, et al: Spinal cord sarcoidosis: a new finding at MR imaging with Gd-DTPA enhancement, *Radiology* 1989;173:839-843.

64. Kelly RB, Mahoney PD, Cawley KM: MR demonstration of spinal cord sarcoidosis: report of a case, *AJNR* 1988;9:197-199.

65. Miller DH, Kendall BE, Barter S, et al: Magnetic resonance imaging in central nervous system sarcoidosis. *Neurology* 1988;38:378-383.

66. Garrod AE: A treatise on rheumatism and rheumatoid arthritis. London, Griffin, 1890.

67. Morizono Y, Sakou T, Kawaida H: Upper cervical involvement in rheumatoid arthritis. *Spine* 1987;12:721-725.

68. Pellicci PM, Ranawat CS, Tsairis P, Bryan WJ: A prospective study of the progression of rheumatoid arthritis of the cervical spine. *J Bone Joint Surg [Am]* 1981;63:342-350.

69. Redlund-Johnell I, Petterson H: Radiographic measurement of the cranio-vertebral region. *Acta Radiol [Diagn]* 1984;25:23-28.

70. Ranawat CS, O'Leary P, Pellicci P, et al: Cervical spine fusion in rheumatoid arthritis. *J Bone Joint Surg [Am]* 1979;61:1003-1010.

71. Kawaida H, Sakou T, Morizono Y, Yoshikuni N: Magnetic resonance imaging of upper cervical disorders in rheumatoid arthritis. *Spine* 1989;14(11):1144-1148.

72. Kramer J, Jolesz F, Kleefield J: Rheumatoid arthritis of the cervical spine. *Rheum Dis Clin North Am* 1991;17(3):757-772.

73. Weisman BNW, Aliabadi P, Weinfeld MS, et al: Prognostic features of atlantoaxial subluxation in rheumatoid arthritis patients. *Radiology* 1982;144:745-751.

74. Halla JT, Harden JG, Uitek J, Alarcon GS: Involvement of the cervical spine in rheumatoid arthritis. *Arthritis Rheum* 1989;32:652-659.

75. Wolfe BK, O'Keeffe D, Mitchell DM, Tchang SPK: Rheumatoid arthritis of the cervical spine: early and progressive radiographic features. *Radiology* 1987;165:145-148.

76. Snelling JP, Pickard J, Wood SK, Prouse PJ: Reversible cortical blindness as a complication of rheumatoid arthritis of the cervical spine. *Br J Rheumatol* 1990;29:228-230.

77. Katz JN, Liang MH: Differential diagnosis and conservative treatment of rheumatic disorders. In Frymoyer JW (ed): *The adult spine: principles and practice*. New York, Raven, 1991.

78. Ball J: Enthesopathy of rheumatoid and ankylosing spondylitis. *Ann Rheum Dis* 1971;30:213-223.

79. Martel W: Pathogenesis of cervical discovertebral destruction in rheumatoid arthritis. *Arthritis Rheum* 1977;20:1217-1225.

80. Bell GR, Stearns KL: Flexion-extension MRI of the upper rheumatoid cervical spine. *Orthopedics* 1991;14(9):969-974.

81. Dvorak J, Grob D, Baumgartner H, et al: Functional evaluation of the spinal cord by magnetic resonance imaging in patients with rheumatoid arthritis and instability of upper cervical spine. *Spine* 1989;14(10):1057-1063.

82. Krodel A, Refior HJ, Westermann S: The importance of functional magnetic resonance imaging (MRI) in the planning of stabilizing operations on the cervical spine in rheumatoid patients, *Arch Orthop Trauma Surg* 1989;109:30-33.

83. Petterson H, Larsson EM, Holtas S, et al: MR imaging of the cervical spine in rheumatoid arthritis. *AJNR* 1988;9:573-577.

84. Bundschuh CV, Modic MT, Kearny F, et al: Rheumatoid arthritis of the cervical spine: surface-coil MR imaging. *AJNR* 1988;9:565-571.

85. Beltran J, Caudill JL, Herman LA, et al: Rheumatoid arthritis: MR imaging manifestations. *Radiology* 1987;165:153-157.

86. Larsson E, Holtas S, Zygmunt S: Pre- and postoperative MR imaging of the craniocervical junction in rheumatoid arthritis. *AJR* 1989;152(3):561-566.

87. Mirvis SE, Geisler F, Joslyn JN, Zrebeet H: Use of titanium wire in cervical spine fixation as a means to reduce MR artifacts. *AJNR* 1988;9:1229-1231.

88. Zygmunt SC, Ljunggren B, Alund M, et al: Realignment and surgical fixation of atlanto-axial and subaxial dislocations in rheumatoid arthritis (RA) patients. *Acta Neurochir Suppl* 1988;43:79-84.

89. Zygmunt S, Saveland H, Brattstrom H, et al: Reduction of rheumatoid periodontoid pannus following posterior occipito-cervical fusion visualised by magnetic resonance imaging. *Br J Neurosurg* 1988;2:315-320.

90. Crockard HA, Pozp JL, Ransford AO, et al: Transoral decompression and posterior fusion for rheumatoid atlanto-axial subluxation. *J Bone Joint Surg [Br]* 1986;68:350-356.

7

Spinal Tumors

THOMAS J. MASARYK

The crux of the diagnostic imaging evaluation of spinal tumors lies with their physical location vis à vis the neuraxis. In conjunction with such information as age and past medical history, tumor location often enables the radiologist to predict a brief differential diagnosis and thus the mode of therapy and prognosis with a reasonable degree of confidence. Myelography has long been the diagnostic mainstay in evaluating spinal neoplasms, providing an indirect image of the spinal cord and nerve roots from the foramen magnum to the sacrum. Visualization of the negative shadow margins of the cord and its coverings as well as direct assessment of the integrity of the bony canal frequently enabled radiologists to predict the location of a mass lesion as intramedullary, extramedullary-intradural, and extramedullary-extradural.[1] In addition, the use of water-soluble intrathecal contrast material in conjunction with high-resolution computed tomography provided a second imaging plane to define the suspected location and thus increase the specificity of the radiographic workup.[2-4]

Magnetic resonance imaging combines the best of both modalities with few (if any) of the disadvantages. Many early reports[5-14] documenting the utility of MRI in the spine commented on its ability to image the cord in multiple planes and thus accurately pinpoint neoplastic disease. Additionally, MRI characterizes lesions based on morphology and location not only with respect to the cord but also according to signal-intensity characteristics that reflect tissue T_1, T_2, and spin-density as well as paramagnetic or chemical-shift effects and motion. The subsequent implementation of surface coil technology, cardiac gating, gradient refocusing, and paramagnetic contrast agents has done much to improve visualization of the spinal cord and surrounding tissues as well as increase both the sensitivity and the specificity to disease.[15-36] Innovations in pulse-sequence design such as saturation pulses, gradient echo imaging,

and rapid acquisition with relaxation enhancement (RARE)—also known as "fast spin echo" and "turbo spin echo" imaging—are likely to refine further the utility of MR imaging of spinal neoplasia.[37-39]

EPIDEMIOLOGY

Tumors of the spinal cord and its coverings are, fortunately, rare; their frequency varies among different clinical series depending on histologic classification and whether masses related to congenital defects, vascular anomalies, and spinal extension of intracranial tumors and extraspinal metastases have been excluded. The annual incidence of primary spinal neoplasms has been estimated[40] at 2.5/100,000 population per year. Overall, there is no significant sex difference for the development of spinal neoplasia.[41]

In a review of numerous series, Nittner[42] suggested that approximately one fifth of all CNS tumors occur in the spine. The frequency at various levels of the spinal canal (cervical, thoracic, lumbar) is roughly proportionate to the number (and length) of segments at that level.[43] Only 1% of primary spinal cord tumors involve multiple separate levels, a finding that should suggest the possibility of neurofibromatosis.[44,45] In his 1976 review of 4885 adult spinal cord tumors presented in the literature, Nittner[42] found nerve sheath tumors (i.e., neurilemomas and schwannomas) (23%), meningiomas (22%), glial (intramedullary) tumors (13.2%) and (extramedullary) ependymomas (2.5%), sarcomas (8.2%), and metastases (6%) to be most common. The remaining 25% were dispersed among a variety of miscellaneous mass lesions. Pain is often the significant presenting complaint among adults with spinal tumors.[43]

Differences exist among spinal neoplasms in series dealing with adults compared to those dealing with children. As might be expected, lipomas, dermoids, and other embryonal tumors are more common earlier in life, increasing the percentage of lesions found in the lumbosacral region of pediatric patients.[46,47] In addition to developmental lesions, primary intramedullary (glioma) and extradural (sarcoma) tumors occur more commonly in children whereas intradural extramedullary masses (schwannoma, meningioma) are uncommon.[48,49] Clinical presentation in children likewise differs from that in adults, with a preponderance of motor findings (gait disturbance, sphincter dysfunction), possibly related to the inability of very young patients to articulate their symptoms.[50]

INTRAMEDULLARY NEOPLASMS
Gliomas

The most common intramedullary neoplasms are the gliomas: ependymoma, astrocytoma (grades 1 to 4), ganglioglioma, and, rarely, primitive neuroectodermal tumors (PNET). Astrocytomas and ependymomas comprise the overwhelming majority of these lesions. Ependymomas are often cited[43,44,51] as the most frequent in adults (65%), particularly at the conus medullaris and filum terminale. Conversely, astrocytomas appear to be slightly more common in the pediatric population (59%).[52,53]

Astrocytoma. Intramedullary astrocytomas account for only 6% to 8% of all primary spinal tumors.[47,54,55] Peak incidence is estimated to be in the third to fourth decades of life.[55]

Astrocytomas appear as soft tissue masses within the substance of the spinal cord, producing a focal enlargement and rarely exophytic growth.[56] Occasionally they present as massive lesions involving the entire length of the spinal cord.[52,53] The vast majority (75% to 92% of cord astrocytomas) are relatively benign (grades I and II).[57,58] Rarely, malignant lesions may spread intracranially via the cerebrospinal fluid pathways.[57] Unlike ependymomas, they seldom have a surgically identifiable cleavage plane between tumor and cord substance.[59] This fact, coupled with their relative resistance to radiotherapy, accounts for the guarded prognosis associated with these lesions.[59,60]

Magnetic resonance imaging findings for intramedullary astrocytomas are as follows: T_1-weighted sagittal examinations typically demonstrate a fusiform enlargement of the spinal cord over one or several segments by a soft tissue mass of normal or slightly decreased signal intensity (Figs. 7-1 and 7-2). T_2-weighted sagittal and axial studies demonstrate focal areas of increased signal within the enlarged cord segment that represent neoplastic and edematous cord tissue.* The use of cardiac gating, even echo rephasing, or additional refocusing gradients during the acquisition of T_2-weighted images will improve the visualization of these intramedullary signal derangements. It has been our continued preference to employ spin-echo techniques for the evaluation of intramedullary disease despite reports of equal or superior results with T_2^* gradient echo sequences.[38] Early experience with RARE sequences[39] suggests that they can provide T_2 contrast with significant reductions in imaging time and thus may also be valuable for the study of intramedullary tumors.

The MR appearance of intramedullary gliomas may vary from the foregoing description with the presence of intramedullary cysts or cavitations. In the series of Sloof et al.[43] 38% of astrocytomas demonstrated "syringomyelic" cavities at autopsy. Cysts located rostral or caudal to the tumor are typically nonneoplastic, with gliotic linings, and filled with fluid similar to cerebrospinal fluid; by contrast, those within neoplastic masses are lined by abnormal glia and are xanthochromic or blood filled.[53,63] In an effort to avoid confusion between benign syringohydromyelia and neoplastic cysts, Gay et al.[62] defined the rostral and caudal cavities as tumor cysts and the central cavitations as intratumoral cysts (Fig. 7–1). Reports of the accuracy of MR in demonstrating such cysts (long T_1, long T_2) vary depending on pulse sequence and the presence of protein within the cysts (which may alter relaxation times of the cyst fluid).[62-65] Also, in the case of large intratumoral cysts without an obvious soft tissue mass, one may have difficulty distinguishing a neoplastic lesion from a benign syrinx cavity.[65] Morpho-

---

*References 5-14, 38, 61, 62.

Fig. 7-1. A, This 500 msec TR/17 msec TE midline sagittal image through the distal spinal cord demonstrates an intramedullary cystic mass lesion *(arrow)* in a young boy who presented only with paresthesia in one thigh. **B** and **C,** 500 msec TR/17 msec TE axial images through a level of the lesion show its cystic nature *(arrows)*. **D,** A 2000 msec TR/120 msec TE midline sagittal image through the cystic mass in the conus demonstrates high signal intensity emanating from the cyst *(arrow)*. **E,** Note in the intraoperative photograph the diffuse swelling of the distal cord with multiple enlarged vessels *(arrows)* overlying it. **F,** When the cord was opened, a blood-filled "intratumoral cyst" *(arrows)* was found within this astrocytoma.

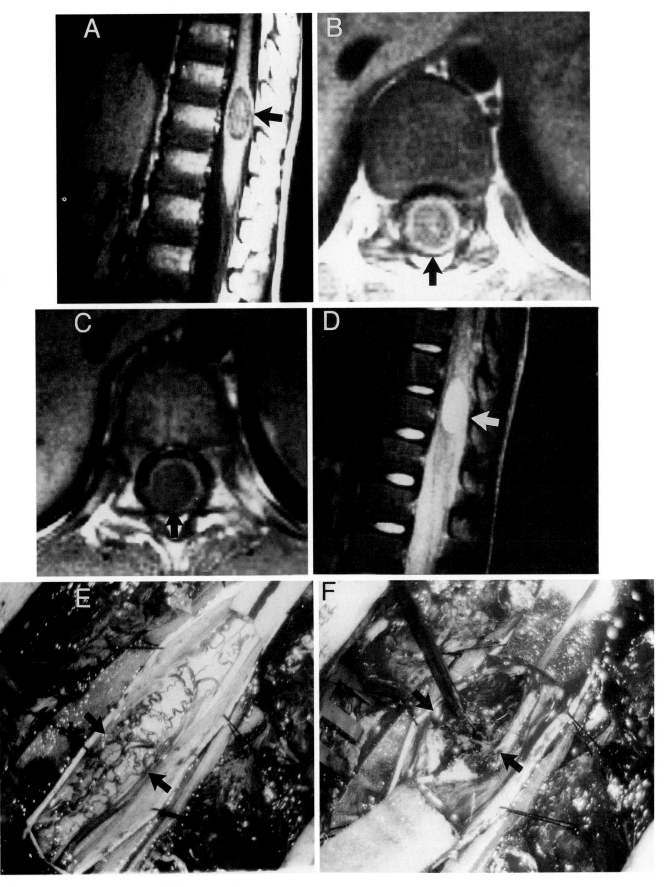

Fig. 7-1. For legend see opposite page.

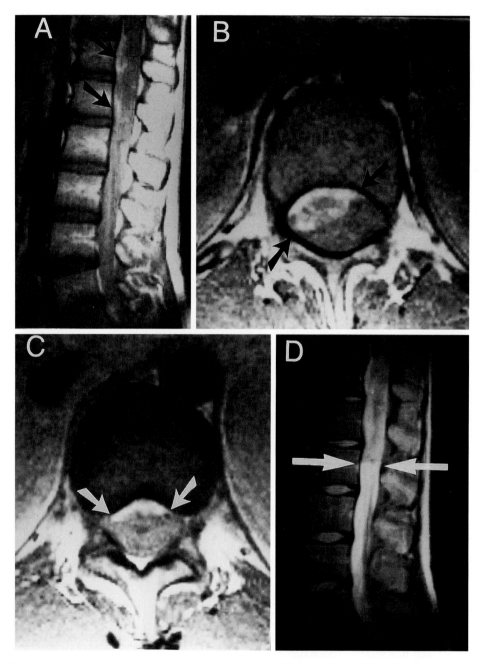

Fig. 7-2. A, A 500 msec TR/17 msec TE midline sagittal image of the thoracolumbar junction demonstrates heterogeneous soft tissue signal in the region of the conus medullaris *(arrows)* but no obvious soft tissue mass. Note that the cord itself is poorly visualized at this level. **B** and **C,** 500 msec TR/17 msec TE axial images through the thoracolumbar junction show heterogeneous areas of signal intensity within the spinal canal *(arrows)* without a discernible cord. Note the enlarged canal in **B.** A 2000 msec TR/90 msec TE midline sagittal image of the thoracolumbar junction, **D,** reveals diffuse soft tissue enlargement of the conus. The CSF space below this level is completely blocked by the mass, as evidenced by its high signal and lack of CSF pulsation artifact in the phase-encoding direction *(arrows).* The diagnosis was astrocytoma.

logically the presence of a distinct sharp and smooth interface as well as cyst fluid that is isointense with CSF favors the diagnosis of benign syrinx.[65]

It must also be noted that motion affects the signal intensity within benign syringomyelic or tumor cysts and may help distinguish them from necrotic intratumoral cysts. It is postulated[66,67] that derangements of intracranial and spinal venous and CSF pressure generate dissecting fluid shifts that both produce and extend these cavities. The motion within nonneoplastic glial-lined syringomyelic and tumor cysts can be recognized by the presence of CSF flow void or signal loss and ghosting on nonrefocused asymmetric-echo T_2-weighted scans.[68,69] Conversely, intratumoral cysts resulting from necrotic cavitation usually do not possess this fluid motion and thus have higher signal intensity (than CSF) on such T_2-weighted sequences.

Paramagnetic contrast has also been used with success* to locate accurately intramedullary mass lesions within the spinal cord on T_1-weighted images, separating tumor from surrounding edema or cystic cavitations. Although most intraspinal gliomas are histologically low grade, the overwhelming majority of reported cases[26,29-34] have demonstrated some evidence of contrast enhancement, which tends to be fairly focal. Intravenous contrast enhancement can aid in the differentiation of benign glial-lined cysts from areas of neoplastic cavitation. As just noted, spinal cord cysts are thought to arise and extend on the basis of fluid or pressure shifts, which can also produce local cord gliosis. This gliosis may be difficult to distinguish from neoplasm on unenhanced MR since it too may demonstrate long T_1 and T_2 relaxation characteristics.[70] Fortunately, neoplastic cysts more frequently demonstrate a surrounding area of enhancement.[70] Despite these differential characteristics, Brunberg et al.[71] have reported that the preoperative delineation of tumor from adjacent intramedullary cysts can be difficult and may require intraoperative sonography.[71]

Ependymoma. Ependymomas may involve any portion of the spinal cord but are particularly noteworthy at the conus medullaris and filum terminale (Figs. 7-3 and 7-4). They are the most common primary tumor of the lower spinal cord, conus medullaris, and filum terminale, representing over 50% of all tumors at this location.[55,72] The myxopapillary subtype is particularly common. Although they comprise only about 30% of all ependymomas, Sonneland et al.[73] reported that of 77 cases of myxopapillary ependymoma 95% either were limited to or involved the filum and conus medullaris and only 4% were located in the cervicothoracic spinal cord. Indeed, so strong is this association between the distal cord and myxopapillary ependymoma that there are reports[74,75] of subcutaneous sacrococcygeal lesions, which

most likely arise from extradural embryonic remnants of the filum terminale.

Ependymomas usually present in the fourth to fifth decade of life (much later than the more common intracranial ependymomas), typically with complaints of back pain.[76] Often they are amenable to surgical removal both within the cord and at the filum because of a well-defined capsule.[59] The prognosis following surgery and radiation therapy can be quite good.[59,60,77]

With MR an ependymoma may appear as a fusiform enlargement of the cord itself or as a lobulated extramedullary mass frequently involving the filum terminale and cauda equina (Figs. 7-3 and 7-4). Much like an astrocytoma it is iso- or hypointense to the normal cord on T_1-weighted images and hyperintense on T_2-weighted scans.[26,29-33] Following the administration of paramagnetic contrast it typically enhances quite vigorously because it is often vascular. In addition, Nemoto et al.[78] have reported areas of hypointensity within or around eight of 35 intramedullary tumors that on T_2-weighted scans were believed to represent a susceptibility effect of hemosiderin or ferritin from prior hemorrhage. Seven of these lesions were surgically proved to be ependymoma, and this finding was appreciated in 64% of all ependymomas in the series. The authors indicated that this finding is strongly suggestive of the diagnosis of ependymoma and may be helpful in delineating a tumor capsule and thus the margin of resection.[78] It is important to recognize, however, that this finding may not be as apparent on RARE-type spin-echo pulse sequences. Also noteworthy, in the series of Sloof et al.,[43] is the fact that 46% of ependymomas were associated with cystic cavities of the spinal cord. The same imaging caveats regarding intratumoral and syrinx cysts noted for astrocytomas apply also to ependymomas.[62,70,71]

Ganglioglioma. Gangliogliomas are an uncommon neoplasm composed of both neural and glial cells that occur in the first three decades of life. They usually affect the temporal lobe, cerebellum, and parietooccipital lobe; in the spinal cord they comprise only 1.1% of spinal neoplasms.[79,80] The most common location in the spine is the cervical cord.[81] The tumors are slow growing with a rather prolonged clinical course although isolated cases of malignant transformation with CSF spread have been reported.[51,82-84]

Johannsson et al.[85] found that the prognosis was related not to histologic appearances but to tumor extent and resectability. The prognosis is usually good, and long-term survival can be achieved after local resection.

Cheung et al.[86] reported two cases of spinal ganglioglioma, both presenting as so-called "holocord" mass lesions. The ability of MR to define the superior-inferior extent of the tumor was thought to be important in planning complete surgical extirpation. The findings on MRI were similar to those with other types of gliomas: the

---

*References 26, 29, 30, 32-34, 36.

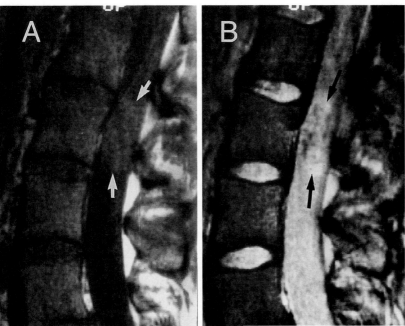

Fig. 7-3. A, A 500 msec TR/17 msec TE midline sagittal image of the lumbar spine demonstrates a rounded globular soft tissue mass present near the conus medullaris *(arrows)* of approximately the same signal intensity as the spinal cord. **B,** The 2000 msec TR 90/msec TE sagittal midline image again demonstrates a globular soft tissue mass *(arrows),* now of increased signal intensity at the conus. **C,** An axial T$_1$-weighted image reveals the mass *(T)* within the canal. Surgery confirmed the presence of an ependymoma of the conus medullaris.

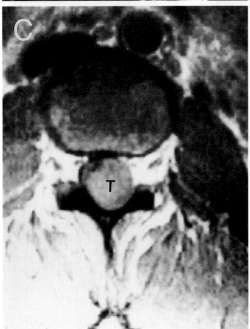

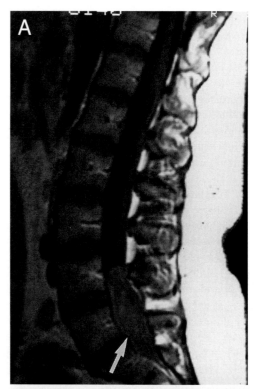

Fig. 7-4. A and B, 500 msec TR/15 msec TE gadolinium-DTPA—enhanced sagittal and axial images of the lower lumbar spine demonstrate a well-circumscribed, heterogeneously enhancing mass at the distal thecal sac that slightly expands the spinal canal. Biopsy and excision demonstrated this lesion to be an ependymoma of the filum terminale.

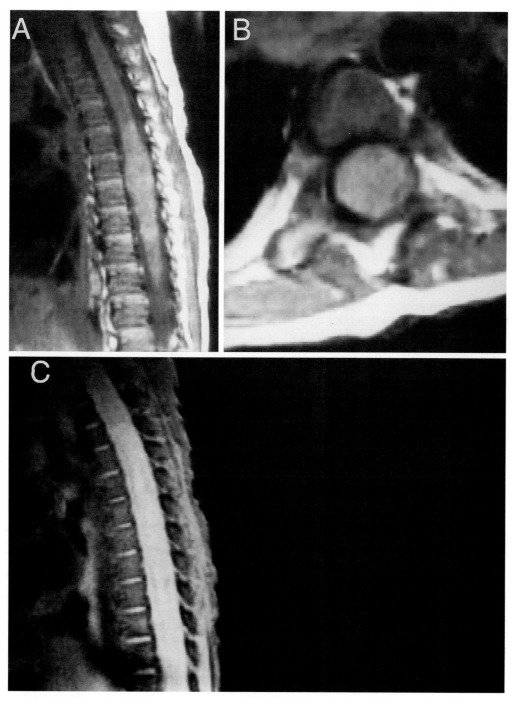

Fig. 7-5. A, This 500 msec TR/17 msec TE midline sagittal slice through the thoracic spine in a child demonstrates fusiform enlargement of the cord. **B,** A 500 msec TR/17 msec TE axial image confirms the enlargement. **C,** A 2000 msec TE midline sagittal T$_2$-weighted image (nonrefocused) shows homogeneously increased signal intensity of the cord and surrounding CSF that masks the lesion. Surgery and histology confirmed the presence of a thoracic ganglioglioma.

tumors appeared hypointense to the cord on T_1 images and hyperintense on T_2 images and were mainly solid at exploration[86] (Fig. 7-5).

Hemangioblastoma

Hemangioblastomas are uncommon. Frequent confusion with vascular malformations and other vascular tumors, as well as the lack of uniformity in classification, has in the past made assessment of their incidence relative to other spinal tumors difficult. In the review of Sloof et al.[43] of 1322 primary spinal canal tumors, there were 300 intramedullary lesions and only four of these were hemangioblastomas. They usually present in the third or fourth decade of life.[43,87]

Whereas they can occur as isolated masses, hemangioblastomas are frequently multiple and seen in association with posterior fossa tumors as part of the von Hippel–Lindau syndrome (VHL)[88] (Fig. 7-6). This autosomal dominant complex has been linked to a defect on chromosome 3 and features hemangioblastomas of the posterior fossa and spinal neuraxis; retinal angiomas; cysts or cystadenomas of the pancreas, adrenals, kidneys, and ovaries; pheochromocytomas; and renal cell carcinomas.[88-91] Although previously thought to be relatively rare, spinal hemangioblastomas may be much more common in association with this disorder, are frequently asymptomatic, and can be either intramedullary or intradural-extramedullary in location[92] (Fig. 7-7). It has been estimated[90,93,94] that approximately one in four patients with brain and spinal cord hemangioblastomas has underlying VHL and approximately a third of patients with known VHL have hemangioblastomas.

Hemangioblastomas are histologically similar to angioblastic meningiomas and apparently arise as small nodules from the pia.[89] They most often present as intramedullary cysts containing a vascular nodule; cyst formation is seen in up to 67% of intramedullary spine lesions[87,95] (Figs.7-6 and 7-8). Another unique feature of hemangioblastomas reported by Solomon and Stein[96] is the striking intramedullary edema seen with these relatively well-circumscribed lesions. Usually the thoracic cord is involved (51%), followed by the cervical cord (41%).[87,97]

Because there are no significant external manifestations of the disease and no readily available genetic tests, imaging plays an important role in the screening and management of these patients.[94] Magnetic resonance is particularly well suited to the evaluation of these lesions because of its superior ability to image not only the spinal cord but also posterior fossa structures (Fig. 7-6). Unenhanced MR studies typically demonstrate extensive widening of the cord with or without associated cysts.[95,96] Whereas the cord typically demonstrates prolongation of T_1 and T_2 relaxation times, the cysts may vary in signal intensity depending on their contents.[95] Signal characteristics can parallel those of CSF or may be of greater intensity as a result of increased protein content.[64,95] Because these tumors are typically quite vascular, serpentine areas of signal void may be seen that represent feeding arteries or draining veins associated with the tumor nidus.[87,97] The administration of paramagnetic contrast dramatically improves visualization of the tumor nidus, often allowing its differentiation from the adjacent edematous spinal cord.[29-31,94-96]

Fig. 7-6. A, A midline sagittal 500 msec TR/15 msec TE image through the brain and cervicomedullary junction demonstrates hydrocephalus secondary to a cystic mass positioned at the inferior aspect of the fourth ventricle that is obstructing CSF outflow. Most of the mass is cystic, but a small heterogeneous nodule *(arrow)* has primarily soft tissue signal with multiple small foci of flow void. **B** and **C,** 2000 msec TR/20 msec TE coronal images demonstrate high signal intensity within the cystic component of the mass *(arrowhead)*, which is of significantly higher signal than the CSF within the lateral ventricles *(curved arrows)*. The nodule itself is rather heterogeneous and of low signal intensity *(solid black arrow)*. Additionally, multiple suspected feeding vessels and draining veins can be seen in the form of a flow void defect near the mass *(curved white arrow)*. **D** and **E,** Corresponding TR 2000 msec/TE 90 msec images again demonstrate obstructive hydrocephalus secondary to the heterogeneous mass *(black arrow)* with a cystic component. The multiple areas of flow void are suspicious for increased vascularity. **F** and **G,** Sagittal and axial 500 msec TR/20 msec TE T_1-weighted images after intravenous administration of gadolinium-DTPA show the avidly enhancing mass within a large cyst, producing obstructive hydrocephalus at the inferior aspect of the fourth ventricle *(arrow)*. **H** and **I,** AP and lateral left vertebral angiograms demonstrate the posterior fossa mass with a disproportionate amount of mass effect. These findings were consistent with a pathologic diagnosis of hemangioblastoma.

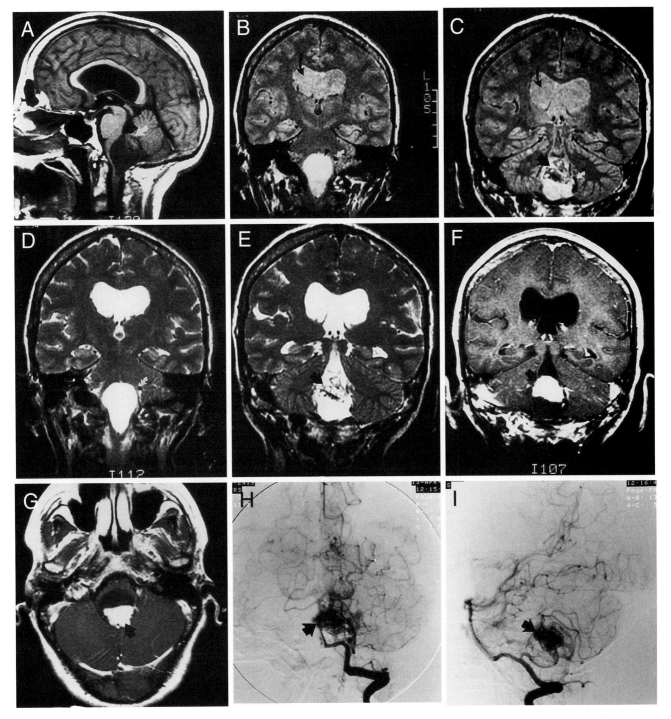

Fig. 7-6. For legend see opposite page.

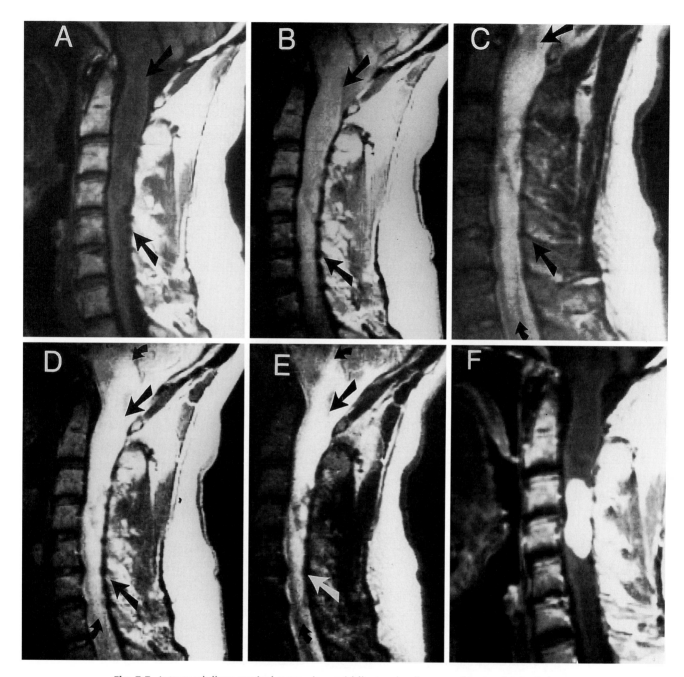

Fig. 7-7. Intramedullary cervical tumor in a middle-aged college professor who had signs and symptoms of cervical myelopathy. The initial MR examination, **A** to **E,** suggested this diagnosis. **A,** A 500 msec TR/17 msec TE midline sagittal image shows diffuse enlargement of the upper cervical spinal cord *(arrows).* **B** to **E,** 2000 msec TR/30, 60, 90, and 120 msec TEs demonstrate spinal cord enlargement *(slanted arrows)* with increased signal in the mass and high-signal edema extending above and below it *(small curved arrows).* Follow-up examination performed with intravenous Gd-DTPA over 1 year after the initial onset of symptoms. A midline sagittal 500 msec TR/17 msec TE image of the cervical spinal cord, **F,** again demonstrates diffuse enlargement, suggesting extensive involvement of the cord, but after the administration of gadolinium the actual tumor nidus is seen to be confined to a small focal area of increased signal at the C3-4 level only. The diagnosis was hemangioblastoma.

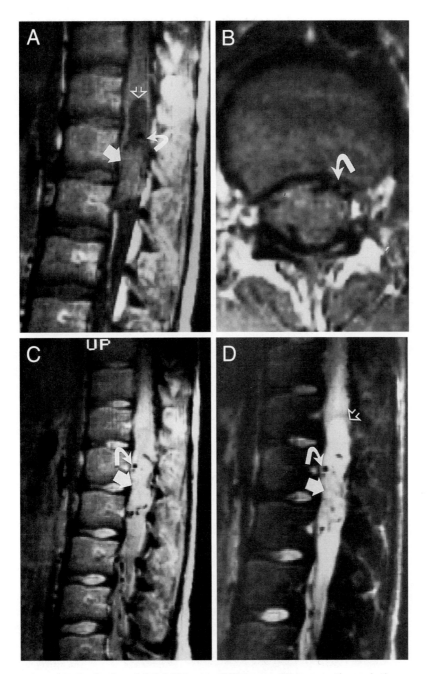

Fig. 7-8. A and **B,** Sagittal and axial 500 msec TR/20 msec TE images through the thoracolumbar junction demonstrate a heterogeneous soft tissue mass *(solid arrow)* surrounded by a superiorly placed cyst at the conus medullaris *(open arrow)*. Multiple areas of flow void suggest increased vascularity *(curved arrow)*. **C** and **D,** 200 msec TR/20 and 90 msec TE images corresponding to the same location and show a heterogeneous soft tissue mass *(solid white arrow)* with multiple focal areas of flow void around it, suggesting increased vascularity *(curved arrow)*. On the T_2-weighted image, note the high signal intensity within the cystic component greater than that of the surrounding edema or CSF *(open arrow)*.   *Continued.*

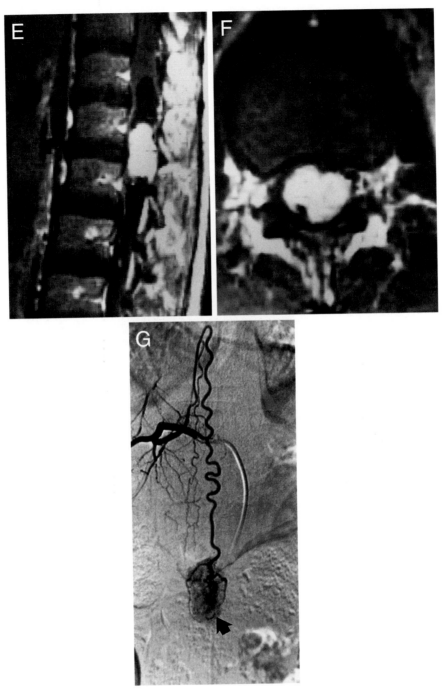

Fig. 7-8, cont'd. E and **F,** 500 msec TR/20 msec TE sagittal and axial images through the soft tissue mass following intravenous gadolinium demonstrate avid uptake of contrast material, suggesting increased vascularity. **G,** A spinal angiogram shows the markedly enhancing mass *(solid arrow)*, consistent with a surgical diagnosis of spinal hemangioblastoma.

Embryonal Tumors

Lipomas, dermoids, and epidermoids may present as primary intramedullary mass lesions at any level of the spine[98-100] (Figs. 7-9 and 7-10). They are most frequently recognized, however, as intradural-intramedullary lesions at or near the conus medullaris in conjunction with dysraphic complexes. They are congenital tumors arising from the implantation of embryonic rests secondary to incomplete separation of neural ectoderm from cutaneous ectoderm during neural tube closure between the sixth and eighth week of intrauterine life. In their report and review of the literature, Roux et al.[101] indicate that the incidence of intraspinal dermoid and epidermoid tumors is approximately 1% or less of all spinal neoplasms; purely intramedullary masses with-

out associated dermal sinus or extramedullary extension are much rarer. Clinical presentation is typically that of myelopathy dominated by motor weakness.

Lipomas are composed of fat and thus are characterized by their high signal intensity on T_1-weighted images, which becomes less intense with more T_2 weighting[7,102] (Fig. 7-9). Central nervous system dermoids and epidermoids display a variety of noncharacteristic signal-intensity patterns on T_1- and T_2-weighted images between different lesions and within one tumor[101,103,104] (Fig. 7-10). This may be related to the physical state (solid vs liquid) and lipid content (cholesterol vs fatty acid) of the cyst.[101] In their report of an intramedullary spinal epidermoid, Roux et al.[101] describe a well-circumscribed focal intramedullary mass that demon-

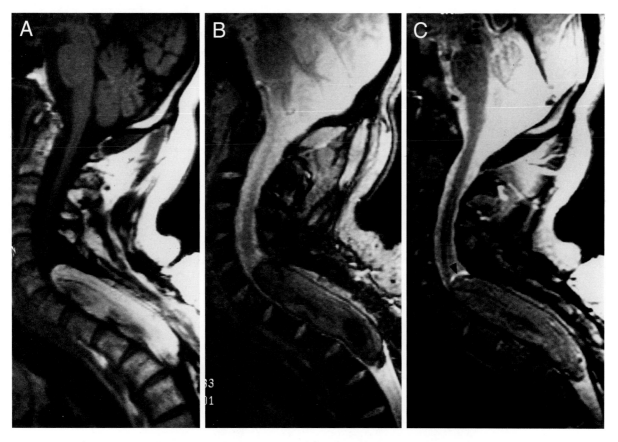

Fig. 7-9. A, A 500 msec TR/17 msec TE T_1-weighted sagittal image through the upper thoracic spine demonstrates an oblong area of heterogeneous (albeit prominently high) signal intensity located within the cord. **B,** A 500 msec TR/10 msec TE steady-state free precession gradient echo image shows the intramedullary mass (note the flaring of of the spinal cord margins to surround the lesion), which is much more heterogeneous. The larger areas of low signal intensity on this study may represent susceptibility artifacts secondary to calcification, or (less likely) hemorrhage. **C,** A sagittal 200 msec TR/90 msec TE image through the cervical thoracic spine again shows the intramedullary mass. Note the high-signal halo along the superior aspect of the mass *(arrowhead)* consistent with chemical-shift artifact secondary to a large amount of fatty material. This image helped make the diagnosis of an intramedullary thoracic lipoma.

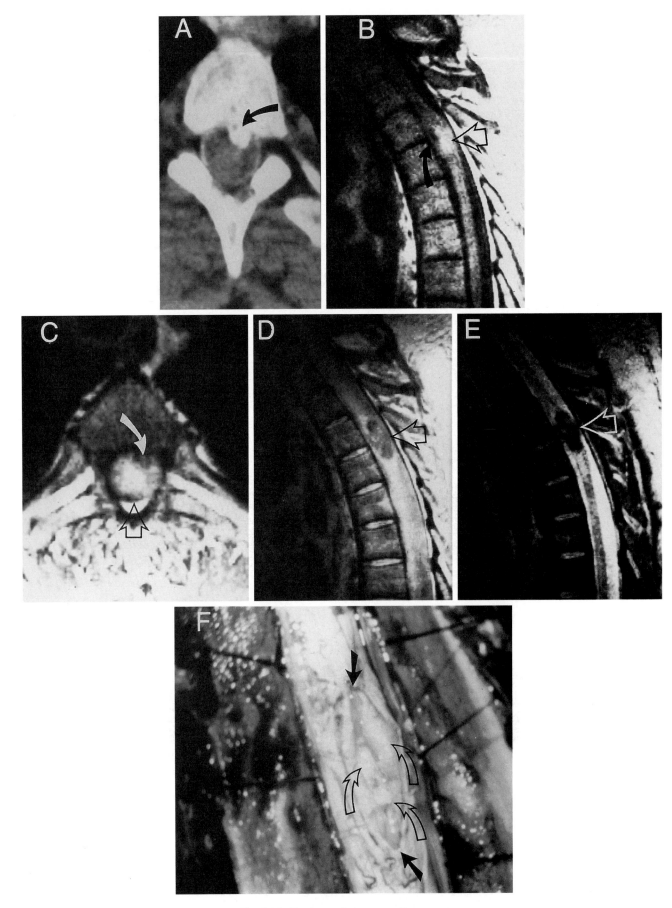

Fig. 7-10. For legend see opposite page.

Fig. 7-10. Myelopathy at the thoracic sensory level in a middle-aged man who was originally evaluated with myelography followed by high-resolution CT. **A,** An axial image from the CT scan at the level of the sensory deficit demonstrates enlargement of the thoracic cord by a partially calcified mass located anteriorly *(arrow).* **B,** On this 500 msec TR/17 msec TE sagittal scan subsequently acquired, the focal intramedullary lesion is well demonstrated. It is primarily of high signal intensity *(open arrow)* with a smaller focal area of decreased signal anteriorly, probably representing the calcification noted on the CT scan. **C,** A 500 msec TR/17 msec TE axial image through the level of the lesion again demonstrates the area of high signal intensity in the central portion of the thoracic cord *(open arrow)* with a small focal area of decreased signal *(curved arrow)* in the region of the calcification. **D,** A 2000 msec TR/60 msec TE sagittal scan through the thoracic spine shows the intramedullary mass, which now appears to be of decreased signal relative to the cord *(open arrow).* **E,** The 2000 msec TR/120 msec TE midline sagittal image demonstrates a focal low-signal enlargement of the cord at the level of the mass lesion *(open arrow)* with a small amount of edema in the cord above and below it. The intraoperative photograph, **F,** demonstrates focal enlargement of the cord *(solid arrows)* that at myelotomy produced a collection of white material *(open arrows).* This was histologically proved to be an intramedullary epidermoid.

---

strated prolongation of T_1 and T_2 relaxation times without adjacent edema but with peripheral enhancement when paramagnetic contrast was used.

Primary Spinal Cord Lymphoma

Primary non-Hodgkin's lymphoma of the CNS is uncommon, with a reported incidence of 0.8% to 1.5% of all primary intracranial tumors.[105,106] The spinal cord is much less frequently involved; only a small number of cases have been reported in the medical literature.[107] Previous reports[51] have referenced this tumor as "microgliomatosis," "perivascular sarcoma," "reticulum cell sarcoma," and "malignant reticuloendothelioma." Bluemke and Wang[108] report a single elderly male presenting with myelopathic symptoms and lower extremity motor weakness who was found to have a fusiform intramedullary mass demonstrating low signal on T_1- and high signal on T_2-weighted images with intense enhancement following intravenous paramagnetic contrast. These findings are nonspecific, however. Metastatic secondary involvement of the cord has also been reported with similar imaging findings, although this too is rare and much less common than lymphoma involving the brain.[109]

Primary Intramedullary Melanoma

Primary melanoma originating in the spinal cord is rare and is presumed to arise either from melanoblasts accompanying the pial sheaths of vascular bundles or from congenital neuroectodermal rests.[110,111] The finding of pial deposits within intramedullary melanomas, the occurrence of an exophytic component, an occasional extradural extension, and the suggestion of metastatic seedings via the CSF or intraaxial pathways support this concept—known as the "chromatophore" or "mesodermal" theory of origin[110,111]—which has also been invoked to explain melanomas of the dura mater.[111,112] The competing hypothesis proposes that during embryogenesis a few neuroectodermal rest cells migrate to reside within the neural tube and its coverings and later undergo neoplastic change.[111] There are criteria for making a diagnosis of primary spinal cord melanoma[110]: (1) no malignant melanoma can be outside the central nervous system (metastatic or primary); and (2) the lesion must be confirmed pathologically.

Different series[110,113,114] document both insidious and abrupt onset of symptoms, occasionally masquerading as another myelopathic entity. Back pain is a frequent complaint.[113,114] CSF analysis may reveal coal-black or grossly bloody fluid.[111,113] MR may be highly suggestive on the basis of a high-signal mass within the spinal cord on unenhanced T_1-weighted images reflecting the paramagnetic effect of melanin or frequently associated hemorrhage (Fig. 7-11).

Metastases

Metastatic disease may also (rarely) present as an intramedullary mass lesion. Autopsy series[115-117] estimate the incidence of cord involvement at 8.5% of patients with systemic disease, although symptomatic disease is probably much less frequent. Primary tumors outside the CNS may spread to the cord hematogenously, either via arterial seeding or transvenously via Batson's plexus.[115,117-119] Carcinomas of the lung and breast are the most frequently identified, with melanoma, lymphoma, and adenocarcinoma also reported.[115,117-119] Intracranial neoplasms such as medulloblastoma, ependymoma, and glioma are known to spread via CSF seeding to the leptomeninges, which may lead to direct invasion of the spinal cord.[120-125] The thoracic spine is most commonly involved.[119] Also, whereas leptomeningeal disease may coexist with intramedullary foci, concomitant osseous metastatic implants are uncommon.[115,117,118]

Like primary intramedullary tumors, metastatic lesions typically produce enlargement (best appreciated on T_1-weighted images) and signal-intensity alterations (low signal on T_1- and high signal on T_2-weighted images) of the cord[126] (Fig. 7-12). Following the administration of contrast, metastases typically enhance vigorously.[26,30]

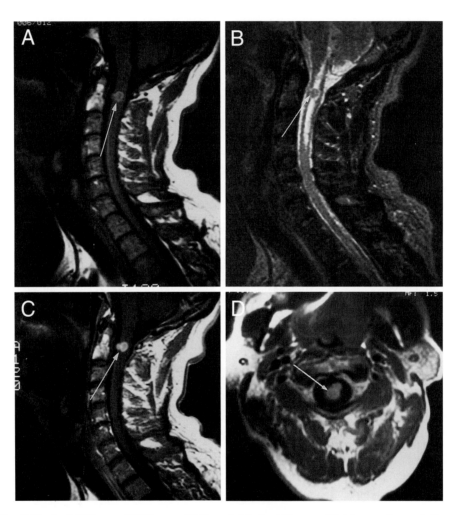

Fig. 7-11. A, A 500 msec TR/15 msec TE T_1-weighted midline sagittal image through the cervical spine demonstrates an area of high signal intensity within the cord at C2 (arrow). **B,** This 2000 msec TR/90 msec TE midline sagittal T_2-weighted image through the cervical spine shows the mass with low signal intensity and a large flame-shaped area of high signal extending both superiorly and inferiorly from it. **C and D,** Sagittal and axial 500 msec TR/20 msec TE images following intravenous gadolinium reveal intense enhancement within the lesion. The paramagnetic effect heralded by this signal intensity characteristic of the mass on an unenhanced study suggests the possibility of hemorrhage and/or melanin. No other lesions were found, and a diagnosis of primary melanoma of the spinal cord was made.

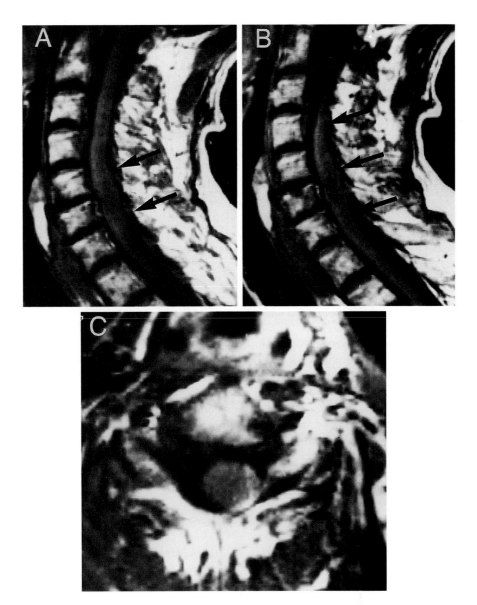

Fig. 7-12. A and **B,** 500 msec TR/17 msec TE sagittal images demonstrate focal enlargement of the cervical cord in a patient with known metastatic carcinoma of the breast. **C,** This 500 msec TR/17 msec TE axial image confirms the enlargement, which proved to be an intramedullary metastatic focus.

EXTRAMEDULLARY-INTRADURAL MASS LESIONS

Extramedullary-intradural tumors are primarily benign and comprise the largest single group of spinal mass lesions; meningiomas and nerve sheath tumors alone account for roughly half of all adult spinal tumors. Typically the lesions are isolated, well-circumscribed, and readily identified solid masses recognized by their soft tissue signal on short-TR T_1-weighted spin-echo pulse sequences relative to the low-signal surrounding CSF.[102,127] On the basis of size and contrast characteristics, secondary neoplasms involving the intradural-extramedullary compartment may be exceptionally difficult to detect by unenhanced MR studies alone.[128-130] However, the use of intravenous paramagnetic contrast agents dramatically improves the conspicuousness of both primary and secondary lesions and is essential for adequate imaging evaluation of suspected intradural masses.[26-28,30-34]

Meningiomas

Meningiomas are unique in that there is a 4:1 female:male predominance, with most patients being over 40 years of age.[42] Some 80% of lesions can be found in the thoracic spine.[42] They are often located anterolaterally or posterolaterally in the canal, being thought to arise in the region of the denticulate ligaments.[43,51] Meningiomas are also the most common tumor of the foramen magnum, where they frequently appear anteriorly or laterally.[42] Rarely, they will be both intradural and extradural (6%) or purely extradural (7%); when extradural, they are often malignant.[42,131] Rarely, also, they may be multiple.[132] The most common presentation is local or radicular pain that is typically ipsilateral to the side of the lesion.

There are four histologic subtypes of meningiomas[42,43,47,51]: meningothelial, fibroblastic, psammomatous, and angiomatous. The tissue of origin for most meningiomas is the covering cell of the arachnoid (the "cap cell" layer). The angiomatous (angioblastic) form differs from the other types of meningiomas in lacking arachnoid cap cells.[133] It is subdivided into hemangioblastic and hemangiopericytic categories. The hemangioblastic form arises from capillary walls and is similar histologically to the cerebellar hemangioblastoma. Meningiomas are calcified in up to 72% of the cases.[133,134]

Magnetic resonance evaluation of possible spinal meningiomas requires special attention to imaging technique. Because of the high frequency of meningiomas in the thoracic spine, care must be taken to reduce or eliminate the ghosting artifact secondary to respiratory and cardiac motion that commonly plagues this region. Possible solutions include switching direction of the phase- and frequency-encoding axes, cardiac and respiratory gating, refocused or symmetric multiecho sequences, and saturation pulses. Additionally, one must be aware of the order in which images are acquired in the axial plane. Cerebrospinal fluid pulsations can produce entry-slice artifact on the initial superiormost image that may strongly resemble an intradural-extramedullary soft tissue mass.

Like meningiomas of the cranial cavity, those in the spinal canal can have variable appearance. Sagittal and axial T_1-weighted images typically demonstrate a small soft tissue mass within the spinal canal that is isointense to the spinal cord and can be seen displacing it[26-28,127] (Figs. 7-13 to 7-15). There may be widening of the adjacent neural foramen. T_2-weighted images most commonly depict the tumor as a low-signal (isointense with spinal cord) intradural defect surrounded by high-signal CSF (Fig. 7-13). Personal experience, however, has proved that this may not always be the case, since there have been instances in which signal from these lesions was relatively high on long–repetition time (TR)/echo time (TE) images[26] (Fig. 7-14). Following the administration of contrast, there is typically uniform and intense enhancement[26-28,127] (Fig. 7-15). Uncommonly, there may be cystic syrinx changes in the adjacent spinal cord secondary to local derangements in CSF flow.[135]

Nerve Sheath Tumors

Nerve sheath tumors appear under a variety of titles: schwannoma, neuroma, neurilemoma, perineural fibroblastoma, and neurofibroma. Classically, there are two main types or categories. Neurofibromas consist of both Schwann cells and fibroblasts, arise as a fusiform mass among dorsal sensory nerve rootlets, and are seen in association with *neurofibromatosis type I* (NF-I, also known as von Recklinghausen's or "peripheral" neurofibromatosis).[42,47,136-139] Schwannomas (also referred to as neurinomas or neurilemomas) are lobulated soft tissue masses, composed solely of Schwann cells, that arise eccentrically from peripheral sensory nerves.[42,47,140] Schwannomas can arise de novo as solitary mass lesions or may be seen in multiples with *neurofibromatosis type II* (NF-II, bilateral acoustic or "central" neurofibromatosis).[137-139]

Although there are a number of neurofibromatosis variants, these two distinct types (NF-I and NF-II) have been recognized by the National Institutes of Health (NIH) Consensus Development Conference.[141] NF-I is an autosomal dominant, single gene, disorder related to chromosome 17.[142,143] It may be inherited or can arise by spontaneous mutation, with an incidence of approximately 1:2000 to 3000 live births.[144] The NIH consensus committee diagnostic criteria include at least two of the following[137,141]: (1) six or more café-au-lait macules >5 mm before puberty or >15 mm after puberty, (2) two or more neurofibromas, (3) one or more plexiform neurofibromas, (4) axillary or inguinal freckling, (5) op-

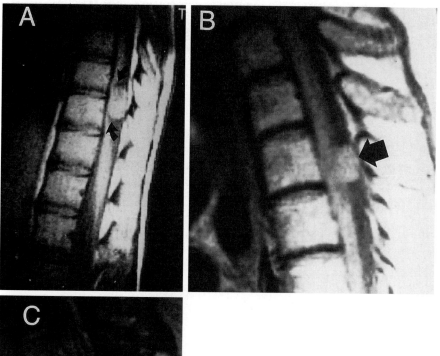

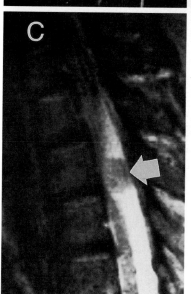

Fig. 7-13. 500 msec TR/17 msec TE sagittal, **A,** and parasagittal, **B,** images through the thoracic spine demonstrate a soft tissue mass posterolateral to the cord that is isointense in signal intensity with the cord *(arrows).* **C,** A 2000 msec TR/120 msec TE parasagittal scan through the region of the mass *(arrow)* again shows it to be isointense with the cord (i.e., low signal). These MR findings suggest a thoracic meningioma, which was confirmed at histology.

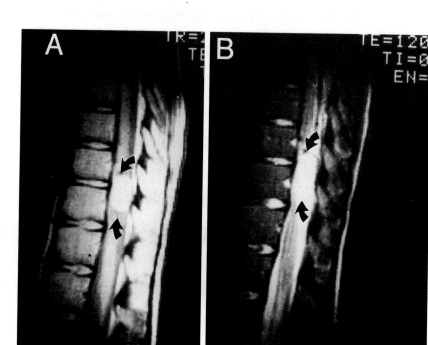

Fig. 7-14. A, A 2000 msec TR/30 msec TE parasagittal image of the thoracic spine demonstrates a soft tissue mass posterolateral to the cord and of approximately the same signal intensity as the cord *(arrows).* **B,** A 2000 msec TR/120 msec TE image through the region of the mass *(arrows)* demonstrates increased signal relative to the cord. On this image, the mass is obscured by the surrounding increased signal of the CSF. Surgery and histology confirmed the presence of a meningioma.

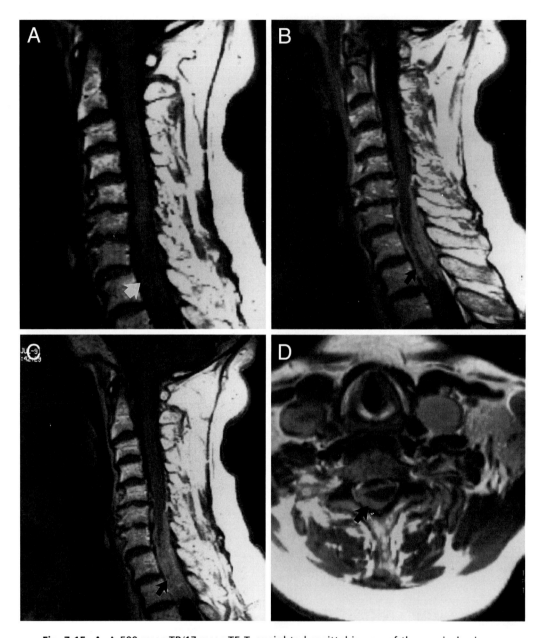

Fig. 7-15. A, A 500 msec TR/17 msec TE T_1-weighted sagittal image of the cervical spine demonstrates what appears to be irregular enlargement of the lower cervical cord. **B** to **D,** 500 msec TR/17 msec TE sagittal, parasagittal, and axial scans following intravenous administration of gadolinium demonstrate a diffuse and cloaking enhancement, suggestive of thickened meninges about the cervical cord. The differential diagnosis included sarcoidosis, pachymeningitis, and en plaque meningioma. Surgery disclosed the presence of meningioma.

tic nerve glioma, (6) two or more iris hamartomas (Lisch nodules), (7) one or more distinctive bone lesions (e.g., sphenoid dysplasia, pseudarthrosis, thinning of long bone cortex), and (8) a first-degree relative with diagnosed NF-I.

As just noted, neurofibromas are uncommon sporadic tumors seen most often in multiples associated with NF-I[145,146] (Figs. 7-16 to 7-18). In the review of 42 sporadic nerve sheath tumors by Halliday et al.[146] only two were neurofibromas. All fourteen patients with NF-I in their series had spinal neurofibromas exclusively.[146] Additionally, none of seven patients with NF-II had a pure neurofibroma, although one had both a schwannoma and a "mixed" tumor. Other spinal findings seen with NF-I include variable degrees of scoliosis and dysplastic enlargement of the subarachnoid space (i.e., lateral meningoceles) that may produce widening of the neural foramina and scalloping of the posterior vertebral

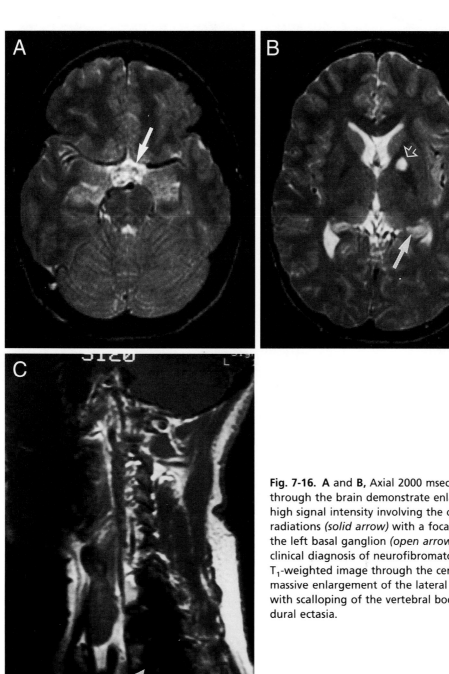

Fig. 7-16. A and **B,** Axial 2000 msec TR/90 msec TE images through the brain demonstrate enlargement and abnormal high signal intensity involving the optic chiasm and radiations *(solid arrow)* with a focal area of high signal in the left basal ganglion *(open arrow),* which confirmed the clinical diagnosis of neurofibromatosis-I. **C,** A parasagittal T₁-weighted image through the cervical spine shows massive enlargement of the lateral subarachnoid space with scalloping of the vertebral bodies consistent with dural ectasia.

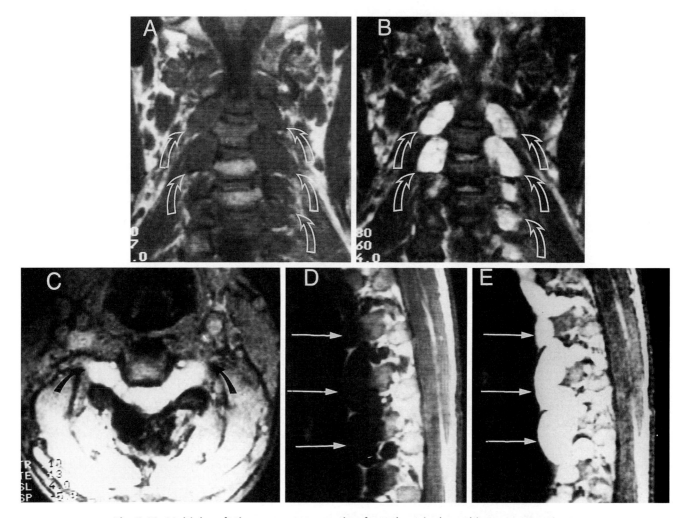

Fig. 7-17. Multiple soft tissue masses emanating from the spinal canal in a young patient with a known history of von Recklinghausen neurofibromatosis. **A,** A 500 msec TR/17 msec TE coronal image through the cervical spine shows that the masses are both intradural and extradural in location *(arrows).* **B,** An 1800 msec TR/60 msec TE image through the same region demonstrates increased signal within the lesions. Some have ill-defined areas of decreased signal, characteristic of neurofibromas *(arrows).* **C,** A 100 msec TR/13 msec TE 10-degree FISP* shows widening of the cervical neural foramina by the high-signal lesions *(arrows).* **D,** A 500 msec TR/17 msec TE parasagittal image through the thoracic spine reveals multiple septated cavities just lateral to the canal *(arrows).* **E,** An 1800 msec TR/60 msec TE scan in the same plane now shows the cyst as having homogeneously increased signal consistent with a thoracic meningocele.

*FISP fast imaging with steady-state precession.

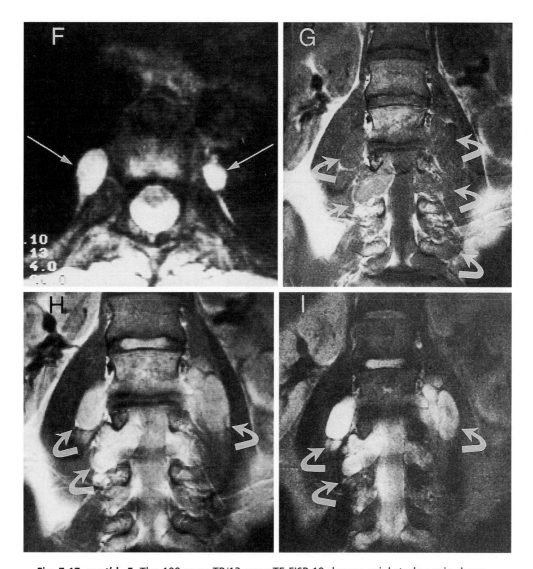

Fig. 7-17, cont'd. F, The 100 msec TR/13 msec TE FISP 10-degree axial study again shows the lateral meningocele. **G,** A 500 msec TR/17 msec TE coronal image through the lumbar spine demonstrates multiple intradural and extradural "dumbbell" neurofibromas that have the signal intensity of soft tissue *(arrows).* **H,** A 2000 msec TR/30 msec TE coronal scan through the lumbar spine shows the dumbbell shape of the neurofibromas, which now are of increased signal intensity *(arrows).* **I,** A 2000 msec TR/120 msec TE coronal scan through the lumbar spine reveals the high-signal neurofibromas, some of which have a lower signal intensity within *(arrows).*

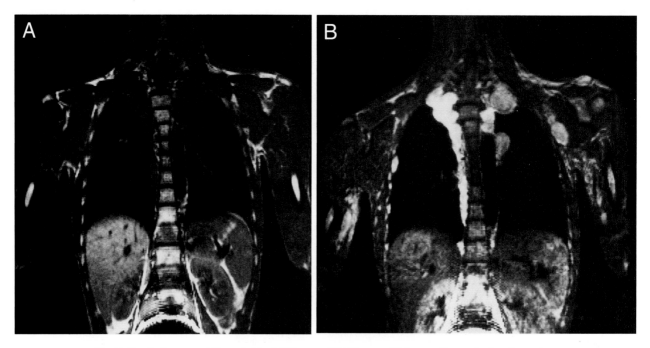

Fig. 7-18. **A,** A coronal T$_1$-weighted 500 msec TR/17 msec TE image through the thoracic spine demonstrates multiple paraspinal soft tissue masses. **B,** A 2000 msec TR/90 msec TE coronal scan through the same plane shows these lesions to have high signal intensity. Note, additionally, the multiple masses at the axillae and along both arms. The clinical diagnosis was neurofibromatosis-I.

bodies.[147] Furthermore, intramedullary gliomas as well as hamartomas (analogous to those seen in the basal ganglia of such patients) have been reported.[139,148]

NF-II is also an autosomal dominant disorder (although much less common than NF-I), related to chromosome 22.[149-152] The NIH consensus committee diagnostic criteria[137,141] for NF-II include (1) bilateral masses of the eighth cranial nerve, and (2) a first-degree relative with NF-II and either a single eighth nerve mass or any two of the following: schwannoma, neurofibroma, meningioma, glioma, or juvenile posterior subcapsular lens opacity.[137,141]

Schwannomas are the principal neoplasms of NF-II, centrally and peripherally (Figs. 7-19 to 7-22). They are more vascular than neuromas; both hemorrhage and "cystic change" are more common than in neurofibromas and are not necessarily reflective of malignant degeneration[137] (Figs. 7-19 to 7-21). Schwannomas generally enhance vigorously on imaging studies.[139] Other findings seen in the spine of patients with NF-II include meningiomas as well as intramedullary mass lesions, notably ependymomas.[139] The proportion of patients with disease involving the spine has been noted[139] to be higher with NF-II than with NF-I.

Isolated nerve sheath tumors are seen most commonly in adults between the ages of 20 and 50 years, with no predilection for either sex[42] (Figs. 7-19 to 7-21 and 7-23). They may occur anywhere in the spine, the thoracic column being most often implicated.[42] The majority of lesions are intradural-extramedullary, 10% are intradural and extradural, and 11% are strictly extradural.[42]

Malignant degeneration is uncommon in nerve sheath tumors and is seen in 2% to 12% of cases.[153-155] Malignant neoplasms arise either from neoplastic degeneration of preexisting nerve sheath tumors or de novo. Smirniotopoulos and Murphy[137] note that most malignant tumors of nerve sheath derivation have features that overlap the traditional boundaries between schwannoma and neurofibroma. Therefore, the less specific term *malignant nerve sheath tumor* is preferable to "malignant schwannoma" or "neurofibrosarcoma." The 5-year survival is poor, between 15% and 30%.[154,156-158] Cases associated with neurofibromatosis tend to occur at a younger age and have a worse prognosis. The most frequent symptoms of nerve sheath tumors are pain and radiculopathy.[136]

Magnetic resonance imaging is particularly helpful in the diagnosis of these lesions, by virtue of its ability to depict the extent of extradural disease. Like meningiomas, nerve sheath tumors appear as a soft tissue mass outlined by low-signal CSF within the spinal canal on T$_1$-weighted images. Often there is displacement of the

Text continued on p. 277.

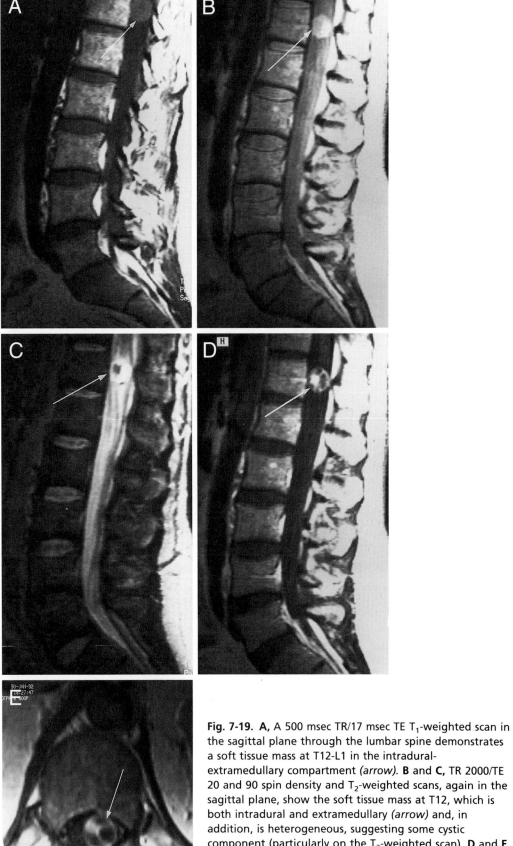

Fig. 7-19. A, A 500 msec TR/17 msec TE T$_1$-weighted scan in the sagittal plane through the lumbar spine demonstrates a soft tissue mass at T12-L1 in the intradural-extramedullary compartment *(arrow).* **B** and **C,** TR 2000/TE 20 and 90 spin density and T$_2$-weighted scans, again in the sagittal plane, show the soft tissue mass at T12, which is both intradural and extramedullary *(arrow)* and, in addition, is heterogeneous, suggesting some cystic component (particularly on the T$_2$-weighted scan). **D** and **E,** Sagittal and axial 500 msec TR/17 msec TE T$_1$-weighted scans after IV gadolinium demonstrate a heterogeneously enhancing, multicystic, lobulated solitary schwannoma.

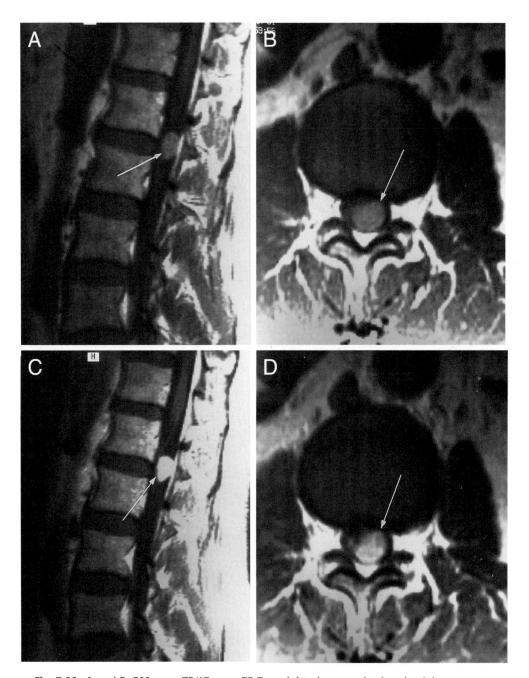

Fig. 7-20. A and **B,** 500 msec TR/17 msec TE T$_1$-weighted parasagittal and axial scans through the upper lumbar spine demonstrate a high-signal intradural-extramedullary mass (possibly a schwannoma) that has hemorrhaged. **C** and **D,** T$_1$-weighted sagittal and axial scans following IV gadolinium show intense enhancement, again consistent with a solitary schwannoma.

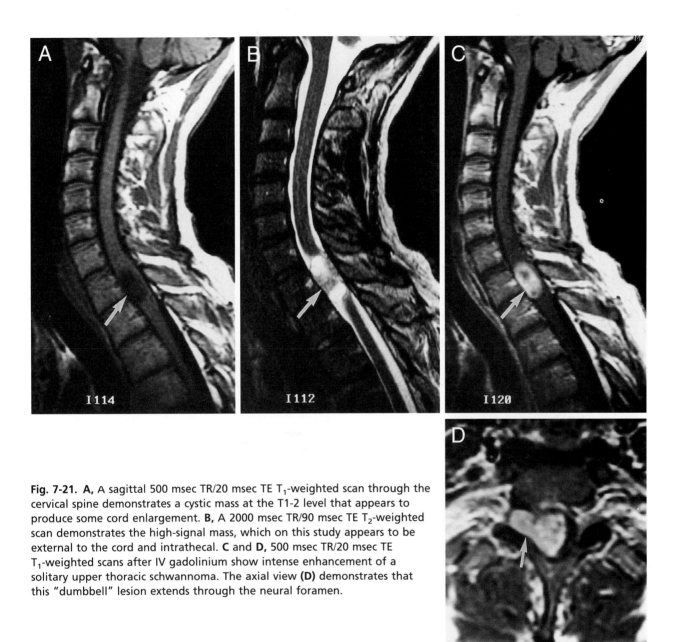

Fig. 7-21. A, A sagittal 500 msec TR/20 msec TE T$_1$-weighted scan through the cervical spine demonstrates a cystic mass at the T1-2 level that appears to produce some cord enlargement. **B,** A 2000 msec TR/90 msec TE T$_2$-weighted scan demonstrates the high-signal mass, which on this study appears to be external to the cord and intrathecal. **C** and **D,** 500 msec TR/20 msec TE T$_1$-weighted scans after IV gadolinium show intense enhancement of a solitary upper thoracic schwannoma. The axial view **(D)** demonstrates that this "dumbbell" lesion extends through the neural foramen.

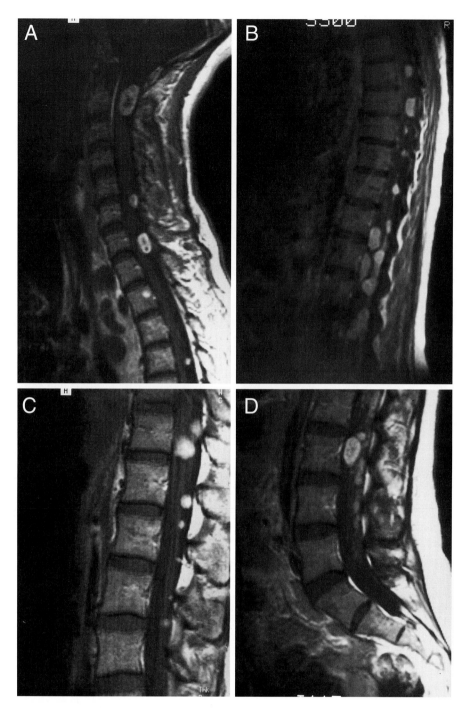

Fig. 7-22. Sagittal 500 msec TR/20 msec TE T₁-weighted sagittal and parasagittal scans through the cervical, **A,** thoracic, **B,** and lumbosacral, **C** and **D,** spine following IV gadolinium demonstrate multiple intradural-extramedullary mass lesions consistent with multiple schwannomatosis (or neurofibromatosis-II).

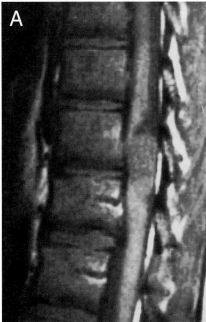

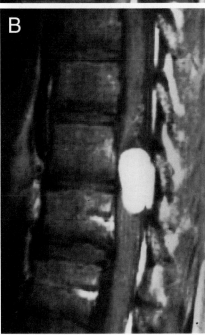

Fig. 7-23. A, A 500 msec TR/17 msec TE sagittal image in a patient with an intradural extramedullary schwannoma demonstrates the soft mass adjacent to and hypointense with the thoracic cord. **B,** Following administration of IV gadolinium, there is a marked increase in signal on this 500 msec TR/17 msec TE image.

cord. More T_2-weighted images typically demonstrate the lesions as high-signal masses outlined by lower-signal spinal and paraspinal soft tissues[159,160] (Figs. 7-17 and 7-18). These foci of high signal may have a central area of lower signal intensity that distinguishes them from lateral meningoceles commonly found with neurofibromatosis.[159] Alternatively, on intermediate scans (long TR/short TE), the masses will often have higher signal than CSF within the canal whereas meningoceles should remain isointense with CSF. Unfortunately, signal intensity characteristics in nerve sheath tumors do not appear to be sensitive for the recognition of malignant degeneration.[160]

As just noted, nerve sheath tumors demonstrate prominent paramagnetic contrast enhancement on T_1-weighted MR images that may be homogeneous when the tumor is small and heterogeneous when the tumor is large* (Figs. 7-19 to 7-23). Also, as with meningiomas, syringomyelic cavities may occur locally in the spinal cord secondary to these lesions—a complication that MR is ideally suited to detect.[135,162] Much as with tumoral cysts found in intramedullary lesions, CSF pulsations in regions of microcystic degeneration produced by the tumor can lead to enlargement of such cord cavities.[135]

Embryonal Tumors

The developmental tumors (epidermoid, dermoid, lipoma, teratoma) have been previously discussed but are reintroduced here to reinforce their association with the lower spine, midline closure (i.e., neurulation) defects, or lumbar puncture and thus their frequent intradural extramedullary location.[98,103,163] Such tumors may be suggested by their associated congenital cutaneous stigmata (subcutaneous lipoma, hairy patch, sacral dimple, or sinus tract and unusual pigmentation) although these need not necessarily be present.[163,164] The lesions typically present in children or young adults with progressive lower extremity or sphincter dysfunction, often the result of some element of cord tethering. Evidence suggests that early diagnosis and treatment often limit the extent of permanent neurologic deficit.[165]

Lipomas possess the most characteristic MR appearance[102]: high signal intensity, globular mass on T_1-weighted images (less intense on T_2), and frequent association with a tethered cord or some form of lipomyelomeningocele (Fig. 7-24). It is noteworthy that fat may be present within the distal conus medullaris and filum terminale in normal subjects (5%).[166] Thus it is likely that lipomas represent a developmental spectrum whose significance lies with the level of the conus (normally L1-2 in adults) and the clinical history. Pierre-Kahn et al.[165] reported their experience with lipomas in

*References 26-28, 138, 139, 161.

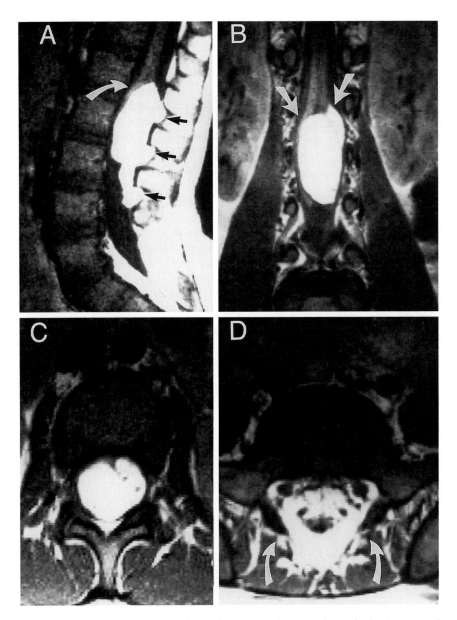

Fig. 7-24. A, A 500 msec TR/17 msec TE midline sagittal image through the lower lumbar spine demonstrates a lipomeningocele *(open arrows)* that extends into the thecal sac and is attached to a tethered conus medullaris *(curved arrow).* **B,** A 500 msec TR/17 msec TE coronal image shows the intradural location of this high-signal lipoma *(arrows).* **C,** An axial 500 msec TR/17 msec TE image reveals that the spinal canal is completely occupied by the high-signal lesion. **D,** A 500 msec TR/17 msec TE axial image through the level of S1 shows spina bifida *(arrows),* emphasizing the frequent association of these lesions with dysraphic states.

association with definite spina bifida, stating that the risk of neurologic deterioration exists at all ages and increases with time. The series of adult patients reported by Petit et al.[167] showed the highest rate of deterioration whereas the Pierre-Kahn series,[165] which included a larger proportion of infants, showed the lowest (35.5%). Furthermore, although neurologic deficits resulting from tethering are usually the sole reason for pre-

sentation in adolescents and adults, most infants are seen for evaluation of lumbosacral abnormalities.[168]

Epidermoids, dermoids, and teratomas have a variable appearance on MRI, reflecting the variety of tissues comprising a single mass* (Figs. 7-25 and 7-26). Epidermoids arise from heterotopic ectoderm, dermoids from

---

*References 103, 104, 169-171.

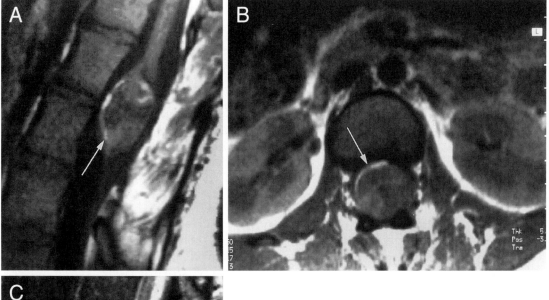

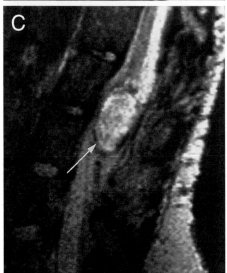

Fig. 7-25. **A** and **B** are sagittal and axial unenhanced 500 msec TR/17 msec TE T$_1$-weighted scans showing a heterogeneous intradural-extramedullary mass that appears to be closely applied to the conus medullaris (arrow). Note the peripheral areas of high signal intensity, suggesting hemorrhage (or, in this case, lipid material). **C,** A sagittal 2000 msec TR/90 msec TE T$_2$-weighted scan demonstrates the heterogeneous signal. Such findings are consistent with an epidermoid of the conus.

Fig. 7-26. A, A 600 msec TR/20 msec TE T$_1$-weighted parasagittal scan through the thoracolumbar junction demonstrates a heterogeneous mass at the distal spinal cord of predominantly high signal intensity but with multiple cystic and solid components. **B,** A TR 2000/90 msec TE T$_2$-weighted scan shows the heterogeneous mass. At surgery a recurrent epidermoid was discovered.

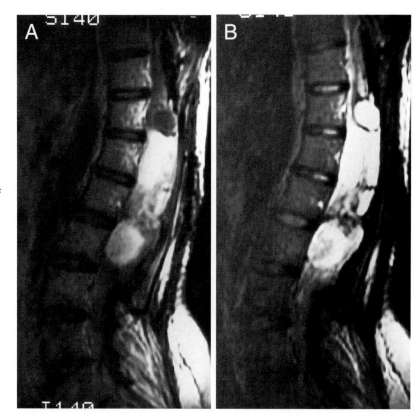

embryonic rests of ectoderm and mesoderm, and teratomas from all three germ layers. Liquid fat, solid keratin or cholesterol, fibrous tissue, muscle, and bone may be present within a single lesion.[169-171] Most epidermoids are nearly isointense with CSF (long T_1, long T_2), whereas dermoids mimic fat (short T_1, short T_2) on spin-echo images (Figs. 7-25 and 7-26). Nevertheless, epidermoids with both short T_1 and short T_2 relaxation times have been described.[172,173] In a study by Barkovich et al.[171] that focused on such lesions in association with dermal sinus tracts, all the dermoids and epidermoids were nearly isointense with CSF on both long TR and short TR spin-echo images. Intramedullary tumors could be contrasted with the adjacent spinal cord and were easily identified, although the identification of intradural-extramedullary tumors was reported to be difficult.[171] Hatfield et al.[170] reported a case of iatrogenic intradural epidermoid secondary to remote lumbar puncture and noted significant ring enhancement on MR with paramagnetic contrast (which can be used to increase the conspicuousness of these lesions).

Paragangliomas

Paragangliomas are tumors of the accessory organs of the sympathetic nervous system or paraganglia.[174] They occur most often in the adrenal medulla (pheochromocytomas), carotid body, glomus jugulare, mediastinum, and paraaortic regions. Typical CNS locations include the petrous ridge, pineal region, and sella turcica. Paragangliomas may rarely arise from paraganglia located in the cauda equina.[140,175-177a] Cystic and multinodular lesions have been identified; and because of similar histologic features, the tumor can be confused with an ependymoma.[178] The most frequent presentation is low back pain with associated sciatica. Motor or sensory deficits in the lower extremities, as well as bowel or bladder symptoms, have also been reported.

Overall, malignancy is found in 6.5% of all extraadrenal paragangliomas. Local tumor recurrence is described in approximately 12%, with late recurrences even after 30 years. Distant metastases are rare, but the tumor may be multifocal in a small percentage of cases.[174] Most tumors are limited to the filum terminale, although secondary involvement of the conus and caudal nerve roots can occur.[178] Because paragangliomas are encapsulated, they are generally totally excised at surgery.

Hayes et al.[179] reported an MR appearance not dissimilar to that of intraspinal nerve root neoplasms: extramedullary soft tissue masses on T_1-weighted scans with very high signal on T_2-weighted studies. When performed, preoperative angiography demonstrates a highly vascular tumor that (although not reported) is likely to enhance avidly with paramagnetic contrast.[174]

Intradural-Extramedullary (Leptomeningeal) Metastases

As does the spinal cord, the spinal subarachnoid space lends itself to secondary invasion by malignancy, primarily CSF seeding from cranial ependymomas, glioblastomas, and medulloblastomas (especially in the pediatric population).[129,180] In the report by Bryan[181] of leptomeningeal tumors resulting from primary intracranial neoplasms, malignant astrocytoma was the most frequent (representing 61% of the cases) (Fig. 7-27). Other series[182] have reported metastatic medulloblastoma as the most frequent; 33% of patients with intracranial recurrence of medulloblastoma will have leptomeningeal spread into the spine at the time of diagnosis of the recurrence.[182] Other CNS malignancies known to spread via the cerebrospinal fluid include ependymoma, oligodendroglioma, pinealoma, retinoblastoma, and malignant choroid plexus papilloma.[181,183,184]

If tumor is present within the spinal canal, spinal axis radiation is employed.[182] Two age peaks for leptomeningeal carcinomatosis are seen in the pediatric population. The first occurs at age 6, and the second at 14 to 15 years.[56] The second peak occurs in patients who have received radiation and have either a delayed spread of primary tumor to the spine or a secondary recurrence intracranially with subsequent subarachnoid spread.[56] Leptomeningeal tumor most often metastasizes to the lumbosacral region (73%), probably because of the effects of gravity, with most tumor cells settling in this area.[182]

Only a small percentage of metastatic lesions arising outside the CNS spread to the subarachnoid space. Carcinoma of the lung and breast as well as lymphoma, leukemia, and melanoma may present in this fashion[185] (Fig. 7-28). Spread to the spinal subarachnoid space may occur by (1) direct extension (although the dura provides a formidable barrier), (2) the lymphatic system, (3) a hematogenous route, or (4) the CSF.[186] This last route is thought to be the most common. There is also evidence[185] that spinal subarachnoid metastases frequently develop as tertiary deposits after the passage of malignant cells in the CSF from secondary lesions elsewhere in the CNS and meninges.

Clinical presentation may be nonspecific: head, neck, or back pain; or there may be focal deficits, including cranial nerve palsies, sphincter dysfunction, or motorsensory deficits. The hallmark of leptomeningeal metastatic disease is positive CSF cytology, which varies in sensitivity depending on the number of samples taken and the extent of disease (i.e., diffuse vs focal).[187,188]

T_1-weighted images often demonstrate nodular masses of soft tissue signal intensity in the distal thecal sac or diffuse thickening of the cauda equina. Intravenously administered paramagnetic contrast greatly increases the conspicuousness of such lesions. Particularly

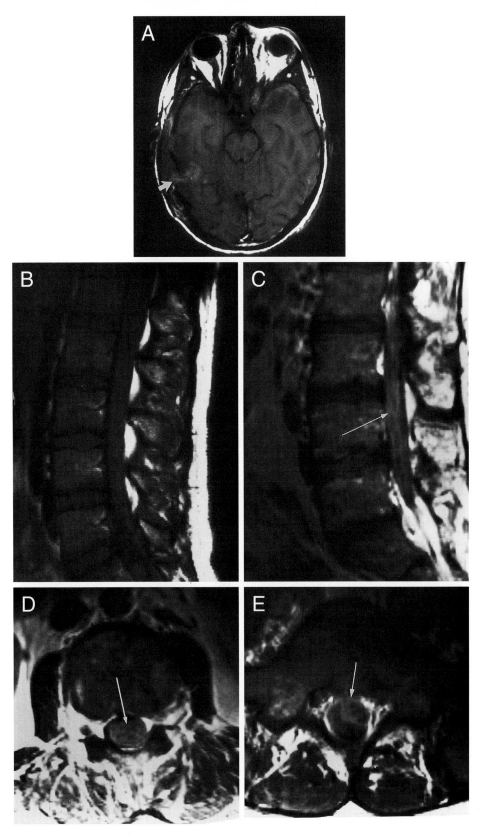

Fig. 7-27. A, A 500 msec TR/20 msec TE postgadolinium scan through the right temporal lobe, status post–craniotomy and biopsy of a glioblastoma multiforme, demonstrates linear enhancement *(arrow)*. **B,** A 500 msec TR/20 msec TE T₁-weighted sagittal scan through the lumbar spine fails to show any mass lesion, although the signal intensity within the thecal sac is slightly higher than what would be expected from CSF alone and is somewhat heterogeneous. **C to E,** 500 msec TR/17 msec TE sagittal and axial scans through the lumbar spine reveal diffuse and somewhat nodular enhancement in the subarachnoid space consistent with CSF seeding of a malignant glioma.

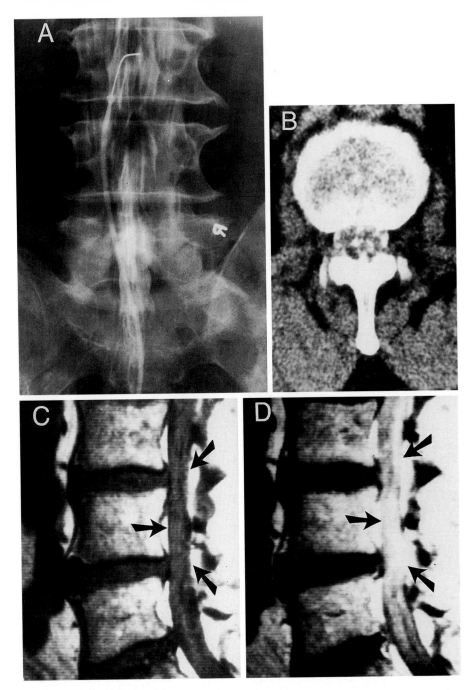

Fig. 7-28. Diffuse thickening of the cauda equinal nerve roots in an elderly retiree who experienced acute sciatica following a round of golf. **A,** The initial evaluation included a water-soluble contrast myelogram. **B,** The follow-up high-resolution CT scan shows thickened nerve roots within the distal thecal sac. **C,** A 400 msec TR/15 msec TE midline sagittal image of the lumbar spine reveals some heterogeneity of signal intensity within the thecal sac *(arrows)*. **D,** A 400 msec TR/15 msec TE midline sagittal image through the lumbar spine following IV gadolinium shows diffuse and intense enhancement of the intrathecal nerve roots. **E,** A 600 msec TR/15 msec TE axial image through the midline lumbar spine is essentially normal. The *arrow* points to nerve roots within the thecal sac. **F,** A 600 msec TR/15 msec TE axial image through the level of **E** again shows diffuse and intense enhancement of the cauda nerve roots *(arrow)*. Histologic examination of the spinal fluid obtained at the time of myelography was positive for histiocytic lymphoma.

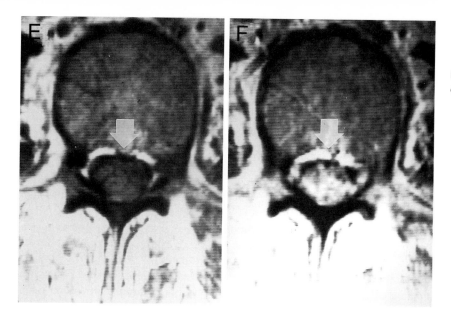

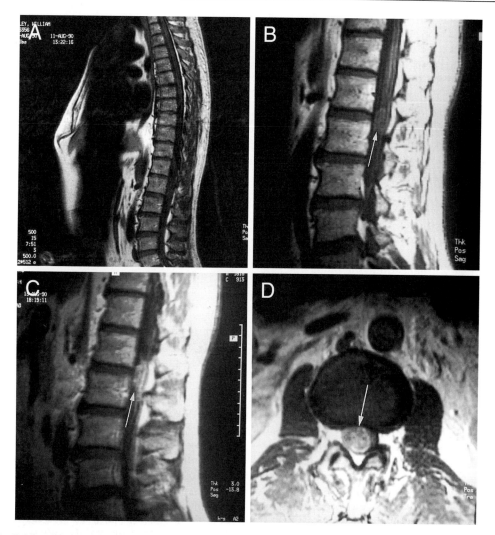

Fig. 7-28, cont'd. For legend see opposite page.

Fig. 7-29. A, A sagittal TR 500 msec/TE 15 msec high-resolution body coil image fails to demonstrate any significant osseous metastatic disease despite a history of significant lower extremity radiculopathy in this patient with known primary malignancy. Note the ghosting from respiratory motion and the signal from the anterior abdominal wall. **B,** A parasagittal surface coil 500 msec TR/15 msec TE image through the same region shows a small soft tissue nodule in the subarachnoid space *(arrow)*. **C** and **D** are 500 msec TR/15 msec TE sagittal and axial scans after IV gadolinium demonstrating enhancement of the nodule, which ultimately was found to be a metastatic adenocarcinoma of the breast to the subarachnoid space.

when there is a diffuse covering of pial metastases rather than an obvious focal mass, gadolinium-enhanced MR scans are superior to myelography[189] (Figs. 7-27 to 7-29). Since the pial enhancement is quite intense, it is rarely confused with benign arachnoiditis, which typically does not (or does only minimally) enhance.[190] T_2-weighted images are less helpful, not only because of their lower signal-to-noise but also because there is low contrast resolution between tumors (long T_2) and CSF (long T_2).

It is important to note that, although myelography and gadolinium-enhanced MRI may be roughly comparable in most cases, in the report by Yousem et al.[185] examination of the CSF is still the most sensitive diagnostic test for determining the presence of leptomeningeal tumor spread. These authors found that, whereas gadolinium administration increased the ability of MR to detect leptomeningeal metastases to the brain and spine, the overall sensitivity of unenhanced and enhanced MR examinations was low (19.3% and 36.1%) in patients with proved cytologic evidence of neoplastic seeding. When specifically addressing the spine in this population, they found only 37.5% of gadolinium-enhanced spine studies to be positive.[185] Studies were most likely to be positive in patients with a non-CNS primary malignancy and least accurate in cases of lymphoma or leukemia.

EXTRADURAL TUMORS

Extradural tumors consist of primary or metastatic, benign and malignant, neoplasms involving the vertebrae, adjacent soft tissue, nerve roots, and dura. The lesions account for approximately 30% of all spinal neoplasms.[42] The primary benign soft tissue tumors include the small minority of extradural meningiomas, neurinomas, and developmental tumors that have already been discussed. Thus this section will focus specifically on a few benign tumors arising from the vertebrae and a range of malignant neoplasms.

Unlike plain film radiographs, myelography, and computed tomography (which focus primarily on the bony architecture of the spinal canal and its adjacent soft tissues), magnetic resonance images the vertebral marrow space and its nearby soft tissues. To some extent, this puts MR at a disadvantage when primary vertebral tumors (which are best known to radiologists on the basis of location, integrity of cortical bone, pattern of cancellous bone involvement, and the presence and type of calcified matrix) are evaluated. The terms *osteolytic* and *osteoblastic* have no meaning with MRI. Nonetheless, certain primary lesions involving the vertebrae have been noted to present a unique appearance with MR. Vertebral lesions are usually well defined as low-intensity masses surrounded by the higher intensity of normal fat-

containing marrow on short TR images.[191] Although often nonspecific, this finding has been determined[192,193] to be more sensitive to marrow abnormalities than radionuclide bone scans. The typical MR parameters for the sensitive detection of vertebral body lesions generally consist of T_1-weighted spin-echo sequences.[191,193-197] Occasionally marrow uninvolved by neoplasm will appear to have low signal, especially in young patients, in whom the vertebral body marrow does not contain much fat, or in patients with chronic disease.[194,196-199] Alternative acquisitions, such as T_2-weighted spin-echo sequences, STIR sequences,* or gradient echo sequences, may help for further evaluation.[200,201]

Enhancement by extradural neoplasms can vary to such a degree that the utility of paramagnetic contrast in evaluating extradural disease is reserved for particular clinical questions. Specifically, tumors can enhance markedly (to become hyperintense relative to normal marrow) or minimally (to remain hypointense). Most disturbing, however, are those that enhance modestly (to become isointense with normal marrow) and thus go undetected.[202] This variability of enhancement has been reported to occur among different lesions within a single patient. Nevertheless, paramagnetic contrast administration may be useful for defining epidural tumor extension.[202]

Vertebral Hemangioma

Vertebral hemangiomas are slow-growing benign lesions that have been demonstrated in 11% of spines at autopsy but are only rarely symptomatic.[203-205] They appear to be solitary in 66% of cases, increasing in incidence with age to become multiple in 34% of cases.[206] Some 60% occur in the thoracic region, 29% in the lumbar region, and fewer in the cervical region and sacrum. They are slightly more common in women.

The majority are discovered incidentally.[206-208] Symptomatic lesions tend to occur in the thoracic region, usually presenting with localized pain and tenderness that often is associated with muscle spasm.[208] Radiculopathy may result from impingement on a nerve root.[208] Myelopathic symptoms are frequently attributed to pathologic vertebral body collapse, epidural extension of tumor, epidural hematoma, or bony expansion resulting in cord compression.[206,208]

Histologically, vertebral hemangiomas appear as collections of thin-walled blood vessels or sinuses lined by endothelium that are interspersed among bony trabeculae and abundant adipose tissue.[209] On plain film studies they produce a corduroy appearance within the affected vertebra because of their vertically oriented bony

---

*Short time-to-inversion recovery.

trabeculae.[206] On axial CT these trabeculae are often surrounded by low-attenuation fat, producing a spotted appearance within the lesion when the trabeculae are viewed end on.[210] They have a relatively distinctive MR appearance.[207] On T_1-weighted images the intraosseous portions appear mottled and of increased signal intensity secondary to the adipose tissue interspersed among thickened bony trabeculae[207] (Figs. 7-30 to 7-32); an extraosseous matrix often displays lower (soft tissue) signal on T_1-weighted images[207] (Fig. 7-32). On T_2-weighted images both intraosseous and extraosseous tumor demonstrates increased signal intensity, possibly related to more cellular components of the tumor.[207] Flow-related effects are not thought to contribute significantly to the MR appearance of the lesions. Focal fat deposition within the spine may mimic a vertebral hemangioma on T_1-weighted images but fail to have the same increased signal on T_2-weighted studies.[211] In the experience of Laredo et al.,[212] fatty vertebral hemangiomas may represent an inactive form, whereas the increased soft tissue content at CT and the low signal intensity on T_1-weighted MR images may indicate a more active vascular lesion with the potential for spinal cord compression.

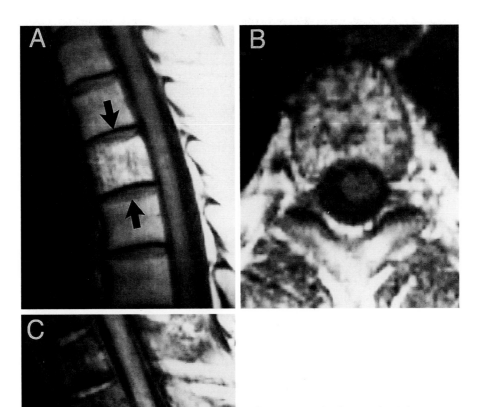

Fig. 7-30. Sagittal, **A,** and axial, **B,** 500 msec TR/17 msec TE images demonstrate heterogeneous increased signal intensity from the thoracic vertebral body *(arrows).* **C,** A more T_2-weighted 2000 msec TR/17 msec TE sagittal examination shows increased signal *(arrows).* These findings are consistent with the diagnosis of vertebral hemangioma.

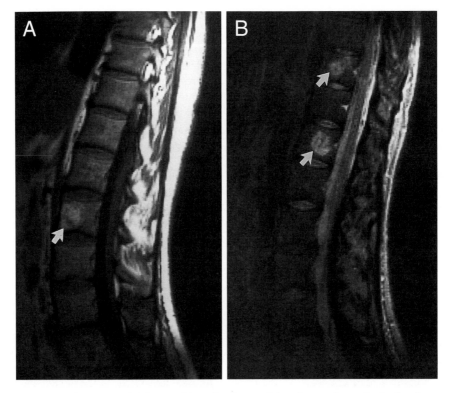

Fig. 7-31. A, A 500 msec TR/15 msec TE sagittal T₁-weighted scan through the lumbar spine demonstrates a rounded area of high signal within L2. **B,** A sagittal 2000 msec TR/90 msec TE scan demonstrates only a faint hint of the L2 lesion, although at L1 and T11 there are two additional focal areas of high signal *(arrows)*. These findings are consistent with multiple vertebral body hemangiomas.

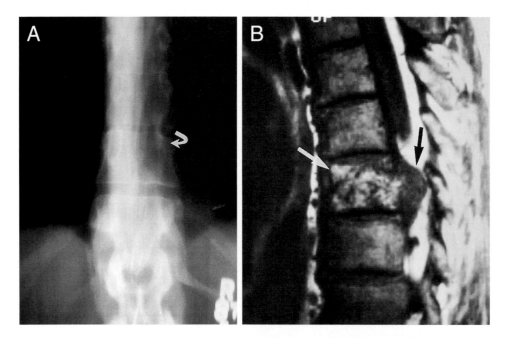

Fig. 7-32. A, A linear tomogram through the lower thoracic spine shows erosion of the pedicle at T10. **B,** A parasagittal 500 msec TR/15 msec TE scan demonstrates heterogeneous high signal within the vertebra *(white arrow)* with low-signal soft tissue extension posteriorly and into the thecal sac *(black arrow)*. These findings are consistent with an osseous and extradural vertebral body hemangioma.

Aneurysmal Bone Cyst

Aneurysmal bone cysts (ABCs) are benign osseous tumors representing only a small fraction (1.4% to 2.3%) of primary bone neoplasms.[213,214] Although most often arising de novo, in approximately a third of the cases they have been reported to occur[215-217] with other bone lesions (giant cell tumor, chondroblastoma, chondromyxoid fibroma, fibrous dysplasia, and nonossifying fibroma). Patients typically present in the first two decades of life and are equally divided between males and females.[213,217-219] Giant cell tumors, which are frequently confused with ABCs, usually occur in patients older than 30 years of age.[216,217,219,220]

The lesions affect the spine in up to 20% of cases, more often involving the posterior elements than the vertebral bodies.* Although thought to be benign, when anterior they have been reported[218] to cross the intervertebral disk space and involve an adjacent vertebra. There may be an associated soft tissue mass. Of those located in the spine, an estimated 44% occur in the lumbosacral region, 34% in the thoracic spine, and 22% in the cervical spine. Presenting symptoms usually consist of localized pain and/or swelling.[216-218] Large lesions may expand to compress the spinal cord, resulting in a clinical presentation of myelopathy.[218,223]

ABCs consist of large anastomosing cavernous spaces or cysts filled with unclotted blood and contained by thinly calcified or noncalcified periosteal membranes.[220,224,227] Giant cells present within the trabeculae of these lesions often lead to confusion with the tumor of the same name.[219,220] Plain films of the spine demonstrate an expanding, radiolucent, or lytic lesion usually involving the posterior elements with marked thinning of adjacent cortical bone.[218,228] Lesions involving the vertebral body may be destructive and produce collapse.[218,219] CT can confirm the geographic expansion of such lesions, delineate multicystic components with fluid-fluid levels, and define soft tissue extension.[224,227,228] As do vertebral hemangiomas, aneurysmal bone cysts have a somewhat unique MR appearance. MRI typically demonstrates numerous well-defined cystic cavities that are surrounded by a rim of low signal intensity and may demonstrate multiple fluid-fluid levels.[229-232] These cavities often show a wide range of signal intensities on both T_1- and T_2-weighted images depending on the various blood products present, their paramagnetic properties, and the field strength of the magnet utilized[231,232] (Fig. 7-33). Tsai et al.[233] have subsequently observed that other bony lesions can mimic this appearance of multiple blood-fluid levels on MR—including telangiectatic osteosarcoma, chondroblastoma, and giant cell tumor of bone as well as fibrous dysplasia, simple bone cyst, recurrent malignant fibrous histi-

ocytoma of bone, two "classic" osteosarcomas, and four "classic" aneurysmal bone cysts. The soft tissue tumors that they found mimicking aneurysmal bone cysts included soft tissue hemangioma and two synovial sarcomas.[233]

Giant Cell Tumor

Giant cell tumors comprise 4% to 5% of all primary bone tumors and are typically seen after the second decade of life.[213,234,235] There is no sex predilection.[234] In Dahlin and Unni's series[213] they were the second most common benign spinal tumor, after vertebral hemangiomas. Additionally, they are the most common benign neoplasm involving the sacrum.[236] Local pain (occasionally with swelling) is the usual presentation.[234,236-238]

Plain films show a geographically expansile lytic lesion, rarely with a sclerotic border.[234] CT may be useful in demonstrating any soft tissue mass.[238] With MR, unenhanced short-TR images demonstrate low-signal tumor within the higher-signal marrow space. The extraosseous extent of the lesion can be delineated with more T_2-weighted images, or alternatively, the administration of contrast with T_1-weighted images.[237] As noted, both the MR and the histologic findings may be similar to those seen with aneurysmal bone cysts.[233]

Osteochondroma

Osteochondromas are believed to arise through lateral displacement of a portion of the epiphyseal growth cartilage. This results in a bonelike outgrowth capped by cartilage whose cortex and medullary cavity are contiguous with those of its bone of origin. Hence, osteochondromas do not occur in bones that develop through membranous ossification (e.g., the cranial vault). Whereas osteochondromas are the most common benign bone tumor, only a fraction (1% to 4%) occur within the spine[239-242]; but because they are so common, they often are found in this location, usually in the posterior elements of the thoracic and lumbar region.* Most osteochondromas are discovered in patients less than 20 years of age, and there is a slight male preponderance.[240] Two patterns of presentation occur: solitary lesions, which are not inherited, and multiple lesions, which are (in hereditary exostosis). The incidence of malignant degeneration is rare in cases of solitary osteochondroma and can be seen in up to one fourth of cases of multiple hereditary exostosis; rapid growth should raise this suspicion.[240] Clinical presentation is nonspecific: although pain is common, neurologic symptoms are rare.

Osteochondromas, often referred to as mushroomlike projections arising from adjacent bone via a pedicle at a site of ligamentous insertion,[240] consist of cancellous bone filled with normal marrow surrounded by cortical

---

*References 214, 216, 218, 220, 222.

*References 240, 241, 243-245.

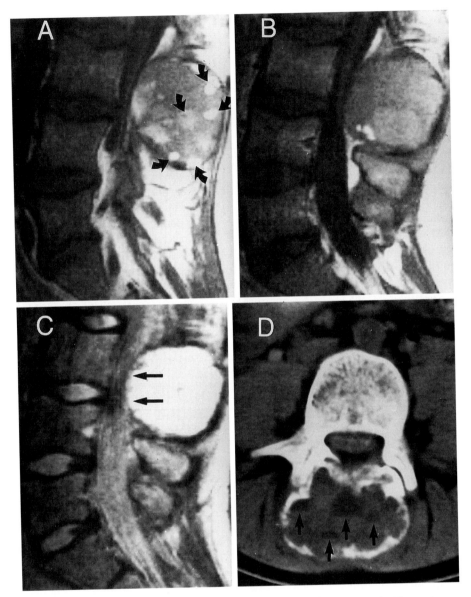

Fig. 7-33. A, A 500 msec TR/17 msec TE parasagittal image of the lower lumbar spine demonstrates diffuse enlargement of the posterior elements of L3. Heterogeneous and focal cystic areas of high signal are evident within this expansile lesion *(arrows).* **B,** A 500 msec TR/17 msec TE midline sagittal image shows the enlarged expansile mass within the spinous process of L3 compressing the thecal sac. **C,** A 2000 msec TR/90 msec TE with more T_2-weighting demonstrates that the lesion has increased signal intensity. Note the compressed thecal sac *(arrows).* **D,** An axial CT scan through the region of the lesion demonstrates an expansile, cystic mass within the posterior elements of L3. *Arrows* point to fluid-fluid levels within multiple cysts of the lesion. Surgery and histology confirmed an aneurysmal bone cyst.

bone.[241] A thin layer of hyaline cartilage caps the tumor. Plain films often show a lesion attached to the posterior elements of the spine, either a pedunculated or a sessile projection of bone with its cortex a direct extension of the adjacent normal bone.[240,246] CT can precisely delineate the site of attachment and the cartilaginous cap.[240] CT can also be helpful in distinguishing between benign osteochondromas and those that have undergone sarcomatous degeneration.[246] The MR characteristics are relatively nonspecific, although T_2-weighted images may permit demonstration of the cartilaginous cap as a rim of high signal intensity relative to the lower-signal osseous portions of the tumor. In rare cases of spinal canal compromise, MR may be advantageous in delineating the relationship of the mass to underlying neural structures.

Osteoid Osteoma

Osteoid osteomas comprise just over 10% of all benign bone tumors and occur with approximately the same incidence in the spine as elsewhere in the body.[213,249-250] The most common spinal locations are the lumbar (59%), followed by the cervical (27%), and less frequently the thoracic and sacral regions.[249] As do osteochondromas, osteoid osteomas involve the posterior elements in most cases.[249,251] They typically occur before age 30 and are more common in males.[247,248,252] The lesions almost always present with pain and/or tenderness localized to the site of the lesion that classically is worse at night and relieved by aspirin.[247,248] Radicular pain is seen in approximately half the patients and can occur if the lesion encroaches on the neural foramina.[247,251] Scoliosis may also result because of muscle spasm and pelvic tilt.[247,251-253]

Histologically the tumor contains multinucleated giant cells with a nidus consisting of vascular fibrous connective tissue surrounded by calcifying osteoid matrix.[250,253,254] Plain films reflect this pathology as a lucent nidus with a small central calcification surrounded by bony sclerosis.* If extensive reactive sclerosis is present, plain films alone may fail to localize the nidus.[248] The nidus can, however, often be seen on cross-sectional imaging. CT shows a small rounded area of low attenuation, with or without calcification, surrounded by sclerotic bone.† On MRI, osteoid osteomas demonstrate a heterogeneous appearance. The calcification within the nidus and the surrounding bony sclerosis are of low signal intensity on T_1-weighted images whereas the noncalcified portions of the nidus itself are of increased signal on T_2-weighted images.[250] Interestingly, Houang et al.[258] have anecdotally reported one case in which the central portion of the lesion was low in signal on both

the T_1- and T_2-weighted scans but a halo of high signal was detected on the T_2-weighted study. They attributed this appearance to calcification of the nidus and inflammatory changes in the surrounding cancellous bone. Because of its inherent vascularity the administration of gadolinium causes intense enhancement within the nidus, which may aid in preoperative localization.

Osteoblastoma

Osteoblastomas are uncommon benign bone tumors (<1%) that usually are encountered in the posterior elements of the spine.[259-266] The lumbar spine is most often involved, followed by the thoracic and the cervical.[260,263,266] The tumors are more common in men, and most occur before the age of 30.* As do osteoid osteomas, they present with pain and local tenderness and scoliosis or torticollis may result.[248,262,263,265]

Osteoblastomas are vascular and friable, with histologic similarities to both osteoid osteoma and osteosarcoma, although they lack the identifiable central nidus and have less surrounding sclerosis than osteoid osteomas do.† On plain films and CT they tend to be geographically expansile with either a lucent or a calcified center and thinned surrounding cortex.[261,266] As noted, they usually involve the posterior elements; CT may show them to be associated with a soft tissue mass and epidural extension,[258,263,265] and MR readily shows them, along with any associated soft tissue mass, to compromise the thecal sac. As with most bone tumors, osteoblastomas are of low signal intensity relative to adjacent soft tissue on T_1-weighted scans. Typically, on long-TR images, they are of high signal intensity. If areas of hemorrhage or calcification are present, the lesions may be heterogeneous on both T_1- and T_2-weighted sequences (Fig. 7-34). There is often generous enhancement on T_1-weighted scans following the administration of paramagnetic contrast. Crim et al.[267] have described an enhancing inflammatory phenomenon (similar to that seen with osteoid osteoma) that may be very misleading because it can extend for several segments above and below the true lesion. It has high signal on T_2-weighted scans (Fig. 7-34).

Osteosarcoma

Osteosarcomas are one of the most common primary malignant bone tumors.[213] Nevertheless, they are unusual as primary tumors of the spine (metastases from osteogenic sarcoma arising elsewhere being more common).[268,269] They occur most often in the first and second decades, with a slight male preponderance,[269-271] and may arise either de novo or within bone that has been previously irradiated.[269] There is usually a 5- to 25-year

*References 248, 252, 253, 255.
†References 249, 250, 256-258.

*References 248, 260, 261, 263, 264, 266.
†References 248, 260-263, 266.

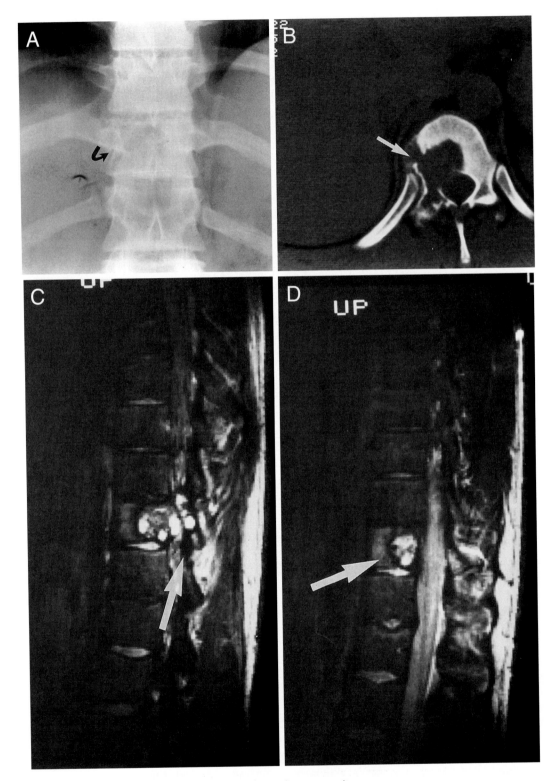

Fig. 7-34. For legend see opposite page.

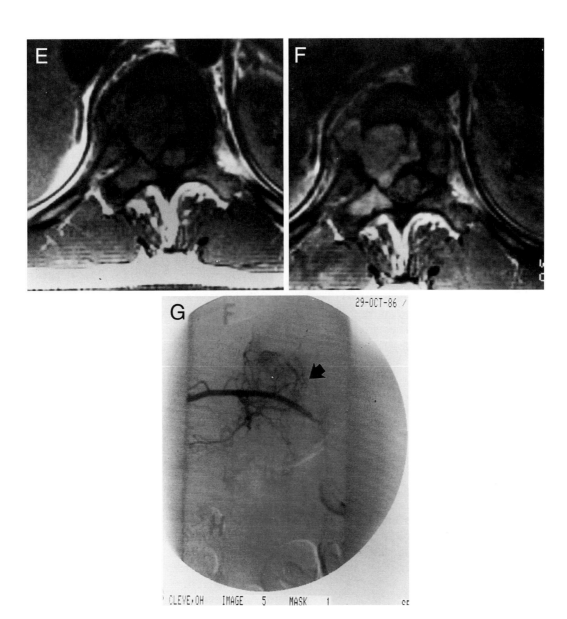

Fig. 7-34. A, An AP plain film of T11 demonstrates slight lucency along the lateral aspect of the vertebral body as well as faint erosion of the right pedicle. **B,** An axial CT scan shows geographic erosion of the cortical margin *(arrow)* and vertebral canal. Note that there is involvement of the pedicle and spinous process. **C** and **D,** 2000 msec TR/90 msec TE sagittal and parasagittal scans through T11 reveal a focal multicystic mass involving the vertebral body and right posterior elements. Note also the high signal intensity within the body, posterior elements, and surrounding soft tissues *(arrows).* **E,** An axial 500 msec TR/15 msec TE T_1-weighted scan, again, shows the mass encroaching on the thecal sac. **F,** A 500 msec TR/15 msec TE axial scan after IV gadolinium demonstrates intense enhancement of the lesion. Note, however, that the cord is intact with no evidence of compression. **G,** A spinal angiogram reveals the highly vascular lesion involving T11 *(arrow).* Surgery and histology confirmed an osteoblastoma.

latent period after the radiation before the tumor develops.[269] They can also arise in osteochondromas or from bone affected by Paget's disease, an event heralded by the new onset of pain and swelling.[268,269]

Osteosarcomas are hard calcified lesions composed primarily of sarcomatous connective tissue that forms a variable amount of osteoid or bone.* Plain films typically show a poorly defined destructive mass involving the spine, often with extensive periosteal reaction. CT can also show osteoblastic or osteolytic changes, the bony margins of the tumor, and any associated paraspinal or epidural soft tissue effects.[274,275] On T_1-weighted sequences the intraosseous tumor appears as a low-signal mass compared to the high signal in the marrow cavity.[270] On T_2-weighted scans the intraosseous tumor can display low, high, or a combination of signal intensities depending on the composition of the underlying matrix. When the bony cortex is infiltrated by tumor, a mottled soft tissue signal will replace the expected signal void of cortical bone; concomitant periosteal reaction and/or cortical expansion will be depicted as areas of low signal.[270,275] Contrast-enhanced studies are not as useful as unenhanced T_1-weighted images in defining the intraosseous component, since the lesion can become isointense with normal marrow. However, they may aid in delineating epidural or intramuscular disease.[277] On unenhanced T_1-weighted images the only changes produced by extraosseous tumor may be displacement or obliteration of fat planes.[270,277,278] On T_2-weighted images, extraosseous tumor can be of high signal relative to adjacent muscle.[278] Several groups[279,280] have recently attempted to use MR to help predict therapeutic response to presurgical chemotherapy. In the series of Holscher et al.[279] involving 57 patients, poor responders could be identified by an increase in tumor size and increased or unchanged soft tissue edema. It was not possible to identify good responders.

Chondrosarcoma

Chondrosarcomas are malignant cartilaginous neoplasms that rarely affect the spine, although they account for up to 20% of all primary malignant bone tumors.[281-284] They may arise de novo or as secondary tumors from a preexisting cartilaginous tumor (e.g., osteochondroma or enchondroma).[285] The peak incidence is between 30 and 60 years of age, and most patients are men.[286] Cases are evenly distributed throughout the spine[284]; pain is the usual presenting symptom.[282]

Chondrosarcomas are characterized by histologic sections revealing malignant chondroblasts that produce a calcified myxoid matrix. On plain films they cause lytic destruction and demonstrate a calcified matrix typified by radiodense swirls, rings, or arcs.[282,284] Frequently

there is an associated soft tissue mass, which may be better demonstrated by CT scan. The MR signal intensity of chondrosarcomas is heterogeneous: focal areas of decreased signal intensity on T_2-weighted images when the calcifications are prominent, cartilaginous lobulations in foci of high signal intensity.[287,288] Areas of hemorrhage can also occur, producing paramagnetic or susceptibility signal changes within the lesions. As with other sarcomas, MR is capable of defining soft tissue masses and possible compromise of the vertebral canal on T_2-weighted images.[288] Additionally, Geirnaerdt et al.[289] have reported that the pattern of gadolinium enhancement may be prognostically significant: thin "arc-and-ring" septa of enhancement correlate better histopathologically with lower-grade neoplasms than with higher-grade lesions, which demonstrate a more diffuse homogeneous or heterogeneous enhancement pattern.

Chordoma

Chordomas are uncommon aggressive extradural lesions of the bony spine arising from remnants of the primitive notochord and representing approximately 3% to 5% of primary bone tumors.[213] They typically present in middle-aged adults with local pain secondary to a destructive or expansile lesion.[292] There is a 2:1 male preponderance.[293] Although notochordal remnants are found distributed equally along the neuraxis, chordomas are found predominantly in the sacrococcygeal area (50%), with 30% to 40% arising from the basisphenoid region and the remainder from the vertebral bodies[294] (Fig. 7-35). Chordomas arising in the vertebral bodies are more malignant than their counterparts in the sacrum or the clivus.[292] Ectopic notochordal tissue may be present intradurally (2% of all autopsies) as small nodules (known as enchondrosis physaliphora) that have only rarely been reported to degenerate into purely intradural chordomas.[295]

The intervertebral disk and two or more adjacent vertebrae are commonly affected, and there is often a paraspinal soft tissue mass that may possess a calcified matrix.[293] Such lesions are composed of vacuolated physaliferous cells arranged in cords. Fibrous septa may divide the tumors into numerous lobules. Plain films show bony destruction with areas of amorphous calcification in a high percentage of cases.[293] As expected, CT better demonstrates the calcification and paravertebral soft tissue masses, including the epidural component.[290] Sze et al.[296] have reviewed the MR findings in 20 cases of histologically verified chordoma. On T_1-weighted images they found such lesions isointense (75%) or hypointense (25%). On T_2-weighted studies all chordomas demonstrated increased signal intensity, and the majority (70%) possessed low-signal septa. Whereas MR is superior to CT scanning in delineating the extent of chordomas and their relationship to adjacent vasculature or

---

*References 268, 269, 272, 273.

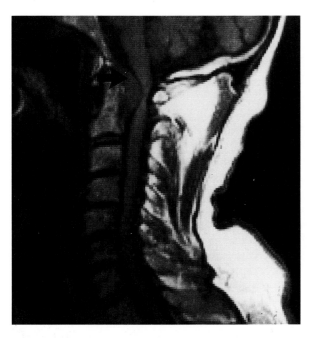

Fig. 7-35. This 500 msec TR/17 msec TE midline sagittal image through the cervical spine demonstrates a soft tissue mass arising from the body of C2 and compressing the cervicomedullary junction *(arrow)*. Diagnostic considerations would include meningioma versus chordoma. Surgery and histology confirmed the presence of a C2 chordoma. (Courtesy A. Smith, M.D., Cleveland.)

neural structures, it was inferior to CT in its ability to detect bone destruction and/or calcification. The authors also pointed out that MR may be able to distinguish chondroid chordomas from typical chordomas based on the shorter T_1 and T_2 relaxation times of chondroid chordomas.[296] This is of some clinical significance inasmuch as chondroid chordomas have a significantly better prognosis than typical chordomas do.

Eosinophilic Granuloma

Eosinophilic granulomas are a nonneoplastic condition of unknown etiology, most often seen in the first two decades of life.[297] There is a male preponderance.[297] The disease can affect the skull, pelvis, vertebrae, ribs, and long bones as single or multiple lesions.[297] Symptoms range from nonspecific systemic complaints (e.g., fever and weight loss) to focal pain.[297] With spinal lesions, collapse of the vertebral body (vertebra plana) can result in spinal cord compression, nerve root impingement, and deformity of the spine.[297,298]

Histologically the lesions are collections of eosinophils, lymphocytes, and in later phases of the disease large macrophages.[297,299] During recovery these inflammatory cells are replaced by connective tissue, which ul-

timately is transformed to bone. Plain films show elliptical, well-marginated, lytic lesions that may have an associated soft tissue mass.[298,299] CT is advantageous only in its ability to demonstrate the soft tissue component. With MR, lesions are similar to the other osseous lesions just discussed, showing decreased signal intensity on T_1-weighted and increased signal on T_2 scans. Spinal cord compression is readily visualized. A kyphosis may develop secondary to vertebra plana (Fig. 7-36).

Peripheral Primitive Neuroectodermal Tumor, Neuroblastoma, Ganglioneuroma, and Ganglioneuroblastoma

Tumors originating from primitive neural crest cells belong in a class of neoplasms that includes peripheral primitive neuroectodermal tumors (PPNETs), neuroblastoma, ganglioneuroblastoma, and ganglioneuroma. If located in the thoracopulmonary region PPNETs are called Askin tumors.[300] They are one of the small blue round-cell malignancies (traditionally including neuroblastoma) that may be morphologically indistinguishable from embryonal and alveolar rhabdomyosarcoma, small cell osteogenic sarcoma, extranodal lymphoma of soft tissue, and skeletal and extraskeletal Ewing sarcomas.[301] Immunohistologic findings show variability as well as similarities in marker expression. These tumors can originate in the adrenal medulla or the paravertebral sympathetic chain. Ganglioneuroma and ganglioneuroblastoma arise from the same cells as neuroblastoma and PPNET but are histologically more differentiated. Ganglioneuroma is the more differentiated of the two and is composed almost entirely of mature ganglion cells. Traditionally neuroblastoma is a disease of infancy, primarily children under 5 years of age, and is one of the more common neoplasms of childhood.[302] Both ganglioneuroma and ganglioneuroblastoma present slightly later (5-to-8-year-olds).[302,303] There is a slight male preponderance.[302] Most often these soft tissue masses originate in a paraspinal location, where they can insinuate themselves into the vertebral canal via the neural foramina to compress the spinal cord.[304-306] Involvement of the spine occurs more frequently in the thoracic and lumbar regions but is rare in the cervical area.[56,305,306] The most common presenting symptoms are local pain and spinal cord dysfunction.[300,301,305]

As just noted, neuroblastoma and PPNETs are composed of primitive small round cells with hyperchromatic dense nuclei often confused with Ewing's sarcoma.[301] Calcifications are seen in 10% of cases. Ganglioneuroma is composed primarily of mature neurons whereas ganglioneuroblastoma is a mixture of immature neuroblastoma and more mature elements. The nuclei are large, and there is more cytoplasm within the cells than in neuroblastoma or PPNETs. Calcifications are seen in 20% of cases.[56] Despite the malignant nature of neuroblas-

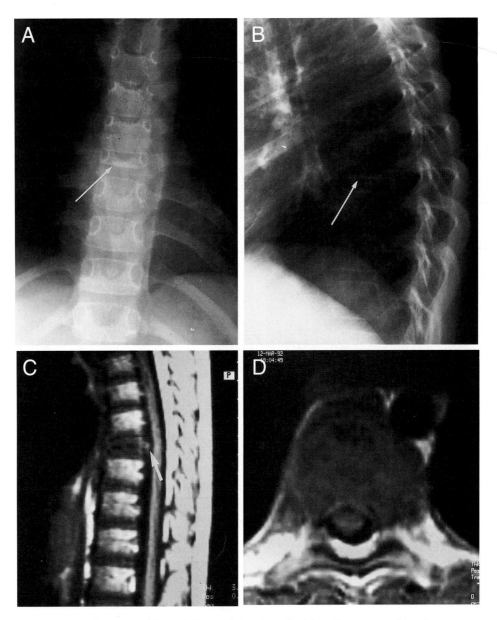

Fig. 7-36. **A** and **B,** AP and lateral views of the thoracic spine show a vertebra plana deformity at the T7 level *(arrows).* **C** and **D,** Sagittal and axial 500 msec TR/20 msec TE scans demonstrate the deformity with displacement of the posterior margin of T7 into the cord. **E** and **F,** 2000 msec TR/20 and 90 msec TE images through T7 show the vertebra plana with a high-signal fragment displaced posteriorly *(arrows).* **G,** Axial 500 msec TR/20 msec TE scans after IV gadolinium show diffuse enhancement of T7 as well as some posterior displacement of the normal vertebral body margin against the thecal sac. Surgery and histology confirmed an eosinophilic granuloma involving T7.

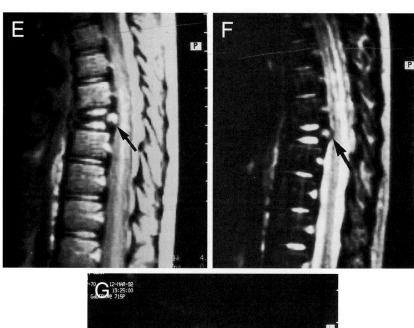

Fig. 7-36, cont'd. For legend see opposite page.

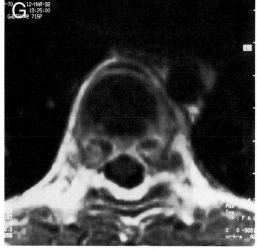

toma, long-term survival can occur, presumably through spontaneous regression or maturation to a benign non-progressive state.[307] As tumor extends through the neural foramina, plain films disclose erosion of the pedicles, widening of the foramina, scalloping of the vertebral bodies, thinning of the ribs, or widening of the spinal canal.[56,302,306] The intraspinal component can spread over several levels, resulting in cord block remote from the site of the paravertebral mass.[301] Although commonly appearing as an extension from a paraspinal mass in the sympathetic chain or adrenal medulla, neuroectodermal tumors may also arise primarily from primordia of the intramedullary posterior root ganglion. Thus it is often difficult, if not impossible, to discern whether the mass has arisen from the spinal canal or secondarily invaded it. CT is useful in delineating the full extent of the mass and is very sensitive to the presence of calcification. MR is excellent for delineating paraspinal dis-

ease, intraspinal extension of disease, and/or a block[304] (Fig. 7-37). Necrosis is not uncommon, producing cystlike areas with low signal intensity on T_1-weighted images and increased signal on T_2-weighted studies. Hemorrhagic necrosis may have a more variable appearance. Unlike radiographs and CT, MR does not show calcification well; large areas of calcification are seen as punctate foci of low or absent signal intensity. Paramagnetic contrast can help to separate epidural disease from the normal thecal sac and spinal cord.[308]

Ewing Sarcoma

Ewing sarcoma is a primary malignancy of bone affecting children and young adults that, as noted, is histologically similar to the PPNETs.[301,309,310] Although it is the second most common primary malignant bone tumor (after osteogenic sarcoma), it does not commonly arise in the vertebral column. Metastatic disease,

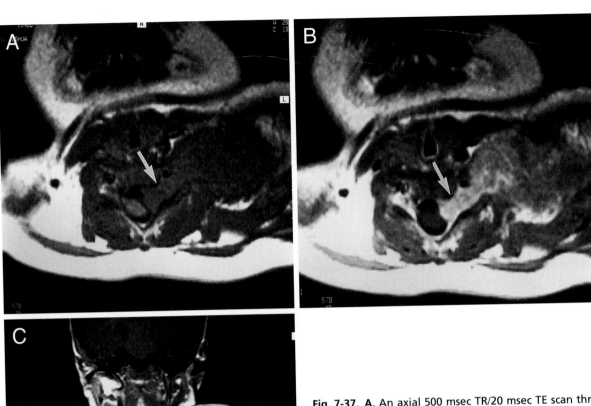

Fig. 7-37. A, An axial 500 msec TR/20 msec TE scan through the upper thoracic spine demonstrates a large dumbbell-shaped lesion extending from the canal through the neural foramen and into the left axilla. **B** and **C,** 500 msec TR/17 msec TE axial and coronal scans after gadolinium show the lesion, which enhances heterogeneously *(arrows).* Surgery revealed the presence of an Askin tumor.

however, often will involve the spine.[310] Clinically the lesions usually present with focal pain and tenderness.[309-311]

Histologically a Ewing sarcoma is composed of small primitive round cells that produce a diffuse, permeative, lytic lesion on plain film examination.* An associated soft tissue mass is common. The "onion peel" periosteal reaction is classic.[309] CT shows a soft tissue mass associated with the bony lesion but has no real advantage over plain film in detecting marrow space disease.[312] MR is better suited for depicting marrow involvement, which appears as low signal on short T_1-weighted images and increased signal on T_2-weighted scans. Soft tissue paravertebral masses are also readily assessed with MRI.

Leukemia

Leukemia is the most common malignancy in childhood, and the ninth most common malignancy in adults.[313-315] Acute lymphoblastic leukemia (ALL) represents 80% of all childhood leukemias and is most common in the 2-to-5-year-old age group.[313,316] There is a slight male preponderance.[316] Children with leukemia are systemically ill with fatigue, migratory myalgias, fever, and weight loss.[313,314]

Plain films may demonstrate osteoporosis with or without vertebral compression fracture.[315] MR in patients with leukemia shows homogeneous decreased signal on T_1-weighted images secondary to the replacement of the high-signal fatty marrow by leukemic cells.*

*References 50, 301, 309-311.

*References 196, 197, 317-322.

Compression deformities of the vertebral bodies can also be seen. Foci of leukemic infiltration display increased signal on T_2-weighted scans.[319] In patients with myelogenous leukemia, chloromas can occur paraspinally. They appear as expanding masses, isointense with adjacent soft tissues on T_1-weighted scans.

It is noteworthy that very young children normally have a little fat within their vertebral marrow space. Thus leukemic infiltration may be more difficult to detect. A variety of techniques, including chemical shift imaging, has been used to improve the sensitivity of MR signal changes in diffuse vertebral marrow disease. In magnetic resonance imaging, T_1 and T_2 are different for each subpopulation of protons (e.g., water protons, methylene protons, lactate protons). Relaxation times for tissues containing methylene (fat) and water protons are composite values resulting from both components.[323,324] T_1 and T_2 relaxation times for vertebral marrow normally decrease with age because the hematopoietic elements are replaced by fat.[325,326] The hematopoietic bone marrow usually reaches an adult distribution and maturation by age 25 years and subsequently continues to evolve.[326] The phenomenon is more pronounced in women and is exaggerated in patients who have undergone radiation therapy.[325-328] By contrast, neoplastic invasion of a vertebra significantly prolongs T_1 and T_2 as a result of the replacement of marrow fat by increasing amounts of tissue water protons.* In addition to the difference in relaxation times, tissue water and methylene (fat) protons actually resonate at slightly different frequencies within the same applied magnetic field secondary to differing local fields induced by nearby nuclei and electrons. Although conventional imaging uses the total signal generated by the spectrum of resonance frequencies, numerous methods exist that selectively image certain hydrogen spectral peaks.[324,325] These techniques are collectively known as chemical-shift imaging.[324,325] Chemical-shift imaging has been applied to the study of axial bone marrow in normal subjects and in patients with neoplastic disease.[331] To date such methods appear to be most helpful for the detection of diffuse, sometimes insidious, changes in bone marrow signal over time. For example, McKinstry et al.[319] have serially studied patients with chronic granulocytic leukemia and aplastic anemia with chemical-shift imaging and were able to demonstrate marrow response to therapy effectively using this technique. Moore et al.[317] examined T_1 relaxation times in 17 children with ALL in different stages—newly diagnosed, in relapse, or in remission. A significant increase in T_1 relaxation times occurred in the marrow of patients with newly diagnosed ALL or ALL in relapse compared to those in healthy age-matched children or patients in remission.

*References 196, 317, 318, 329, 330.

Lymphoma

Non-Hodgkin's lymphoma (or reticulum cell sarcoma) is an adult disease that can involve the spine primarily or (more commonly) secondarily.[313,332] The vast majority of cases occur after 20 years of age, and more commonly in men.[313,333,334] Patients frequently present with local pain.[313,333,334]

Typically the lesions are highly cellular and very vascular. Plain films show a wide spectrum of radiographic manifestations, from a permeative moth-eaten appearance to a more geographic, lytic, area of destruction.[313,315] On MR, infiltration of the normal high-signal fatty marrow of the vertebral bodies results in focal or diffuse areas of low signal on T_1-weighted images.[318,335] On T_2-weighted images areas of tumor infiltrate have increased signal intensity, a nonspecific finding.

Multiple Myeloma

Multiple myeloma is defined by a progressive neoplastic proliferation of plasma cells resulting in marrow plasmacytosis, a monoclonal protein band (i.e., Bence Jones protein) at urine or serum electrophoresis, and permeative or geographic lesions of the axial skeleton. It is a disease of older people, with a yearly incidence of approximately 3 per 100,000.[336] Patients may present with nonspecific constitutional symptoms, back pain, renal failure, or recurrent infections (especially pneumococcal pneumonia). The prognosis is believed to correlate with tumor cell mass and renal function.[337] In the past, serum β_2 microglobulin levels were considered to be the single most powerful determinant of outcome.[338]

It is recognized that bone marrow involvement in multiple myeloma takes two forms: diffuse infiltration and nodular deposits of malignant plasma cells.[338] Plain film examination is predictably variable from case to case and may reveal diffuse osteoporosis secondary to widespread marrow infiltration, numerous small geographic lytic lesions involving primarily the axial skeleton that result from multiple nodules, and pleural or paraspinal soft tissue masses (i.e., the solitary plasmacytoma). As with other paraspinal tumors, CT and CT-myelography can demonstrate the degree of bony destruction and compromise of the spinal cord respectively. Libshitz et al.[339] reported the clinical and MR findings in 32 patients with multiple myeloma. On T_1-weighted images signal intensity of the vertebrae was approximately that of muscle in 14 cases and was intermediate between those of muscle and fat in 18; definite foci of decreased signal were seen in eight cases (25%). On T_2-weighted images the marrow signal approximated that of muscle in 17 cases and was intermediate in 15. Definite foci of increased signal intensity were seen in 17 (53%) patients. The authors reported that only 50% of compression fractures demonstrated a definite pattern consistent with neoplastic disease and concluded that foci of tumor were better

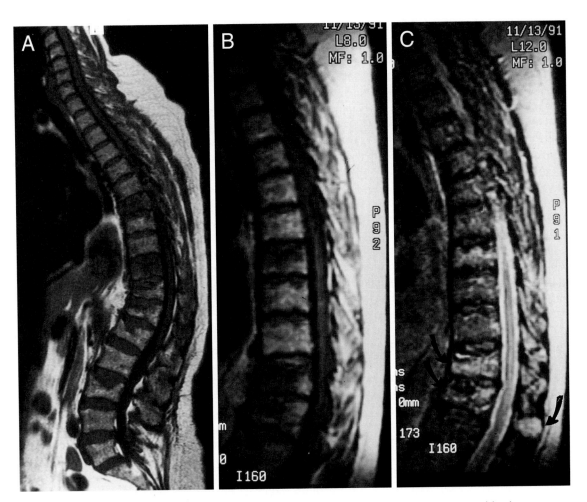

Fig. 7-38. A, A 500 msec TR/15 msec TE T$_1$-weighted scout using a 300 cm FOV and body coil demonstrates heterogeneous signal intensity with multiple compression fractures throughout the thoracolumbar spine. T7 and T10 in particular are of low signal intensity although some focal areas of high signal remain. These are suspicious for metastatic disease. **B** and **C,** 2000 msec TR/20 and 90 msec TE parasagittal scans through the thoracolumbar junction show vague signal intensity changes without complete marrow replacement in the thoracic spine. However, on the T$_2$-weighted scan T10 and T11 demonstrated focal high signal, especially of the T11 spinous process *(curved arrows).* These findings were consistent with a diagnosis of myeloma, which was confirmed by serum protein electrophoresis.

demonstrated on T$_2$-weighted images in patients with focal disease[339] (Fig. 7-38). Other suggestions of multiple myeloma on T$_1$-weighted images were the absence of fatty replacement and/or a generalized decrease in signal intensity. No correlation was found between MRI findings and the severity of laboratory or bone marrow findings.[339] Although chemical-shift techniques were not employed, the findings on conventional spin-echo spinal examinations were nonspecific and relatively insensitive to the full range of disease.[194,339] Fat-suppressed dynamic T$_1$-weighted contast-enhanced studies do not appear to improve sensitivity of MR in the presence of myeloma above that achieved by traditional T$_1$-weighted studies.[339a]

Secondary (Metastatic) Extradural Tumor

Spinal metastases occur frequently in neoplastic disease; 5% to 10% of cancer patients develop spinal metastases with neurologic manifestations.[340,341] Involvement of the spine or epidural soft tissues is most commonly seen with breast carcinoma, prostate and uterine carcinoma, lung carcinoma, myeloma, and lymphoma.[341] Constans et al.[342] reviewed 600 cases of spinal metastases and classified the lesions as (1) purely intradural (1.16%), (2) purely epidural (5.00%), (3) purely osseous (10.34%), and complex (83.50%). Gilbert et al.[341] state that the site of epidural tumor is thoracic in approximately 68%, lumbar or sacral in 16%, and cervical in 15%. The most frequent symptoms of spinal cord compression are pain, weakness, autonomic dysfunction, and sensory loss.[341] Back pain, which may be radicular, is the initial symptom in 61% to 96% of patients.[341,343] In the series of Constans et al.,[342] 27.67% of patients presented with an acute onset of symptoms (less than 48 hours) and 61.00% with a subacute onset (within 7 to 10 days).

Although MRI is sensitive in detecting most primary or secondary extradural spinal neoplasms, their appearance is generally nonspecific.* Typically the lesions are recognized by their involvement with one or more vertebrae and the adjacent soft tissues (Figs. 7-39 to 7-43). Most possess a long T_1 relative to the fat normally present within the bone marrow and are thus recognized as focal areas of decreased signal on T_1-weighted images within the bony spine. On T_2-weighted studies the lesions demonstrate variably increased signal and consequently may be less conspicuous relative to the adjacent normal marrow than on T_1-weighted studies (Figs. 7-39 to 7-43). In adults the vast majority of such lesions are represented by metastatic foci that frequently involve the bony canal (e.g., lung, breast, prostate). Malignant lymphoma (Hodgkin's disease and reticulum cell sarcoma) may also manifest in this fashion; however, most of these cases have minimal vertebral body involvement compared to epidural and paravertebral disease.[347] Addi-

tional, more subtle findings of spinal malignancy include diffuse changes in marrow signal intensity, which can cause the disks to have relatively high signal on T_1-weighted images[322] (Figs. 7-44 and 7-45); or a tumor confined strictly to the vertebral canal may present only as a subtle interruption of normal epidural fat (i.e., the "fat-cap sign").[348]

The role of paramagnetic contrast in evaluating malignant extradural disease is less clearly defined than are the indications for its use with intradural mass lesions. The preliminary experience of Sze et al.[202] suggests that intravenous Gd-DTPA may actually mask osseous spinal implants by making them isointense with normal vertebral marrow (Fig. 7-46). Contrast, however, may increase the specificity of MR for extradural masses (e.g., distinguishing metastases from disk fragment) and aid in directing needle biopsy.[202]

Whereas primary or metastatic tumors of the spine are evaluated in terms of their biologic activity, they are also (and possibly more urgently) evaluated with respect to the degree of mechanical compression they exert on the cord. Classically, the clinical manifestations of spinal cord compression have been divided into three stages[51,349]: The first (neuralgic) stage is characterized by root pain and segmental sensory and motor loss. The second (transitional) stage, or incomplete transection, is

---

*References 195, 202, 344, 346.

Text continued on p. 305.

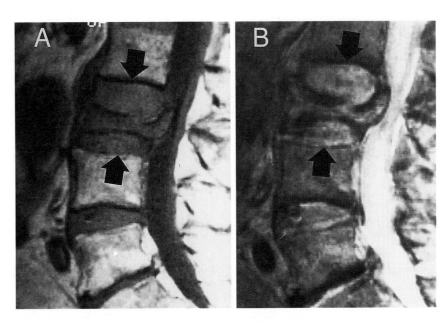

Fig. 7-39. A, A 500 msec TR/17 msec TE midline sagittal image through the lumbar spine demonstrates compression of L3 *(open arrows),* which is of low signal intensity on this T_1-weighted image. These findings are most consistent with a pathologic fracture due to metastatic disease. **B,** The 2000 more T_2-weighted msec TR/120 msec TE sagittal image shows a pathologic compression fracture with somewhat higher signal intensity.

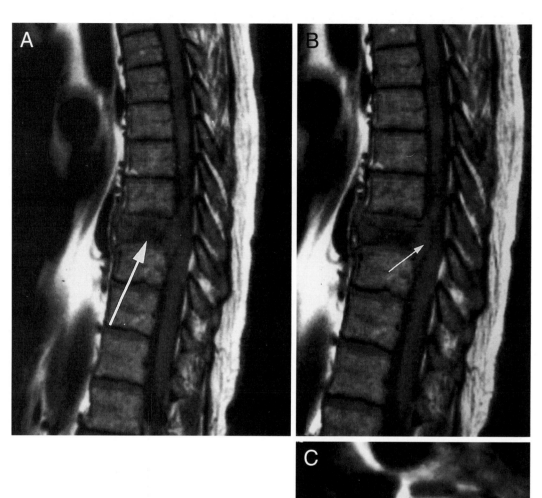

Fig. 7-40. A, A 500 msec TR/15 msec TE 300 cm FOV body coil image with a 512 × 512 matrix demonstrates complete marrow replacement of T9 *(arrow).* **B,** A magnified image from the same acquisition shows a metastatic lesion with pathologic fracture of the vertebral body. **C,** The axial T$_1$-weighted 500 msec TR/15 msec TE surface coil image demonstrates displacement of the spinal cord *(arrows)* although spinal fluid is identified around the cord. No definite block can be appreciated.

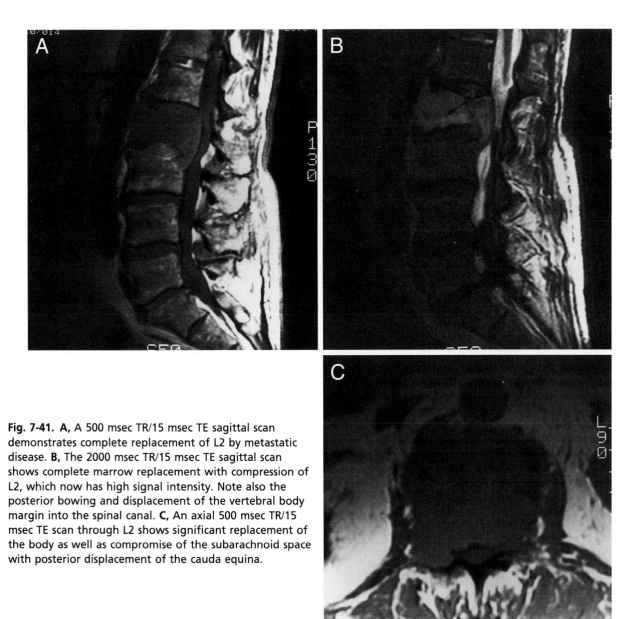

Fig. 7-41. A, A 500 msec TR/15 msec TE sagittal scan demonstrates complete replacement of L2 by metastatic disease. **B,** The 2000 msec TR/15 msec TE sagittal scan shows complete marrow replacement with compression of L2, which now has high signal intensity. Note also the posterior bowing and displacement of the vertebral body margin into the spinal canal. **C,** An axial 500 msec TR/15 msec TE scan through L2 shows significant replacement of the body as well as compromise of the subarachnoid space with posterior displacement of the cauda equina.

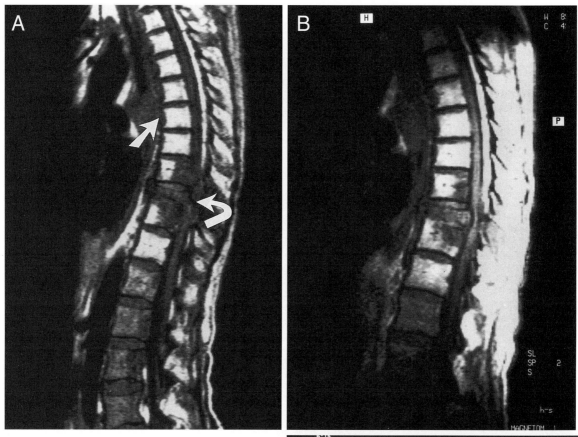

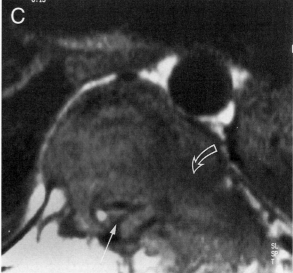

Fig. 7-42. A, A 500 msec TR/15 msec TE 300 cm FOV scout demonstrates metastatic foci at the T9 and T11 levels with a compression fracture and compromise of the subarachnoid space at T10 *(curved arrow)*. Note the high signal intensity within the thoracic vertebral bodies *(angled arrow)* consistent with previous radiation therapy for carcinoma of the lung. **B** and **C,** Surface coil sagittal and axial 500 msec TR/15 msec TE scans through the level of compromise show cord compression secondary to epidural metastases *(straight arrow)*. Note also the paraspinal mass *(open arrow)*.

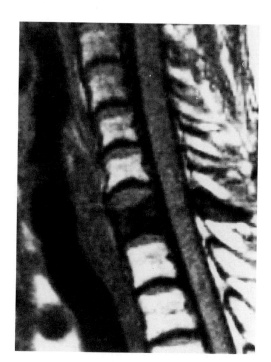

Fig. 7-43. A T_1-weighted midline sagittal 500 msec TR/17 msec TE image through the cervical spine shows diffuse replacement of the marrow of C6 by a metastatic osteoblastic carcinoma of the breast. Consequently, the vertebral body and spinous process are of diffusely low signal intensity.

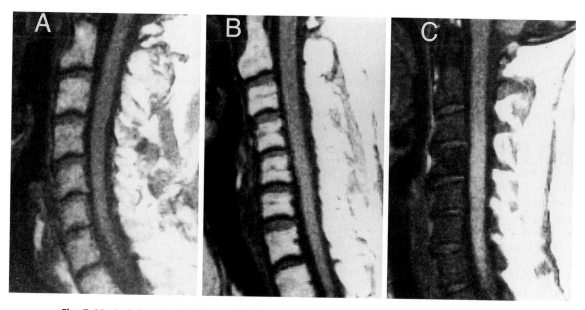

Fig. 7-44. Serial sagittal 500 msec TR/17 msec TE T_1-weighted images in three patients demonstrate the variability of marrow signal in normal subjects and various disease states. **A,** Normal signal intensity from the cervical body marrow space in a patient with cervical disk disease. **B,** Increased signal intensity within the cervical vertebrae indicative of previous radiation therapy. Radiotherapy leads to replacement of normal hematopoietic elements by vertebral body fat. **C,** A diffuse decrease in signal intensity of the vertebral body marrow space in this patient with leukemia suggests neoplastic invasion.

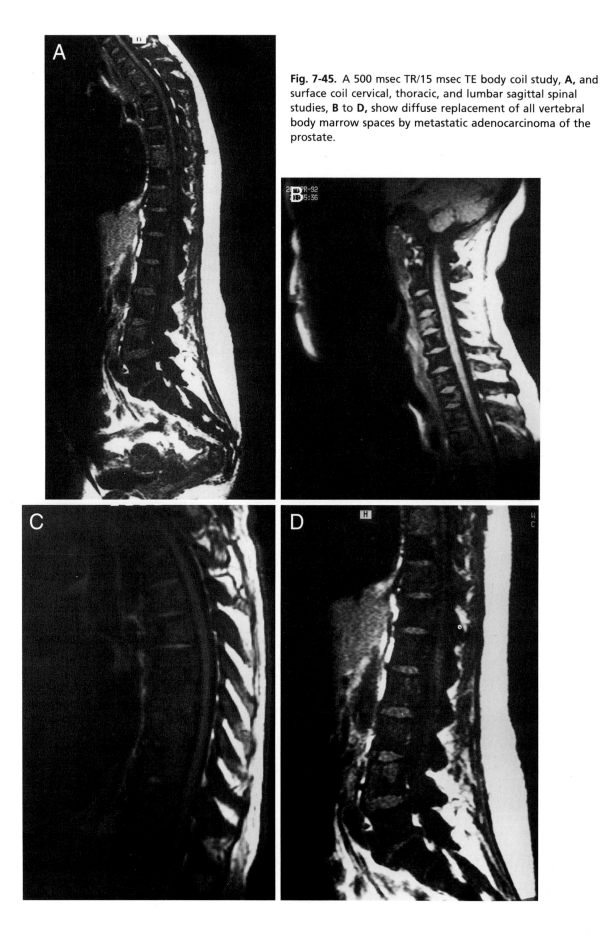

Fig. 7-45. A 500 msec TR/15 msec TE body coil study, **A,** and surface coil cervical, thoracic, and lumbar sagittal spinal studies, **B** to **D,** show diffuse replacement of all vertebral body marrow spaces by metastatic adenocarcinoma of the prostate.

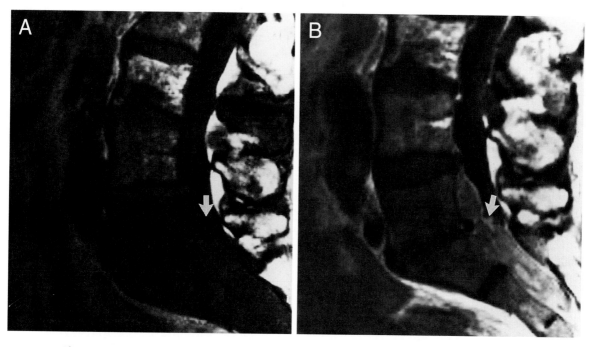

Fig. 7-46. A, A 500 msec TR/15 msec TE sagittal scan through the lumbosacral junction shows diffuse replacement of the marrow signal at L5 and the first two sacral levels. Note the faint suggestion of a soft tissue mass within the thecal sac *(arrow)*. **B,** A 500 msec TR/15 msec TE sagittal scan through the same level demonstrates enhancement of extensive epidural metastases from adenocarcinoma of the colon. Note, however, that there has been some normalization of the signal intensity in the vertebral body marrow space, which could mask the presence of bony metastases in the absence of an unenhanced study.

heralded by the onset of a Brown-Séquard syndrome. In the third stage, or complete transection, there is total deficit, usually beginning in the distal extremities and ascending as the lesion progresses. Unfortunately, it may be difficult to determine clinically what stage of compression a patient is experiencing at the time of presentation; and it is certainly impossible to predict the rate of progression from stage to stage (and thus the eminent risk of permanent neurologic deficit).

Historically, such clinical questions have been answered by myelography (occasionally aided by CT) and the complete obstruction to flow of contrast in the subarachnoid space was considered to be an indication for emergency therapy.[1] Unfortunately, CSF pressure shifts induced by lumbar puncture in the presence of complete subarachnoid block may lead to rapid neurologic deterioration in a significant percentage of these patients.[350] Other potential pitfalls include (1) puncture site hematoma, (2) inability to examine the entire spine in the presence of multiple compression sites, and (3) inability to demonstrate paravertebral disease.[351-353] In a prospective review of 70 patients with suspected epidural metastases and cord compression, Carmody et al.[195] found

MR to have a sensitivity of 0.92 and a specificity of 0.90 compared to 0.95 and 0.88 for myelography in the diagnosis of cord compression. For extradural masses and osseous metastases MR was found to be far superior to myelography; and because it is also noninvasive, it was considered the examination of choice in evaluating spinal metastases and possible cord compression. Additional, retrospective, studies[346,347] have reached similar conclusions. Frank et al.,[193] likewise, compared the sensitivities of spin-echo and inversion recovery MR to technetium 99m scintigraphy in 106 patients with suspected spinal metastasis and found MR statistically more sensitive.

The MR examination may be tailored specifically to particular clinical questions. With respect to cord compression, obtaining a localizing sagittal T_1 body coil image through the midline, followed by rapid serial sagittal and axial studies over the length of the spinal cord, may expeditiously detect "block" (Figs. 7-40 and 7-42). This is especially effective with a large field of view and additional K_y lines to improve spatial resolution and signal-to-noise.[354] New coil designs may permit rapid single-acquisition studies of the spine with comparable quality to that obtained by multiple surface coil studies.[355]

If tumor is found but the clinical question of a "complete block" lingers, it may be possible to perform a magnetic resonance version of the Queckenstedt test. More specifically, a nongated nonrefocused long TR/long TE sagittal image through a suspected compressive lesion will not demonstrate ghosting artifact secondary to CSF pulsation in the presence of complete block.[356] This will be more apparent when the phase-encoding direction is oriented perpendicular to the spine. Finally, several studies[357,358] have attempted to define criteria for distinguishing between benign senile osteoporotic compression fractures and pathologic fractures resulting from underlying tumor. Although they implemented a variety of T_1- and T_2-weighted pulse sequences, these studies have generally stressed the complete replacement of normal high-signal marrow fat within the vertebral body only on T_1-weighted images as a useful sign of malignancy, especially if the suspected lesion was subacute or chronic (Figs. 7-39 to 7-41). However, even acute benign fractures will demonstrate some residual high signal within the affected body, and, additionally, paraspinal fat planes are usually undisturbed by a paraspinal mass (unlike some neoplastic fractures) (Fig. 7-47).

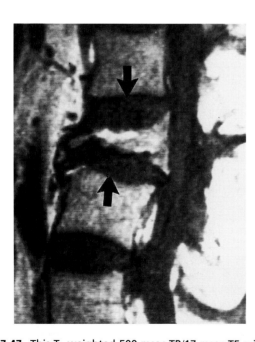

Fig. 7-47. This T_1-weighted 500 msec TR/17 msec TE midline sagittal image through the lumbar spine demonstrates a wedge-compression fracture of one of the upper lumbar vertebrae. Note that it has relatively high signal intensity. Such findings are most consistent with a compression fracture resulting from senile osteoporosis rather than a pathologic fracture secondary to metastatic disease, which more typically has diffuesly low signal on T_1-weighted images.

REFERENCES

1. Shapiro R: Tumors. In Shapiro R (ed): *Myelography*. Chicago, Year Book, 1984, pp 345-421.
2. Aubin ML, Jardin C, Bar D, et al: Computerized tomography in 32 cases of intraspinal tumor. *J Neuroradiol* 1979; 6:81-92.
3. Hammerschlag SB, Wolpert SM, Carter BL: Computed tomography of the spinal canal. *Radiology* 1976;121:361-367.
4. Nakagawa H, Haung YP, Malis LI, et al: Computed tomography of intraspinal and paraspinal neoplasm. *J Comput Assist Tomogr* 1977;1:377-390.
5. Modic MT, Weinstein M, Pavlicek W, et al: Nuclear magnetic resonance imaging of the spine. *Radiology* 1983; 147:757-762.
6. Modic MT, Weinstein M, Pavlicek W, et al: Magnetic resonance imaging of the cervical spine: technical and clinical observations. *AJR* 1983;141:1129-1136.
7. Han JS, Kaufman B, El Yousef SJ, et al: NMR imaging of the spine. *AJR* 1983;141:1137-1145.
8. Norman D, Mills CM, Brant-Zawadzki M, et al: Magnetic resonance imaging of the spinal cord and canal: potentials and limitations. *AJR* 1983;141:1147-1152.
9. Modic MT, Hardy RW Jr, Weinstein MA, et al: Nuclear magnetic resonance of the spine: clinical potential and limitation. *Neurosurgery* 1984;15:582-592.
10. Bradley WG, Waluch V, Yadley RA, Wycoff RR: Comparison of CT and MR in 400 patients with suspected disease of the brain and cervical spinal cord. *Radiology* 1984; 152:695-702.
11. Hyman RA, Edwards JH, Vacirca SJ, Stein HL: 0.6 T MR imaging of the cervical spine: multislice and multiecho techniques. *AJNR* 1985;6:229-236.
12. Kucharczyk W, Brant-Zawadzki M, Sobel D, et al: Central nervous system tumors in children: detection by magnetic resonance imaging. *Radiology* 1985;155:131-136.
13. Di Chiro G, Doppman JL, Dwyer AJ, et al: Tumors and arteriovenous malformations of the spinal cord: assessment using MR. *Radiology* 1985;156:689-697.
14. Haughton VM, Rimm AA, Sobocinski KA, et al: A blinded clinical comparison of MR imaging and CT in neuroradiology. *Radiology* 1986;160:751-755.
15. Axel L: Surface coil magnetic resonance imaging. *J Comput Assist Tomogr* 1984;8:381-384.
16. Fisher MR, Barker B, Amparo EG, et al: MR imaging using specialized coils. *Radiology* 1985;157:443-447.
17. Kulkarni MV, Patton JA, Price RR: Technical considerations for the use of surface coils in MRI. *AJR* 1986; 147:373-378.
18. Enzman DR, Rubin JB, Wright A: Use of cerebrospinal fluid gating to improve T_2 weighted images. I. The spinal cord. *Radiology* 1987;162:763-767.
19. Enzman DR, Rubin JB, Wright A: Cervical spine MR imaging: generating high signal CSF in sagittal and axial images. *Radiology* 1987;163:233-238.
20. Rubin JB, Enzman DR: Optimizing conventional MR imaging of the spine. *Radiology* 1987;163:777-783.
21. Rubin JB, Enzman DR, Wright A: CSF-gated MR imaging of the spine: theory and clinical implementation. *Radiology* 1987;163:784-792.

22. Rubin JB, Enzman DR: Harmonic modulation of proton MR precessional phase by pulsative motion: origin and spinal CSF flow phenomena. *AJR* 1987;148:938-994.

23. Haacke EM, Lenz GW: Improving MR image quality in the presence of motion by using rephasing gradients. *AJR* 1987;148:1251-1258.

24. Brasch RC: Contrast enhancement in NMR imaging. In Newton TH, Potts DG (eds): *Advanced imaging techniques: modern neuroradiology.* San Anselmo Calif, Clavadel, 1983, vol 2, pp 63-79.

25. Bydder GM, Kingsley DP, Brown J, et al: MR imaging of meningiomas including studies with and without gadolinium-DTPA. *J Comput Assist Tomogr* 1985;9:690-697.

26. Bydder GM, Brown J, Niendorf HP, Young IR: Enhancement of cervical intraspinal tumors in MR imaging with intravenous gadolinium-DTPA. *J Comput Assist Tomogr* 1985;9:847-885.

27. Schroth G, Thron A, Guhl L, et al: Magnetic resonance imaging of spinal meningiomas and neurinomas: improvement of imaging by paramagnetic contrast enhancement. *J Neurosurg* 1987;66:695-700.

28. Sze G, Abramson A, Krol G, et al: Gadolinium-DTPA in the evaluation of intradural extra-medullary spinal disease. *AJNR* 1988;9:153-163.

29. Sze G, Krol G, Zimmerman RD, Deck MDF: Intramedullary disease of the spine: diagnosis using gadolinium-DTPA enhanced MR imaging. *AJNR* 1988;9:847-858.

30. Valk J: Gadolinium-DTPA in MR of spinal lesions. *AJNR* 1988;9:345-350.

31. Dillon WP, Norman D, Newton TH, et al: Intradural spinal cord lesions: Gd-DTPA-enhanced MR imaging. *Radiology* 1989;170:229-237.

32. Parizel PM, Baleriaux D, Rodesch G, et al: Gd-DTPA-enhanced MR imaging of spinal tumors. *AJNR* 1989;10:249-258.

33. Breger RK, Williams AL, Daniels DL, et al: Contrast enhancement in spinal MR imaging. *AJNR* 1989;10:633-637.

34. Sze G, Stimac GK, Barlett C, et al: Multicenter study of gadopentetate dimeglumine as an MR contrast agent: evaluation in patients with spinal tumors. *AJNR* 1990;11:967-974.

35. Greco A, McNamara MT, Lanthiez P, et al: Gadodiamide injection: nonionic gadolinium chelate for MR imaging of the brain and spine-phase II-III clinical trial. *Radiology* 1990;176:451-456.

36. Runge VM, Bradley WG, Brant-Zawadzki MN, et al: Clinical safety and efficacy of gadoteridol: a study in 411 patients with suspected intracranial and spinal disease. *Radiology* 1991;181:701-709.

37. Edelman RR, Atkinson DJ, Silver MS, et al: FRODO pulse sequences: a new means of eliminating motion, flow and wraparound artifacts. *Radiology* 1988;166:231-236.

38. Katz BH, Quencer RM, Hinks RS: Comparison of gradient-recalled-echo and T_2-weighted spin-echo pulse sequences in intramedullary spinal lesions. *AJNR* 1989;10:815-822.

39. Hennig J, Naureth A, Friedburg H: RARE imaging: a fast method for clinical MR. *Magn Reson Med* 1986;3:823-833.

40. Kurland LT: The frequency of intraspinal neoplasms in the resident population of Rochester, Minnesota. *J Neurosurg* 1958;15:627-641.

41. Percy AK, Elveback LR, Okazaki H, Kurland LT: Neoplasms of the central nervous system: epidemiologic considerations. *Neurology* 1972;22:40-48.

42. Nittner K: Spinal meningiomas, neurinomas and neurofibromas and hourglass tumors. In Vinken PJ, Bruyn GW (eds): *Handbook of clinical neurology.* New York, Elsevier North-Holland, 1976, vol 20, pp 177-322.

43. Sloof JL, Kernohan JW, MacCarty CS: *Primary intramedullary tumors of the spinal cord and filum terminale.* Philadelphia, Saunders, 1964.

44. Kernohan JW, Sayre GP: Tumors of the central nervous system. In National Research Council: *Atlas of tumor pathology.* Washington DC, Armed Forces Institute of Pathology, 1952.

45. Lombardi G, Passerini A: Spinal cord tumors. *Radiology* 1962;76:381-392.

46. Mosberg WH Jr: Spinal tumors diagnosed during the first year of life. *J Neurosurg* 1951;8:220-224.

47. Okazaki H: *Fundamentals in neuropathology.* New York, Igaku-Shoin, 1983.

48. Alter M: Statistical aspects of spinal cord tumors. In Vinken PJ, Bruyn GW (eds): *Handbook of clinical neurology.* New York, Elsevier–North Holland, 1975, vol 19, pp 1-22.

49. DiLorenzo N, Giuffre R, Fortuna A: Primary spinal neoplasms in childhood: analysis of 1,234 published cases (including 56 personal cases) by pathology, sex, age, and site: differences from the situation in adults. *Neurochirurgia* 1982;25:153-164.

50. DeSousa AL, Kalsbeck JE, Mealey J Jr, et al: Intraspinal tumors in children. *J Neurosurg* 1979;51:437-445.

51. Russell DS, Rubinstein LJ (eds): *Pathology of tumors of the nervous system.* Baltimore, Williams & Wilkins, 1989.

52. Epstein F, Epstein N: Intramedullary tumors of the spinal cord. In Shillito J Jr, Matson DD (eds): *Pediatric neurosurgery of the developing nervous system.* New York, Grune & Stratton, 1982, pp 529-539.

53. Epstein F, Epstein N: Surgical treatment of spinal cord astrocytomas of childhood. *J Neurosurg* 1982;57:685-689.

54. Connelly ES: Spinal cord tumors in adults. In Youmans JR (ed): *Neurological surgery,* ed 2. Philadelphia, Saunders, 1982, pp 3196-3214.

55. Reimer R, Onofrio BM: Astrocytomas of the spinal cord in children and adolescents. *J Neurosurg* 1985;63:669-675.

56. Harwood-Nash DC, Fitz CR: *Neuroradiology in infants and children.* St Louis, Mosby, 1976, pp 1167-1226.

57. Johnson DL, Schwarz S: Intracranial metastases from malignant spinal-cord astrocytoma. *J Neurosurg* 1987;66:621-625.

58. Cohen AR, Wisoff JH, Allen JC, Epstein F: Malignant astrocytomas of the spinal cord. *J Neurosurg* 1989;70:50-54.

59. Guidetti B, Mercuri S, Vagnozzi R: Long-term results of surgical treatment of 129 intramedullary spinal gliomas. *J Neurosurg* 1981;54:323-330.

60. Kopelson G, Linggood RM, Kleinman GM, et al: Management of intramedullary spinal cord tumors. *Radiology* 1980;135:473-479.

61. Packer RJ, Zimmerman RA, Bilaniuk LT, et al: Magnetic resonance imaging of lesions of the posterior fossa and upper cervical cord in childhood. *Pediatrics* 1985;76:84-90.

62. Goy AMC, Pinto RS, Raghavendra BN, et al: Intramedullary spinal cord tumors: MR imaging with emphasis on associated cysts. *Radiology* 1986;161:381-386.

63. Poser CM: The relationship between syringomyelia and neoplasm. In *American lecture series* no. 262: *American lectures in neurology.* Springfield Ill, Thomas, 1956.

64. Rubin JM, Hisen A, DiPietro MA: Ambiguities in MR imaging of tumoral cysts in the spinal cord. *J Comput Assist Tomogr* 1986;10:395-398.

65. Williams AL, Haughton VM, Pojunas KW, et al: Differentiation of intramedullary neoplasms and cysts by MR. *AJR* 1987;149:159-164.

66. Williams B: On the pathogenesis of syringomyelia: a review. *J R Soc Med* 1980;73:798-806.

67. Ball MJ, Dayan AD: Pathogenesis of syringomyelia. *Lancet* 1972;2:799-801.

68. Sherman JL, Barkovich AJ, Citrin CM: The MR appearance of syringomyelia: new observations. *AJR* 1987;148:381-391.

69. Enzmann DR, O'Donohue J, Rubin JB, et al: CSF pulsations within nonneoplastic spinal cord cysts. *AJR* 1987;149:149-157.

70. Slasky BS, Bydder GM, Niendorf HP, Young IR: MR imaging with gadolinium DTPA in the differentiation of tumor, syrinx, and cysts of the spinal cord. *J Comput Assist Tomogr* 1987;11:845-850.

71. Brunberg JA, DiPietro MA, Venes JL, et al: Intramedullary lesions of the pediatric spinal cord: correlation of findings from MR imaging, intraoperative sonography, surgery, and histologic study. *Radiology* 1991;181:573-579.

72. Kernohan JW, Fletcher-Kernohan EM: Ependymomas: a study of 109 cases. *Assoc Res Nerv Ment Dis* 1935;16:182-209.

73. Sonneland PR, Scheithauer BW, Onofrio BM: Myxopapillary ependymoma: a clinicopathologic and immunocytochemical study of 77 cases. *Cancer* 1985;56:883-893.

74. Barone BM, Elridge AR: Ependymomas: a clinical survey. *J Neurosurg* 1970;33:428-438.

75. Domingues RC, Mikulis D, Swearingen B: Subcutaneous sacrococcygeal myxopapillary ependymoma: CT and MR findings. *AJNR* 1991;12:171-172.

76. Rawlings CE, Giangaspero F, Burger PC, Bullard DE: Ependymomas: a clinicopathologic study. *Surg Neurol* 1988;29:271-281.

77. Wen BC, Hussey DH, Hitchon PW, et al: The role of radiation therapy in the management of ependymomas of the spinal cord. *Int J Radiat Oncol Biol Phys* 1991;20(4):781-786.

78. Nemoto Y, Inoue Y, Tashiro T, et al: Intramedullary spinal cord tumors: significance of associated hemorrhage at MR imaging. *Radiology* 1992;82:793-796.

79. Zimmerman H: Introduction to tumors of the central nervous system. In Minckler J (ed): *Pathology of the nervous system.* New York, McGraw-Hill, 1971, vol 2, pp 1947-1951.

80. Henry JM, Heffner RR, Easle KM: Ganglioglioma of CNS: a clinicopathological study of 50 cases. [Abstract.] *J Neuropathol Exp Neurol* 1978;37:626.

81. Lichtenstein BW, Zeitlin H: Ganglioglioneuroma of the spinal cord associated with pseudosyringomyelia: a histology study. *Arch Neurol Psychiatry* 1937;37:1356-1370.

82. Bell WO, Packer RJ, Seigel KR, et al: Leptomeningeal spread of intramedullary spinal cord tumors. Report of three cases. *J Neurosurg* 1988;69:295-300.

83. Russel DS, Rubinstein LJ, Gangliogliomas: a case with long history and malignant evolution. *J Neuropathol Exp Neurol* 1962;21:185-193.

84. Kitano M, Takayama S, Nagao T, Yoshimura O: Malignant ganglioglioma of the spinal cord. *Acta Pathol Jpn* 1987;37:1000-1018.

85. Johannsson JH, Rekate HL, Roessmann U: Gangliogliomas: pathological and clinical correlation. *J Neurosurg* 1981;54:58-63.

86. Cheung YK, Fung CF, Chan FL, Leong LLY: MRI features of spinal ganglioglioma. *Clin Imaging* 1991;15:109-112.

87. Browne TR, Adams RD, Roberson GH: Hemangioblastoma of the spinal cord: review and report of five cases. *Arch Neurol* 1976;33:435-441.

88. Sato Y, Waziri M, Smith W: et al: Hippel-Lindau disease: MR imaging. *Radiology* 1988;166:241-246.

89. Wyburn Mason R: *The vascular abnormalities and tumors of the spinal cord and its membranes.* London, Kimpton, 1943.

90. Horton WA, Wong V, Eldridge R: Von Hippel–Lindau disease: clinical and pathological manifestations in nine families with 50 affected members. *Arch Intern Med* 1976;136:769-777.

91. Hosoe S, Brauch H, Latif F, et al: Localization of von Hippel–Lindau disease to a small region of chromosome 3. *Genomics* 1990;6:634-640.

92. Ismail SM, Cole G: Von Hippel–Lindau syndrome with microscopic hemangioblastomas of the spinal nerve roots. *J Neurosurg* 1984;60:1279-1281.

93. Neumann HP, Eggert HR, Weigel K, et al: Hemangioblastomas of the central nervous system: a 10 year study with special reference to von Hippel–Lindau syndrome. *J Neurosurg* 1989;70:24-30.

94. Elster AD: Radiologic screening in the neurocutaneous syndromes: strategies and controversies. *AJNR* 1992;13:1078-1082.

95. Kaffenberger DA, Sah CP, Murtagh FR, et al: MR imaging of spinal cord hemangioblastoma: associated with syringomyelia. *J Comput Assist Tomogr* 1988;12:495-498.

96. Solomon RA, Stein BM: Unusual spinal cord enlargement related to intramedullary hemangioblastoma. *J Neurosurg* 1988;68:550-553.

97. Enomoto H, Shibata T, Ito A, et al: Multiple hemangioblastomas accompanied by syringomyelia in the cerebellum and the spinal cord. *Surg Neurol* 1984;22:197-203.

98. Thomas JE, Miller RH: Lipomatous tumors of the spinal canal. *Mayo Clin Proc* 1973;48:393-400.

99. Alves AM, Norrell H: Intramedullary epidermoid tumors of the spinal cord. *Int Surg* 1970;54:239-243.

100. Bailey IC: Dermoid tumors of the spinal cord. *J Neurosurg* 1970;33:676-681.

101. Roux A, Mercier C, Larbrisseau A, et al: Intramedullary epidermoid cysts of the spinal cord. *J Neurosurg* 1992;76:528-533.

102. Barnes PD, Lester PD, Yamanashi WS, Prince JR: Magnetic resonance imaging in infants and children with spinal dysraphism. *AJNR* 1986;7:465-472.

103. Phillips J, Chiu L: Magnetic resonance imaging of intraspinal epidermoid cysts. *J Comput Assist Tomogr* 1987;11:181-183.

104. Davidson HD, Ouchi T, Steiner RE: NMR imaging of congenital intracranial germ layer neoplasms. *Neuroradiology* 1985;27:301-303.

105. Jellinger K, Radaskiewicz TH, Slowik F: Primary malignant lymphomas of the central nervous system in man. *Acta Neuropathol (suppl)* 1975;6:95-102.

106. Zimmerman HM: Malignant lymphomas of the nervous system. *Acta Neuropathol (suppl)* 1975;6:69-74.

107. Itami J, Mori S, Arimizu N, et al: Primary intramedullary spinal cord lymphoma: report of a case. *Jpn J Clin Oncol* 1986;16:407-412.

108. Bluemke DA, Wang H: Case report. Primary spinal cord lymphoma: MR appearance. *J Comput Assist Tomogr* 1990; 14(5):812-814.

109. Wong Chung ME, van Heesewijk JP, Ramos LM: Intramedullary non-Hodgkin's lymphoma of the spinal cord; a case report. *Eur J Radiol* 1991;12:226-227.

110. Hayward RD: Malignant melanoma and the central nervous system: a guide for classification based on the clinical findings. *J Neurol Neurosurg Psychiatry* 1976;39:526-530.

111. Pappenheim E, Bhattacharji SK: Primary melanoma of the central nervous system. *Arch Neurol* 1962;7:101-113.

112. Ozden B, Barlas O, Hacihanefioglu U: Primary dural melanomas: report of two cases and review of the literature. *Neurosurgery* 1984;15:104-107.

113. Hirano A, Carton CA: Primary malignant melanoma of the spinal cord. *J Neurosurg* 1960;17:935-944.

114. Larson TC III, Houser OW, Onofrio BM, Piepgras DG: Primary spinal melanoma. *J Neurosurg* 1987;66:47-49.

115. Costigan DA, Winkelman MD: Intramedullary spinal cord metastasis: a clinicopathological study of 13 cases. *J Neurosurg* 1985;62:227-233.

116. Edelson RN, Deck MD, Posner HB: Intramedullary spinal cord metastases. *Neurology* 1972;22:1222-1231.

117. Jellinger K, Kothbauer P, Sunder-Plassmann E, Weiss R: Intramedullary spinal cord metastases. *J Neurol* 1979; 22:31-41.

118. Benson DR: Intramedullary spinal cord metastasis. *Neurology* 1960;10:281-287.

119. Grem JL, Burgess J, Trump DL: Clinical features and natural history of intramedullary spinal cord metastases. *Cancer* 1985;56:2305-2314.

120. Wood EH, Taveras JM, Pool JL: Myelographic demonstration of spinal cord metastases from primary brain tumors. *AJR* 1953;69:221-230.

121. Sagerman RH, Bayshaw MA, Hanbery J: Considerations in treatment of ependymoma. *Radiology* 1965;84:401-408.

122. Smith DR, Hardman JM, Earle KM: Metastasizing neuroectodermal tumors of the central nervous system. *J Neurosurg* 1969;31:50-58.

123. Puljic S, Batnitzky S, Yang WC, Schechter MM: Metastases to the medulla of the spinal cord: myelographic features. *Radiology* 1975;117:89-91.

124. Erlich SS, Davis RL: Spinal subarachnoid metastasis from primary intracranial glioblastoma multiforme. *Cancer* 1978; 42:2854-2864.

125. Deutsch M, Reigel DH: The value of myelography in the management of childhood medulloblastoma. *Cancer* 1980; 45:2194-2197.

126. Donovan Post JM, Quencer RM, Green BA, et al: Intramedullary spinal cord metastases, mainly of non-neurogenic origin. *AJR* 1987;48:1015-1022.

127. Scotti G, Scialfa G, Columbo N, Landoni L: MR imaging of intradural extramedullary tumors of the cervical spine. *J Comput Assist Tomogr* 1985;9:1037-1041.

128. Davis PC, Hoffman JC, Ball TI, et al: Spinal abnormalities in pediatric patients: MR imaging findings compared with clinical, myelographic, and surgical findings. *Radiology* 1988;166:679-685.

129. Krol G, Sze G, Malkin M, Walker R: MR of cranial and spinal meningeal carcinomatous comparison with CT and myelography. *AJNR* 1988;9:709-714.

130. Davis PC, Griedman NC, Fry SM, et al: Leptomeningeal metastasis: MR imaging. *Radiology* 1987;163:449-454.

131. Lombardi G, Passerini A: *Spinal cord disease, a radiologic and myelographic analysis.* Baltimore, Williams & Wilkins, 1964.

132. Levy WJ, Bay J, Dohn D: Spinal cord meningioma. *J Neurosurg* 1982;57:804-812.

133. Earle KM, Richany SF: Meningiomas: a study of the histology, incidence and biologic behavior of 243 cases from the Frazier-Grant collection of brain tumors. *Med Ann DC* 1969; 8:353-356.

134. Levy WJ, Bay J, Dohn D: Spinal cord meningioma. *J Neurosurg* 1982;57:804-812.

135. Quencer RM, El Gammal T, Cohen G: Syringomyelia associated with intradural extramedullary masses of the spinal canal. *AJNR* 1986;7:143-148.

136. Hughes JT: *Pathology of the spinal cord tumors.* London, Lloyd-Luke, 1966, pp 160-180.

137. Smirniotopoulos JG, Murphy FM: The phakomatoses. *AJNR* 1992;13:725-746.

138. Lewis TT, Kingsley DP: Magnetic resonance imaging of multiple spinal neurofibromata: neurofibromatosis. *Neuroradiology* 1987;29:562-564.

139. Egelhoff JC, Bates DJ, Ross JS, et al: Spinal MR findings in neurofibromatosis types 1 and 2. *AJNR* 1992;13:1071-1077.

140. Reference deleted in proofs.

141. National Institutes of Health Consensus Development Conference: Neurofibromatosis: conference statement. *Arch Neurol* 1988;45:575-578.

142. Barker D, Wright E, Nguyen K, et al: Gene for von Recklinghausen neurofibromatosis is in the pericentromeric region of chromosome 17. *Science* 1987;236:1100-1102.

143. Seizinger BR, Rouleau GA, Ozelius LF, et al: Genetic linkage of von Recklinghausen neurofibromatosis to the nerve growth factor receptor gene. *Cell* 1987;49:589-594.

144. Gardeur D, Palmieri A, Mashaly R: Cranial computed tomography in the phakomatoses. *Neuroradiology* 1983; 25:293-304.

145. Harkin JC, Reed RJ: Tumours of the peripheral nervous system. In *Atlas of tumor pathology,* Fascicle 3, Series 2. Washington DC, Armed Forces Institute of Pathology, 1969, pp 29-97.

146. Halliday AL, Sobel RA, Martuza RL: Benign spinal nerve sheath tumors: their occurrence sporadically and in neurofibromatosis types 1 and 2. *J Neurosurg* 1991;74:248-253.

147. Laws JW, Dallis CP: Spinal deformities in neurofibromatosis. *J Bone Joint Surg [Br]* 1963;451:674-682.

148. Katz BH, Quencer RM: Hamartomatous spinal cord lesion in neurofibromatosis. *AJNR* 1989;10:S101.

149. Martuza RL, Eldridge R: Neurofibromatosis 2 (bilateral acoustic neurofibromatosis). *N Engl J Med* 1988;318:684-688.

150. Wertelecki W. Rouleau GA, Superneau DW, et al: Neurofibromatosis 2: clinical and DNA linkage studies of a large kindred. *N Engl J Med* 1988;319:278-283.

151. Seizinger BR, Martuza RL, Gusella JF: Loss of genes on chromosome 22 in tumorigenesis of human acoustic neuroma. *Nature* 1986;322:644-647.

152. Rouleau GA, Wertelecki W, Hains JL, et al: Genetic linkage of bilateral acoustic neurofibromatosis to a DNA marker on chromosome 22. *Nature* 1987;329:246-248.

153. Brasfield RD, Das Gupta TK: Von Recklinghausen's disease: a clinical pathologic study. *Ann Surg* 1972;175:86-104.

154. Sordillo PP, Helson L, Hajdu SI, et al: Malignant schwannoma: clinical characteristics, survival, and response to therapy. *Cancer* 1981;10:2503-2509.

155. Herman J: Sarcomatous transformation in multiple neurofibromatosis (von Recklinghausen's disease). *Ann Surg* 1950;131:206-217.

156. Levine E, Huntrakoon M, Wetzel LH: Malignant nerve-sheath neoplasms in fibromatosis neuro: distinction from benign tumors by using imaging techniques. *AJR* 1987;149:1059-1064.

157. Herrman J: Sarcomatous transformation in multiple neurofibromatosis (von Recklinghausen's disease). *Ann Surg* 1950;131:206-217.

158. White HR: Survival in malignant schwannoma: an 18-year study. *Cancer* 1971;3:720-729.

159. Burk DL Jr, Brumberg JA, Kanal E, et al: Spinal and paraspinal neurofibromatosis: surface coil MR imaging at 1.5 T. *Radiology* 1987;162:797-801.

160. Levine E, Huntrakoon M, Wetzel LH: Malignant nerve sheath neoplasms in neurofibromatosis: distinction from benign tumors using imaging techniques. *AJR* 1987;149:1059-1064.

161. Chui MC, Bird BL, Rogers J: Extracranial and extraspinal nerve sheath tumors: computed tomographic evaluation. *Neuroradiology* 1988;30:47-53.

162. Castillo M, Quencer RM, Grenn BA, Montalvo BM: Syringomyelia as a consequence of compressive extra-medullary lesions: postoperative clinical and radiological manifestations. *AJNR* 1987;8:973-978.

163. Choremis C, et al: Intraspinal epidermoid tumors (cholesteatoma) in patients treated for tuberculous meningitis. *Lancet* 1956;2:437-439.

164. Sachs E, Horrax G: A cervical and lumbar pilonidal sinus communicating with intraspinal dermoids: report of 2 cases and review of the literature. *J Neurosurg* 1949;6:97-112.

165. Pierre-Kahn A, Lacombe J, Pichon J, et al: Intraspinal lipomas with spina bifida. *J Neurosurg* 1986;65:756-761.

166. Okumura R, Minami S, Asato R, Konishi J: Fatty filum terminale: assessment with MR imaging. *J Comput Assist Tomogr* 1990;14(4):571-573.

167. Petit H, Jomin M, Julliot JP, et al: Dysraphie lombosacrée et "moelle longue" de révélation tardive (neuf observations). *Rev Neurol* 1979;135:427-438.

168. Yamade S, Zinke DE, Sanders D: Pathophysiology of "tethered cord syndrome." *J Neurosurg* 1981;54:494-503.

169. Monajati A, Spitzer RM, Wiley JL, Heggeness L: MR imaging of a spinal teratoma. *J Comput Assist Tomogr* 1986;10:307-310.

170. Hatfield, MK, Udesky RH, Strimling AM, et al: MR imaging of a spinal epidermoid tumor. *AJNR* 1989;10:95-96.

171. Barkovich AJ, Edwards MSB, Cogen PH: MR evaluation of spinal dermal sinus tracts in children. *AJNR* 1991;12:123-129.

172. Newton DR, Larson TC, Dillon WP, Newton TH: Magnetic resonance characteristics of cranial epidermoid and teratomatous tumors. *AJNR* 1987;8:S945.

173. Awwad EE, Backer R, Archer CR: The imaging of an intraspinal cervical dermoid tumor by MR, CT, and sonography. *Comput Radiol* 1987;11:169-173.

174. Boker D-K, Wassmann H, Solymosi L: Paragangliomas of the spina canal. *Surg Neurol* 1983;19:461-468.

175. Miller CA, Torack RM: Secretory ependymoma of the filum terminale. *Acta Neuropathol* 1970;15:240-250.

176. Binkley W, Vakili ST, Worth R: Paraganglioma of the cauda equina: case report. *J Neurosurg* 1982;56:275-279.

177. Anderson J, Gullan R: Paraganglioma of the cauda equina: a case report. *J Neurol Neurosurg Psychiatry* 1987;50:100-103.

177a. Silverstein AM, Quint DJ, McKeever PE: Intradural paraganglioma of the thoracic spine. *AJNR* 1990;11:614-616.

178. Sonneland P, Scheithauer B, LeChago J, et al: Paraganglioma of the cauda equina region: clinicopathologic study of 31 cases with special reference to immunocytology and ultrastructure. *Cancer* 1986;58:1720-1735.

179. Hayes E, Lippa C, Davidson R: Paragangliomas of the cauda equina. *AJNR* 1989;10:45-47.

180. Barloon TJ, Yuh WT, Yang CJ, Schulz DH: Spinal subarachnoid tumor seeding from intracranial metastasis: MR findings. *J Comput Assist Tomogr* 1987;11:242-244.

181. Bryan P: CSF seeding of intracranial tumors: a study of 96 cases. *Clin Radiol* 1974;25:355-360.

182. Dorwart RH, Wara WM, Norma D, Levin VA: Complete myelographic evaluation of spinal metastasis from medulloblastoma. *Radiology* 1981;139:403-408.

183. Meli FJ, Boccaleri CA, Manzitti J, Lylyk P: Meningeal dissemination of retinoblastoma: CT findings in eight patients. *AJNR* 1990;11:983-986.

184. Mathews V, Broome D, Smith R, et al: Neuroimaging of disseminated germ cell neoplasms. *AJNR* 1990;11:319-324.

185. Yousem DM, Patrone PM, Grossman RI: Leptomeningeal metastases: MR evaluation. *J Comput Assist Tomogr* 1990;14(2):255-261.

186. West GH: Spinal subarachoid metastatic spread from non-neuraxial primary neoplasms. *J Neurosurg* 1979;51:251-253.

187. Little JR, Dale AJD, Okazaki H: Meningeal carcinomatosis: clinical manifestations. *Arch Neurol* 1974;30:138-143.

188. Glass JP, Melamed M, Chernik NL, Posner JB: Malignant cells in the cerebrospinal fluid (CSF): the meaning of positive CSF cytology. *Neurology* 1979;29:1369-1375.

189. Lim V, Sobel D, Zyroff J: Spinal cord pial metastases: MR imaging with gadopentetate dimeglumine. *AJNR* 1990;11:975-982.

190. Johnson CE, Sze G: Benign lumbar arachnoiditis: MR imaging with gadopentetate dimeglumine. *AJNR* 1990;11:763-770.

191. Beltram J, Noto AM, Chakeres DW, Christoforidis AJ: Tumors of the osseous spine: staging with MR imaging versus CT. *Radiology* 1987;162:565-569.

192. Avrahami E, Tadmor R, Dally O, et al: Early MR demonstration of spinal metastases in patients with normal radiographs and CT and radionuclide bone scans. *J Comput Assist Tomogr* 1989;13:598-602.

193. Frank JA, Ling A, Patronas NJ, et al: Detection of malignant bone tumors: MR imaging vs scintigraphy. *AJR* 1990; 155:1043-1048.

194. Vogler JB, Murphy WA: Bone marrow imaging. *Radiology* 1988;168:679-693.

195. Carmody RF, Yankg DJ, Seeley GW, et al: Spinal cord compression due to metastatic disease: diagnosis with MR imaging versus myelography. *Radiology* 1989;173:225-229.

196. Daffner RH, Lupetin AR, Cash N, et al: MRI in the detection of malignant infiltration of bone marrow. *AJR* 1986; 146:353-358.

197. Ruzal-Shapiro C, Berdon WE, Cohen MD, Abramson SJ: MR imaging of diffuse bone marrow replacement in pediatric patients with cancer. *Radiology* 1991;181:587-589.

198. Geremia GK, McCluney R, Adler SS, et al: The magnetic resonance hypointense spine of AIDS. *J Comput Assist Tomogr* 1990;14:785-789.

199. Steinbach LS, Tehranzadeh J, Fleckenstein JL, et al: Human immunodeficiency virus infection: musculoskeletal manifestations. *Radiology* 1993;186:833-838.

200. Stimac GK, Porter BA, Olson DO, et al: Gadolinium-DTPA–enhanced MR imaging of spinal neoplasms: preliminary investigation and comparison with unenhanced spin-echo and STIR sequences. *AJNR* 1988;9:839-846.

201. Gusnard DA, Grossman RI, Hackney DB. The differential utility of gradient-echo and spin-echo MRI of the abnormal spine. ASNR, 1988, p 15.

202. Sze G, Abramson A, Krol G, et al: Gadolinium-DPTA: malignant extradural spinal tumors. *Radiology* 1988;67:217-233.

203. Feuerman T, Divan PS, Young RF: Vertebrectomy for treatment of vertebral hemangioma without preoperative embolization. *J Neurosurg* 1986;65:404-406.

204. Mohan V, Gupta SK, Tuli SM, Sanyal B: Symptomatic vertebral hemangiomas. *Clin Radiol* 1980;31:575-579.

205. Paige ML, Hemmati M: Spinal cord compression by vertebral hemangioma. *Pediatr Radiol* 1977;6:43-45.

206. McAllister VL, Kendall BE, Bull JW: Symptomatic vertebral hemangiomas. *Brain* 1975;98:71-80.

207. Ross JS, Masaryk TJ, Modic MT: Vertebral hemangiomas: MR imaging. *Radiology* 1987;165:165-169.

208. Krueger EG, Sobel GL, Weinstein C: Vertebral hemangiomas: radiologic evaluation. *J Neurosurg* 1961;18:331-338.

209. Murray RO, Jacobson HG: *Radiology of skeletal disorders*, ed 2. New York, Churchill Livingstone, 1977, p 578.

210. Wilmer D: *Radiology of bone tumors and allied disorders*. Philadelphia, Saunders, 1982, p 664.

211. Hajek PC, Baker LL, Goobar JE, et al: Focal fat deposition in axial bone marrow: MR characteristics. *Radiology* 1987; 162:245-249.

212. Laredo JD, Assouline E, Gelbert F, et al: Vertebral hemangiomas: fat content as a sign of aggressiveness. *Radiology* 1990;177:467-472.

213. Dahlin DC, Unni KK: *Bone tumors: general aspects and data on 8,542 cases*. Springfield Ill, Thomas, 1986, pp 62-69.

214. Cory DA, Fritsch SA, Cohen MD, et al: Aneurysmal bone cysts: imaging findings and embolotherapy. *AJR* 1989; 153:369-373.

215. Spjut HJ, Ayala AG: *Skeletal tumors in childhood and adolescence: pathology of neoplasia in children and adolescents*. Philadelphia, Saunders, 1984.

216. Dahlin DC, McLeon RA: Aneursymal bone cyst and other non-neoplastic conditions. *Skeletal Radiol* 1982;8:243-250.

217. Biescker JL, Marcove RC, Huvos AG, Mike V: Aneurysmal bone cyst, a clinical pathologic study of 66 cases. *Cancer* 1970;26:615-625.

218. Hay MC, Paterson D, Taylor TK. Aneurysmal bone cysts of the spine. *J Bone Joint Surg [Br]* 1978;60:406-411.

219. Tillman BP, Dahlin DC, Lipscomb PR, Stewart JR: Aneurysmal bone cyst: an analysis of 95 cases. *Mayo Clin Proc* 1968;43:478-495.

220. Gunterberg B, Kindblom LG, Laurin S: Giant cell tumor of bone and aneurysmal bone cyst. *Skeletal Radiol* 1977;2:65-74.

221. Kozlowski K, Beluffi G, Masel J, et al: Primary vertebral tumours in children: report of 20 cases with brief review of the literature. *Pediatr Radiol* 1984;14:129-139.

222. Hay MC, Paterson D, Taylor TKF: Aneursymal bone cysts of the spine. *J Bone Joint Surg [Br]* 1978;60:406-411.

223. Ameli NO, Abbassioun K, Saleh H, Eslamdoost A: Ancurysmal bone cysts of the spine. *J Neurosurg* 1985;63:685-690.

224. Wang A, Lipson S, Hay Kal HA, et al: Computed tomography of aneurysmal bone cyst of the vertebral body. *J Comput Assist Tomogr* 1984;8:1186-1189.

225. Banna M: *Clinical radiology of the spine and spinal cord*. Rockville Md, Aspen, 1985.

226. Hudson TJ: Fluid levels in aneurysmal bone cysts: a CT feature. *AJR* 1984;142:1001-1004.

227. Beltran J, Simon D, Levey M, et al: Aneurysmal bone cysts: MR imaging at 1.5 T. *Radiology* 1986;158:689-690.

228. Munk PL, Helms CA, Holt RG, et al: MR imaging of aneurysmal bone cysts. *AJR* 1989;153:99-101.

229. Zimmer WD, Berquist TH, McLeod RA, et al: Bone tumors: magnetic resonance imaging versus computed tomography. *Radiology* 1985;155:709-718.

230. Zimmer WD, Berquist TH, Sim FH, et al: Magnetic resonance imaging of aneurysmal bone cysts. *Mayo Clin Proc* 1984;59:633-636.

231. Hudson TM, Hamlin DJ, Fitzsimmons JR: Magnetic resonance imaging of fluid levels in an aneurysmal bone cyst and in anticoagulated human blood. *Skeletal Radiol* 1985; 13:267-270.

232. Beltran J, Simon DC, Levy M, et al: Aneurysmal bone cysts: MR imaging at 1.5 T. *Radiology* 1986;158:689-690.

233. Tsai JC, Dalinka MK, Fallon MD, et al: Fluid-fluid level: a nonspecific finding in tumors of bone and soft tissue. *Radiology* 1990;175:779-782.

234. McInerney DP, Middlemiss JH: Giant cell tumor of bone. *Skeletal Radiol* 1978;2:195-204.

235. Jacobs P: The diagnosis of osteoclastoma (giant cell tumours): a radiological and pathological correlation. *Br J Radiol* 1972;45:121-136.

236. Goldenberg RR, Campbell CJ, Bonfiglio M: Giant cell tumor of bone, an analysis of 218 cases. *J Bone Joint Surg [Am]* 1970;52:619-664.

237. Brady TJ, Gebhardt MC, Pickett IL: NMR imaging of forearms in healthy volunteers and patients with giant cell tumor. *Radiology* 1982;144:549-552.

238. Aisen AM, Martel W, Braunstein EM, et al: MRI and CT evaluation of primary bone and soft tissue tumors. *AJR* 1986;146:749-756.

239. Albrecht S, Crutchfield S, SeGall GK: On spinal osteochondromas. *J Neurosurg* 1992;77:247-252.

240. Malat J, Virapongse C, Levine A: Solitary osteochondroma of the spine. *Spine* 1986;11:625-628.

241. Karian JM, DeFilipp G, Buchheit WA, et al: Vertebral osteochondroma causing spinal cord compression. *Neurosurgery* 1984;14:483-484.

242. Twersky J, Kassner EG, Tenner MS, Camera A: Vertebral and costal osteochondromas causing spinal cord compression. *AJR* 1978;124:124-128.

243. Novick GS, Pavlov H, Bullough PG: Osteochondroma of the cervical spine: report of two cases in preadolescent males. *Skeletal Radiol* 1982;8:13-15.

244. Ingilis AE, Rubin RM, Lewis RJ, Villacin A: Osteochondroma of the cervical spine, case report. *Clin Orthop* 1977; 126:127-129.

245. Palmer FJ, Blum PW: Osteochondroma with spinal cord compression, report of three cases. *J Neurosurg* 1980; 52:842-845.

246. Kenney PJ, Gilula LA, Murphy WA: The use of computed tomography to distinguish osteochondroma and chondrosarcoma. *Radiology* 1981;139:129-137.

247. MacLellan DI, Wilson FC: Osteoid osteoma of the spine. *J Bone Joint Surg* 1967;49:111-121.

248. Jackson RP, Reckling FW, Mantz FA. Osteoid osteoma and osteoblastoma. *Clin Orthop* 1977;128:303-313.

249. Gamba JL, Martinez S, Apple J, et al: CT of axial skeletal osteoid osteoma. *AJR* 1984;142:769-772.

250. Glass RB, Poznanski AK, Fisher MR, et al: Case report. MR imaging of osteoid osteoma. *J Comput Assist Tomogr* 1986;10:1065-1067.

251. Heiman ML, Cooley CJ, Bradford DS: Osteoid osteoma of a vertebral body: report of a case with extension across the intervertebral disk. *Clin Orthop* 1976;118:159-163.

252. Swee RG, McLeod RA, Beabout JW: Osteoid osteoma. *Radiology* 1979;130:117-123.

253. Freiberger RH: Osteoid osteoma of the spine. *Radiology* 1960;75:232-235.

254. Resjo IM, Harwood-Nash D, Fitz CR, Chuang S: CT metrizamide myelography for intraspinal and paraspinal neoplasms in infants and children. *AJR* 1979;132:367-372.

255. Omojola MF, Cockshott P, Beatty EG: Osteoid osteoma: an evaluation of diagnostic modalities. *Clin Radiol* 1981; 32:199-204.

256. Bell RS, O'Connor GD, Waddell JP: Importance of magnetic resonance imaging in osteoid osteoma: a case report. *Can J Surg* 1989;32:276-278.

257. deSantos LA, Goldstein HM, Murray JA, Wallace S: Computed tomography in the evaluation of musculoskeletal neoplasms. *Radiology* 1978;128:89-94.

258. Houang B, Grenier N, Greselle JF, et al: Osteoid osteoma of the cervical spine: misleading features about a case involving the uncinate process. *Neuroradiology* 1990;31:549-551.

259. De Souza Dias L, Frost HM: Osteoblastoma of the spine, a review and report of 8 new cases. *Clin Orthop* 1973;91:141-151.

260. Reference deleted in proofs.

261. Tonai M, Campbell CJ, Ahn GH, et al: Osteoblastoma: classification and report of 16 patients. *Clin Orthop* 1982; 167:222-235.

262. Doron Y, Gruszkiewicz J, Gelli B, Peyser E: Benign osteoblastoma of vertebral column and skull. *Surg Neurol* 1977; 7:86-90.

263. Myles ST, MacRae ME: Benign osteoblastoma of the spine in childhood. *J Neurosurg* 1988;68:884-888.

264. Steiner GC: Ultrastructure of osteoblastoma. *Cancer* 1977; 39:2127-2136.

265. Omojola MF, Fox AJ, Vinuela FV: Computed tomography metrizamide myelography in the evaluation of thoracic osteoblastoma. *AJNR* 1976;126:321-335.

266. McCleod RA, Dahlin DC, Beabout JW: The spectrum of osteoblastoma. *AJR* 1976;126:321-335.

267. Crim JR, Mirra JM, Eckardt JJ, Seeger LL: Widespread inflammatory response to osteoblastoma: the flare phenomenon. *Radiology* 1990;177:835-836.

268. Dahlin DC, Coventry MB: Osteogenic sarcoma, a study of 600 cases. *J Bone Joint Surg* 1967;49:101-110.

269. McKenna RJ, Schwinn CP, Soong KY, Higinbotham NL: Sarcoma of the osteogenic series (osteosarcoma, fibrosarcoma, chondrosarcoma, parostealosteogenic sarcoma, and sarcomata arising in abnormal bone). *J Bone Joint Surg* 1966;48:1-26.

270. Redmond OM, Stack JP, Dervan PA, et al: Osteosarcoma: use of MR imaging and MR spectroscopy in clinical decision making. *Radiology* 1989;172:811-815.

271. Marcove RC, Mike V, Hajeck JV, et al: Osteogenic sarcoma under the age of twenty one. *J Bone Joint Surg* 1970; 52:411-423.

272. Felson B, Wiot J: Osteogenic sarcoma: an update. *Semin Roentgenol* 1989;24:143-200.

273. Fielding JW, Fietti VG, Hughes JE, Gabriellian JC: Primary osteogenic sarcoma of the cervical spine. *J Bone Joint Surg [Am]* 1976;58:892-894.

274. Berger PE, Kuhn JP: Computed tomography of tumors of the musculoskeletal system in children. *Radiology* 1978; 127:171-175.

275. Zimmer WD, Berguist TJ, McLeod RA: Bone tumors: MR imaging versus CT. *Radiology* 1985;155:709-718.

276. Zimmer WD, Berguist TH, McLeod RA, et al: Magnetic resonance imaging of osteosarcomas, comparison with computed tomography. *Clin Orthop* 1986;208:289-299.

277. Erlemann R, Reiser MF, Peters PE, et al: Musculoskeletal neoplasms: static and dynamic Gd-DTPA-enhanced MR imaging. *Radiology* 1989;171:767-773.

278. Sundaram M, McGuire MH, Herbold DR. Magnetic resonance imaging of osteosarcoma. *Skeletal Radiol* 1987; 16:23-29.

279. Holscher HC, Bloem JL, Vanel D, et al: Osteosarcoma: chemotherapy-induced changes at MR imaging. *Radiology* 1992;182:839-844.

280. Erlemann R, Sciuk J, Bosse A, et al: Response of osteosarcoma and Ewing's sarcoma to preoperative chemotherapy: assessment with dynamic and static MR imaging and skeletal scintigraphy. *Radiology* 1990;175:791-796.

281. Huvos AG, Marcove RC: Chondrosarcoma in the young: a clinicopathologic analysis of 79 patients younger than 21 years of age. *Am J Surg Pathol* 1987;11:930-942.

282. Barnes R, Catto M: Chondrosarcoma of bone. *J Bone Joint Surg* 1966;48:729-764.

283. Marcove RC: Chondrosarcoma: diagnosis and treatment. *Orthop Clin North Am* 1977;8:811-820.

284. Camins MB, Duncan AW, Smith J, Marcove RC: Chondrosarcoma of the spine. *Spine* 1978;3:202-209.

285. Garrison RC, Unni KK, McCleod RA, et al: Chondrosarcoma arising in osteochondroma. *Cancer* 1982;49:1890-1897.

286. Henderson ED, Dahlin DC. Chondrosarcoma of bone. A study of 288 cases. *J Bone Joint Surg [Am]* 1963;45:1450-1458.

287. Cohen EK, Kressel HY, Frank TS, et al: Hyaline cartilage-origin bone and soft tissue neoplasms: MR appearance and histologic correlation. *Radiology* 1988;167:477-481.

288. Chan SL, Turner-Gomes SO, Chuang SH, et al: A rare cause of spinal cord compression in childhood from intraspinal mesenchymal chondrosarcoma. *Neuroradiology* 1984;26:323-327.

289. Geirnaerdt MJA, Bloem JL, Eulderink F, et al: Cartilaginous tumors: correlation of gadolinium-enhanced MR imaging and histopathologic findings. *Radiology* 1993;186:813-817.

290. Krol G, Sundaresan N, Deck M: Computed tomography of axial chordomas, *J Comput Assist Tomogr* 1983;7:285-289.

291. Higinbotham NL, Phillips RF, Farr HW, Hustu HO: Chordoma; thirty-five year study at Memorial Hospital. *Cancer* 1967;20:1841-1850.

292. Heffelfinger MJ, Dahlin DC, McCarty CS, Beabout JW: Chordomas and cartilaginous tumors at the skull base. *Cancer* 1973;32:410-420.

293. Firooznia H, Pinto RS, Lin JP, Zausner J: Chordoma: radiologic evaluation of 20 cases. *AJR* 1976;127:797-805.

294. Higinbothan NL, Phillips RF, Farr HW, Hustu HO: Chordoma: thirty-five-year study at Memorial Hospital. *Cancer* 1967;20:1841-1850.

295. Mapstone TB, Kaufman B, Ratcheson RA: Intradural chordoma without bone involvement: nuclear magnetic resonance (NMR) appearance. *J Neurosurg* 1983;59:535-537.

296. Sze G, Vichan LS, Brant-Zawadzki M, et al: Chordomas: MR imaging. *Radiology* 1988;166:187-191.

297. McGavran MH, Spady HA: Eosinophilic granuloma of bone, a study of 28 cases. *J Bone Joint Surg [Am]* 1960;42:979-992.

298. Oschsner SF: Eosinophilic granuloma of bone; experience with 20 cases. *AJR* 1966;97:719-726.

299. Arcomano JP, Barnett JC, Wunderlich HO: Histiocytosis. *AJR* 1961;85:663-679.

300. Askin FB, Rosai J, Sibley RK, et al: Malignant small cell tumor of the thoracopulmonary region in childhood: a distinctive clinicopathologic entity of uncertain histogenesis. *Cancer* 1979;43:2438-2451.

301. Dehner LP: Soft tissue carcinomas of childhood: the differential diagnosis dilemma of the small blue cell. *Natl Cancer Inst Monogr* 1981;56:43-59.

302. Balakrishnan V, Rice MS, Simpson DA: Spinal neuroblastomas: diagnosis, treatment, and prognosis. *J Neurosurg* 1974;40:431-438.

303. Miller JH, Sato JK: *Adrenal origin tumors: imaging in pediatric oncology.* Baltimore, Williams & Wilkins, 1985, pp 305-339.

304. Reed JC, Hallet KK, Feign DS: Neural tumors of the thorax: subject review from the AFIP. *Radiology* 1978;126:9-17.

305. Siegel MJ, Jamroz GA, Glazer HS, Abramson CL: MR imaging of intraspinal extension of neuroblastoma. *J Comput Assist Tomogr* 1986;10:593-595.

306. Punt J, Pritchard J, Pincott JR, Till K: Neuroblastoma: a review of 21 cases presenting with cord compression. *Cancer* 1980;45:3095-3101.

307. Koop CE, Hernandez JR: Neuroblastoma experience with 100 cases in children. *Surgery* 1964;56:726-733.

308. Faubert C, Inniger R: MRI and pathological findings in two cases of Askin tumors. *Neuroradiology* 1991;33:277-281.

309. Bhansali SK, Desai PB: Ewing's sarcoma: observations of 107 cases. *J Bone Joint Surg [Am]* 1963;45:541-553.

310. Pritchard DJ, Dahlin DC, Dauphine RT, et al: Ewing's sarcoma: a clinicopathological and statistical analysis of patients surviving five years or longer. *J Bone Joint Surg [Am]* 1975;57:10-16.

311. Dahlin DC, Coventry MB, Scanlon PW: Ewing's sarcoma: a critical analysis of 165 cases. *J Bone Joint Surg* 1961;43:185-193.

312. Ginaldi S, deSantos LA: Computed tomography in the evaluation of small round cell tumors of bone. *Radiology* 1980;134:441-446.

313. Parker BR, Marglin S, Castellino RA: Skeletal manifestations of leukemia, Hodgkin disease, and non-Hodgkin lymphoma. *Semin Roentgenol* 1980;15:302-315.

314. Pinkel D: Treatment of acute leukemia. *Pediatr Clin North Am* 1976;23:117-130.

315. Pear BL: Skeletal manifestations of the lymphomas and leukemias. *Semin Roentgenol* 1974;9:229-240.

316. Pierce MI, Borges WH, Heyn R, et al: Epidemiological factors and survival experience in 1770 children with acute leukemia. *Cancer* 1969;6:1296-1304.

317. Moore SG, Gooding CA, Brasch RC, et al: Bone marrow in children with acute lymphocytic leukemia: MR relaxation times. *Radiology* 1986;160:237-240.

318. Olson DO, Shields AF, Scheurick CJ, et al: Magnetic resonance imaging of the bone marrow in patients with leukemia, aplastic anemia and lymphoma. *Invest Radiology* 1986;21:540-546.

319. McKinstry CS, Steiner RE, Young AT, et al: Bone marrow in leukemia and aplastic anemia: MR imaging before, during and after treatment. *Radiology* 1987;162:701-707.

320. Cohen MD, Klatte EC, Baehner R, et al: Magnetic resonance of bone marrow disease in children. *Radiology* 1984; 151:715-718.

321. Kangarloo H, Dietrich RB, Taira RT, et al: MR imaging of bone marrow in children. *J Comput Assist Tomogr* 1986; 10:205-209.

322. Castillo M, Malko JA, Hoffman JC Jr: The bright intervertebral disk: an indirect sign of abnormal spinal bone marrow on T1-weighted MR images. *AJNR* 1990;11:23-26.

323. Rosen BR, Carter EA, Pykett IL, et al: Proton chemical shift imaging: an evaluation of its clinical potential using an in vivo fatty liver model. *Radiology* 1985;154:469-472.

324. Brateman L: Chemical shift imaging: a review. *AJR* 1986; 146:971-980.

325. Dooms GC, Fisher MR, Hricak H, et al: Bone marrow imaging: magnetic resonance studies related to age and sex. *Radiology* 1985;155:429-432.

326. Weinreb JC: MR imaging of bone marrow: a map could help. *Radiology* 1990;177:23-24.

327. Ramsey RG, Zacharias CE: MR imaging of the spine after radiation therapy: easily recognizable effects. *AJR* 1985; 144:1131-1135.

328. Yankelevitz DF, Henschke CJ, Knapp PH, et al: Effect of radiation therapy on thoracic and lumbar bone marrow: evaluation with MR imaging. *AJR* 1991;157:87-92.

329. Sugimura K, Yamasaki K, Kitagaki H, et al: Bone marrow disease of the spine: differentiation with T1 and T2 relaxation times in MR imaging. *Radiology* 1987;165:541-544.

330. Smith SR, Williams CE, Davies JM, et al: Bone marrow disorders: characterization with quantitative MR imaging. *Radiology* 1989;172:805-810.

331. Wismer GL, Rosen BR, Buxton R, et al: Chemical shift imaging of bone marrow: preliminary experience. *AJR* 1985; 145:1031-1037.

332. Young JL, Miller RW: Incidence of malignant tumors in U.S. children. *J Pediatr* 1975;86:245-258.

333. Steinback HL, Parker BR: Primary bone tumors. In Parker BR, Castellino RA (eds): *Pediatric oncologic radiology.* St Louis, Mosby, 1977, pp 378-386.

334. Dahlin DC: Reticulum cell sarcoma of bone. *J Bone Joint Surg* 1953;35:835-842.

335. Weaver GR, Sandler MP: Increased sensitivity of magnetic resonance imaging compared to radionuclide bone scintigraphy in the detection of lymphoma of the spine. *Clin Nucl Med* 1987;12:333-334.

336. Longo DL: Plasma cell disorders. In Wilson JD, Braunwald E, Isselbacher KJ, et al (eds): *Harrison's Principles of internal medicine,* ed 12. New York, McGraw-Hill, 1991, pp 1412-1416.

337. Durie BGM, Salmon SE: A clinical staging system for multiple myeloma. *Cancer* 1975;36:842-854.

338. Galton DAG: Myelomatosis. In Hoffbrand AV, Lewin SM (eds): *Postgraduate haematology,* ed 3. Oxford, Heinemann, 1989, pp 474-501.

339. Libshitz HI, Malthouse SR, Cunningham D, et al: Multiple myeloma: appearance at MR imaging. *Radiology* 1992; 182:833-837.

339a. Rahmouni A, Divine M, Mathieu D, et al: Detecting multiple myeloma of the spine: efficacy of fat suppression and contrast-enhanced MR imaging, *AJR* 1993;160:1049-1052.

340. Barron KD, Hirano A, Araki S, et al: Experiences with metastatic neoplasms involving the spinal cord. *Neurology* 1959;9:91-106.

341. Gilbert RW, Kim JH, Posner JB: Epidural spinal cord compression from metastatic tumour: diagnosis and treatment. *Ann Neurol* 1978;3:40-51.

342. Constans JP, de Divitiis E, Donzelli R, et al: Spinal metastases with neurological manifestations: review of 600 cases. *J Neurosurg* 1983;59:111-118.

343. Livinston KE, Perrin RG: The neurosurgical management of spinal metastases causing cord and cauda equina compression. *J Neurosurg* 1978;49:839-843.

344. Smoker WRK, Godersky JC, Knutzon RK, et al: The role of MR imaging in evaluating metastatic spinal disease. *AJNR* 1987;8:901-908.

345. Lien HH, Blomlie V, Heimdal K: Magnetic resonance imaging of malignant extradural tumors with acute spinal cord compression. *Acta Radiol* 1990;31:187-190.

346. Williams MP, Cherryman GR, Husband JE: Magnetic resonance imaging in suspected metastatic spinal cord compression. *Clin Radiol* 1989;40:286-290.

347. Friedman M, Kim TH, Panahon A: Spinal cord compression in malignant lymphoma. *Cancer* 1976;37:1485-1491.

348. Horner NB, Pinto RS: The fat-cap sign: an aid to MR evaluation of extradural spinal tumors. *AJNR* 1989;10:S93.

349. Oppenheim H: Lehrbuch der Nervenkrankheiten fur Arzte und Studierende, ed 6. Berlin, Karger, 1923, vol 1.

350. Hollis PM, Malis LI, Zappulla RA: Neurologic deterioration after lumbar puncture below complete spinal subarachnoid block. *J Neurosurg* 1986;64:253-256.

351. Mapstone TB, Rekate HL, Shurin SB: Quadriplegia secondary to hematoma after lateral C1-2 puncture in a leukemic child. *Neurosurgery* 1983;12:230-231.

352. Rengachary SS, Murphy D: Subarachnoid hematoma following lumbar puncture causing compression of the cauda equina: case report. *J Neurosurg* 1974;41:252-254.

353. Rogers LA: Acute subdural hematoma and death following lateral cervical spinal puncture: case report. *J Neurosurg* 1983;58:284-286.

354. Anderson CM, Lee R: Large FOV spine screening with 512 matrix and body coil: contrast to noise comparison with surface coil imaging. SMRM, 1990.

355. Yousem DM, Schnall MD: MR examination for spinal cord compression: impact of a multicoil system on length of study. *J Comput Assist Tomogr* 1991;15(4):598-604.

356. Quint DJ, Patel SC, Sanders WP, et al: Importance of absence of CSF pulsation artifacts in the MR detection of significant myelographic block at 1.5 T. *AJNR* 1989;10:1089-1095.

357. Yuh WT, Zachar CK, Barloon TJ, et al: Vertebral compression fractures: distinction between benign and malignant causes with MR imaging. *Radiology* 1989;172:215-218.

358. Baker LL, Goodman SB, Perkash I, et al: Benign versus pathologic compression fractures of vertebral bodies: assessment with conventional spin-echo, chemical shift, and STIR MR imaging. *Radiology* 1990;174:495-502.

8

Spinal Trauma

THOMAS J. MASARYK

Although the estimated annual incidence of spinal cord injury in the United States is only 40 to 50 cases per million, the resultant hardship placed on patients, their families, and society can hardly be overemphasized.[1-4] This chapter reviews fundamental pathologic and diagnostic concepts of spinal trauma with respect to present and future roles of magnetic resonance imaging in the management of these injuries.

PATHOLOGIC SEQUELAE

In 1980 the National Head and Spinal Cord Injury Survey (under the auspices of the National Institute of Neurological and Communicative Disorders and Stroke [NINCDS]) reported on the morbidity and socioeconomic impact of significant trauma to the head and spine. Most of the patients were young (under 44 years of age), the majority were male, and a large percentage of the injuries resulted from motor vehicle accidents or falls (i.e., closed trauma). This report also documented the enormous resources dedicated to the medical and surgical management of such cases. As expected, care of these patients is directed toward preventing the progression of injury to the spinal cord. Important to the appropriate planning and institution of therapy is the diagnostic recognition of spinal instability and/or the characterization of direct injury to the spinal cord itself.

Spinal Instability

Stability of the spinal column is an often discussed, but poorly defined, clinical concept regarding the structural integrity (both static and dynamic) of the bony canal and ligaments relative to their ability to protect the spinal cord from present or future compromise. Denis[5] addresses the issue of stability by dividing the spine into three columns, stating that instability requires disruption

of at least two of these columns. The anterior column consists of the anterior longitudinal ligament, anterior anulus, and anterior half of the vertebral body. The middle column consists of the posterior half of the vertebral body, posterior anulus, and posterior longitudinal ligament. The posterior column consists of bony elements posterior to the vertebral body and includes the (facet) capsular, interlaminar, interspinous, and supraspinous ligaments. Holdsworth[6] divides the spine into an anterior and a posterior column and suggests that injuries isolated to the posterior ligaments produce instability. The anterior group consists of the vertebral bodies, intervertebral disks, and anterior and posterior longitudinal ligaments. The posterior apparatus is formed from the spinous processes and interspinous ligaments, laminae and ligamentum flavum, facet joints, and vertebral body pedicles. White and Panjabi[7] and White et al.[8] define clinical instability as the loss of relationships between the vertebrae such that there is damage or subsequent irritation to the spinal cord or nerve roots or, in addition, the development of incapacitating deformity or pain from structural changes. More objective criteria include the displacement of two adjacent vertebrae greater than 3.5 mm and angulation greater than 11 degrees.[7]

Spinal Cord Concussion, Contusion, and Compression

The reactions of the spinal cord, roots, coverings, and vasculature to penetrating and closed injuries are wide ranging. Primary spinal cord lesions can be related to the site, intensity, and distribution of impact, to biochemical and electrophysiologic derangements, and to hemodynamic changes.[9,10]

Concussion of the cord implies a purely functional derangement, attributed to a variety of conditions and etiologies. It is a reversible disorder of the spinal cord that has been attributed to temporary changes in the function of interneuronal transmitters or, possibly, to transient deficiencies in the cord's microcirculation.[11-14]

Contusion of the cord includes all injuries (in the absence of continuing compression by epidural blood, bone, or disk) that exceed the reversible functional disturbance known as concussion.[15] Grossly contusion injuries range in severity from mild intramedullary (petechial) hemorrhage with edema to extensive pulverization and rhexic bleeding to complete transection. Of note is the role played by the cord microvasculature in the pathophysiology of such lesions.[16-19] The early stages feature intramedullary hemorrhage involving the central gray matter that extends centrifugally with the severity of trauma.[16,17] Edema, in conjunction with hemorrhagic necrosis and liquefaction necrosis, is also present within the central gray matter.[16,17] Although edema, necrosis, and hemorrhage are often localized to the region of direct trauma, the bleeding may extend in a tapering fashion cephalocaudad over several segments to produce the condition known as hematomyelia. Whereas alterations in cord microcirculation with bleeding and hemorrhagic necrosis maximize at 24 to 48 hours, posttraumatic edema peaks at 3 to 6 days.

After 1 to 2 weeks the edema has subsided and blood pigments are absorbed while the damaged segment undergoes demyelination. Eventually there is cystic dissolution of the central necrotic area.[18] The margins of the injured region are characterized by reactive gliosis and vascular proliferation. As with open wounds, there may be dense fibrous scarring of the leptomeninges at the site of fracture-dislocation that may adhere to the damaged cord.

Compression of the cord can result from any of the following: fracture-dislocation, dislocation, traumatic disk herniation, epidural hematoma, preexisting exostoses, or spondylitic bars. Although compression in the thoracic and lumbar spine most frequently results from direct persistent mechanical impingement, it may be a transitory "pinching" event in the cervical spine. A sudden or permanent loss of up to 50% of the anterior-posterior dimension of the spinal canal is necessary for cord compression,[20] which may be aggravated by extensive intramedullary hemorrhage as described previously with cord contusion. The pathologic changes in the cord caused by pressure may be transient or permanent, including necrosis with or without hemorrhage. If the cord is compressed for a short period, the pathologic findings will be the same as those of a simple concussion; however, longer more intense compression will result in more severe damage.

■ ■ ■

Several experimental models[21,22] have given information concerning the separate and sometimes additive effects of compression and contusion. The cause of reversible neurologic deficit produced by cord compression has been attributed[23-25] to direct mechanical distortion of the tissue as well as to impairment of the spinal cord circulation.

MANAGEMENT OF SPINAL TRAUMA
Clinical Assessment

The management of spinal cord injury begins at the scene of the accident. When spinal injury is suspected, instability is assumed and immediate immobilization of the spine is mandatory. Optimal oxygen and blood flow to the spinal cord should be provided; strict attention must be paid to maintaining a good airway and oxygenation, as well as providing the support necessary to maintain blood pressure within normal limits. Nasogastric and urinary catheters are often inserted to minimize distention. A neurologic examination must be performed to assess motor and sensory function of the cord as well as reflex changes and autonomic function.

Various clinical classification schemes of spinal cord injury have been developed as a means with which to document efficacy of treatment.[26,27] For example, in the Frankel classification[26] a grade A lesion is synonymous with complete cord interruption (i.e., no sensory or motor function below that level) whereas grades B through E describe broad categories of increasing motor and sensory function, which, for a particular patient, may change with time. However, it should be noted that several of the grades are difficult to compare given subjective differences in evaluating purposeful, useful, or functional voluntary motion.[26] Additionally, it is difficult to correlate the extent of spinal cord pathologic impairment from physical examination or assessment of an initial neurologic deficit, and hence such classifications have little predictive value with respect to ultimate recovery of neurologic function. In view of the possible etiologies of spinal cord dysfunction following significant trauma (concussion, contusion, transection, compression), this is not surprising.

As a consequence of the lack of specificity and predictive value in clinically evaluating, diagnosing, and treating spinal cord injury, it is clear that diagnostic imaging (and particularly MRI) will continue to gain importance in patient selection and follow-up as new and promising methods of surgical and medical therapy are developed.[28,29]

Imaging Assessment and the Role of MRI
Spinal stability

Diagnostic imaging of patients with spine injury is directed to recognition and treatment of instability and cord compression. Historically and for practical purposes, the evaluation of potential spine trauma victims begins in the emergency department with plain film radiographs. The routine application of cervical spine immobilizers in the field as well as rising concerns about potential litigation have led to a marked increase in requests for cervical radiographs.[30] The incidence of significant cervical spine injury in such patients is low (as little as 2%).[31] The low yield of "screening" x-ray examinations has resulted in efforts to identify risk factors that would correlate with cervical spine abnormality.[31-33] Virtually all patients with cervical spine injuries and a normal level of consciousness have symptoms or signs referable to the cervical spine, in particular local pain.[5,30,31] In patients with concomitant head injury, diminished level of consciousness, alcohol intoxication, or multisystem injury, cervical spine injuries cannot be reliably excluded on the basis of a physical examination.[34] Radiographs should be obtained for all patients with pain or neurologic deficit referable to the cervical spine as well as for patients who are not fully alert and cooperative at the time of their initial evaluation.[33]

Although the American College of Surgeons Committee on Trauma recommends obtaining cross-table lateral views of the cervical spine in all major trauma victims, controversy exists regarding which views constitute an adequate examination of the cervical spine.[32] It has been estimated[30,31,35] that the cross-table lateral cervical spine has a maximum sensitivity of only 82% and thus should not be considered an adequate screening examination. The addition of AP and open-mouth odontoid views increases the maximum sensitivity of the plain radiographic examination to 93%.

Equivocal radiographic findings or indirect indicators of trauma (e.g., soft tissue swelling) warrant further investigation. For example, a prevertebral hematoma is typical of injuries involving the anterior bony and ligamentous structures but is much less common in injuries of the posterior elements.[36] (Although 5 mm is frequently considered the maximum width of prevertebral soft tissue swelling anterior to the upper cervical spine, there is considerable variability among trauma victims and between trauma victims and normals; Templeton et al.[37] have proposed 7 mm as the upper limit of normal.)

Should the preliminary studies prove negative, flexion-extension radiographs may reveal otherwise nascent ligamentous disruption. Positive or suspicious findings (with or without neurologic deficit) on the plain film examination often warrant further delineation with computed tomography directed to the region of interest. A number of studies[38-53] have documented the ability of CT to demonstrate fractures to better advantage than plain film radiographs as well as MRI (particularly complex injuries to the posterior elements).

With respect to the role of MR in evaluating spinal instability, an early report of 14 patients with vertebral fractures[52] indicated a sensitivity of 100% for vertebral body fractures but of only 57% for posterior element fractures. Additional experience,[48,51,53] however, has provided even less favorable results regarding the ability of MR imaging to detect both anterior and posterior spinal fractures. Nevertheless, Flanders et al.[53] found the predictive values of positive MR imaging studies acceptable (88% and 100% for vertebral body and posterior element defects respectively). Conventional spin-echo images offer the best detail of cortical surface interruptions. Sagittal scans are optimal for demonstrating posttraumatic deformities of the vertebral bodies. An additional ancillary finding with MR imaging is the demonstration of compressive injury to the medullary space of the vertebral body—visualized as increased signal of the vertebra relative to adjacent segments on the T_2-weighted image and relatively decreased signal on T_1-weighted images.[48,54-57] The change in vertebral body signal characteristics is thought to represent hemorrhage into the marrow elements. These findings should suggest the presence of a fracture even when a cortical defect is not visualized with MR.

Unlike other conventional imaging modalities, MR is capable of directly demonstrating ligamentous tears[48-51,57,58] (Fig. 8-1). Typically these are visualized during the acute period as interruption of the normally low–signal intensity ligamentous structures (e.g., the longitudinal and the inter- and supraspinous ligaments) on both T_1- and T_2-weighted scans surrounded by or with intervening areas of high signal on the T_2-weighted studies, representing soft tissue edema.

It should be noted that the impact of variable K space sampling and associated filtering phenomena (i.e., RARE spin-echo imaging) on the sensitivity of MR in detecting spinal fracture lines and ligamentous disruption, and thus instability, is not yet known.

Injury to the spinal cord

The importance of distinguishing traumatic cord contusion from direct cord compression, and of correctly diagnosing it, can be assessed by reviewing numerous case series[59,60] in which improvement or resolution is described of both acute and chronic neurologic deficits following surgical decompression of an offending compressive lesion. Some experimental evidence[61-64] indicates that the degree of permanent neurologic deficit may be a direct function of the duration of cord compression. Conversely, it is noteworthy that analogous clinical series[65-67] have failed to demonstrate significant change in clinical outcome between operative and nonoperative cases. Such discrepancies in treatment philosophy are not trivial, inasmuch as early surgery has been associated with increased risk of neurologic deterioration. Possible explanations for the acute operative versus nonoperative treatment controversy include the following: (1) inaccu-

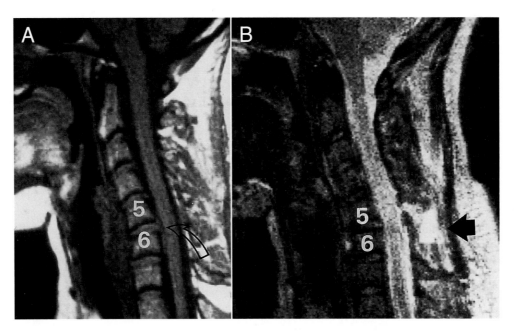

Fig. 8-1. A, Sagittal 500 msec TR/17 msec TE image in a patient with a flexion injury and anterior cord syndrome. The point of flexion was at C5-6. Note the traumatic disk herniation at this level *(open arrow).* A less prominent disk herniation is also visible at C4-5. **B,** Midline sagittal 2000 msec TR/120 msec TE scan. The traumatic disk herniation is not as well demonstrated as in the T_1-weighted study. However, this T_2-weighted image points out a previously unsuspected disruption of the intraspinous ligaments, which can be seen as a wedge-shaped area of increased signal intensity behind C5-6 *(arrow).*

rate criteria were used to define significant cord compression and/or satisfactory decompression; (2) the type of operative procedure performed (anterior vs posterior, stabilizing vs decompressing) is distinctly different; (3) the initial assessment of neurologic deficit secondary to concomitant head injury was inaccurate; and (4) the preoperative imaging studies could not accurately characterize the type and extent of cord trauma (i.e., concussion vs contusion vs compression).

Although it is agreed that plain film radiography and computed tomography are essential to the diagnosis of posttraumatic spinal instability, several series indicate that these studies do not correlate with the patient's presenting or future neurologic status. Kulkarni et al.[54] described patients with vertebral burst fractures (65% of whom had an acute neurologic deficit), with no apparent correlation between radiographic appearance and neurologic status. Furthermore, the presence of posterior element fractures, subluxation, and spinal canal narrowing did not appear to predict the neurologic deficit. In a series of patients with hyperextension injuries producing central cord syndrome with neurologic deficit, Goldberg et al.[50] reported that 75% had no demonstrable fracture whereas 96% had severe spondylosis. Flanders et al.[53] have reported a similar lack of correlation between ra-

diographic findings and neurologic condition in 78 spinal trauma victims.

Several studies[53,54,68-71] describe spinal cord MR signal intensity patterns on T_1- and T_2-weighted images that not only have proved reliable in discriminating cord edema and hemorrhage but also reflect the neurologic deficit and its prognosis for improvement. Kulkarni et al.[54] initially reported three patterns of intramedullary signal changes observable by MRI in patients with acute trauma. In the *first* pattern traumatic lesions acutely demonstrate tapering foci of hypointensity on T_1- and T_2-weighted images that are consistent with cord contusion, intramedullary hemorrhage (composed of deoxyhemoglobin), and a poor prognosis. Subsequently the degradation of deoxyhemoglobin to intracellular methemoglobin produces high signal on T_1-weighted images (beginning at the periphery) and low signal on T_2-weighted images. Eventually red blood cell lysis and the release of extracellular methemoglobin produce high signal on both T_1- and T_2-weighted images (Fig. 8-2). The *second* pattern is recognized as low or normal signal on T_1-weighted images and a spindle-shaped region of high signal on T_2-weighted images.[54,68,71] Such lesions are consistent with the edema of cord concussion and carry a more favorable prognosis. The *third* pattern represents

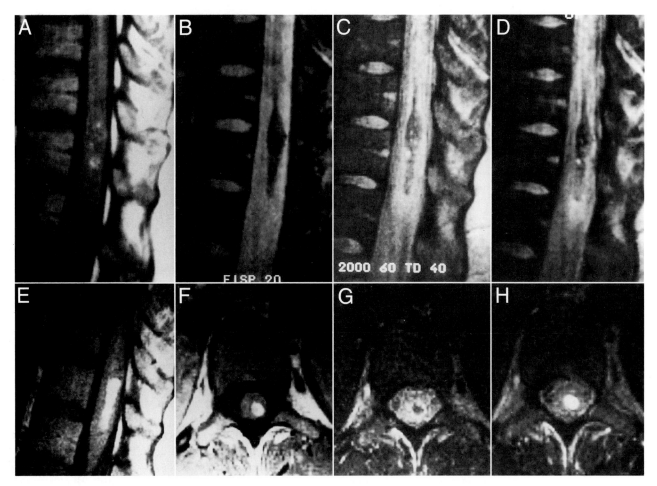

Fig. 8-2. A and **B,** Sagittal 500 msec TR/17 msec TE spin-echo and 20-degree FISP gradient echo scans demonstrating focal areas of low signal intensity within the conus medullaris of a young woman following spinal cord trauma. The findings are consistent with subacute intramedullary hemorrhage. In particular, the loss of signal from this region on the gradient echo study is highly suggestive of magnetic susceptibility effect secondary to hemorrhage. **C** and **D,** 2000 msec TR/60 and 120 msec TE images. The focal area of decreased signal represents intramedullary hemorrhage whereas the peripheral area of increased signal within the conus suggests edema. Another MR image obtained 1 week after the initial study, **E,** a 500 msec TR/17 msec TE sagittal through the level of the conus, demonstrates the focal area of increased signal consistent with intracellular methemoglobin. **F,** This axial 500 msec TR/17 msec TE through the same region shows a focal hematoma composed of intracellular methemoglobin. **G,** 2000 msec TR/120 msec TE. Note the focal area of low signal within the cord at the site of the hematoma, again consistent with the signal-intensity characteristics of intracellular methemoglobin. **H,** Follow-up 2000 msec TR/20 msec TE axial image several weeks after the initial injury. Note the focal area of increased signal intensity within the cord, consistent with extracellular methemoglobin.

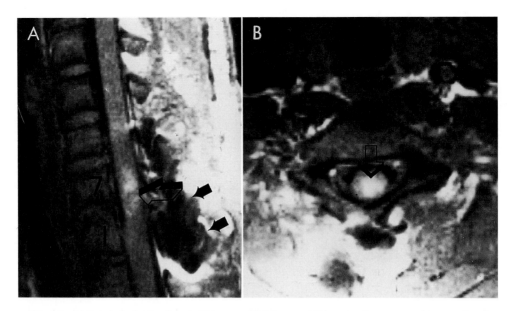

Fig. 8-3. Sagittal, **A,** and axial, **B,** 500 msec TR/17 msec TE images in a man who sustained a flexion-dislocation injury at C7-T1 several weeks earlier. The patient has undergone posterior wire fusion for stabilization *(solid arrows).* Residual petechial hemorrhage within the spinal cord *(open arrows)* is represented as ill-defined areas of increased signal intensity on these T_1-weighted images.

a mixture of the first two, the low-signal center surrounded by a peripheral ring of high signal on T_2-weighted images. Patients with these lesions may be capable of neurologic improvement with appropriate treatment (Fig. 8-3). Note that the T_2 filtering effect of variable K space sampling is known to alter the signal characteristics of hemorrhage on spin-echo MR; however, it is as yet unknown whether this significantly affects its prognostic value relative to spinal cord trauma.

In the past the presence of an acute incomplete traumatic neurologic deficit (with or without fracture-dislocation) justified the administration of intrathecal contrast to evaluate cord integrity and exclude potentially reversible cord compression. Computed tomographic myelography was preferred over plain film myelography because of its ability to outline the anterior spinal cord, determine the etiology of block, and visualize the vertebral canal beyond points of obstruction.[72] Axial and sagittal MR scans are valuable in their ability to detect and quantify cord compression secondary to bone fragments, hematoma, or acutely herniated disk material—with the added advantage of being noninvasive.* Flanders et al.[53] reported that the overall prevalence of traumatic disk herniation was quite high (51%), ranging from 20% in the incomplete Frankel grade C patients to 100% in the incomplete Frankel grade B patients. Among patients with a complete neurologic deficit, 48% had traumatic disk

herniations and a similar percentage of neurologically intact Frankel E patients had disk herniations (42%). Thus, although the presence of a herniated disk fragment did not necessarily indicate a negative clinical consequence, it would be reasonable to consider any patients with a significant neurologic deficit, cord compression by traumatic extradural mass, and little or no intramedullary hemorrhage as the candidates most likely to benefit from acute surgical decompression and stabilization.[53]

Technical considerations

Despite agreement that accurate noninvasive imaging of ligamentous disruption and of traumatic disk herniation with cord compression, cord concussion, and cord contusion is desirable, the potential for ferromagnetic interactions between imager and spine stabilization instruments, electronic monitoring equipment, and respiratory support devices has limited the enthusiasm for MR in evaluating acute spinal cord trauma. Fortunately, significant progress has been made in overcoming these obstacles.

The potential risks and problems associated with performing MR imaging in a patient with metallic implants or metallic materials are related to the induction of an electrical current within metallic stabilizing loops or struts, as well as the heating, movement, or dislodgment of such implants, along with the creation of an image-degrading artifact or the misinterpretation of such artifact as abnormality.[74,75] A typical example is the halo fixation device, commonly used as a means of closed sta-

---

*References 41, 46, 48, 49, 51-53, 57, 69, 70, 73.

TABLE 8-1
Cervical spine devices: physical characteristics and image quality

Device	Alterations	Ferrous components	Image quality — Spine T₁	T₂	Gradient echo	Brain T₁
EXO adjustable collar	None	Yes	NI			NI
Philadelphia collar	Plastic fasteners	No	ACC			NI
S.O.M.I. cervical orthosis	None	Yes	NI			NI
Guilford cervical orthosis	None	Yes	UNAC			NI
Modified Guilford orthosis	Monel rivets, plastic fasteners	No	ACC			NI
PMT halo cervical orthosis	None	No	ACC			NI
Bremer halo cervical orthosis	None	No	ACC			UNAC
MR-compatible Bremer orthosis	Split crown, plastic spacers, titanium fasteners	No	ACC	ACC	ACC	ACC*
Modified PMT halo orthosis	Graphite-carbon rods and halo, plastic ball-and-socket joints	No	AC	ACC	ACC	LQ†

*Body-coil image.
†Surface-coil image.
Code: *NI,* not imaged; *ACC,* acceptable; *UNAC,* unacceptable; *LQ,* limited quality.
From Clayman DA, Marakami ME, Vines FS: *AJNR* 1990; 11:385-390. Copyright the American Society of Neuroradiology.

bilization.[76] The halo thoracic brace consists of a "halo" ring that is fixed to the skull by four pins. The ring is attached to a removable vest. The vest has two halves, anterior and posterior, lined with synthetic sheepskin. Vests range in size from 28 to 42 inches and are available to fit the contour of the patient's chest. Not only have isolated components such as snaps and buckles of some of these devices been constructed of ferromagnetic material, but in one instance[77] the halo itself has been shown to conduct MR-generated current by Faraday induction. Claymen et al.[78] have reviewed these devices and determined that the risks involved can be reduced by appropriate selection of materials. Cervical orthoses with aluminum or graphite-carbon components that are interconnected with plastic joints (e.g., the plastic ball-and-socket) are, to date, the most successful devices for MR compatibility (Table 8-1). The authors also note that, to make these orthoses CT compatible, low–electron density materials are presently being evaluated to replace the titanium skull pins. Shellock and Slimp[75] describe a device that eliminates the risk of induced current and minimizes image artifact (although it too utilizes titanium alloy skull pins, which do produce minor local artifacts). Additionally, McArdle et al.[79] have described an inexpensive and effective traction system for MR imagers to be used in conjunction with halo devices. We prefer the Trippi-Wells traction device with such vests since it allows for closer application of the surface coils.

It is important to remember that patients with acute spinal cord trauma may be subject to hemodynamic instability and/or ventilatory compromise. Safe and effective imaging of such patients within the confines of high–field strength whole-body imagers requires that monitoring instruments be as remote from the magnet as possible, through the use of either telemetric or fiberoptic transmission.[80,81] Appropriate selection of monitoring equipment operated at frequencies outside the imager's field strength–dependent radiofrequency (RF) spectrum or that are appropriately RF shielded will minimize any distortion of signal.[82] Arterial blood pressure must frequently be monitored outside the scanner by lengthening the pneumatic tubing connected to the blood pressure cuff, since auscultation is usually difficult to perform in the presence of an actively scanning imager.[80,83] Decisions concerning the necessity and/or type of ventilatory support are best left to the anesthesiologist; however, pneumatically driven, volume- and pressure-cycled, MRI-compatible fluidic ventilators are available commercially.[84,85] Similarly, there are numerous reports in the literature describing several ventilatory circuits and anesthesia techniques for use with MRI. (One important note: laryngoscopes are nonmagnetic but can only be employed at an imager when batteries with paper or plastic casings are used.[83])

CLASSIFICATION AND MECHANISM: IMAGING FINDINGS

Spinal trauma can typically be classified as (1) lesions or defects resulting from sharp or penetrating injury and (2) lesions or defects resulting from blunt injury. The pathologist might further characterize traumatic lesions as primary, secondary, late sequelae, and late complica-

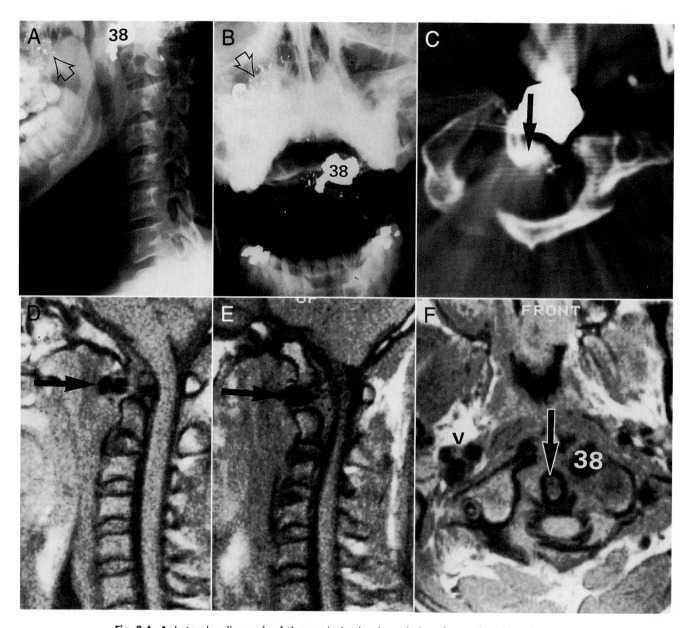

Fig. 8-4. A, Lateral radiograph of the cervical spine in a victim of armed robbery, in which the weapon was fired point-blank into the nose. Lead fragments remain within the nasal cavity *(open arrow)* although most of the .38-caliber slug can be seen against the dens. **B,** Open-mouth view. Again, debris can be seen within the right nasal cavity and maxillary antrum *(open arrow)* as well as the bulk of the bullet *(38)* just to the left of midline. **C,** Axial CT scan performed on the level of the dens. Fracture of the atlas with posterior displacement of the odontoid is evident *(arrow)*. **D,** Similar axial MR scan performed using a 500 msec TR/17 msec TE spin-echo technique. Note the fracture of the atlas, with a signal void immediately anterior to the displaced dens *(arrow)* representing the bullet fragment *(38)*. It is difficult to distinguish the neurovascular bundle *(v)* from additional bullet fragments. **E,** A sagittal 500 msec TR/17 msec TE midline image demonstrates the displaced and fractured dens abutting on the cervicomedullary junction, with the bullet fragment *(arrow)* immediately anterior. Note the significant amount of soft tissue swelling present within the oropharynx. **F,** A parasagittal 500 msec TR/17 msec TE image of the cervical spine just to the left of midline again demonstrates the bulk of the bullet fragment *(arrow)* completely replacing the anterior arch of C1.

tions. Primary lesions are those due to direct mechanical force on tissue. Secondary or reactive alterations are most commonly posttraumatic vascular disruptions. Late sequelae are the natural results of healing (e.g., arachnoid scarring, myelomalacia). Late complications include such entities as infection and syringomyelia.

Penetrating (Open) Trauma

The incidence of open or penetrating spinal trauma ranges from over 75% in wartime to 12% in civilian life.[1,86,87] Most civilian missile injuries are produced by bullets from handguns. Injuries by other types of missiles (e.g., fragments of metal, rocks, debris from explosions) are relatively rare. Classification schemes for such injuries are based on type of damage to the spinal cord (direct vs indirect) and location of the missile after impact.[11,88] Direct lesions result from passage of the missile across the spinal canal. In these circumstances cord transection is common and has been reported even in the absence of significant osseous disruption.[88] More commonly, however, the cord escapes direct damage but is compressed or contused by bony fragments or blast effects (Fig. 8-4). As one might expect, civilian missile injuries are less extensive than wounds inflicted during military combat.[86,87,89]

By contrast, puncture or stab wounds involving the spine are typically well-defined cuts, usually located in the thoracic region (74%).[90] This type of lesion attracts considerable clinical interest owing to the close correlation between lesion and symptoms.[91] The degree of damage to the cord varies according to the level of injury, character of the weapon, and force of delivery. Because the vertebral laminae protect the spinal cord dorsally, stab wounds typically enter lateral to the midline and produce an asymmetric dorsolateral lesion (Fig. 8-5).

Pathologically, penetrating wounds produce a slit or tear in the meninges that is frequently hemorrhagic (Fig. 8-6). The ends of the torn dura tend to approximate, and the margins of the cord wound separate (Fig. 8-5). Histologically there are three zones constituting the spinal cord wound[15,92]: (1) a debris zone of total liquefaction necrosis and hemorrhage; (2) a petechial zone of indirect but irreversible damage, as evidenced by vacuolization and decreased stainability; and (3) a zone of reversible, peritraumatic, intracellular edema composed of swollen astroglia. The central area of primary debris rapidly undergoes dissolution and clearing of blood pigments, while the petechial zone accumulates red blood cells, over the first 24 hours. Astroglial edema is maximal between 2 and 12 hours.

After the immediate posttraumatic necrosis period (36 to 48 hours) there is resorption and organization by phagocytes and microglia, with astroglial and mesenchymal proliferation at the wound margins. Subsequently the damaged spinal cord is replaced by gliofibrous scar at 3 to 4 weeks. Grossly an incompletely transected cord

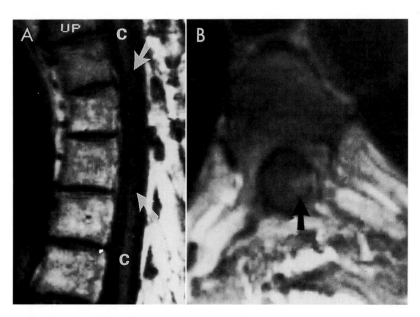

Fig. 8-5. A, Midline sagittal 500 msec TR/17 msec TE image of the thoracic spine in a patient with Brown-Sequard syndrome following a stab wound to the spine. The cord is identified *(c)* above and below an area of extreme cord thinning at the site of the lesion *(arrows).* **B,** An axial 500 msec TR/17 msec TE image demonstrates that the remaining half of the cord is unaffected by the stab wound on the left *(arrow).*

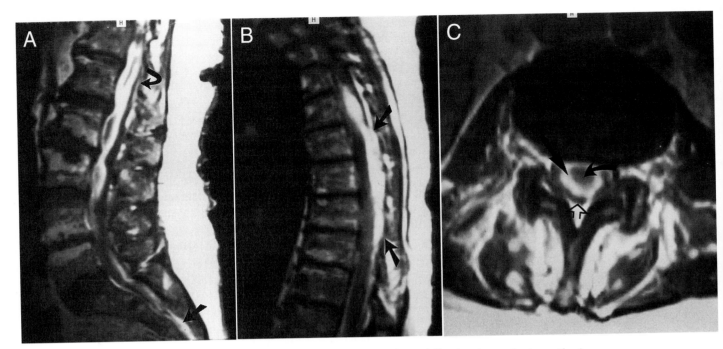

Fig. 8-6. Iatrogenic subarachnoid-subdural hemorrhage following intraspinal anesthesia (penetrating trauma). **A,** A sagittal T$_1$-weighted scan of the lumbar spine (TR 500 msec/TE 17 msec) demonstrates an intrathecal hematoma *(curved arrow)* that is difficult to distinguish from epidural fat *(slanted arrow)*. **B,** A sagittal T$_1$-weighted of the thoracic spine likewise demonstrates blood surrounding the spinal cord *(arrows)*. **C,** The axial T$_1$-weighted confirms this, showing the spinal cord *(curved black arrow)*, subarachnoid blood *(straight black arrow)*, and subarachnoid space *(open arrow)*.

segment is thin and hard secondary to the union of meninges to cord and spinal canal by collagenous scar. The meninges may demonstrate local hemosiderin deposition in this region and may also become thickened to the point of mimicking an extradural mass that extends over several segments.[93,94] Similar cicatrization can occur in the arachnoid, producing CSF cavities and adhesive arachnoiditis. Following complete cord transection there may be dehiscence of the disrupted ends, with thickening of the meninges adherent to the dura and stump.

Late sequelae include intramedullary cysts secondary to remote liquefaction necrosis or dissecting CSF pressure shifts, along with secondary degeneration of the ascending and descending fiber tracts at areas of transection (Fig. 8-5).

Late complications generally are inflammatory lesions (e.g., extradural or subdural empyema), leptomeningitis, and cord infection. However, such sequelae are rare, even in the presence of bullets, knife fragments, or splinters, which are often surrounded by dense collagenous connective tissue with fibrous reactive change.[86,87,95]

Concerning the management of such injuries, surgical intervention rarely changes the neurologic outcome in cases of direct penetrating trauma. In the absence of a communication between the wound, foreign bodies, and skin, the chance of infection is rare with appropriate antibiotic therapy.[5,6,9] Thus, without spinal instability or blunt cord compression, immediate interventional therapy is usually limited to debridement.[89] If a more extensive surgical procedure is required, preoperative imaging beyond plain radiographs and tomography may be necessary. Should MRI be considered, it is necessary for the consulting radiologist to be aware of the presence and composition of metallic foreign bodies.[96,97] For example, bullets may be homogeneous (lead, zinc, magnesium, plastic), "coated" (lead covered by a thin layer of copper or brass), or "jacketed" (core of lead or steel surrounded by a thicker layer of copper or steel). Patients with such metallic foreign bodies may be at risk for ferromagnetic interactions with the imager—including (1) local tissue heating secondary to RF deposition, (2) motion of the foreign fragment related to the static or gradient magnetic fields, and (3) eddy current effects secondary to the applied gradient fields that may locally degrade the image (military ammunition is more commonly ferromagnetic) (Table 8-2 and Fig. 8-7). Reports[98] already exist for complications resulting from ferromagnetic-induced motion of a foreign body within the CNS. Personal experience with imaging a small number of civilian gunshot wounds has indicated that MRI can safely produce valuable information concerning the location of bullet fragments with respect to the spinal cord, without significant artifact (unlike x-ray CT), provided the composition of the projectile is MR compatible (i.e., without nonaustenitic steel or nickel). It is noteworthy that nickel is a frequent trace element in lead bullets.[98]

Closed Trauma

Closed spinal trauma is the result of both blunt forces transmitted to the spine and penetrating injuries that do not pierce the canal. A significant example occurs predominantly at sites of maximum spinal mobility. Hence the lower cervical region and the thoracolumbar junction are the most frequent sites of traumatic damage, although the frequency distribution at the level of the traumatic lesion varies in different series.[99-101] Since no ideal classification of closed spinal cord injuries has been formulated in terms of pathogenesis, the anatomic deformities (with or without neurologic deficit) are usually described in terms of the forces that produced the trauma relative to the salient anatomic features of the vertebral level involved. Thus there are general patterns of spinal trauma that recur and merit separate descriptions. Most commonly an attempt is made to classify an injury as (1) flexion, (2) extension, (3) vertical compression (axial loading), or (4) rotation.[102-104] Frequently the mechanism of insult is actually a combination of these.[105]

Craniovertebral junction: atlantooccipital articulation

Normal physiologic motion of the craniovertebral junction is the most complex of the spinal axis and includes flexion, extension, rotation, axial loading, and lateral bending.[106-108] This versatility is due to the unique anatomic configuration and articulation of the occiput, atlas, and axis.[109]

The atlantooccipital articulation, between the occipital condyles and the lateral masses of C1, consists of paired synovial joints that are primarily responsible for flexion and extension of the head. The atlantooccipital capsular ligaments, the anterior and posterior atlantooccipital membrane ligaments, and the two lateral atlantooccipital ligaments unite the atlas with the cranium. The cruciate ligament (a longitudinally oriented structure associated with the transverse ligament of the atlas) also contributes some strength to this articulation. However, a second group of ligaments is what provides the major structural support for the craniocervical junction. This group of ligaments, which run from the occiput to the axis, includes the apical dental ligament, the paired alar ligaments, and the broad tectorial membrane.

The dynamics of the occipitocervical articulation were elucidated in a comprehensive series of cadaver studies by Werne.[110] This work demonstrated that forward flexion is limited by contact of the dens with the anterior foramen magnum, hyperextension by the tectorial membrane, and lateral flexion by the alar ligaments. Werne also showed that sectioning of the alar ligaments and tectorial membrane will allow dislocation of the cranium with respect to the spine.

Atlantooccipital dislocation. Traumatic atlantooccipital (AO) dislocation is a rare injury. Although traditionally considered fatal, posttraumatic AO dislocation is sometimes compatible with survival.[34,111,112] It is more common in children and typically results from motor vehicle accidents. In the series of Traynelis et al.[113] dealing with AO dislocations, patients who survived over 48 hours were three times more likely to be children than adults. Despite the fact that the mechanism of injury is controversial, some authors[114] think it results from hyperextension and distraction. In cases of nonfatal traumatic AO dislocation, many patients suffer serious head injury in addition to the dislocation. Direct brain stem insult may result in quadriparesis, paraparesis, or cranial nerve palsy.[113] The upper spinal cord may be injured to such a degree that the patient is rendered quadriplegic (although in the literature hemiparesis is a more common occurrence).[113] In conjunction with craniovertebral dislocation a secondary injury may occur to the vertebral arteries—including arterial compression, intimal tearing, and/or thrombosis. Nevertheless, patients with no subsequent deficit have been described.[18,114]

The presence of significant head trauma may make early recognition of the neurologic manifestations of injury to the atlantooccipital spine difficult. Additionally, the plain radiographic findings may be subtle, particularly in children, in whom the common mechanism of injury is thought to be distraction.[113,114] The most obvious finding is retropharyngeal soft tissue swelling. Specific signs of anterior cranial dislocation include displacement of the basion anteriorly from its normal position superior to the odontoid, malalignment between the spinolaminar line of C1 and the posterior margin of the foramen magnum, and failure of the clival line to intersect the odontoid.[18,114,115] If the cranium is distracted superiorly, displacement of the occipital condyles from the superior facets of the atlas and widening of the atlantooccipital articulation more than 5 mm are present.[114] Recently, Goldberg et al.[111] reported such a case in which MR was able to demonstrate not only intraaxial blood products at the craniovertebral junction but also anterior ligamentous disruption at that level (Fig. 8-8).

Nontraumatic AO subluxations (both anterior and posterior) are rare but occasionally are mentioned in refer-

TABLE 8-2
Data summary of the most common projectiles available in the urban setting

	Caliber	Manufacturer	Weight (g)	Deflection (dynes)	Tip	Body	Core	Gild	SMC	FMC
Copper-jacketed nonsteel bullets										
1.	.25 auto	Rem	50	—	Pb(r)	Pb	Pb			Cu
2.	.32 auto	Rem	71	—	Pb(r)	Pb	Pb			Cu
3.	.45	Win				Pb	Pb			Cu
4.	.38 Sp semi-wadcutter	USAC	158	—	Pb(r)	Pb	Pb			Cu
5.	7.38 mm Mauser	Century Arm	86	1691	Pb(r)	Pb	Pb			Cu
6.	.38 Sp	Spur	125	—	Pb(h)	Pb	Pb		Cu	
7.	.38 Sp + P	Rem	125	—	Pb(h)	Pb	Pb		Cu	
8.	.38 Sp	Win SuperX	125	—	Pb(h)	Pb	Pb		Cu	
9.	.38 Glasser Safety Sug	W&W	54	—	Teflon(h)	Pb	Pb Pellet or Teflon		Cu	
10.	.44 Semi-wadcutter	Rem	224	—	Pb(h)	Pb	Pb		Cu	
11.	.22 (rifle)	Rem	40	—	Pb(r)	Pb	Pb		Cu-Gild	
12.	.22 (rifle)	Win	40	—	Pb(r)	Pb	Pb		Luboloy	
Non–copper-jacketed nonsteel bullets										
13.	.38 Sp	CCI (Blazer)	158	—	Pb(h)	Pb	Pb			
14.	.38 Sp wadcutter	Fed	148	—	—	Pb	Pb			
15.	.38 Sp semi-wadcutter	S&W Nyclad	158	—	Pb(h)	Pb	Pb			
16.	.45			—	Pb(h)	Pb				
17.	.22 (rifle)	Win	38	—	Pb(r)	Pb	Pb			
18.	9 mm	BAT		—	Plastic(r)	Cu	Cu			
19.	.38 JSP + P	PMC Tubular	66	—	—	Cu(h)	(None)			
20.	.357 silver-tip H.P.	Win	125	—	Al(h)	Pb	Pb			Al
21.	Slug	Rem	443	—	N/A	Pb				
22.	18 shot	Rem	52	—	N/A	Pb	Pb			
Steel-containing bullets										
23.	.25 auto	Gego	50	514	Steel(r)	Steel	Steel			Steel
24.	.30-06	Win armor piercing	164	5887	Pb(p)	Pb	Steel			Steel
25.	.38 SP	KTW armor piercing	88	10,180	Pb(p)	Pb	Carbide Steel		Cu	
26.	.38	Win armor piercing	66	0	Pb(p)	Pb	Steel			Cu
27.	7.62 × 39 mm	Chinese Military	122	15,504	Pb(p)	Pb	Steel		Cu	
28.	12-gauge shot (0.162 mm)	Rem	3.8	Not tested	N/A		Steel			

Suggested by the Ballistic Section, Cleveland Police Department Forensic Laboratory.
r, Round; *p*, pointed; *h*, hollow; *Gild*, gilding (dry lubricant); *SMC*, semijacketed case; *FMC*, full metal jacket or case; *H.P.*, high power; *Sp*, special; *P*, plus powder; *JSP*, jacketed soft point; *BAT* (USA); *CCI*, Cascade Cartridge Industry (USA); *Fed*, Federal Arms (USA); *Gego* (Germany); *KTW* (USA); *PMC*, Pan Metal Co. (Korea); *Spur* (USA); *REM*, Remington Arms (USA); *S & W*, Smith & Wesson (USA); *W & W*, Winchester & Western (USA); *Win*, Winchester (USA); *USAC*, United States of America Cartridge (USA).
From Smith AS, Hurst GC, Duerk JL, Diaz PJ: *AJNR* 1991;12:567-562. Copyright the American Society of Neuroradiology.

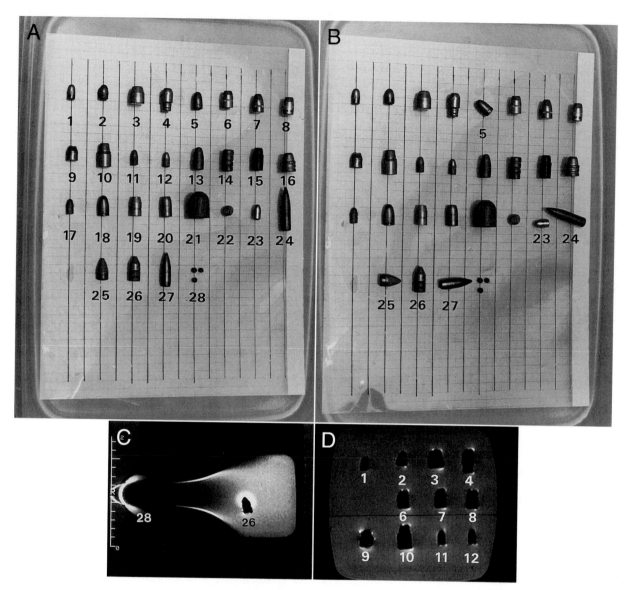

Fig. 8-7. A, Projectiles oriented along the Z axis of the magnet do not move after 30 minutes. **B,** Placement of the projectile axis perpendicular to the Z axis results in a 90-degree rotation for steel-containing projectiles (Gego 25-caliber automatic *[23]*, KTW armor-piercing *[25]*, and 7.62 × 39 mm Chinese military *[27]*) and a 60-degree rotation for the .30-06 Winchester armor-piercing *(24)*. The steel-cored Winchester armor-piercing *(26)* does not rotate, but the nonsteel Century Arm 7.38 Mauser *(5)* does (45 degrees). **C,** A single 0.160 mm 12-gauge steel shot produces an approximately 14 cm of field distortion. The steel shot is on the left. On the right is the .30-06 Winchester armor-piercing bullet *(26)*, which has a steel core but had no deflection. Note the perimeter artifact due to the copper jacket. (MR image 500/30/1.) **D,** Copper-jacketed nonsteel bullets. The composite image shows a minimal bright perimeter artifact on spin-echo MR imaging (550/26/11). (The 7.38 Mauser *[5]* is not shown because of a large artifact.) (Reprinted from Smith AS, et al. *AJNR* 1991;12:567-572.)

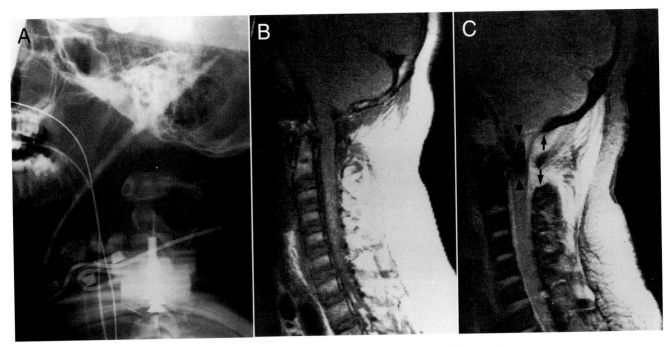

Fig. 8-8. A, A lateral radiograph, obtained following craniocervical fixation by a halo-vest, shows atlantooccipital dislocation. The atlantoaxial articulation is also distracted. **B,** A sagittal T$_1$-weighted spin-echo shows swelling of the high cervical cord (and probably medulla oblongata) with poor delineation of the CSF-cord interface. **C,** Marked hypointensity within the high cervical cord on the gradient echo sagittal image is indicative of acute hemorrhage *(arrowheads)*. Abnormally widened atlantooccipital and atlantoaxial distances *(arrows)*, as well as a prevertebral hematoma, are also evident. (From Goldberg AL, et al: *J Comput Assist Tomogr* 1991;15[1]:174-178.)

ence to trauma.[116,117] They may be secondary to rheumatoid arthritis, massive erosive calcium pyrophosphate dehydrate depositions, congenital skeletal abnormalities (e.g., Down syndrome), or infection.[118]

Axial loading injury. Direct axial loading with forces transmitted through the lateral masses of the atlas typically produces the Jefferson fracture—ipsilateral disruption of both the anterior and the posterior arches[119]—which may be unilateral or bilateral. The lateral view of the cervical spine shows that axial loading of C1 results in ipsilateral disruption of the anterior and posterior arches. It also shows soft tissue swelling and may demonstrate fracture of the posterior arch. The atlantoaxial distance is normal unless there is concomitant rupture of the transverse ligament. The fracture is more readily characterized on open-mouth odontoid views, in which lateral displacement of the lateral masses of the atlas relative to those of the axis can be identified.[120] Although a minimal degree of displacement may be seen in healthy individuals, if there is more than 6 mm of total lateral displacement on this view transverse ligament damage should be suspected.[121]

Extension injuries. The most frequent fracture of C1 involves the posterior arch as it is crushed between the occiput and the posterior arch of C2 in extension.[112,120] This isolated posterior arch fracture is stable and not associated with appreciable soft tissue swelling. It can be differentiated on radiographic studies from the commonly seen congenital cleft of the posterior arch by its lack of corticated borders.

Craniovertebral junction: atlantoaxial articulation

The primary motion at the C1-C2 joint is rotation rather than flexion or extension. The bony ring of C1 does not contain a body or distinct spinous process; thus its articulation with C2 is circular and flat. The atlantoaxial articulation is anterior to the joints below this level and corresponds anatomically to the level of the nonarticulating lateral masses of the remaining cervical vertebrae.[122] C2 also differs anatomically from the remainder of the vertebrae by its larger size and the presence of the odontoid process.[122] This unique anatomy results in a set of injuries specific to this region, typically the result of direct trauma to the head.[112]

Atlantoaxial subluxation. Isolated posttraumatic atlantoaxial subluxation is also a rare injury. Normally the dens is tightly bound to C1 by the dense fibers of the transverse ligament, which is attached bilaterally to the lateral masses of C2.[121] The transverse ligament prevents forward subluxation of the atlas on the axis with flexion. Tears of the transverse ligament or avulsion fractures at its site of insertion allow anterior displacement of C1 relative to C2. The normal distance between the dens and the posterior margin of the anterior arch of C1 is less than 3 mm in adults, being more conspicuous with flexion.[112,121] MR may be particularly valuable in such circumstances through its ability to assess cord compression directly. Alternatively, compromise of the canal and spinal cord may be positional and in these cases the ability of MR to provide dynamic studies is somewhat limited.

Rotary subluxation. Rotary fixation of the atlantoaxial joint often occurs after minor trauma but also may develop spontaneously or after an upper respiratory tract infection. The patient presents with a painful torticollis and the typical head position of slight flexion, cranial rotation, and tilting contralateral to the direction of rotation.[123] Rotary fixation can be diagnosed only when the rotated relationship between the lateral masses of the atlas and axis is shown to be abnormally fixed.[124] On open-mouth odontoid views the dens is positioned eccentrically between the lateral masses of C1, and the anteriorly displaced lateral mass appears wider and closer to midline.[123] This radiographic appearance also is seen in healthy persons with cranial rotation and in patients with torticollis, but in these cases the abnormality is reversible.[112,125] CT scanning both in the resting position and with maximum rotation to the contralateral side is the optimum method of evaluation. Individuals with rotary fixation show no change in the C1-C2 relationship with contralateral rotation whereas healthy persons and patients with torticollis are able to correct the deformity.[125]

Flexion fracture-dislocation. The dens, in conjunction with the anterior arch of C1 and the transverse ligament, prevents anterior subluxation of C1 on C2. The mechanism of injury resulting in odontoid fractures or (less frequently) dislocation is not well understood, although flexion is suspected as a prominent component.[126] Odontoid fractures are classified as type I (avulsion), type II (involving the body), and type III (basilar) (Fig. 8-9).[127] It is worth noting that type II fractures demonstrate the highest incidence of nonunion and delayed instability (26% to 36%)[127,123] (Fig. 8-10). Most survivors have no neurologic deficit and present with minimal upper cervical pain. Fractures of the odontoid are well demonstrated on plain film open-mouth radiographs. Magnetic resonance imaging may demonstrate the fracture line (particularly for types II and III); however, more impressive are compromise of the subarachnoid space and compression of the cord.

Extension fracture-dislocation. Extension injuries

have also been reported to fracture the odontoid, but this is unusual. More commonly extension produced through sudden deceleration results in fracture of the posterior ring of the atlas or bilateral fracture of the pedicles of the axis.[129] Perhaps the most characteristic injury of C2 is the hangman's fracture—bilateral avulsion of the neutral arches from the vertebral body. This injury, also referred to as traumatic spondylolisthesis, accounts for 4% to 7% of all cervical spinal fractures.[130] It typically is the result of axial compression and hyperextension, although other mechanisms of injury can also produce these findings.[130] Anterior avulsion fractures of the axis with severe extension injury may be seen. As one might expect from previous comments on the sensitivity of MR to posterior element fractures, it is not frequently implemented in the evaluation of such injuries.

Lower cervical spine

Flexion fracture-dislocation. Because of the inherent anterior-posterior mobility of the lower cervical spine, serious closed spinal flexion-extension injuries occur with some regularity in this region. Flexion injuries of the lower cervical spine result from significant posterior-to-anterior forces applied to the cervical vertebrae and

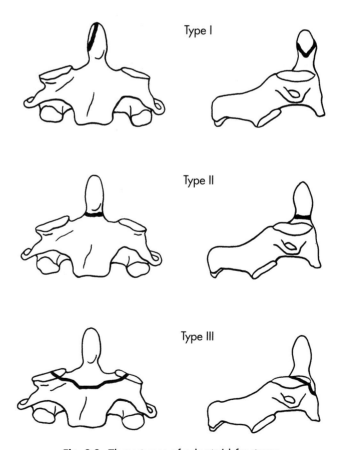

Fig. 8-9. Three types of odontoid fractures.

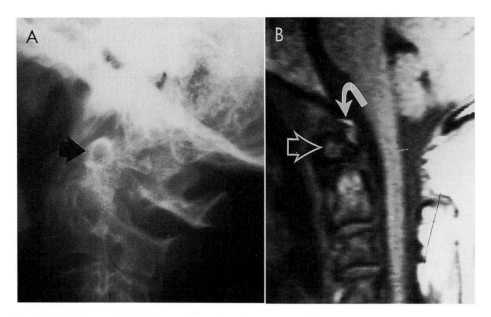

Fig. 8-10. A, Lateral plain film radiograph of a patient with a remote odontoid fracture. The dens is not well visualized, although the body of C2 can be seen directly beneath the anterior arch of C1 *(arrow)*. **B,** The sagittal 500 msec TR/17 msec TE demonstrates nonunion of a remote type II odontoid fracture with partial resorption of the dens *(curved arrow)* and subluxation of the body of C2 beneath the anterior arch of the atlas *(open arrow)*.

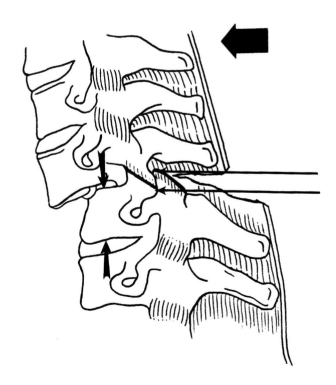

Fig. 8-11. Flexion injury of the cervical spine. Such injuries typically result from force applied in a posterior-to-anterior direction in the upper cervical spine *(thick horizontal arrow)*. As the spine is driven forward, the force may be transmitted vertically to produce compression of a more inferior vertebral body *(vertical arrows)*. With extreme forward motion of the upper spine there may be disruption of the interspinous ligament and/or the joint capsule of the articular facets *(thin horizontal arrows)*.

ligaments (Fig. 8-11). The spectrum of sequelae includes disk protrusion, vertebral body wedge-compression fracture, tearing of the posterior ligaments, subluxation of the articular processes, and fracture-dislocation with potentially severe central cord necrosis or hemorrhage.

The simple "clay shoveler's" and wedge-compression fractures are stable sequelae of significant flexion. The clay shoveler's injury is an avulsion fracture of the spinous process by the supraspinous ligament, typically at the lower two cervical elements. The wedge-compression fracture consists of a comminuted fracture of the anterior-superior vertebral body endplate at the fulcrum of forced flexion but without injury to the posterior elements[120] (Fig. 8-12). As noted previously, flexion-compression fractures are well demonstrated on sagittal T_1- and T_2-weighted images with intermediate and high signal respectively.[48] Axial images display concentric rings of heterogeneous signal, which represent

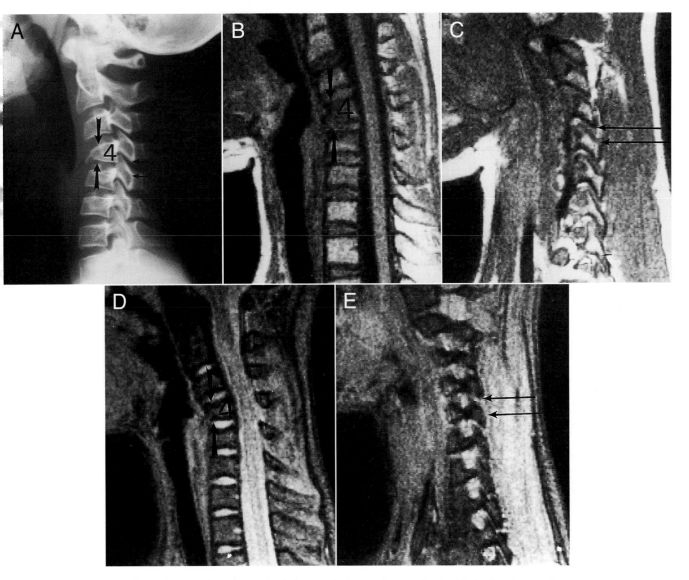

Fig. 8-12. A, Lateral radiograph of the cervical spine in a patient with flexion injury at C4-5. Note the wedge-compression of the C4 vertebral body *(vertical arrows)* and mild distraction of the C4 and C5 facets *(horizontal arrows)*. Flexion films failed to demonstrate any significant instability. **B,** A sagittal 500 msec TR/17 msec TE image demonstrates the wedge-compression of C4 *(vertical arrows)*. **C,** The parasagittal 500 msec TR/17 msec TE image again shows slight distraction of the facet joints at this level *(arrows)*. **D** and **E,** Similar findings on these 10-degree FISP sagittal and parasagittal scans. There is no evidence of posterior ligamentous disruption on the MR examination.

the expanded and fractured body. The outermost ring is the anterior longitudinal ligament and associated fragments; the middle ring, avulsed dark endplate cortex; and the innermost ring, cortex of the superior endplate.[48] Fractured bodies demonstrate diffuse increased signal intensity on T_2-weighted images within the cancellous marrow space but may be isointense (acutely) or of increased signal (subacutely) depending on their age and the presence or absence of traumatic hemorrhage.[48] Actual fracture lines are often demonstrated on high signal-to-noise T_1 or spin-density images as either increased or decreased signal relative to the adjacent cortex or cancellous (marrow-filled) bone.

Subluxation resulting from flexion produces tears of the articular joint capsules, posterior ligaments, and posterior anulus and longitudinal ligament. In the past these were infrequently recognized by radiologists, but they are significant for their relatively high incidence of delayed instability[131] (Figs. 8-1 and 8-12). More dramatic forward displacement may result in bilateral interfacet dislocation (bilateral "locked" or "perched" facets). These dislocated facets pass upward and forward over the inferior facets of the joint and come to lie in the intervertebral foramina, an occurrence facilitated by the relatively horizontal orientation of the cervical facets.

Bilateral facet dislocation is associated with a high incidence of cord damage, resulting from compression between the posterior part of the inferior vertebral body and the dislocated or fractured posterior arch of the upper vertebra.[132,133] Simple disruption of the articular joint capsules and posterior longitudinal and spinous ligaments may be suspected on the basis of increased interspinous and interfacet distances associated with local high signal intensity on T_2-weighted sagittal MR scans in the acute and subacute phases following trauma[48,51,57] (Fig. 8-1). Actual facet subluxation can easily be seen on plain film studies as well as on parasagittal MR scans or, alternatively, on axial MR and CT acquisitions by the apparently "naked" facets. Associated abnormalities include posterior disk space *narrowing* and avulsion fractures of the laminae; however, characterization of posterior element fractures with axial MR studies may be inferior to that possible with CT.[48]

A flexion teardrop fracture-dislocation is the most severe injury of the lower cervical spine.[134] It consists of a sagittal vertebral body fracture and anterior wedging in conjunction with forward subluxation or dislocation of the posterior elements secondary to ligamentous disruption (Fig. 8-13). The name "teardrop fracture" derives from the triangularly shaped fragment at the

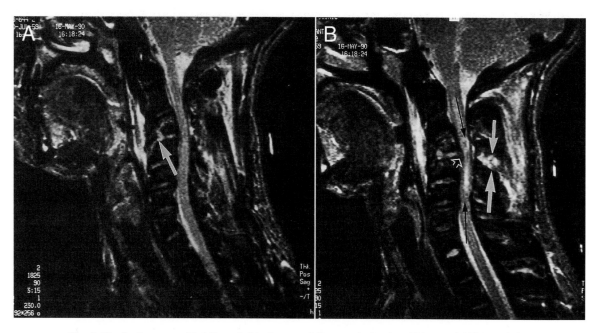

Fig. 8-13. A, A parasagittal T_2-weighted scan of the cervical spine (TR gated 1825/TE 90) demonstrates a flexion teardrop fracture of C3 *(white arrow)* with a prevertebral hematoma anteriorly as well as a suggestion of high signal intensity along the supraspinous and interspinous ligaments posteriorly, possibly representing posterior ligamentous disruption. **B,** A midline sagittal T_2-weighted of the cervical spine demonstrates cord contusion with surrounding edema *(long black arrows)* from C1 to C5. Again note the disruption of supraspinous and interspinous ligaments *(solid white arrows)* and the prevertebral hematoma. Also, there is a traumatic disk herniation with compromise of the canal *(open arrow)*.

anterior-inferior margin of the vertebral body, which resembles a dripping tear. In addition to widening of the interspinous and interfacet distances as well as narrowing of the posterior disk space, signs of ligamentous disruption include in a high percentage of cases kyphotic deformities, with backward displacement of the upper column of the divided cervical spine causing malalignment of the posterior laminar line.[135] Flexion teardrop fracture-dislocation is often associated with the anterior cord syndrome, defined as complete motor paralysis with loss of pain and temperature sensation but with sparing of the sense of position, vibration, and motion in the posterior column[136] (Fig. 8-14).

Flexion rotation fracture-dislocation. In conjunction with rotational forces, flexion may produce unilateral facet dislocation. The rotational force is directed about one facet, which acts as a pivot point, while flexion causes the contralateral facet to dislocate. This condition is characterized by mechanical stability, even though the posterior ligament complex and single facet joint are disrupted.[137] Descriptions of plain film findings include loss of superimposition of the facets at and superior to the injury in conjunction with mild anterior subluxation on lateral views as well as rotation of the spinous processes at and superior to the injury on anteroposterior

views.[33,120] Nevertheless, even slightly rotated cervical spine films can make definitive diagnosis difficult and multiplanar imaging with CT or MR may be needed to exclude flexion-rotational injuries with certainty. Typically, rotational fractures involve the tip of the superior articulating facet on the side toward which the rotational force is directed (Fig. 8-15).

Extension fracture-dislocation. Hyperextension trauma to the cervical spine results from severe anterior-posterior forces that drive the spinous and articular processes of the midcervical vertebrae together. The posterior column becomes a fulcrum separating the anterior vertebral body and subjacent intervertebral disk (Fig. 8-16) and resulting in dislocation or ventral fracture-dislocation with concomitant compression or fracture of the articular processes and disruption (and displacement) of the disk. With sufficient force the separation may rupture the anterior and posterior longitudinal ligaments, resulting in so-called extension teardrop fractures from anterior longitudinal ligament avulsion. Unlike the flexion teardrop, this injury is most often small, located at the anterior-inferior aspect of an upper cervical vertebra (C2), and not associated with posterior displacement.[138] The buckling of the *posterior longitudinal ligament* may decrease the anterior-posterior dimensions of the spinal

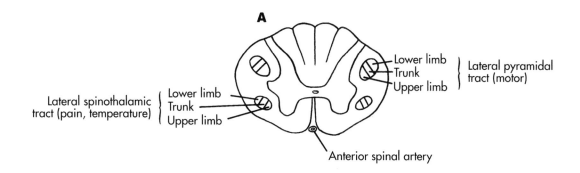

Fig. 8-14. A, Cross section of the cervical spinal cord demonstrating the relative positions of the ascending and descending fiber tracts. **B,** The affected portions of the cord in the so-called anterior cord syndrome.

Anterior Cord Syndrome

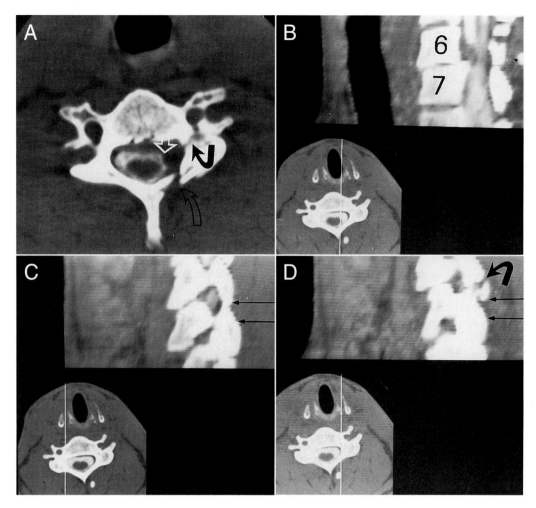

Fig. 8-15. Flexion-rotation injury. **A,** Axial CT scan through the level of the C6 pedicle in a patient with a flexion-rotation injury. As the patient's head and upper cervical spine were flexed over C6, additional right-to-left rotation forces were applied, causing the spine to pivot (and thus crush) the left C6 pedicle and facet while producing subluxation on the contralateral side. This scan demonstrates fractures of the left pedicle and lamina *(curved black arrows)* as well as a traumatic disk herniation *(open white arrow)* in the lateral recess on the left. **B,** Sagittal reconstruction of the postmyelogram CT demonstrates C6-C7 subluxation as well as a soft tissue mass anterior to the thecal sac. **C,** Right parasagittal reconstruction of this examination demonstrating subluxation of the right C6 and C7 facets *(arrows)*. **D,** Left parasagittal reconstruction demonstrating the fractured C6 facet *(curved arrow)* and distraction of the joint itself *(straight arrows)*, indicating instability. **E,** The midline sagittal 500 msec TR/17 msec TE image demonstrates a traumatic disk herniation at C6-7 with an anterior extradural mass immediately behind the body of C6 *(open arrow)*. Note that there has been disruption of the anterior longitudinal ligament at C6-7 *(curved arrow)*. **F,** A left parasagittal 500 msec TR/17 msec TE image again demonstrates the traumatic disk herniation at C6-7 *(open arrow)*. **G,** A parasagittal 500 msec TR/17 msec TE image at C6-7 on the left shows some distraction of the facet joints *(horizontal arrows)* as well as a fracture of the C6 facet *(curved arrow)* secondary to pivoting of the flexion-rotation force. **H,** An axial 500 msec TR/17 msec TE image through C6 demonstrates the fractured lamina *(open curved arrow)*, disrupted facet joint *(solid curved arrow)*, and traumatic disk herniation *(open straight arrow)*.

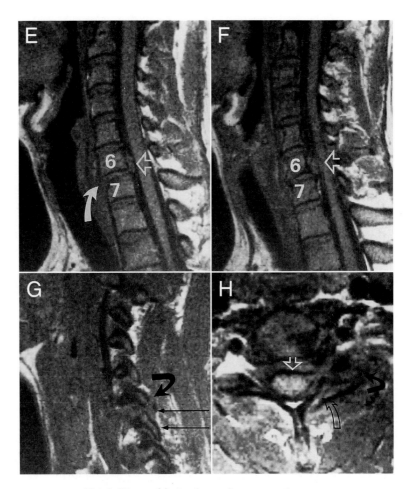

Fig. 8-15, cont'd. For legend see opposite page.

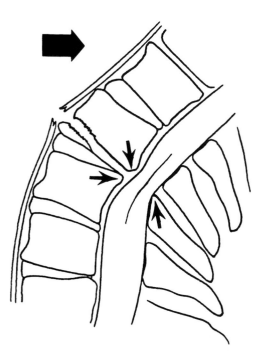

Fig. 8-16. Cervical extension injury. With the force of the injury directed from anterior to posterior *(thick horizontal arrow)* there can be disruption of the anterior longitudinal ligament and disk, with pinching of the spinal cord as the superior vertebral body is driven toward the posterior elements at the lower level *(smaller arrows).*

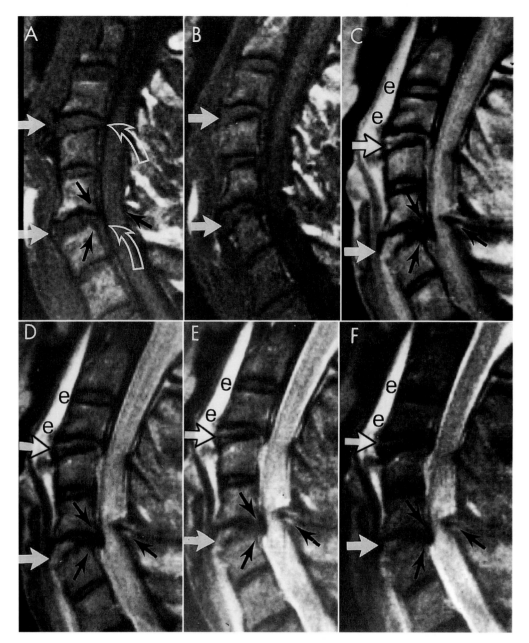

Fig. 8-17. A, 500 msec TR/17 msec TE sagittal image in a patient who sustained a cervical extension injury. Note the disruption of the anterior longitudinal ligament at multiple levels *(solid white arrows)* as well as the traumatic disk herniations *(open arrows)*. Pinching occurs at the C5-6 level *(black arrows)*. **B,** A parasagittal 500 msec TR/17 msec image shows the anterior longitudinal ligamentous disruption *(arrows)*. There is prevertebral soft tissue swelling as well. **C,** The midline sagittal 2000 msec TR/30 msec TE 7 mm image demonstrates ligamentous disruption *(white arrows)*, prevertebral edema *(e)*, and pinching at C5-6 *(black arrows)*. The canal compromise appears more serious on this 7 mm sagittal image, most likely because of partial volume effect from the lamina laterally. **D,** A 2000 msec TR/60 msec TE midline sagittal image shows similar findings, again with prevertebral edema *(e)*, ligamentous disruption *(white arrows)*, and some increase in signal intensity of the spinal cord at the site of compression *(black arrows)*. **E** and **F,** 2000 msec TR/90 and 120 msec TE images. Similar findings, although the increased signal intensity within the spinal cord secondary to edema is more obvious on these more T₂-weighted scans. The absence of any significant focal areas of decreased signal intensity indicates a relative absence of intramedullary hemorrhage (contusion) and a more favorable prognosis. Despite the initially severe neurologic deficit, this patient went on to recover significant function.

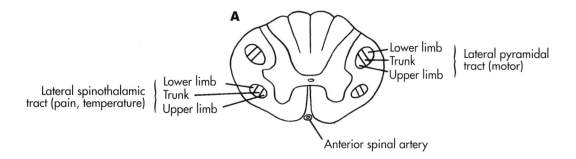

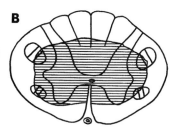

Fig. 8-18. A, Relative positions of the ascending and descending fiber tracts of the cervical spinal cord. **B,** The tracts involved in the central cord syndrome, frequently the result of a severe cervical extension injury. This may be aggravated by preexisting cervical spondylosis or posterior osteophytes.

Central Cord Syndrome

canal, producing simple compression or cord transection[139] (Fig. 8-17). This squeezing mechanism frequently causes the most extensive hemorrhage and necrosis to occur within the central part of the cord[140] (Fig. 8-18). Ironically, although such injuries can be associated with significant neurologic deficit, the musculoskeletal trauma is often radiographically nascent. Goldberg et al.[50] have described their experience using MRI for the evaluation of adult hyperextension injuries. Common findings include prevertebral hematoma in association with anterior longitudinal ligament and disk disruption, preexisting spondylosis, and cord contusion-concussion.[50]

Significant extension injury has also been reported in neonates,[141] producing acute hemorrhage or hemorrhagic cord necrosis even in the absence of fracture (Fig. 8-19). Avulsion of the spinal cord during vaginal delivery is a well-documented, though uncommon, obstetric complication. Over 75% of these cases occur with breech presentation. With fetal hyperextension and breech presentation, the incidence of avulsion of the cord is greater than 20%.[142-144] The prevalence of injury to the lower cervical and upper thoracic area is believed to be related to the relative resistance of the cervical area to stretching enlargement, leaving most of the stretch to be taken up by the more attenuated thoracic region.[145] The occurrence of cord transection during cephalic delivery involves torsion of the fetus in

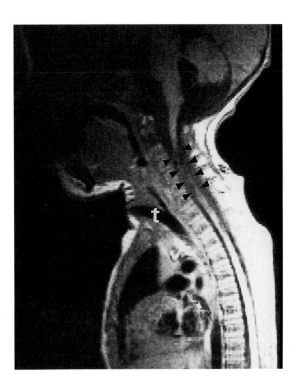

Fig. 8-19. An example of extension birth injury demonstrated on this 500 msec TR/17 msec TE midline sagittal image. There appears to be complete transection of the cervical spinal cord *(arrowheads).* Note the tracheostomy tube in place *(t).*

addition to traction, and the resulting injury is primarily in the upper cervical segments of the cord.[146] Mathis et al.[147] have described the MR findings in such patients. Characteristic of cord avulsion, there was associated dural interruption, with approximately 1 cm separation of the attenuated adjacent ends of the thecal sac, and fibrous bands (scarring) bridging the defect on T_2-weighted images.

Extension-rotation trauma. Rotation in conjunction with extension can cause unilateral facet and/or pillar fractures. These common injuries (3% to 11% of all cervical fractures) may be difficult to detect on conventional radiographs. The facet fractures are particularly troublesome since they often are comminuted and involve the neural foramina to produce cervical radiculopathy.[148]

Thoracic spine

Axial loading injuries. In general, because of the stability provided by the rib cage, costovertebral ligaments, and intervertebral disks, the thoracic spine is resistant to all but the most violent trauma.[149] As mentioned previously, injuries are more commonly seen in the upper cervical spine or thoracolumbar junction, although between T2 and T10 flexion and axial loading are more common. Compressive (axial loading) forces secondary to vertical impact (e.g., diving or jumping accidents) are often absorbed by the thoracic vertebral bodies, resulting in vertical or burst fractures (Figs. 8-20 and 8-21). Ligaments are typically intact. Even in the presence of fracture or fracture-dislocation resulting from a severe flexion injury, the upper thoracic spine remains quite stable by virtue of its supporting structures and also because its sagittally placed facets limit the potential for rotational forces to produce trauma.

Lumbosacral spine

Flexion-compression injuries. Unlike the upper thoracic spine, which is braced by adjacent ribs, the thoracolumbar junction acts as a fulcrum for spinal motion and is thus susceptible to unstable traumatic injury. Whereas rotational components of injury may be minimized by the thick sagittally oriented facets, flexion (or flexion-dislocation) and axial loading are common (Figs. 8-21 to 8-23). These forces frequently combine to produce flexion-compression injury or the so-called "burst fractures," which are significant for (1) motion instability and (2) a predisposition toward displacing fracture fragments and causing cord compromise respectively[104,106] (Figs. 8-21 to 8-23). AP and lateral radiographs supply adequate information for screening such injuries. Some 40% of the injuries incur neurologic deficit, however; and if compromise of the canal by displaced fragments or instability due to posterior ligament disruption is suspected, CT or MR may be invaluable for defining the full extent of the lesion.[150]

Another common, purely flexion, lumbar spinal injury associated with rapid-deceleration motor vehicle accidents is the so-called "seat-belt" or "Chance" fracture. Hyperflexion occurs at the level of the seat belt while the upper lumbar spine experiences tensile loading. The result is an injury that, at minimum, manifests as posterior ligamentous disruption but may extend as a horizontal fracture through both the anterior and the posterior elements (Fig. 8-24) with posterior instability or facet subluxation.[151,152]

Sacral stress fractures. MR is frequently employed for the diagnostic evaluation of low back pain, often in older patients predisposed to degenerative disk disease as well as metastatic neoplasm. Of particular interest in

Text continued on p. 345.

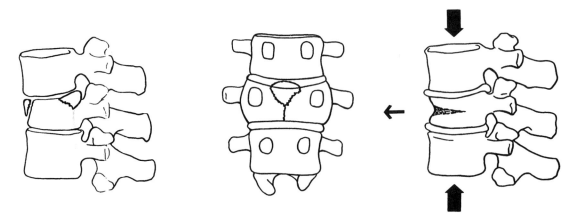

Fig. 8-20. Axial loading injury. With the application of vertical or axial force the nucleus pulposus above is driven through the endplate and into the vertebral body below, resulting in a so-called burst fracture. Typically this produces fragmentation of the superior endplate, often with compromise of the vertebral canal.

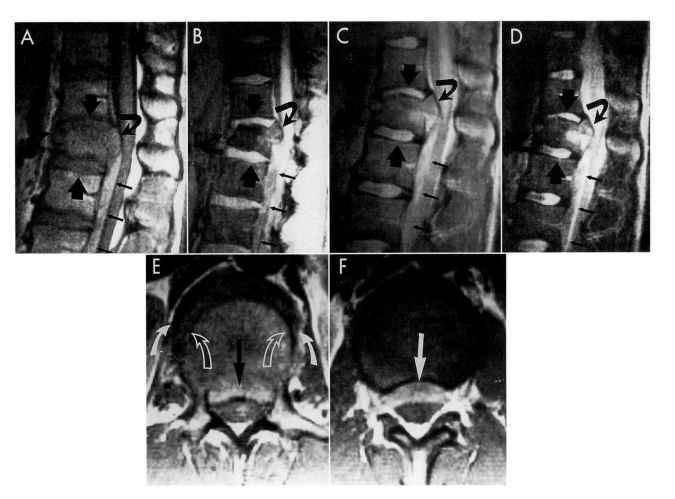

Fig. 8-21. A, A 500 msec TR/17 msec TE sagittal image at the thoracolumbar junction following axial loading *(vertical arrows)*. Note the displaced fracture fragments *(curved arrows)* as well as the soft tissue immediately anterior to the canal, probably an epidural hematoma *(thin straight arrows)*. **B,** FLASH 60-degree midline sagittal image following axial loading *(vertical arrows)*. Again, note the displaced fracture fragments *(curved arrows)* as well as an anterior epidural mass *(small straight arrows)*. The low signal intensity of the hemorrhage on this gradient echo scan is probably related to a magnetic susceptibility effect. **C** and **D,** 2000 msec TR/30 and 120 msec TE images. With more T_2 weighting the signal intensity from the fractured vertebral body increases compared to the relatively low signal on the T_1-weighted image. This is characteristic of acute fractures. Again, note the displaced fragment *(curved arrow)* and epidural hematoma. **E,** Axial 500 msec TR/17 msec TE image through the region of the fragment. The central fragment is retropulsed *(black arrow)*. The outer dark ring represents the anterior longitudinal ligament *(curved white arrow)*, the inner ring the cortex of the superior endplate *(open arrows)*. **F,** An axial 500 msec TR/17 msec TE image through a lower intervertebral disk continues to demonstrate what was believed to be an epidural hematoma *(solid arrow)*.

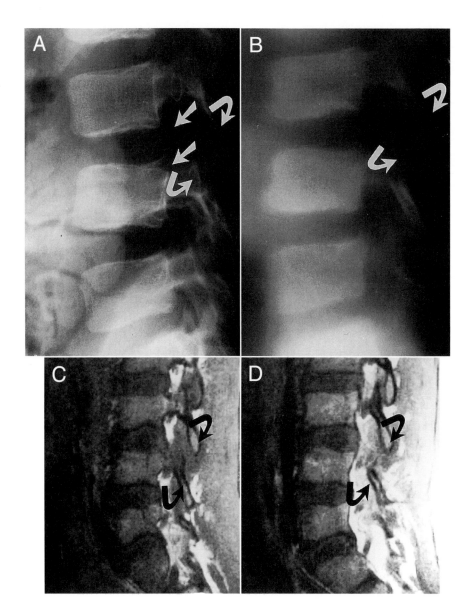

Fig. 8-22. For legend see opposite page.

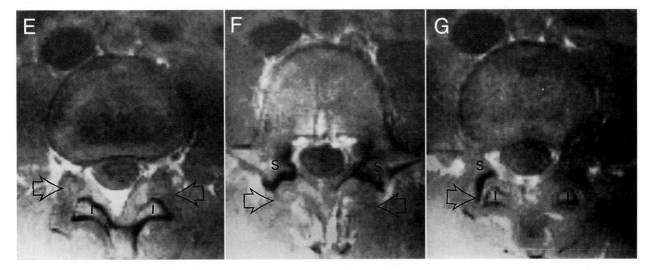

Fig. 8-22. A, Lateral radiograph of the lumbar spine in a patient with a flexion-dislocation injury. Note the separation of the intervertebral disk posteriorly *(straight arrows)* as well as the distraction of the facet joints posteriorly *(curved arrows)*. These injuries result from the same forces and produce defects analogous to those observed in the cervical spine. **B,** A parasagittal tomogram of the lumbar spine demonstrates the marked distraction of facet joints at this level *(curved arrows)*. **C** and **D,** Parasagittal 500 msec TR/17 msec TE images of the lumbar spine show widely separated facet joints at the L3-4 level bilaterally *(curved arrows)*. **E,** An axial 500 msec TR/17 msec TE image through the L3-4 intervertebral disk demonstrates the inferior facet *(I)* of L3 posteriorly but no superior facets of L4 articulating with it anteriorly, only soft tissue and hemorrhage *(open arrows)*. **F,** An axial 500 msec TR/17 msec TE image through the upper L4 vertebral body shows the inferior facets of L3 barely articulating with the superior facets of L4 *(S)*. Note that the joint is just barely maintained *(open arrows)*. **G,** An axial 500 msec TR/17 msec TE image through the L4 vertebral body demonstrates the superior facets of L4 *(S)*, which no longer articulate with the distracted inferior facets of L3 *(I)*. This gives the appearance of the so-called "naked facets" *(open arrows)*.

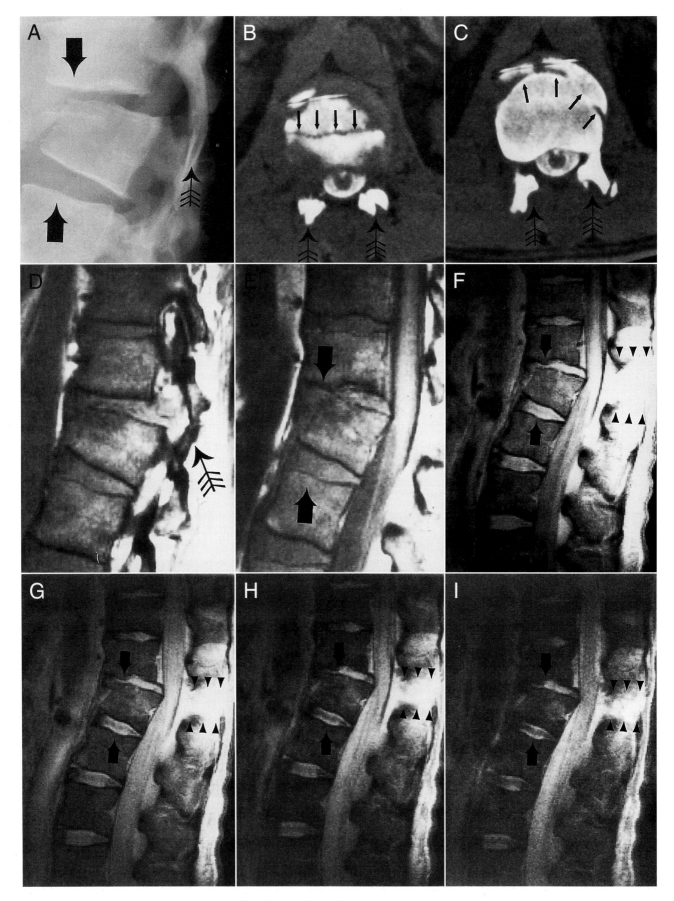

Fig. 8-23. For legend see opposite page.

Fig. 8-23. A, Lateral radiograph from a flexion-dislocation injury at the thoracolumbar junction. There is mild compression of the L1 vertebral body *(solid arrows)* as well as distraction of the facets posteriorly *(tailed arrow)*. **B,** The axial CT scan following a myelogram at the level of the T12-L1 disk demonstrates a horizontal fracture of the endplate *(arrows)* and minimal articulation of the facets as well as facet malalignment *(tailed arrows)*. **C,** A more inferior axial scan demonstrates the naked facets of L1 *(tailed arrows)* and the adjacent endplate fractures anteriorly *(arrows)*. **D,** A parasagittal 500 msec TR/17 msec TE image shows malalignment and dislocation of the facet joints *(tailed arrow)*. **E,** Midline sagittal 500 msec TR/17 msec TE. Note the dislocation and compression at T12-L1 *(arrows)*. **F** to **I,** 2000 msec TR/30, 60, 90, and 120 msec TE images, respectively, demonstrate vertical compression and dislocation of T12-L1 *(arrows)*. More important in these T₂-weighted studies, however, is the ability to detect disruption of the interspinous ligaments posteriorly *(arrowheads)* with increasing T₂ weighting.

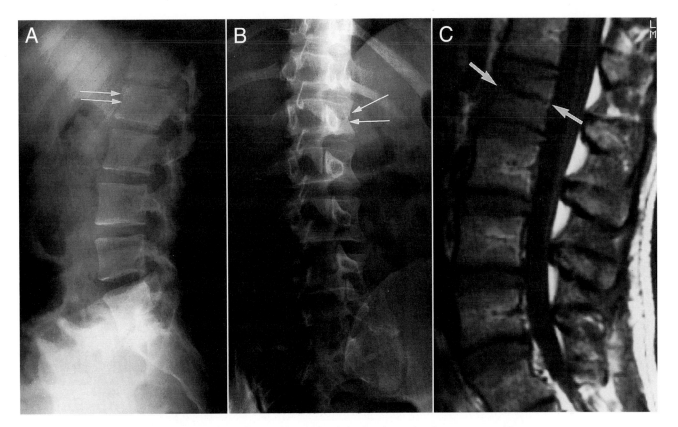

Fig. 8-24. A, Lateral plain film radiograph of the lumbar spine in a 19-year-old man status posttrauma demonstrating a slight step-off of the anterior cortical margin of the L1 vertebral body *(arrows)*. **B,** The RAO oblique examination, likewise, demonstrates a small fracture along the anterolateral margin of L1. **C,** A T₁-weighted 500 msec TR/17 msec TE sagittal spin-echo pulse image of the lumbar spine demonstrates generalized signal loss from L1 as well as a Chance fracture through the midportion breaking the anterior cortical margin *(arrows)*.

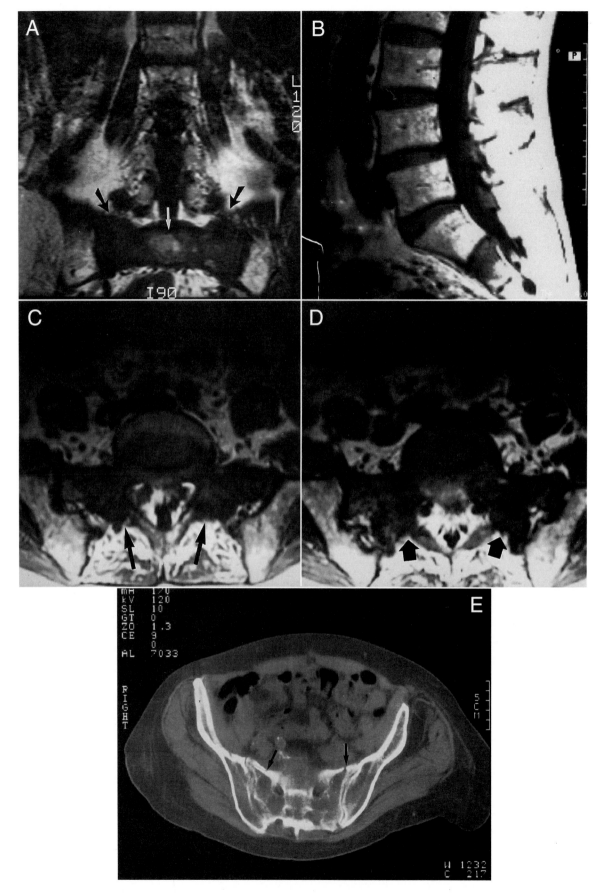

Fig. 8-25. For legend see opposite page.

Fig. 8-25. A, Coronal T_1-weighted scout of the lumbar spine (500 msec TR/15 msec TE) demonstrating normal signal intensity from the sacral promontory *(white arrow)* with signal loss diffusely from the sacral ala *(black arrows)*. **B,** The midline sagittal T_1-weighted of the lumbar spine is essentially normal. **C** and **D,** Serial axial T_1-weighted scans (500 msec TR/15 msec TE) of the S1 vertebral body demonstrate, again, generalized signal loss from the sacral ala with a suggestion of mild irregularity and a possible fracture line. **E,** Confirmatory CT scan showing bilateral stress fractures of the sacrum *(arrow)*.

---

the differential diagnosis of the latter is the MR appearance of insufficiency fractures of the sacrum, which have a similar clinical presentation. Such lesions typically occur as the result of chronic axial loading in the presence of senile osteoporosis, rheumatoid arthritis, radiation therapy, or chronic corticosteroid treatment. There is often no history of overt closed spinal trauma. T_1-weighted sequences demonstrate bands of decreased signal, usually paralleling the sacral aspect of the sacroiliac joints and at times occurring as a horizontal band across the vertebral body (Fig. 8-25). (A similar pattern of uptake has been reported on nuclear medicine bone scans.) Lee and Yao[153] have described a temporal pattern related to the appearance on T_2-weighted studies of a stress fracture that had high signal at the same location but was usually more prominent within 3 weeks of the onset of symptoms. Brahme et al.[154] have also described low signal involving the sacral and ileal aspects of the sacroiliac joints on T_1-weighted scans in such patients.

LATE COMPLICATIONS

The sequelae or complications of cord contusion (particularly in the cervical spine) may result in posttraumatic myelopathy.[155,156] Potential etiologies include (1) narrowing of the spinal canal (e.g., cervical spondylosis) with cord compression, (2) secondary arachnoid adhesions, (3) cystic degeneration leading to syringomyelia, and (4) late-onset vascular compromise. For a patient who has incurred spinal cord injury with permanent neurologic deficit, the acquisition of new and debilitating symptoms can be catastrophic. This clinical entity has been termed posttraumatic progressive myelopathy, and it may be classified as posttraumatic "cystic myelopathy" (i.e., syringohydromyelia) or a noncystic lesion such as myelomalacia.[157] The distinction is significant inasmuch as the cystic form of myelopathy may be remediable by surgical shunting.[157-161]

In 1966 Barnett et al.[162] drew attention to a progressive posttraumatic spinal cord syndrome that, on the basis of clinical presentation and surgical findings, closely resembled syringomyelia. Numerous clinical series[163-166] have provided an estimated incidence of 2%

or less in all posttraumatic spinal cord injuries. Patients typically present with spinothalamic symptoms (i.e., pain and/or sensory loss) that occur months or years following the injury. This cystic degeneration does not appear to be related to the site or severity (incomplete or complete) of the original cord lesion[157-166] (Fig. 8-26). Cysts may occur either above or below the level of the lesion.[159]

The exact mechanism of posttraumatic cyst formation and extension is not known. McLean et al.[167] have suggested that at the time of traumatic contusion a necrotic blood-filled space develops within the spinal cord that in the course of normal healing results in a cavity lined with glial cells. Alternatively, posttraumatic arachnoid adhesions at the site of injury may so tether the cord that it becomes subject to unusual stresses by common CSF pressure changes associated with Valsalva maneuvers, coughing, sneezing, or motion above or below the site of injury.[161,166,167]

Until recently, delayed high-resolution CT scanning with water-soluble contrast material was the examination of choice for preoperative detection of posttraumatic spinal cord cystic myelopathy.[160,161,168] It could determine the presence of cysts within enlarged or atrophic spinal cords, locate them dorsally or ventrally above or below the lesion, and help determine whether they were single or multiple.[160,161,168] Unfortunately, delayed-contrast CT suffers from its invasiveness and nonspecificity (i.e., inability to distinguish some spinal cord cysts from myelomalacia).[157,160,161]

More recently, T_1- and T_2-weighted MR images have been shown[157,169,170] to be the examination of choice for evaluating posttraumatic myelopathy. Yamashita et al.[170] described five major MR patterns to the chronic (mean 13.6 months ± 9) spinal cord injury: (1) normal signal on T_1- and T_2-weighted images, (2) normal cord signal on T_1-weighted images with high signal on T_2 (seen in 83% of patients with cord compression), (3) low signal on T_1-weighted scans with high signal on T_2, (4) cord atrophy, and (5) syrinx cavitation with low signal on T_1 and high signal on T_2 studies. When correlated with neurologic dysfunction, patients with normal cord signal had minimal deficit (low on T_1, high on T_2) and

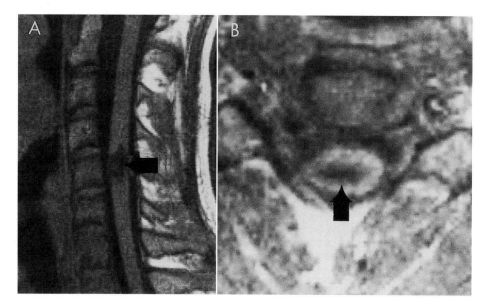

Fig. 8-26. A, Sagittal and, **B,** axial 500 msec TR/17 msec TE images in a patient with previous cervical spinal trauma. There was no evidence of bony disruption or fracture at the time of the original injury, which rendered the patient quadriparetic. A neurologic deficit persisted, however, and this subsequent MR examination demonstrated a focal cystic region within the spinal cord *(arrow).*

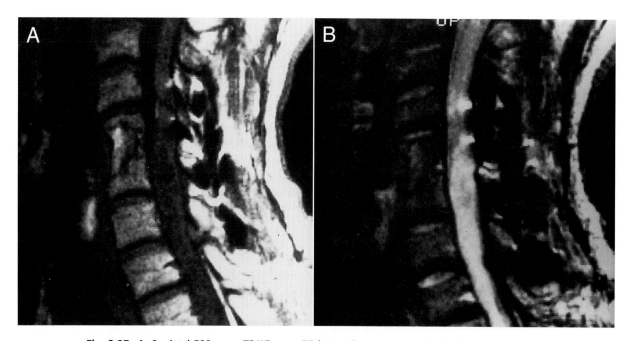

Fig. 8-27. A, Sagittal 500 msec TR/17 msec TE image in a woman who had a remote cervical spinal cord injury. She underwent an anterior and posterior interbody fusion (wiring) procedure. Note the cystic area within the spinal cord immediately posterior to the fusion. **B,** An axial 500 msec TR/17 msec TE image through this region demonstrates what appears to be a cystic region within the spinal cord. In the presence of worsening clinical symptoms there was a clinical suspicion of posttraumatic syringomyelia. **C,** On this 2000 msec TR/30 msec image, however, it can be seen that the area of traumatic cord damage has increased signal intensity, consistent with the diagnosis of myelomalacia rather than syringomyelia.

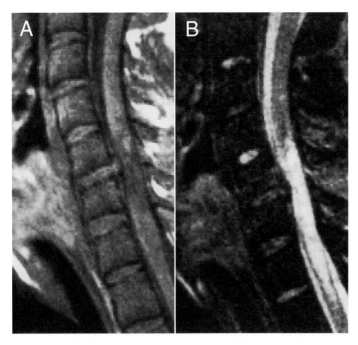

Fig. 8-28. A, 500 msec TR/17 msec TE image in a patient who has sustained flexion-dislocation injury remotely at C5-6. Note the persistent cord compression by the traumatic disk. There also are ill-defined areas of low signal intensity within the spinal cord in this region. **B,** Sagittal 2000 msec TR/120 msec TE image through the region of chronic cord damage demonstrates increased signal intensity, consistent with the diagnosis of myelomalacia.

mild neurologic dysfunction; patients with a spinal cord showing low signal on T_1 and high signal on T_2 had the worst prognosis.

Perhaps MR's greatest advantage is its ability to distinguish myelomalacia from treatable posttraumatic cysts. On T_1-weighted images both myelomalacia and posttraumatic syringes are of low signal intensity with respect to the surrounding cord parenchyma. On spin-density (short TE, long TR) images, true posttraumatic syringes continue to have a low signal with respect to the cord (paralleling CSF), whereas myelomalacia is isointense or of higher signal compared to normal cord parenchyma (Fig. 8-27). On T_2-weighted images both posttraumatic cysts and myelomalacia may have hyperintense signal with respect to normal cord parenchyma but the syringes should follow CSF signal on all pulse sequences[157,169] (Fig. 8-28). Occasionally, sagittal and axial imaging will fail to confirm this "characteristic" progression of signal-intensity changes because of CSF pulsation–induced signal loss seen in some large cysts on T_2-weighted images.[171] Such cyst fluid motion may also be recognized on single-slice axial gradient echo scans by the flow-related enhancement it produces.[171] Absence of these motion-induced signal changes following surgical shunting could have prognostic significance (i.e., indicate successful decompression).

REFERENCES

1. Kraus JF, Franti CE, Riggins RS, et al: Incidence of traumatic spinal cord lesions. *J Chron Dis* 1975;28:471-492.
2. Bracken MB, Freeman DH, Hellenbrand K: Incidence of acute traumatic hospitalized spinal cord injury in the United States, 1970-1977. *Am J Epidemiol* 1981;113:615-622.
3. Anderson DW, McLauren RL (eds): The national head and spinal cord injury survey. *J Neurosurg* 1980;53(suppl):S1-S43.
4. Young JS, et al: *Spinal cord injury statistics systems.* Phoenix, Good Samaritan Medical Center, 1982.
5. Denis F: The three column spine and its significance in the classification of acute thoracolumbar spinal injuries. *Spine* 1983;8:817-831.
6. Holdsworth FW: Fractures, dislocations and fracture-dislocations of the spine. *J Bone Joint Surg [Am]* 1970;52:1534-1551.
7. White AA, Panjabi MM: *Clinical biomechanics of the spine.* Philadelphia, Lippincott, 1978.
8. White AA, Southwick WO, Panjabi MM: Clinical instability in the lower cervical spine: a review of past and current concepts. *Spine* 1976;1:15-27.
9. Saul TB, Ducker TB: Treatment of spinal cord injury. In Cowley RA, Trump B (eds): *Cellular injury in shock, anoxia, and ischemia: pathophysiology, prevention, and treatment.* Baltimore, Williams & Wilkins, 1981.
10. De La Torre JA: Spinal cord injury: review of basic and applied research. *Spine* 1981;6:315-335.

11. Guttman L: *Spinal cord injuries: comprehensive management and research.* Oxford, Blackwell, 1973.

12. Dohrmann GJ, Wagner FC, Buey PC: The microvasculature in transitory traumatic paraplegia: an election microscopic study in the monkey. *J Neurosurg* 1971;35:263-271.

13. Dohrmann GJ, Wick KM, Buey PC: Blood flow patterns in the intrinsic vessels of the spinal cord following contusion. *Trans Am Neurol Assoc* 1972;97:189-192.

14. Dohrmann GJ, Wick KM, Buey PC: Spinal cord blood flow patterns in experimental traumatic paraplegia. *J Neurosurg* 1973;38:52-58.

15. Jellinger K: Neuropathology of cord injuries. In Vinken PJ, Bruyn GW (eds): *Handbook of clinical neurology,* vol 25, Amsterdam, Elsevier, 1976, pp 43-121.

16. Ducker TB, Assenmacher D: Microvascular response to experimental spinal cord trauma. *Surg Forum* 1969;20:428-430.

17. Ducker TB, Kindt GW, Kempe LG: Pathological findings in acute experimental spinal cord trauma. *J Neurosurg* 1971;35:700-708.

18. Assenmacher DR, Ducker TB: Experimental traumatic paraplegia. The vascular and pathological changes seen in reversible and irreversible spinal cord lesions. *J Bone Joint Surg [Am]* 1971;53:671-680.

19. Wolman L: The disturbances of circulation in traumatic paraplegia in acute and late stages. A pathological study. *Paraplegia* 1965;2:231-236.

20. Scarff JE: Injuries of the vertebral column and spinal cord. In Brock S (ed): *Injuries of the brain and spinal cord and their coverings,* ed 4. London, Cassell, 1960, pp 530-589.

21. Tarlov IM: *Acute spinal cord compression.* Springfield Ill, Charles C Thomas, 1957.

22. Bohlman HH, Bahniuk E, Raskulinecz G, Field G: Mechanical factors affecting recovery from incomplete spinal cord injury: a preliminary report. *Johns Hopkins Med J* 1979;145:115-125.

23. Tarlov IM: Acute spinal cord compression paralysis. *J Neurosurg* 1972;36:10-20.

24. Doppman JL, Girton M: Angiographic study of the effect of laminectomy in the presence of acute anterior epidural masses. *J Neurosurg* 1976;45:195-202.

25. Hukuda S, Wilson CB: Experimental cervical myelopathy. *J Neurosurg* 1972;37:631-652.

26. Frankel HL, Hancock DO, Hyslop G, et al: The value of posteral reduction in the initial management of closed injuries of the spine with paraplegia and tetraplegia. *Paraplegia* 1969;7:179-192.

27. Lucas JT, Ducker TB: Motor classification of spinal cord injuries with mobility, morbidity, and recovery indices. *Am Surg* 1979;45(3):151-158.

28. Hackney DM: Denominators of spinal cord injury. *Radiology* 1990;177:18-20.

29. Bracken MB, Shepard MJ, Collins WF, et al: A randomized, controlled trial of methylprednisolone or naloxone in the treatment of acute spinal-cord injury. *N Engl J Med* 1990;322(20):1405-1411.

30. Vandemark RM: Radiology of the cervical spine in trauma patients: practice pitfalls and recommendations for improving efficiency and communication. *AJR* 1990;155:465-472.

31. Bachulis BL, Long WB, Hynes GD, Johnson MC: Clinical indications for cervical spine radiographs in the traumatized patient. *Am J Surg* 1987;153:473-478.

32. Mirvis SE, Diaconis JN, Chirico PA, et al: Protocol-driven radiologic evaluation of suspected cervical spine injury: efficacy study. *Radiology* 1989;170:831-834.

33. Wales LR, Knopp RK, Morishima MS: Recommendations for evaluation of the acutely injured cervical spine: A clinical radiologic algorithm. *Ann Emerg Med* 1980;9:422-428.

34. Bohlman HH: Acute fractures and dislocations of the cervical spine: an analysis of three hundred hospitalized patients and a review of the literature. *J Bone Joint Surg [Am]* 1979;61:1119-1142.

35. Streitwieser DR, Knopp R, Wales LR, et al: Accuracy of standard radiographic views in detecting cervical spine fractures. *Ann Emerg Med* 1983;12:538-542.

36. Penning L: Prevertebral hematoma in cervical spine injury: Incidence and etiologic significance. *AJR* 1981;136:553-561.

37. Templeton PA, Young JW, Mirvis SE, Buddemeyer EU: The value of retropharyngeal soft tissue measurements in trauma of the adult cervical spine. *Skeletal Radiol* 1987;16:98-104.

38. Brant-Zawadzki M, Miller EM, Federle MP: CT in the evaluation of spine trauma. *AJR* 1981;136:369-375.

39. Donovan Post MJ, Green BA, Quencer RM, et al: The value of computed tomography in spinal trauma. *Spine* 1982;7:417-431.

40. Keene JS, Goletz TH, Lilleas F, et al: Diagnosis of vertebral fractures: a comparison of conventional radiography convention tomography and computed axial tomography. *J Bone Joint Surg [Am]* 1982;64:586-594.

41. McAfee PC, Yuan HA, Fredrickson BE, Lubicky JP: The value of computed tomography in thoracolumbar fractures. *J Bone Joint Surg [Am]* 1982;65:461-473.

42. Kilcoyne RF, Mack LA, King HA, et al: Thoracolumbar spine injuries associated with vertical plunges: reappraisals with computed tomography. *Radiology* 1983;146:137-140.

43. Handel SF, Lee Y: Computed tomography of spinal fractures. *Radiol Clin North Am* 1981;19:69-89.

44. Cooper PR, Cohen W: Evaluation of cervical spinal cord injuries with metrizamide myelography-CT scanning. *J Neurosurg* 1984;61:281-289.

45. Faerber EN, Wolpert SM, Scott RM, et al: Computed tomography of spinal fractures. *J Comput Assist Tomogr* 1979;3:657-661.

46. Kalfas I, Wilberger J, Goldberg A, Prostko ER: Magnetic resonance imaging in acute spinal cord trauma. *Neurosurgery* 1988;23:295-299.

47. Goldberg AL, Rothfus WE, Deeb ZL, et al: The impact of magnetic resonance on the diagnostic evaluation of acute cervicothoracic spinal trauma. *Skeletal Radiol* 1988;17:89-95.

48. McArdle CB, Crofford MJ, Mirfakhraee M, et al: Surface coil MR of spinal trauma: preliminary experience. *AJNR* 1986;7:885-893.

49. Manelfe C: Magnetic resonance imaging of the spinal cord. *Diagn Intervent Radiol* 1989;1:3-14.

50. Goldberg AL, Rothfus WE, Deeb ZL, et al: Hyperextension injuries of the cervical spine: magnetic resonance findings. *Skeletal Radiology* 1989;18:283-288.

51. Mirvis SE, Geisler FH, Jelinek JJ, et al: Acute cervical spine trauma: evaluation with 1.5 T MR imaging. *Radiology* 1988;166:807-816.

52. Tarr RW, Drolshagen LF, Kerner TC, et al: MR imaging of recent spinal trauma. *J Comput Assist Tomogr* 1987;11:412-417.

53. Flanders AE, Schaefer DM, Doan HD, et al: Acute cervical spine trauma: correlation of MR imaging findings with degree of neurologic deficit. *Radiology* 1990;177:25-33.

54. Kulkarni MV, McArdle CB, Kopanicky D, et al: Acute spinal cord injury: MR imaging at 1.5 T. *Radiology* 1987;164:837-843.

55. Kulkarni MV, Bondurant FJ, Rose SL, Narayana PA: 1.5 tesla magnetic resonance imaging of acute spinal trauma. *Radiographics* 1988;8:1059-1082.

56. Baker LL, Goodman SB, Perkash I, et al: Benign versus pathologic compression fractures of vertebral bodies: assessment with conventional spin-echo, chemical shift, STIR MR imaging. *Radiology* 1990;174:495-502.

57. Beers GJ, Raque GH, Wagner GG, et al: MR imaging in acute cervical spine trauma. *J Comput Assist Tomogr* 1988;12:755-761.

58. Emery SE, Pathria MN, Wilber RG, et al: Magnetic resonance imaging of posttraumatic spinal ligament injury. *J Spinal Disorders* 1989;2:229-233.

59. Larson SJ, Holst RA, Hemmy DC, et al: Lateral extracavitary approach to traumatic lesions of the thoracic and lumbar spine. *J Neurosurg* 1976;45:628-637.

60. Brodkey JS, Miller CF, Harmody RM: The syndrome of acute cervical spinal cord injury revisited. *Surg Neurol* 1980;14:251-257.

61. Marshall LF, Knowlton S, Garfin SR, et al: Deterioration following spinal cord injury: a multicenter study. *J Neurosurg* 1987;66:400-404.

62. Dolan EJ, Tator CH, Endrenyi L: The value of decompression for acute experimental spinal cord compression injury. *J Neurosurg* 1980;53:749-755.

63. Tarlov IM, Klinger H: Spinal cord compression studies. II. Time limits for recovery after acute compression in dogs. *Arch Neurol Psychiatr* 1954;71:271-290.

64. Tarlov IM: Spinal cord compression studies. III. Time limits for recovery after gradual compression in dogs. *Arch Neurol Psychiatr* 1954;71:588-597.

65. Maynard FM, Reynolds GG, Fountain S, et al: Neurological prognosis after traumatic quadriplegia. *J Neurosurg* 1979;50:611-616.

66. Harris P, Karmi MZ, McClermont E, et al: The prognosis of patients sustaining severe cervical spine injury. *Paraplegia* 1980;18:324-330.

67. Wagner FC, Chehrazi B: Early decompression and neurological outcome in acute cervical spinal cord injuries. *J Neurosurg* 1982;56:699-705.

68. Hackney DB, Asato R, Joseph PM, et al: Hemorrhage and edema in acute spinal cord compression: demonstration by MR imaging. *Radiology* 1986;161:387-390.

69. Schweitzer ME, Cervilla V, Resnick D: Acute cervical trauma: correlation of MR imaging findings with neurological deficit. *Radiology* 1991;179:287-288.

70. Schaefer DM, Flanders AE, Osterholm JL, Northrup BE: Prognostic significance of magnetic resonance imaging in the acute phase of cervical spine injury. *J Neurosurg* 1992;76:218-223.

71. Schouman-Claeys E, Frija G, Cuenod CA, et al: MR imaging of acute spinal cord injury: results of an experimental study in dogs. *AJNR* 1990;11:959-965.

72. Brant-Zawadzki M, Post MJD: Trauma. In Newton TH, Potts DG (eds): *Computed tomography of the spine and spinal cord: modern neuroradiology,* vol 1. San Anselmo Calif, Clavadel, 1983, pp 149-186.

73. Betz RR, Gelman AJ, DeFilipp GJ, et al: Magnetic resonance imaging (MRI) in the evaluation of spinal cord injured children and adolescents. *Paraplegia* 1987;25:92-99.

74. New PF, Rosen BR, Brady TJ, et al: Potential hazards and artifacts of ferromagnetic and nonferromagnetic surgical and dental materials and devices in nuclear magnetic resonance imaging. *Radiology* 1983;147:139-148.

75. Shellock FG, Slimp G: Halo vest for cervical spine fixation during MR imaging. *AJR* 1990;154:631-632.

76. Chan RC, Schweigel JF, Thompson GB: Halo-thoracic brace immobilization in 188 patients with acute cervical spine injuries. *J Neurosurg* 1983;58:508-515.

77. Letters to the Editor. *Radiology* 1990;177:586-587.

78. Clayman DA, Marakami ME, Vines FS: Compatibility of cervical spine braces with MR imaging: a study of nine nonferrous devices. *AJNR* 1990;11:385-390.

79. McArdle CB, Wright JW, Prevost WJ, et al: MR imaging of the acutely injured patient with cervical traction. *Radiology* 1986;159:273-274.

80. Roth JL, Nugent M, Gray JE, et al: Patient monitoring during magnetic resonance imaging. *Anesthesiology* 1985;62:80-83.

81. Higgins CB, Lanzer P, Stark D, et al: Imaging by nuclear magnetic resonance in patients with chronic ischemic heart diseases. *Circulation* 1984;69:523-531.

82. McArdle CB, Nicholas DA, Richardson CJ, Amparo EG: Monitoring of the neonate undergoing MR imaging: technical considerations. *Radiology* 1986;159:223-226.

83. Geiger RS, Cascorbi HF: Anesthesia in an NMR scanner. *Anesth Analg* 1984;63:622-623.

84. Dunn V, Coffman CE, McGowan JE, Erhardt JC: Mechanical ventilation during magnetic resonance imaging. *Magn Reson Imaging* 1985;3:169-172.

85. Mirvis SE, Borg V, Belzberg H: MR imaging of ventilator-dependent patients: preliminary experience. *AJR* 1987;149:845-846.

86. Wannamaker GJ: Spinal cord injuries: a review of early treatment in consecutive cases during the Korean conflict. *J Neurosurg* 1954;11:517-524.

87. Jacobson SA, Bors E: Spinal cord injury in Vietnamese combat. *Paraplegia* 1970;7:263-281.

88. Klaw R: Beitrag zur pathologischen Anatomie der Verletzungen des Rückenmarks mit besonderer Berücksichtigung der Rückenmarkskontusion. Ein Vergleich zwischen Rückenmarks-und Hirnverletzungen. *Arch Psychiatr Nervemkr* 1948;180:206-270.

89. Yashon D, Jane JA, White RJ: Prognosis and management of spinal cord and cauda equina bullet injury in 65 civilians. *J Neurosurg* 1970;32:163-170.

90. Lipschitz R: Stab wounds of the spinal cord. In Vinken PJ, Bruyn GW (eds): *Handbook of clinical neurology,* vol 25. Amsterdam, Elsevier, 1976, pp 197-207.

91. Brown-Sequard CE: Lectures on the physiology and pathology of the nervous system and on the treatment of organic nervous affections. *Lancet* 1968;2:539, 659, 755, 821.

92. Wolman L: The neuropathology of traumatic paraplegia. A critical historical review. *Paraplegia* 1954;2:233-251.

93. Elsburg CA. *Ann Surg* 1919;69:239. Quoted by Wolman L: *Paraplegia* 1964;1:233-251.

94. Marburg O: Zur Pathologie der Kriegsschädigungen des Rückenmarks. *Arch Neurol Inst Univ Wien* 1919;1:498-556.

95. Wolf SM: Delayed traumatic myelopathy following transfixation of the spinal cord by a knife blade. *J Neurosurg* 1973;38:221-225.

96. Finck PA: Ballistic and forensic pathologic aspects of missile wounds. Conversion between Anglo-American and metri-system units. *Milit Med* 1965;130:545-569.

97. Smith AS, Hurst GC, Duerk JL, Diaz PJ: MR of ballistic materials: imaging artifacts and potential hazards. *AJNR* 1991;12:567-572.

98. Kelly WM, Paglen PG, Pearson JA, et al: Ferromagnetism of intraocular foreign body causing unilateral blindness after MR study. *AJNR* 1986;7:243-245.

99. Adams AE: Über Grundlagen und klinische Beurteilung der stumpfen Traumen des Rückenmarks. *Nervenartz* 1969;40:579-585.

100. Wilcox NE, Staufner EF, Nickel VL: A statistical analysis of 423 consecutive patients admitted to the spinal cord injury center Rancho Los Amigos Hospital. *Paraplegia* 1970;8:27-35.

101. Hardy AG, Rossier AG: Tetra- und Paraplegie. In Nigst H (ed): *Spezielle Fraturen-und Luxationslehre,* vol I/z. Stuttgart, Thieme, 1972, pp 64-140.

102. Beatson TR: Fractures and dislocations of the cervical spine. *J Bone Joint Surg [Br]* 1963;45:21-25.

103. Felding JW, Hawkins RJ: Roentgenographic diagnosis of the injured neck. Instructional course lectures, *American Academy of Orthopedic Surgeons,* vol 25, St Louis, Mosby, 1976, p 149.

104. Holdsworth F: Fractures, dislocations and fracture-dislocations of the spine. *J Bone Joint Surg [Am]* 1970;52:1534-1551.

105. Roaf R: International classification of spine injuries. *Paraplegia* 1972;10:78-84.

106. Felding JW: Cineroentgenography of the normal cervical spine. *J Bone Joint Surg [Am]* 1957;39:1280-1288.

107. Hohl M: Normal motions of the upper portion of the cervical spine. *J Bone Joint Surg [Am]* 1964;46:1777-1779.

108. Hohl M, Baker HR: The atlanto-axial joint. Roentgenographic and anatomic study of normal and abnormal motion. *J Bone Joint Surg [Am]* 1964;46:1739-1752.

109. Goss CM (ed): *Gray's Anatomy of the human body,* ed 29. Philadelphia, Lea & Febiger, 1973, pp 294-297.

110. Werne S: Studies in spontaneous atlas dislocation. *Acta Orthop Scand Suppl* 1957;23:1-150.

111. Goldberg AL, Baron B, Daffner RH: Clinical images. Atlantooccipital dislocation: MR demonstration of cord damage. *J Comput Assist Tomog* 1991;15(1):174-178.

112. Shapiro R, Youngberg AS, Rothman SLG: The differential diagnosis of traumatic lesions of the occipito-atlanto-axial segment. *Radiol Clin North Am* 1973;11:505-526.

113. Traynelis VC, Marano GD, Dunker RO, Kaufman HH: Traumatic atlanto-occipital dislocation. *J Neurosurg* 1986;65:863-870.

114. Kaufman RA, Dunbar JS, Botsford JA, McLaurin RL: Traumatic longitudinal atlanto-occipital distraction injuries in children. *AJNR* 1982;3:415-419.

115. Atlas SW, Regenbogen V, Rogers LF, Kim KS: The radiographic characterization of burst fractures of the spine. *AJR* 1986;147:575-582.

116. Alker GJ, Oh YS, Leslie EV, et al: Postmortem radiology of head and neck injuries in fatal traffic accidents. *Radiology* 1975;114:611-617.

117. Powers B, Miller MD, Kramer RS, et al: Traumatic anterior atlanto-occipital dislocation. *J Neurosurg* 1979;4:12-17.

118. El-Khoury GY, Clark CR, Dietz FR, et al: Posterior atlantooccipital subluxation in Down's syndrome. *Radiology* 1986;159:507-509.

119. Jefferson G: Fractures of the atlas vertebrae: report of four cases and a review of those previously recorded. *Br J Surg* 1920;7:407-422.

120. Harris JR, Edeiken-Monroe B: *The radiology of acute cervical spine trauma.* Baltimore, Williams & Wilkins, 1987.

121. Fielding JW, Cochran G van B, Lawsing JF III, et al: Tears of the transverse ligament of the atlas. *J Bone Joint Surg [Am]* 1974;56:1683-1691.

122. Jacobson G, Adler DC: Examination of the atlanto-axial joint following injury: with particular emphasis on rotational subluxation. *AJR* 1956;76:1081-1094.

123. Fielding JW, Hawkins RJ: Atlanto-axial rotary fixation. *J Bone Joint Surg [Am]* 1977;59:37-44.

124. Rinaldi I, Mullins WJ Jr, Delaney WF, et al: Computerized tomographic demonstration of rotational atlantoaxial fixation. *J Neurosurg* 1979;50:115-119.

125. Kowalski HM, Cohen WA, Cooper P, Wisoff JH: Pitfalls in the CT diagnosis of atlantoaxial rotary subluxation. *AJR* 1987;149:595-600.

126. Schatzker J, Rorabeck CH, Waddell JP: Fractures of the dens (odontoid process): an analysis of thirty-seven cases. *J Bone Joint Surg [Br]* 1971;53:392-405.

127. Anderson LD, D'Alonzo RT: Fractures of the odontoid process of the axis. *J Bone Joint Surg [Am]* 1974;56:1663-1691.

128. Clark CR, White AA. Fractures of the dens: a multicenter study. *J Bone Joint Surg [Am]* 1985;67:1340-1348.

129. Schneider RC, Livingston KE, Cave AJ, et al: "Hangman's fracture" of the cervical spine. *J Neurosurg* 1965;22:141-154.

130. Mirvis SE, Young JW, Lim C, Greenberg J: Hangman's fracture: radiologic assessment in 27 cases. *Radiology* 1987;163:713-717.

131. Cheshire DJ: The stability of the cervical spine following treatment of fractures and fracture-dislocations. *Paraplegia* 1969;7:193-203.

132. Barnes R: Paraplegia in cervical spine injuries. *J Bone Joint Surg [Br]* 1948;30:234-244.

133. Penning L: *Functional pathology of the cervical spine.* Amsterdam, Excerpta Medica, 1968.

134. Schneider RC, Kahn EA: Chronic neurological sequelae of acute trauma to the spine and spinal cord: I. The significance of the acute flexion or "tear-drop" fracture-dislocation of the cervical spine. *J Bone Joint Surg [Am]* 1956;38:958-997.

135. Kim KS, Chen HH, Russell EJ, Rogers LF: Flexion teardrop fracture of the cervical spine: radiographic characteristics. *AJNR* 1988;9:1221-1228.

136. Schneider RC: Chronic neurological sequelae of acute trauma to the spine and spinal cord: V. The syndrome of acute central cervical spine cord injury followed by chronic anterior cervical cord injury (or compression) syndrome. *J Bone Joint Surg [Am]* 1960;42:253-260.

137. Braakman R, Vinken PJ: Unilateral facet interlocking in the lower cervical spine. *J Bone Joint Surg [Br]* 1967;49:249-257.

138. Lee C, Kim KS, Rogers LF: Triangular cervical vertebral body fractures: diagnostic significance. *AJR* 1982;138:1123-1132.

139. Braakman R, Penning L: *Injuries to the cervical spine.* Amsterdam, Excerpta Medica, 1971.

140. Gosch H, Hooding HE, Schneider RC: An experimental study of cervical spine and cord injuries. *J Trauma* 1972;12:510-576.

141. Jellinger K, Schwingshackl A: Birth injury of the spinal cord. *Neuropaediatrie* 1973;4:111-123.

142. Caterine H, Langer A, Sama JC, et al: Fetal risk in hyperextension of the fetal head in breech presentation. *Am J Obstet Gynecol* 1975;123:632-636.

143. Daw E: Hyperextension of the head in breech presentation. *Br J Clin Pract* 1970;24:485-487.

144. Bresnan MJ, Abroms IF: Neonatal spinal cord transection secondary to intrauterine hyperextension of the neck in breech presentation. *Fetal Neonatal Med* 1974;84:734-737.

145. Crothers B: The effect of breech extraction upon the central nervous system of the fetus. *Med Clin North Am* 1922;5:1287-1304.

146. Shulman ST, Madden JD, Esterly JR, Shanklin DR: Transection of the spinal cord. *Arch Dis Child* 1971;46:291-294.

147. Mathis JM, Wilson JT, Barnard JW, Zelenik ME: MR imaging of spinal cord avulsion. *AJNR* 1988;9:1232-1233.

148. Woodring JH, Goldstein SJ: Fractures of the articular processes of the cervical spine. *AJR* 1982;139:341-344.

149. Bohlman HH, Freehafer A, Dejak J: The results of treatment of acute injuries of the upper thoracic spine with paralysis. *J Bone Joint Surg [Am]* 1985;67:360-369.

150. Brant-Zawadski M, Jeffrey RB Jr, Minagi H, Pitts LH: High resolution CT of thoracolumbar fractures. *AJR* 1982;138:699-704.

151. Chance GQ: Note on a type of flexion fracture of the spine. *Br J Radiol* 1948;21:452-453.

152. Smith WS, Kaufer H: Patterns and mechanisms of lumbar injuries associated with lap seat belts. *J Bone Joint Surg [Am]* 1969;51:239-254.

153. Lee JK, Yao L: Stress fractures: MR imaging. *Radiology* 1988;169:217-220.

154. Brahme SK, Cervilla V, Vint V, et al: Magnetic resonance appearance of sacral insufficiency fractures. *Skeletal Radiol* 1990;19:489-493.

155. Dohrmann GJ, Wagner FC, Buey PC: Transitory traumatic paraplegia: electron microscopy of early alteration in myelinated nerve fibers. *J Neurosurg* 1972;367:407-415.

156. Jellinger K: Traumatic vascular disease of the spinal cord. In Vinkin PJ, Bruyn GW (eds): *Handbook of clinical neurology. II. Vascular disease of the nervous system,* vol 12, Amsterdam, Elsevier, 1972, pp 556-630.

157. Gebarski SS, Maynard FW, Gabrielson TO, et al: Posttraumatic progressive myelopathy. *Radiology* 1985;157:379-385.

158. Edgar RE: Surgical management of spinal cord cysts. *Paraplegia* 1976;14:21-27.

159. Tator CH, Meguro K, Rowed DW: Favorable results with syringosubarachnoid shunts for treatment of syringomyelia. *J Neurosurg* 1982;56:517-523.

160. Quencer RM, Green BA, Eisemont FJ: Posttraumatic spinal cord cysts: clinical features and characterization with metrizamide computed tomography. *Radiology* 1983;146:415-423.

161. Quencer RM, Morse BM, Green BA, et al: Intraoperative spinal sonography: an adjunct to metrizamide CT in assessment and surgical decompression of spinal cord cysts. *AJR* 1984;142:593-601.

162. Barnett HJ, Botterell EH, Jousse AT, Wynn-Jones M: Progressive myelopathy as a sequel to traumatic paraplegia. *Brain* 1966;89:159-173.

163. Williams B, Terry AF, Jones F, McSweeney T: Syringomyelia as a sequel to traumatic paraplegia. *Paraplegia* 1981;19:67-80.

164. Griffiths ER, McCormic CC: Posttraumatic syringomyelia (cystic myelopathy). *Paraplegia* 1981;19:96-97.

165. Watson N: Ascending cystic degeneration of the cord after spinal cord injury. *Paraplegia* 1981;19:9-95.

166. Vernon JD, Silver JR, Ohry A: Post-traumatic syringomyelia. *Paraplegia* 1982;20:339-364.

167. McLean DR, Miller JD, Allen PB, et al: Posttraumatic syringomyelia. *J Neurosurg* 1973;39:485-492.

168. Seibert CE, Dreisbach JN, Swanson WB, et al: Progressive posttraumatic cystic myelopathy: neuroradiologic evaluation. *AJR* 1981;136:1161-1165.

169. Quencer RM, Sheldon JJ, Post MJ, et al: MRI chronically injured cervical spinal cord. *AJR* 1986;147:125-132.

170. Yamashita Y, Takahashi M, Matsuno Y, et al: Chronic injuries of the spinal cord: assessment with MR imaging. *Radiology* 1990;175:849-854.

171. Enzmann DR, O'Donohue J, Rubin JB, et al: CSF pulsations within nonneoplastic spinal cord cysts. *AJR* 1987;149:149-157.

9

Pediatric Spine: Normal Anatomy and Spinal Dysraphism

MARILYN J. GOSKE
MICHAEL T. MODIC
SHIWEI YU

The recent advances in neuroimaging of the pediatric spine have dramatically improved our ability to evaluate children noninvasively.[1,2] In the past, infants with minimal skin changes, such as a hairy nevus or skin dimple, often deteriorated neurologically before invasive myelography could be performed. Now (in addition to plain films) ultrasound, CT, and MRI are readily available. Children with spinal cord tumors and infection are diagnosed earlier and more easily[3]; and children with complex congenital anomalies of the brain and spinal cord can be completely evaluated, both before and after surgery.

Although MRI does not offer the portability or low cost of ultrasound and cannot depict bony anatomy as well as CT, it has allowed improved understanding of cross-sectional anatomy and it does provide superior resolution of the spinal cord and surrounding soft tissues.

Nevertheless, other imaging modalities may be preferred in specific clinical circumstances:

Plain films of the spine are more helpful in evaluating trauma, spinal instability, scoliosis, and spina bifida.[4] Certain primary bone tumors of the spine are better detected initially on routine radiographs.

Ultrasound of the spinal contents in infants with a skin dimple or nevus has proved invaluable in assessing for spinal cord anomalies when there is no or only minimal neurologic deficit.[2,4] It may also be used in the operating room for precise localization of intramedullary tumors, cysts, or syringohydromyelia.[5] In patients who have undergone surgery and in whom there is a question

as to retethering of the spinal cord, ultrasound may be performed through the surgical bony defect or congenitally absent posterior elements.[6] Cord retethering is diagnosed when there are diminished or absent nerve root pulsations, an eccentric and nonmovable spinal cord, or a mass.[7]

Computed tomography is excellent in assessing bone pathology and may be used with or without intrathecal contrast to delineate cord anatomy and surrounding soft tissues. It also is useful in evaluating patients with severe scoliosis whose spine may be difficult to observe fully on a single MR scan plane because of marked rotational changes. Subtle areas of tethering, spinal metastases from brain neoplasms, and hydromyelia with severe cord atrophy can be better evaluated with contrast-enhanced CT.[1]

Angiography of the spinal cord is used (rarely) to map the blood supply to vascular malformations or highly vascular neoplasms.

Obtaining a Motionless Examination

Often the most difficult task in performing an MR examination of a child is obtaining a motionless state. The chances of success will be increased if certain steps are followed:

1. The older child and family should be prepared through the use of *prep booklets* (which explain the examination, the appearance of the MRI unit, and the loud knocking noise that occurs during the examination). Parents and child are told ahead of

time that they may remain together during the examination. Families with young children are encouraged to bring stuffed animals, blankets, or pacifiers for the scan. The parents are given a contact person to call if questions arise before the scan or an upper respiratory infection develops in a younger child, which will preclude sedation and necessitate canceling the procedure.

Although most children over the age of 5 are able to cooperate without sedation, children under the age of 8 are kept NPO before the study, in case sedation is required. The American Academy of Pediatrics[8] has recommended that if sedation is necessary children aged 0 to 3 years remain NPO for 4 hours and children 3 to 6 years NPO for 6 hours in advance of planned sedation. Children are encouraged to wear comfortable loose-fitting clothing without snaps or metal.

Upon arrival in the department a child should find toys and books and a friendly atmosphere. A warm greeting, brief history taking and physical, and simple explanation of the study are reassuring to the child and family.

2. Infants less than 18 months of age may be *sedated* with chloral hydrate. Oral chloral hydrate is effective at a standard dosage of 75 to 100 mg/kg for the first 10 kg of body weight and then 50 mg/kg for each kilogram above 10. If the child is still awake after 20 minutes, additional doses up to a total of 2000 mg may be given.[9]

Intravenous pentobarbital (Nembutal) has been shown[10] to be a safe sedative for pediatric imaging when used appropriately. It is useful in children over 18 months of age who do not have hepatic or metabolic disease. In one protocol the dose (5 mg/kg) is drawn up and half (or 2.5 mg/kg) is administered, followed by observation for 30 seconds to 2 minutes; if the child is still awake, half the remaining dose (1.25 mg/kg) is given and the child observed for another 30 seconds to 2 minutes; if still awake, the remainder of the dose is given. Nembutal may also be used in infants. If an IV line is to be started anyway for gadolinium, it may be used to give Nembutal.

This short acting barbiturate, however, carries an uncommon (though real) risk of respiratory depression. Thus persons trained in pediatric life support, as well as emergency equipment, must be readily available.

3. *Monitoring* with a pulse oximeter is a simple and effective means of detecting any drop in oxygen saturation, which is the earliest sign of respiratory depression. Often a drop in oxygen saturation is due to flexion of the neck, causing redundancy of the soft tissues in the pharynx. Straightening the

head or removing the pacifier will allow a return to normal oxygen saturation levels. Another helpful monitoring technique is capnography. With this method exhaled gas is aspirated from the nasopharynx and its carbon dioxide content is measured by infrared absorption in a device remote from the scanner. Such information is limited, however, particularly if the patient is not intubated and the sample gas is mixed with room air. Capnography could be used in conjunction with pulse oximetry.[10]

4. *Supplemental oxygen* may be administered either with a "blow-by" technique or by nasal cannula or mask. This increases the pulmonary oxygen reserve as well as the margin of safety during the examination. It may be contraindicated, however, in premature infants (risk of retinopathy) or children with abnormal ventilatory response but, in most other patients, is a helpful, inexpensive, and safe drug.[11]

Other newer drugs with shorter half-lives—such as midazolam (Versed) and propofol (Diprivan)—are also being investigated. Compared to intravenous pentobarbital, propofol appears to be a safe alternative sedative. It is a continuous intravenous agent (which means constant supervision and meticulous technique), but it has the advantage of being titratable to effect and its recovery time after discontinuation is extremely rapid.[12]

5. When the scan is complete, the parents should be *present* as the child awakes.

Lots of praise for a job well done, and a sticker or toy as a reward, will help ensure a pleasant experience. When the child is alert enough to leave, the radiologist should give the parents written instructions and the names of persons to contact if questions arise.

Embryology

The study of the developing spine has been a source of fascination and argument for well over a century.[13] Recent leaders in the field of pediatric neuroradiology[14] have emphasized the relationship between various developmental anomalies and interruptions or disturbances at particular stages of embryonic growth. Therefore a knowledge of embryonic development is illuminating and necessary for better understanding these often complex malformations.

At about 7 days after conception the three germ layers—endoderm, mesoderm, and ectoderm—are formed.[15]

The ectoderm gives rise to the spinal cord, notochord, and skin; the mesoderm gives rise the vertebral bodies, ribs, and paraspinal musculature.

At about 16 days of fetal life the primitive streak forms from ectodermal cells on the surface of the embryo.[16] In the cranial portion some cells aggregate to form a nodular proliferation (Hensen nodes) that surrounds a pit. Cells migrate cranially into the pit to form the notochordal process, which fuses with endoderm.[9] The notochordal process later separates, having formed the intestinal lining ventrally. The dorsal component separates from the overlying neural tube to form a solid rod of tissue along the axis of the developing embryo, the notochord. The notochord has a most important function[15]: It acts as a primitive framework about which the entire spine is formed and is the inducer for the floor plate of the neural tube.

The primitive streak continues to develop and is now termed the *neural plate*. The neural plate will be transformed through three successive stages into the spinal cord[17]: *neurulation, canalization,* and *retrogressive differentiation*.

Initially the neural plate forms a groove along its dorsal surface in a rostrocaudal direction. Contractile filaments at the base of the neural groove cause the lateral walls to fuse posteriorly at 3 weeks of gestation.[14] This process (of neurulation) results in the formation of a hollow tube of tissue. The tube closes midway along its length initially and then proceeds to close from this point both rostrally (cranially) and caudally at the same time.

This produces two openings, one at the extreme rostral and one at the extreme caudal end of the embryo. The anterior neuropore (rostral end) closes first, followed by the posterior neuropore (caudal end) at 4 weeks of gestation. Neurulation is now complete (Figs. 9-1 and 9-2).

As the neural groove is closing, the overlying ectoderm separates from the underlying neuroectoderm and differentiates into skin, which will fuse in the midline. During this process, termed *disjunction*,[14] mesenchyme insinuates itself between the neuroectoderm and cutaneous ectoderm to form the meninges, bony spinal column, and paraspinal muscles.

The second stage of development of the spinal cord, *canalization*, occurs at 4½ weeks of gestation. The caudal end of the neural tube elongates into a caudal cell mass. Microcysts and groups of cells at this site organize to form an ependymal lined tube that fuses with the neural tube above[14] (Fig. 9-3).

The final stage, *retrogressive differentiation*, results in formation of the conus medullaris, filum terminale, and central canal at 5½ weeks of gestation. Cell necrosis and a diminution of the central lumen lead to an overall decrease in the size of the neural tube at the caudal end of the embryo, resulting in these structures (Fig. 9-3). The conus medullaris is defined as the distal end of the spinal cord; it maintains a conical shape and normally ends at the L1 to L2-3 level. The filum terminale is a small slen-

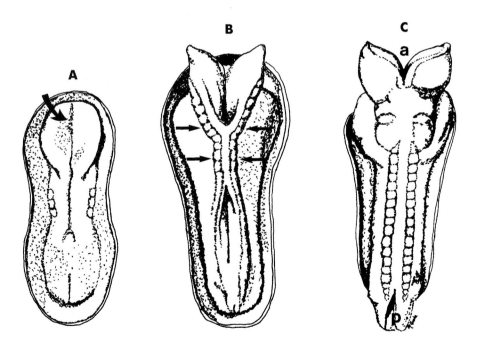

Fig. 9-1. A, Dorsal view of a human embryo at 18 days. The neural plate *(curved arrow)* is forming at the cranial end of the embryo. **B,** At 22 days somites are visible on each side of the neural tube *(arrows).* Neurulation is occurring. **C,** At 23 days the anterior *(a)* and posterior *(p)* neuropores still open to the amniotic cavity. (Modified from Langman J: *Medical embryology,* ed 2. Baltimore, Williams & Wilkins, 1969.)

der strand of glial-ependymal tissue that extends from the conus and courses inferiorly through the dura to attach to the coccyx. It is normally less than 2 mm in diameter. The focal dilation of the central canal within the conus medullaris is known as the terminal ventricle.

Simultaneous with the process of neurulation, the bony spinal column forms from somites.[18] These paired mesodermal segments will give rise to the paraspinal muscles, subcutaneous connective tissue, and vertebral bodies.

During the *membranous* stage, at 25 days of gestation, the notochord separates from endoderm and the overlying neural tube.[15] It is a continuous column of cells that governs the subsequent positions of the spinal ganglia, spinal nerves, segmental vessels, and intervertebral disks. The mesenchyme surrounding the notochord forms the somites (separated by small sclerotomic fissures). The more ventral medial mesenchyme gives rise to the sclerotomes, which later form the vertebral bodies and ribs. The dorsal and lateral dermomyotomes give rise to the paraspinal musculature.[19]

During the second stage, *chondrification*,[9,18] at about 35 days, the sclerotomes divide in half along the intersegmental fissure, which contains feeding vessels. This forms a loosely packed zone of mesenchymal cells in the rostral portion of the canal and a denser zone in the caudal portion. The caudal half

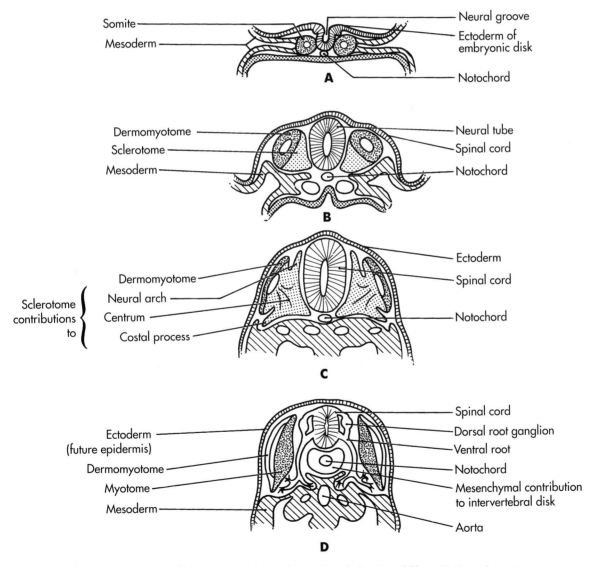

Fig. 9-2. Formation of the neural tube and spinal cord showing differentiation of somites into sclerotomes and dermatomyotomes. Transverse sections depict, **A,** 18 days, **B,** 22 days, **C,** 27 days, and, **D,** 30 days.

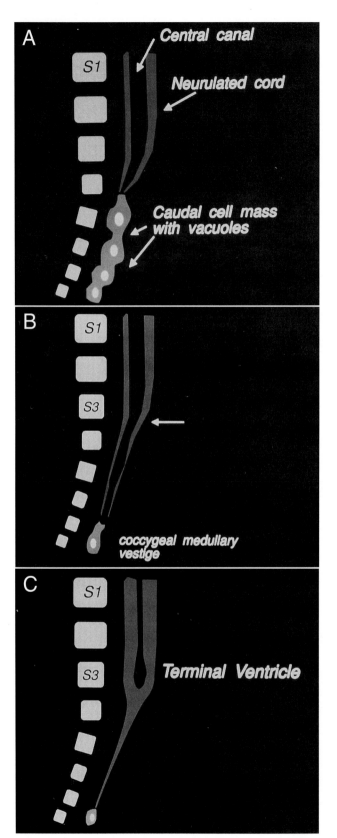

Fig. 9-3. Canalization and retrogressive differentiation. **A,** At 4½ weeks of gestation the caudal end of the neural tube elongates into the *caudal cell mass,* which is formed by fusion of the neural epithelium and notochord. Multiple vacuoles appear in the caudal cell mass. **B,** These cysts and clumps of cells, now termed the *coccygeal medullary vestige,* fuse with the more cranial neural tube *(arrow).* **C,** At 5½ weeks of gestation cell necrosis in the caudal tube decreases the size of this structure, forming the filum terminale, conus medullaris, and terminal ventricle (by a process called retrogressive differentiation).

of one sclerotome fuses with the rostral half of the adjacent sclerotome across the intersegmental vessels and fissure to form a vertebral body (Fig. 9-4). The paired sclerotomes fuse symmetrically so each side forms one half of a vertebral body. The site of fusion, which can be identified on MRI in neonates, is called Hahn's notch (Fig. 9-5). O'Rahilly and Benson[18] have observed the formation of "butterfly" vertebrae in an embryo in which the right and left chondrification centers failed to fuse. Furthermore, they noted a hemivertebra when one of these chondrification centers failed to develop.

During the last stage, *ossification* centers form within the cartilaginous models at 9 weeks of gestation. At birth three ossification centers are present, one for the center of the body and one for each half of the neural arch.

▪ ▪ ▪

The pediatric spine differs from the adult spine in many respects[3,18,20-26]: The vertebral ossification centers are incompletely ossified, the disks are thicker and have a higher water content as well as relatively less collagen, the spinal column and neural foramina are more capacious, and there is less curvature to the spine.

In neonates the spine has a straight or slightly C-shaped configuration because there is less cervical and lumbar lordosis. Once the infant develops head control, a cervical lordosis develops; and the lumbar lordosis appears later, with weight-bearing.

Although the pediatric spine is readily viewed by MRI, few large studies to date have investigated spinal development in the normal infant and young child.[27]

Sze et al.[27] have emphasized the dynamic changes that occur in pediatric spines. Not only are there marked morphologic changes between neonates and 2-year-olds, there are different stages of signal intensity over a brief period that can create significant confusion. The overall signal intensity of the vertebral bodies on T_1-weighted images is noted to be less in young children than in older

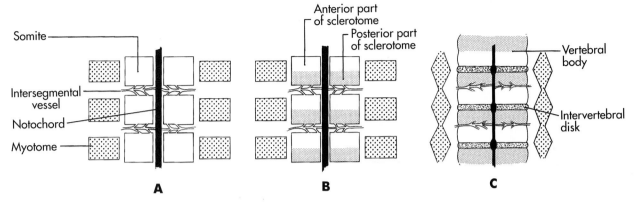

Fig. 9-4. Development of the vertebral body and intervertebral disk. The vertebral bodies are formed by fusion of the adjacent portions of sclerotomes. The intervertebral disks develop from these sclerotomes and from the incorporation of notochordal remnants. The intersegmental vessels are incorporated into these areas of fusion and become the basivertebral vessels.

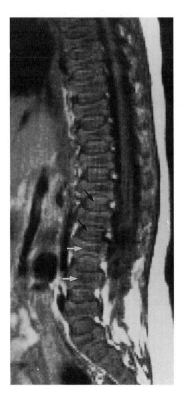

Fig. 9-5. Hahn's notch in a 2-month-old infant. Note the areas of decreased signal intensity in the central portion of the vertebral bodies, which represent the transverse basivertebral venous channels marking the site of fusion of the sclerotomes *(black arrows)*. The intervertebral disks are thick and spherical *(white arrows)*.

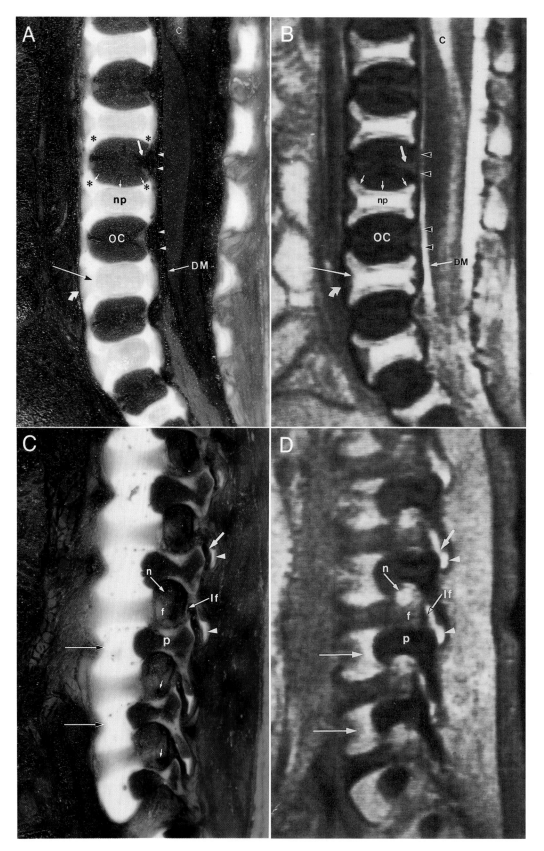

Fig. 9-6. For legend see opposite page.

children or adults, reflecting the more abundant red (hematopoietic) marrow compared to yellow (fat) marrow at this stage of life. With increasing age the vertebral marrow increases its signal intensity on T_1-weighted images until it is of similar intensity to the adult spine. On T_2-weighted images the high signal of the intervertebral disks, which represents greater hydration of the disks, is prominent. Although the signal intensity of a tissue specimen examined by MR may vary with fixation or postmortem changes,[20] the relative intensities from structures in the cadaveric pediatric spine appear to remain similar to those in the living patient. These changes have been carefully studied in cadaveric pediatric spines.

In *full-term infants* (Fig. 9-6) the lumbar vertebral column is nearly straight. The general vertebral body size is small relative to the size of the spinal canal. This is quite obvious on sagittal cryomicrotome sections of the lumbar spine, in which the epidural fat behind L5 and S1 can appear rather prominent and the thecal sac rather capacious against the L5 vertebral body. As the vertebrae grow, this discrepancy becomes less apparent. The spinal cord ends at the level of the second lumbar vertebra. On sagittal cryomicrotome sections the spongy bone of the ossification center in the centrum appears ellipsoidal, occupying a near-central portion of the centrum (Fig. 9-6, *A*). The segmental basivertebral veins indent the posterior borders of the respective ossification centers. Alongside the rostral, ventral, and caudal surfaces of each ossification center is a thick layer of hyaline cartilage with relatively massive-appearing "corners." The cartilaginous intervertebral disk is a relatively narrow band containing notochordal remnants and distinct types of cartilage. The nucleus pulposus is a homogeneous, gelatinous, gray, and translucent structure in the near-central portion of the disk. A thin bright band in its equator represents the residual primitive notochord.[20] The nucleus pulposus may vary in shape with the disk level, being ellipsoidal in the upper region of

the lumbar spine and round in the lower region. It is sharply demarcated from the anulus anteriorly and posteriorly and from the hyaline cartilage of the vertebral bodies superiorly and inferiorly. The anulus is slightly thicker anteriorly than posteriorly. The fibrous lamellae in the outer portion of the anulus, where Sharpey's fibers are developing, have a dark gray color.

A thin layer of ivory-colored fibrocartilage constituting the inner portion of the anulus is shown in Fig. 9-6, *A*. The posterior longitudinal ligament appears as a thin fibrous band attaching to the surfaces of the intervertebral disks and spanning the concave surfaces of the vertebral bodies. In the plane of the neural foramina (Fig. 9-6, *C* and *D*) the neurocentral synchondrosis of the vertebral body and the lateroposterior surface of the disk form the anterior boundary of the foramen, the pedicles form the superior and inferior boundaries, and the facets and ligamentum flavum form the posterior boundary. The channel is ovoid and capacious. It contains the nerve roots, vessels, and fat and is slightly larger superiorly than inferiorly. The nerve roots occupy the upper portion, and the veins the lower portion, of the foramen. The pedicles are well ossified with a flat superior margin and shallow concave inferior border. The ligamentum flavum is thin and fibrous, situated anterior to the facet joints. The facet joint space is wide. Hyaline cartilage at the tips of the inferior articular processes of each facet joint is evident.

On MR images (Fig. 9-6, *B* to *D*) the ossification center has a low and less homogeneous signal intensity because it consists of spongy trabecular bone and red marrow. Deoxyhemoglobin in a cadaveric specimen may alter the signal intensity of the bone marrow or subarachnoid space where CSF has become blood tinged. The transverse basivertebral venous channel in the middle of the ossification center of a vertebral body is of intermediate signal intensity. The anterior and posterior longitudinal ligaments and the outer portion of each anulus

Text continued on p. 364.

Fig. 9-6. Normal lumbar spinal anatomy in a full-term infant. A sagittal midline cryomicrotome section, **A,** and a T_2-weighted MR image, **B,** show the ellipsoidal ossification centers of the vertebral bodies *(OC),* the basivertebral vein *(white arrow),* the outer *(curved arrow)* and inner *(long arrow)* anulus fibrosus, and the hyaline cartilage of the vertebrae *(small arrows).* At the "corners" of each ossification center the hyaline cartilage has a massive appearance *(asterisks).* The posterior longitudinal ligament *(arrowheads)* attaches to the posterior surfaces of the intervertebral disks and spans the posterior convexities of the vertebral bodies. *np,* Nucleus pulposus; *DM,* dura mater; *C,* spinal cord. Another cryomicrotome section in the plane of the neural foramen, **C,** and a T_2-weighted image, **D,** illustrate the ovoid capacious foramen. The bright signal in the facet joint represents the joint space *(large arrow)* and the hyaline cartilage *(arrowheads)* at the tips of the inferior articular processes. *Long arrows* point to the neurocentral synchondrosis of the vertebral body. *n,* Nerve root; *small arrows,* veins; *f,* fat; *lf,* ligamentum flavum; *p,* pedicles.

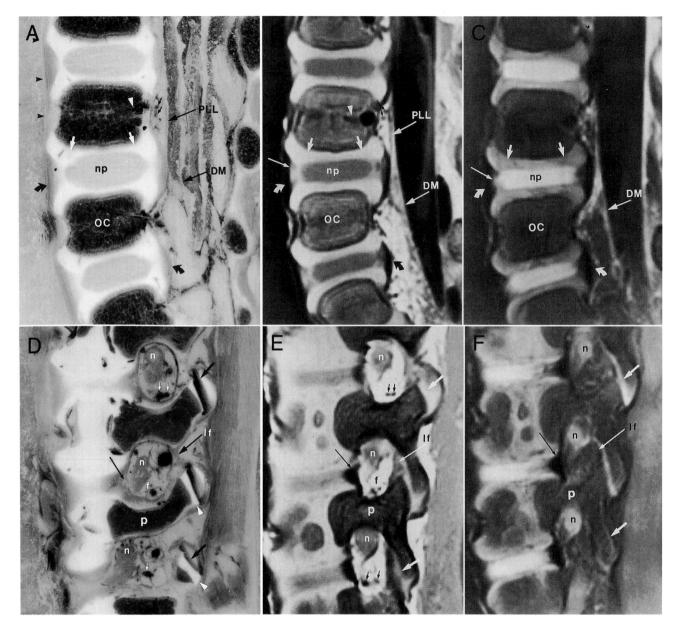

Fig. 9-7. Normal lumbar spinal anatomy in a 3-month-old child. A sagittal cryomicrotome section, **A,** and a T_1-weighted, **B,** and T_2-weighted, **C,** image demonstrate the rectangular ossification centers of the vertebral bodies *(OC),* the basivertebral vein *(white arrowhead),* the retrovertebral venous plexus *(small arrows),* and the translucent nucleus pulposus *(np)* with ivory-colored inner anulus *(long arrow)* and well-laminated outer anulus *(curved arrows).* The posterior longitudinal ligament *(PLL)* is attached to the midsurface of the intervertebral disk but separated from the vertebral bodies and dura mater *(DM). Black arrowheads* point to the anterior longitudinal ligament; the *small white arrow* denotes hyaline cartilage. Another cryomicrotome section in the plane of the neural foramina, **D,** along with a T_1-weighted, **E,** and a T_2-weighted, **F,** image illustrates the capacious neural foramen and concave anular surface *(thin long black arrow). n,* Nerve root; *small arrows,* veins; *f,* fat; *lf,* ligamentum flavum; *p,* pedicles; *thick arrows,* facet joint spaces; *arrowheads,* relatively thick and uniform hyaline cartilage.

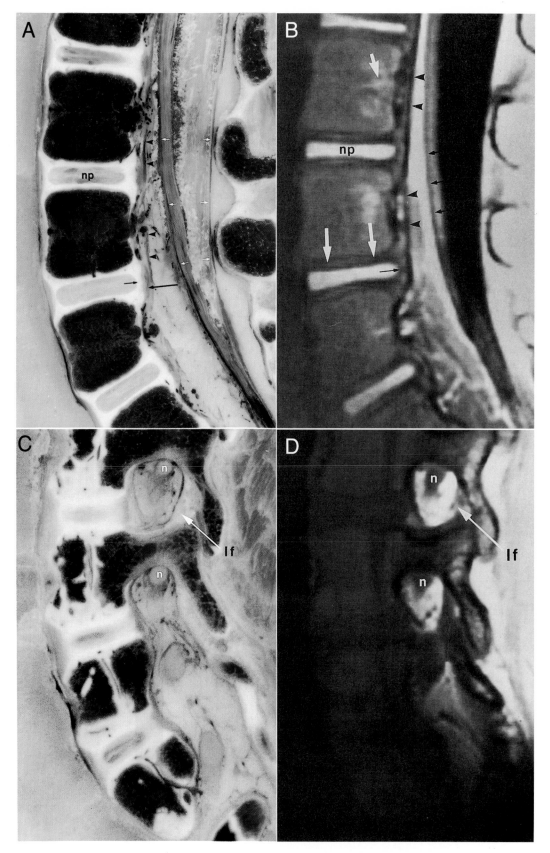

Fig. 9-8. Normal lumbar spinal anatomy in a 2-year-old child. A sagittal midline cryomicrotome section, **A**, and a T$_2$-weighted MR image, **B**, show the square ossification centers quite clearly. Fibers have formed in the nucleus pulposus *(np)*. The ivory-colored inner anulus *(thin arrow),* the compact outer anulus *(long arrow),* the well-developed posterior longitudinal ligament *(arrowheads),* and the dura mater are all visible. Another cryomicrotome section in the plane of the neural foramen, **C**, and a T$_1$-weighted image, **D**, demonstrate the nerve root in the neural foramen *(n)* and the ligamentum flavum *(lf)*. Note that the inferior portion of the neural foramen is narrower than the superior portion.

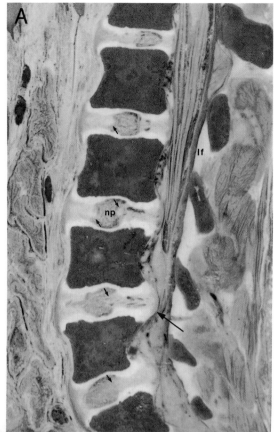

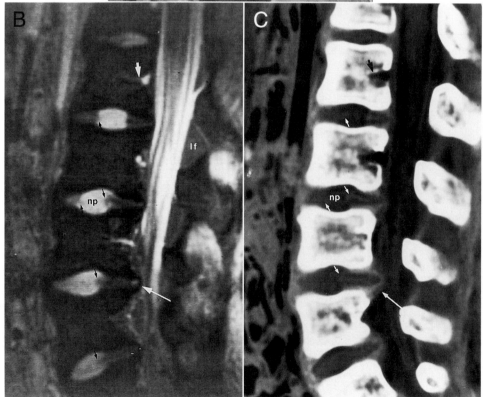

Fig. 9-9. For legend see opposite page.

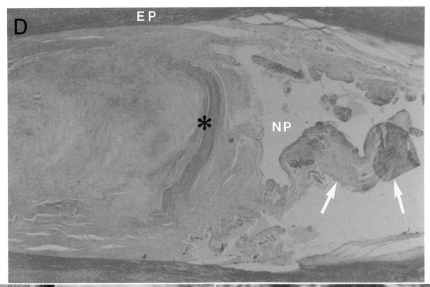

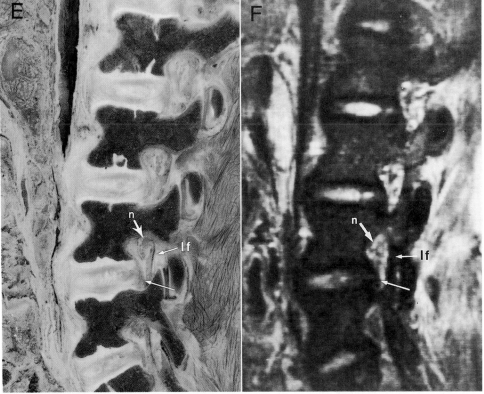

Fig. 9-9. Normal lumbar spinal anatomy in a 10-year-old child. A sagittal midline cryomicrotome section, **A,** a T_2-weighted image, **B,** and a CT image, **C,** illustrate that the superior and inferior surfaces of the vertebral bodies become concave with increasing age. Arcuate fibrous tissue *(small arrows)* indents the amorphous portion of the nucleus pulposus *(np)* anteriorly and posteriorly. Note that the nucleus is eccentrically located. *Thick arrow,* Basivertebral vein; *long arrow,* convex outer anulus. A histologic section of the L1-2 disk, **D,** shows the arcuate *(asterisk)* and clumped *(arrows)* tissue in the nucleus pulposus *(NP).* The hyaline cartilaginous endplate *(EP)* is shown. Another crymicrotome section through the plane of the neural foramina, **E,** and a T_2-weighted MR image, **F,** show the inverted-pear shape of the neural foramen resulting from encroachment by the posterior surface of the intervertevbral disk *(arrow)* and the enlarged ligamentum flavum *(lf). n,* Nerve root.

fibrosus have negligible signal intensity. On T_2-weighted images the nucleus pulposus has a homogeneous and greater signal intensity than the adjacent hyaline cartilage of the vertebral bodies and the inner portion of the anulus, which have a slightly low signal intensity. The segmental portions of the posterior longitudinal ligament posterior to the ossification centers appear as a low-signal line separable from the vertebral bodies and dura mater but indiscernible from the outer anulus of the disk.

By *3 months of age* (Fig. 9-7) the amount of spongy bone in the ossification centers of the vertebral bodies has conspicuously increased and the hyaline cartilage of the vertebral bodies has decreased, resulting in a more rectangular shape of the ossification centers (Fig. 9-7, *A* to *C*). The nucleus pulposus is relatively longer antero-posteriorly than in full-term infants but is still well demarcated from the hyaline cartilage of the vertebral bodies and the fibrocartilage of the anulus. The inner portion of each anulus has the same ivory color as the hyaline cartilage of the vertebral body. The outer portion is better developed and more distinctly laminated. The posterior longitudinal ligament, which is separable from the posterior surfaces of the vertebral bodies and closely juxtaposed to the intervertebral disks, again appears as a thin fibrous structure in the 3-month-old child. The anterior longitudinal ligament appears as a relatively thick fibrous band.

The neural foramina change little, remaining capacious and ovoid (Fig. 9-7, *D* to *F*). The hyaline cartilage on the surfaces of the articular processes appears thick and uniform. The joint spaces are wide.

The ossification centers, hyaline cartilage of the vertebral bodies, nucleus pulposus, and inner and outer anulus are readily differentiated on both T_1- and T_2-weighted images (Fig. 9-7, *B, C, E,* and *F*). On T_1-weighted MR images, although the signal intensity of the ossification centers of the vertebral bodies and the nucleus pulposus is intermediately low, the hyaline cartilage of the vertebral bodies and the inner anulus fibrosus have high signal intensity. The outer portion of the anulus is of negligible signal intensity. The posterior longitudinal ligament appears as a separate intermediate-signal line posterior to the vertebral bodies. A low-signal band in the periphery of the intervertebral disks represents Sharpey fibers and the longitudinal ligaments. A similar appearance is shown on T_2-weighted images, but with the signal intensities of the nucleus pulposus and the hyaline cartilage reversed. On T_2-weighted images the nucleus pulposus has high signal intensity whereas the inner anulus and hyaline cartilage have intermediate signal intensities. The nerve root within the neural foramen is well demonstrated, in contrast to its surrounding fat (which has an opposite signal intensity on T_1- and T_2-weighted images).

By *2 years of age* (Fig. 9-8) the normal spinal curvatures begin to develop as a result of weight-bearing. A mild lordosis appears in the lumbar spine. The ossified portion of the vertebral body increases significantly, producing a square ossification center (Fig. 9-3, *A* and *B*). The intervertebral disk spaces are much thinner, and the nucleus pulposus becomes a long and narrow region. It is no longer uniformly gelatinous, for it now contains fibers that have formed within it. The ivory-colored inner portion of the anulus is thicker than that seen in full-term infants. The outer portion is much more compact. The anterior and posterior longitudinal ligaments are well developed. The attachments of the posterior longitudinal ligament to the midsurfaces of the outer anulus and over the concavities of the posterior vertebral body surfaces are well demonstrated. The ligament does not adhere to the vertebral bodies. Fat both anterior and posterior to the ligament is, again, rather prominent.

The neural foramen remains capacious, with the inferior part distinctly narrower than the superior part (Fig. 9-8, *C* and *D*). The inferior borders of the pedicles become more concave. Ossification of the pedicles and the articular processes is nearly complete. The facet joint spaces are narrower than in young infants, and the ligamentum flavum is thicker. Ossification of the vertebral bodies in this plane has a bipartite appearance.

On T_2-weighted images (Fig. 9-8, *B*) a large region of high signal intensity in the central portion of the intervertebral disk represents the nucleus pulposus and the inner anulus fibrosus. The posterior longitudinal ligament is also well shown. The nerve roots within the neural foramen, however, are better shown on T_1-weighted images (Fig. 9-8, *D*).

By *10 years of age* (Fig. 9-9) the lumbar lordosis is similar to that in adults. Ossification of the vertebral bodies and neural arches is nearly complete (Fig. 9-9, *A*). Because the vertebral bodies are nearly completely ossified, the spinal canal becomes less capacious. The vertebral bodies have a biconcave contour superiorly and inferiorly. The nucleus pulposus becomes smaller and covers about half the area of the disk in the sagittal plane, occupying an eccentric position, more posteriorly in disks of the upper lumbar region and more anteriorly in disks of the lower.

A distinct feature of 10-year-old disks is that the fibrous tissue within the nucleus pulposus increases in a characteristic pattern. The nucleus begins to lose its translucent appearance—showing, instead, an arcuate arrangement of clumped fibers in its anterior aspect (upper disks), its anterior and posterior aspects (middle disks), and its posterior aspect (lower disks). There is no longer a sharp demarcation between nucleus and anulus. The anulus, however, remains distinctly laminated and compact, with lamellae that are oriented in an outwardly convex fashion.

Another development in 10-year-old spines is that the neural foramina take on an inverted pear shape. The inferior portion is much narrower because the posterior surfaces of the disks are convex anteriorly and the ligamentum flavum is enlarged posteriorly. The foramina are less capacious, but the nerve roots are still surrounded by a relatively large amount of fat. The pedicles are shorter superoinferiorly, and the superior and inferior margins become more concave. A thin layer of hyaline cartilage on the surfaces of the articular processes is observable.

The pattern of fibrous distribution within the nucleus pulposus seen in cryomicrotome sections of 10-year-old spines is well shown on MR images, appearing as regions of lower signal intensity within the high-signal nucleus. The signal intensity of the inner anulus is similar to that of the hyaline cartilage of vertebral bodies. The outer anulus also has low signal on all MR sequences. The region of higher signal from the hyaline cartilage of the vertebral bodies and from the inner anulus and nucleus pulposus simulates a "Milk-Bone" appearance. The nerve roots and ganglia within the neural foramina have a higher signal intensity than the adjacent fat. The fibrous portion of the nucleus pulposus, as shown on cryomicrotome and MR images, is also well demonstrated on the correlative CT image (Fig. 9-4, C). The segmented nerves and vessels within the neural foramina are well demonstrated because they contrast well with the surrounding fat. The facet joint space and ligamentum flavum in the plane of the neural foramina are also well evaluated by MRI.

Normal Position of the Conus Medullaris

Early in fetal life the caudal spinal cord extends to the inferior aspect of the bony spinal column. The nerve roots exit the spinal cord horizontally. However, the vertebral bodies grow faster longitudinally than the spinal cord, and this causes the conus medullaris to terminate in the upper lumbar spine at birth and the nerves to course inferiorly and diagonally as they exit the foramina. Although it was thought that the spinal cord "ascends" in early childhood, recent MRI studies[28] have suggested that this is not the case. Instead, a conus level of L2-3 or above is normal at any age and L3-4 is abnormal at any age. A conus level of L3 is indeterminate since a normal or tethered cord could be located at this level. The vast majority of patients with a conus terminating at L3, however, will be abnormal and associated with a thickened filum or mass.[29]

SPINAL DYSRAPHISM

Spinal dysraphism is a general term that encompasses a wide variety of anomalies of the spine resulting from imperfect midline fusion during early embryogenesis.[18]

Failure of the embryonic neural tube to close properly leads to abnormalities of midline mesenchymal, bony, and neural structures. This term, spinal dysraphism, refers to significant defects involving the spine. Small vertical clefts commonly seen in the spinous processes of L5 or S1 are not included in it.[30]

The early medical literature referred to spina bifida aperta ("open") as existing if any portion of the spinal contents visibly protruded through the midline bony defect and lacked a skin covering (i.e., myelomeningocele). Spina bifida cystica ("cyst") was used to refer to large defects that were skin covered (i.e., lipomyelomeningocele).

Occult spinal dysraphism, spina bifida occulta ("hidden"), is a bony discontinuity in the spine associated with a hidden neural defect without an obvious back mass or exposed neural tissue.

Byrd et al.[17] use a classification of spinal dysraphism modified from the works of Harwood-Nash, Naidich, and McLone in which they divide the disorders into three categories, similar to the old classification but without the confusing Latin terminology. The first category consists of spinal dysraphism *associated with a non–skin-covered* back mass (myelocele, myelomeningocele). The second is spinal dysraphism *with a skin-covered* back mass (lipomyelomeningocele, posterior meningocele, myelocystocele). The third is spinal dysraphism *without an associated* back mass. This is the largest category and includes diastematomyelia, dorsal dermal sinus, syringohydromyelia, spinal lipoma, tight filum terminale, anterior sacral and lateral thoracic meningocele, split notochord syndrome (including neurenteric cyst), and caudal regression syndrome. It is this last, extensive, group of lesions that may benefit most from MRI examination.

Dysraphism Associated With a Non–Skin-Covered Back Mass
Myelomeningocele

Myelomeningocele is the most common significant form of spinal dysraphism. It is characterized by overexpansion of the ventral subarachnoid space, which causes herniation of neural tissue through a large bony defect dorsally above the plane of the back (Fig. 9-10) and results in an obvious back mass (Fig. 9-11). The cord is tethered at the defect or at the site of other structural anomalies.

Myelomeningocele is thought to be secondary to lack of closure of the posterior neuropore at approximately 3 weeks of gestation. Many investigators[17,18] believe that there is a lack of normal migration of cells or that hyperplasia of the neural tissue prevents closure of the neural tube, leading to an arrest of the cord in its primitive state. Instead of a hollow tube, the "neural plate" remains with a ventral and a dorsal surface. This primitive configuration is termed the *placode*. The ventral

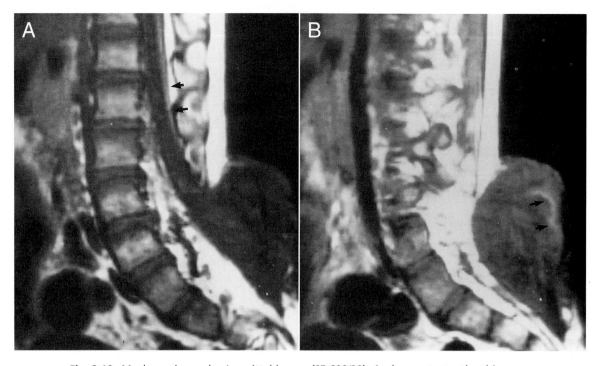

Fig. 9-10. Myelomeningocele. A sagittal image (SE 600/20), **A**, demonstrates the thin, stretched, and posteriorly positioned spinal cord (*arrows*) tethered at the bony defect. A parasagittal image, **B**, shows the neural placode clearly (*arrows*). This study is unique in that most infants born with a myelomeningocele are not examined by magnetic resonance preoperatively but are operated on within the first 48 hours of life. (Courtesy A. James Barkovich, M.D., San Francisco.)

Fig. 9-11. Stillborn infant with a myelomeningocele. Note the absence of skin in the center of the back mass and the clubfoot deformity. (Courtesy Jeffrey Ross, M.D., Cleveland.)

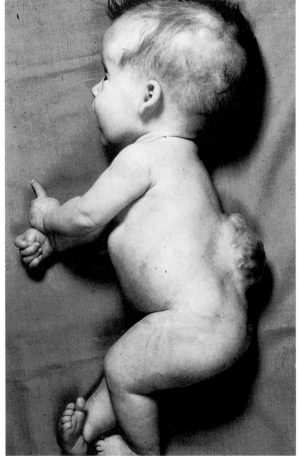

nerve roots continue to exit ventrally. The dorsal nerves however, which in a normal spine would exit posteriorly, now lie ventrally and laterally because the spinal cord is splayed. The dorsal surface of the placode should have been the central canal of the spinal cord and is, therefore, not covered by meninges.

Myelomeningocele occurs at a rate of 1 per 1000 live births. It is slightly more common in girls (1.3:1) than boys and tends to affect firstborn children more frequently. Subsequent siblings are at 7 to 15 times higher risk for neural tube defects than the general population.[31] The defects occur most commonly in the lumbosacral region, followed by the lumbar region and the thoracic region.

Clinically, these patients have severe weakness or paralysis of the lower extremities. Because of abnormal innervation, they are often plagued by a neurogenic bladder, which may result in hydronephrosis and renal compromise. Constipation and soiling are also seen. Progressive scoliosis, identified in 66% of patients, is due to the congenital vertebral anomalies as well as to the abnormal paraspinal musculature.[18]

Patients with myelomeningocele have a high incidence of the Chiari II malformation (99%), resulting in hydrocephalus that requires shunting and inferior displacement of the cerebellar tonsils and cerebellum, medulla, and fourth ventricle. Other anomalies include diastematomyelia (Fig. 9-12), syringohydromyelia, and myelodysplasia or duplication of the central canal.

Diastematomyelia (a cleft spinal cord with or without bony or fibrous spurs, seen in 30% to 40% of patients) may occur at, above, or below the myelomeningocele and may (rarely) be multiple.

Syringohydromyelia is seen in 40% to 80% of patients, possibly secondary to postsurgical obstruction of the central canal after repair or secondary to altered CSF flow from the Chiari II malformation.

Children with myelomeningocele do not usually undergo MRI imaging until after repair of the myelomeningocele, which is done within the first 24 hours of life. However, after repair, a baseline MRI of the brain and entire spinal cord is obtained. In neonates, because of the lack of cervical and lumbar lordosis, often the entire spine can be imaged on one scan.

As children grow older, the tethered cord syndrome is an important delayed consequence of myelomeningocele repair (Fig. 9-13). Follow-up spinal MRIs are obtained in children who exhibit progressive neurologic deterioration or in whom a new deficit is superimposed on an existing one.[32] Worsening of bladder or bowel dysfunction or the loss of previously stable sensory or motor function is a clue to this condition. Back or leg pain as well as progressive scoliosis may be seen and usually occurs during adolescence, coinciding with a linear growth spurt. It may be due to retethering of the cord

by adhesions at the surgical repair site[33] or to associated structural abnormalities (e.g., a thickened filum terminale, diastematomyelia, lipoma). Dermoid tumors secondary to the growth of congenital dermal rests anterior to the placode or incomplete removal of dermal tissue at the initial surgery also may cause tethering.

Retethering occurs in 3% to 15% of patients, and stretching of the cord as well as compression against the vertebral bodies is thought[32] to cause cord ischemia and myelomalacia. The surgical aim is to prevent further progression of dysfunction. Patients may or may not return to their baseline neurologic state.

Not all patients with tethered cord disclosed by MRI have a change in their clinical status; consequently, the decision to operate is based on clinical deterioration.[32] Also, since these patients often have complex neurologic disease involving the entire neural axis, imaging of the brain and entire spine is mandatory to ensure that clinical symptoms and levels of neural change correlate with the planned site of surgery.

Ultrasound may be done through the bony defect to demonstrate pulsation of the cord. If spinal cord motion is present, no tethering exists[34] (Fig. 9-13, *B*).

T_1-weighted spin echo sequences provide excellent contrast between the neural elements, CSF, and lipomatous tissue. Thus they are the mainstay of any evaluation of suspected tethering. Sagittal T_1-weighted spin echo images should be obtained first, with a slice thickness of no greater than 3 mm. The conus medullaris can be identified because of its characteristic appearance (a distinct enlargement) and is almost always low lying with a tethered cord or tight filum. A conus level below L3 is abnormal at any age. Axial images should also be obtained, from the thoracolumbar junction through the lumbosacral region, to supplement the sagittal images and obviate any difficulties with partial volume averaging, which can occur if only the sagittal scan plane is used.

An area of decreased signal intensity within the center of the distal spinal cord has been reported[35] in approximately 25% of patients with tethering. It is not clear whether this represents mild dilation of the normal terminal ventricles, mild hydromyelia, or myelomalacia. The relationship of other abnormalities, such as lipomas, can also be better appreciated in two orthogonal planes. Lipomas appear on MR images as areas of high signal intensity.

The presence or absence of spinal cord motion on MRI is another indicator of tethering. Spinal cord motion can be evaluated with phase contrast methods,[35,36] in which even small pulsations and cephalad-caudad motion of the cord are detectable.

Myelocele

A myelocele is exposed neural tissue that is not skin covered and is flush with the plane of the back.[17] The

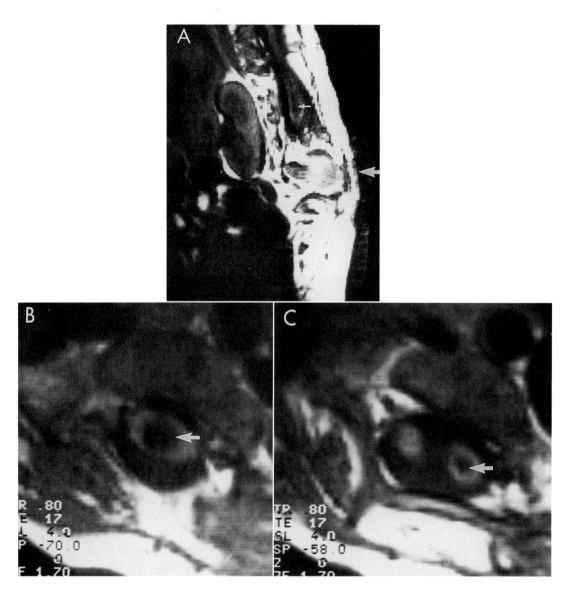

Fig. 9-12.   Postoperative myelomeningocele, diastematomyelia, and syringohydromyelia in a 1-month-old child. **A,** This sagittal T$_1$-weighted spin-echo image demonstrates deformity of the lower thoracic and upper lumbar spine at the site of surgical repair *(large arrow)*. There is a syringohydromyelia within the lower thoracic cord *(small arrow)*. **B** to **E,** Axial T$_1$-weighted spin-echo images passing rostrocaudally to just above the region of the placode show the syringohydromyelia *(arrow in* **B**) of a single cord as it joins the left hemicord **(C)** above the level of a bony spur, producing a diastematomyelia **(D).** Note that there is no evidence of the syringohydromyelia at this level. Below the spur **(E)** the hemicords reunite, again with evidence of syringohydromyelia. **F,** This sagittal T$_1$-weighted image through the cervicomedullary junction demonstrates a Chiari type II malformation *(arrows).*

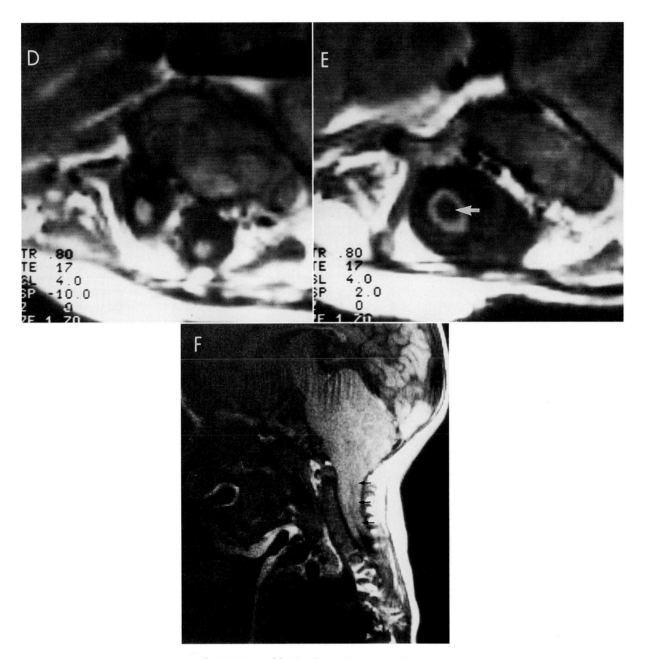

Fig. 9-12, cont'd. For legend see opposite page.

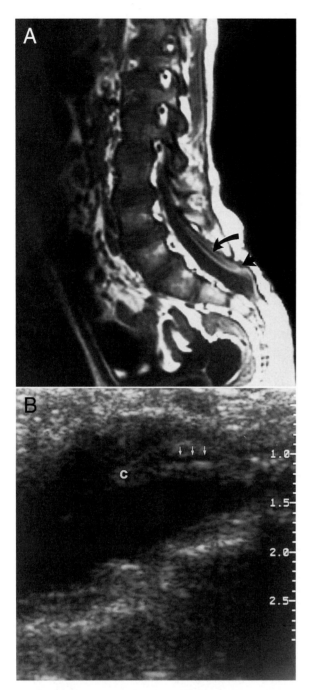

exposed placode in the early embryologic configuration of a split cord is also seen. This is the same lesion embryologically as a myelomeningocele, except that the neural tissue has not been pushed posteriorly by the ventral CSF-filled meninges.

Dysraphism Associated with a Skin-Covered Back Mass
Lipomyelomeningocele

Lipomyeloschisis refers to a dorsal dysraphism with lipoma. It is a general term that includes intradural lipoma and lipomyelomeningocele.[37] Intradural lipoma is discussed later under dysraphism without a skin-covered back mass.

Lipomyelomeningocele consists of a skin-covered back mass characterized by lipomatous tissue that extends from the subcutaneous tissue ventrally through a large bony defect to infiltrate or abut on a tethered placode. It is associated with a meningocele and often is eccentric (Fig. 9-14).

The lesion is thought to be secondary to incomplete closure of the posterior neuropore with associated abnormal separation of neuroectoderm from cutaneous ectoderm. The paraaxial mesoderm or "packing material" is then able to insinuate itself into the spinal cord. Mesoderm is induced at this site to form fat. Another theory is that ectodermal rests overgrow and prevent separation of the neuroectoderm and cutaneous ectoderm. Regardless, the end result is a fatty mass that is contiguous with the subcutaneous fat and splayed spinal cord.

Deep to this mass is a bony defect that most often involves the lumbosacral spine. In addition, the lesion is characterized by a fibrovascular band that joins the lamina of the most cephalic vertebra with other, widened, laminae and is contiguous with the periosteum of these laminae.[37] The meningocele and placode herniate into the subcutaneous lipoma and are kinked at the superior margin by this fibrovascular band, which seems to be the primary site of tethering and can be identified on MRI. As seen in myelomeningocele, there is a dorsal deficiency of dura that allows the lipoma to extend for variable distances superiorly into the bifid spinal canal and become attached to the placode. The lipoma is typically asymmetric; and as it tethers the placode, the placode rotates toward the side of the lipoma. The meningocele then balloons to the side opposite the lipoma.[37]

Lipomyelomeningocele is about one fourth as common as myelomeningocele[33] and represents 20% of skin-covered lumbosacral back masses. It is more common in girls than boys and usually occurs sporadically, although there may be an increased incidence within families. Fifty percent of patients have cutaneous stigmata (e.g., skin tags or dimples, dermoid sinus, hypertrichosis, hemangioma) (Fig. 9-15). Rarely, there may be no superficial manifestations.[33] Depending on the size of the mass, children are sometimes not evaluated until a slightly older age.

Fig. 9-13. Progressive leg weakness developed in a 6-year-old boy following repair of a myelomeningocele. **A,** The sagittal T$_1$-weighted image demonstrates a low-lying tethered spinal cord. Note the syringohydromyelia *(curved arrow)* extending to the site of fixation *(arrow)*. **B,** An ultrasound image with the patient prone shows the posteriorly positioned spinal cord *(c)* and syrinx *(arrows)*. Realtime scanning failed to reveal normal cord pulsations. The cranial cord is outside the scan plane on this image.

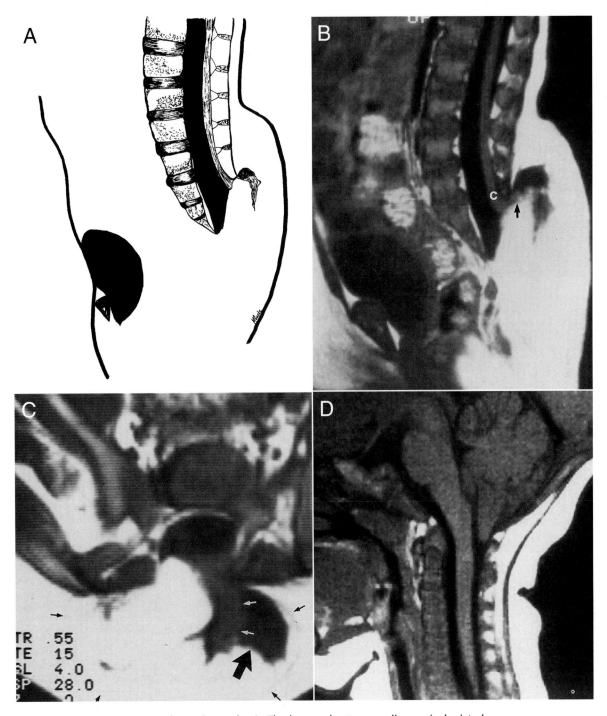

Fig. 9-14. Lipomyelomeningocele. **A,** The large subcutaneous lipoma is depicted as contiguous with a low-lying tethered cord. **B,** On this T$_1$-weighted sagittal scan, note the associated bony defect as well as the posterior herniation of the placode *(arrow).* c, Cord. **C** , A transverse image shows the neural elements *(white arrows)* herniating posteriorly as part of the lipomyelomeningocele *(large arrow). Small black arrows* outline the extent of the sac, which is filled primarily with fat. **D,** A sagittal T$_1$-weighted image through the craniovertebral junction demonstrates an associated Chiari malformation.

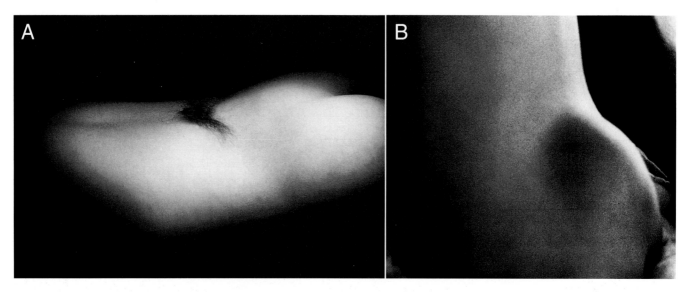

Fig. 9-15. Cutaneous stigmata associated with a lipomyelomeningocele. **A,** Hairy patch or "fawn's tail." **B,** Large lipoma in the lumbosacral region. (Courtesy Arno Fried, M.D., Providence.)

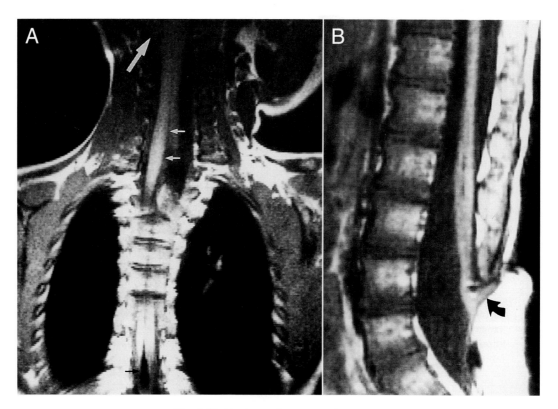

Fig. 9-16. For legend see opposite page.

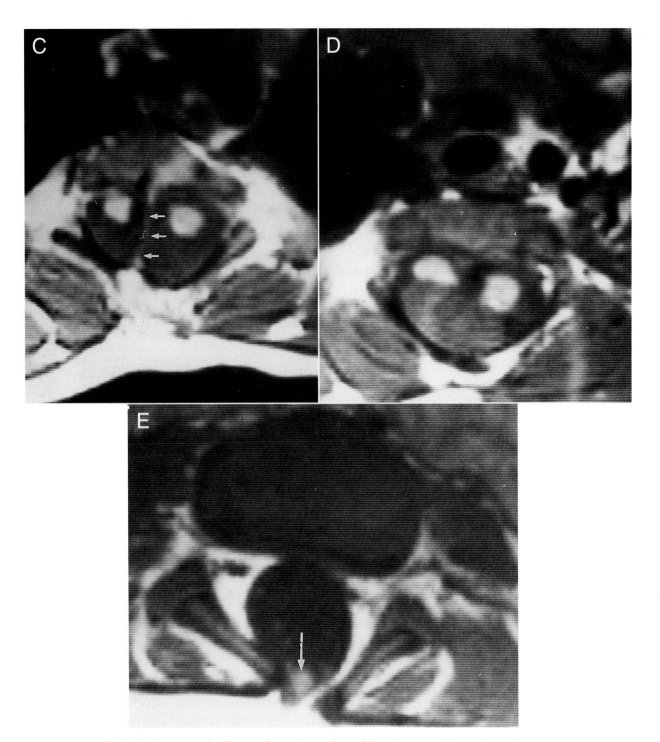

Fig. 9-16. Postoperative lipomyelomeningocele and diastematomyelia. **A,** Coronal T$_1$-weighted spin-echo image of the cervical and thoracic spine. A Chiari malformation is denoted by the *large white arrow.* The cord splits in the lower cervical region *(small white arrows)* and continues down into the thoracic region *(small black arrows).* **B,** Sagittal T$_1$-weighted spin-echo image through the lumbar region. The distal cord is adherent posteriorly to the site of surgical repair of the lipomyelomeningocele at the inferior aspect of L4 *(arrow).* **C,** Axial T$_1$-weighted spin-echo image at the level of the fibrous septum in the upper thoracic region *(arrows).* **D** and **E,** Representative axial images through the midthorax **(D)** and site of the tethered cord distally **(E).** Note the slight asymmetry of the hemicords in **D** and the posterior location of the tethered cord at the level of the spina bifida in **E** *(arrow).*

Typically the patient will be neurologically normal at birth. However, most develop neurologic dysfunction if not repaired early.[38,39]

Associated anomalies are less common than in myelomeningocele. However, a Chiari I malformation (Fig. 9-14, *C*) or hydromyelia may be seen in 10% of cases. Partial sacral agenesis occurs with increased frequency. A Chiari II malformation is not seen.[38]

If repair is not done early, it is theorized[36] that increased fat deposition within a fixed number of fat cells in the spinal canal will cause a greater mass effect over time. Another theory[37] postulates that the lipoma will tether the cord, causing stretching and ischemia. The role of surgery is to debulk the lipoma within the canal and untether the cord.

As with other developmental lesions, T_1-weighted spin-echo imaging remains the method of choice. The soft tissue signal intensity of the neural structures, the decreased signal of the CSF, and the high signal of lipomatous tissue stand out sharply. Orthogonal imaging is especially critical to determine the exact relationship of the lipoma and neural structures. In patients with a lipomyelomeningocele the lipoma may rotate the dorsal surface of the placode, which leads to asymmetry between the size and location of the nerve roots. This aberrant positioning then limits the mobility of the cord; it also makes untethering at the time of sugery more difficult and it increases the risk of direct surgical trauma to the nerve roots.[14] As with other developmental anomalies, one is obligated to screen the spinal axis for any associated abnormalities.

After surgery the caudad displacement of the conus may remain unchanged on MRI studies, despite untethering. The only difference may be a decrease in the size of the lipoma[38] (Fig. 9-16).

Simple posterior meningocele

The simple posterior meningocele is a skin-covered herniated sac of meninges, filled with CSF, that does not contain neural elements although occasionally an adherent nerve root will be present (Fig. 9-17). The conus is in normal position. Typically, this sac is located in the lumbosacral region. It is much rarer than myelomeningocele (10:1) and is seen equally in girls and boys. The bony defect tends to be more limited.[9,17]

Myelocystocele

Myelocystocele is a rare[40] localized dilation of the central canal of the spinal cord, most often in the lumbosacral region,[17,41] that herniates through a large spina bifida and presents as a cystic skin-covered back mass[41] (Fig. 9-18). It may be associated with cloacal exstrophy and typically is lined by ependyma.[41] The spinal cord is tethered and low lying.

Myelocystoceles are associated with a syringohydromyelia within the cord. They also may be associated with

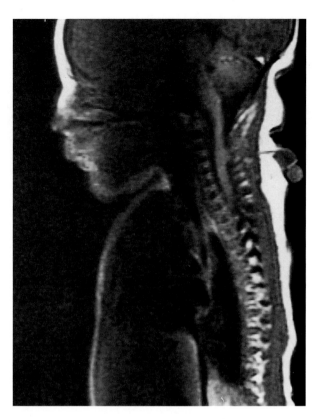

Fig. 9-17. Simple posterior meningocele. This neonate was found to have a simple posterior meningocele at surgery and pathologic examination. It is in an atypical location. The "stalk" is also unusual.

a ventral or dorsal meningocele to form a myelocystomeningocele. Although surrounded by subcutaneous fat, the myelocystocele remains separate and does not invade the cord. Embryologically a myelocystocele is postulated* to result from nonclosure of the posterior neuropore. Clinically patients have a neurogenic bladder and bowel dysfunction.

Besides cloacal exstrophy, other associations include partial sacral agenesis,[17] anomalies of the gastrointestinal or genitourinary tract, and scoliosis. Arnold-Chiari II is not usually associated with myelocystocele.

T_1-weighted images demonstrate splaying of the distal cord as well as the fluid-filled cyst. The fluid in the myelocystocele may be of slighter greater signal than CSF in the remainder of the thecal sac.[17]

Dysraphism Without an Associated Back Mass
Diastematomyelia

Diastematomyelia (*diastema*, space or cleft) is defined as a sagittal splitting of the spinal cord, conus medullaris, or filum terminale into two segments (Fig. 9-19).

---

*References 7, 17, 30, 42, 43, 44.

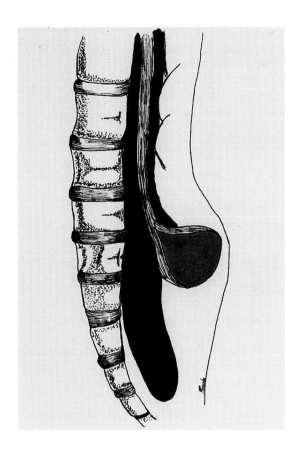

Fig. 9-18. Myelocystocele. A large spina bifida with a skin-covered back mass is depicted. The mass is actually a tethered low-lying cord with marked dilation of the central canal, which herniates through the bony defect.

Fig. 9-19. Diastematomyelia. This intraoperative photograph shows splitting of the spinal cord *(c)*, with two separate dural sacs, by a fibrofatty spur *(s)*. (Courtesy Arno Fried, M.D., Providence.)

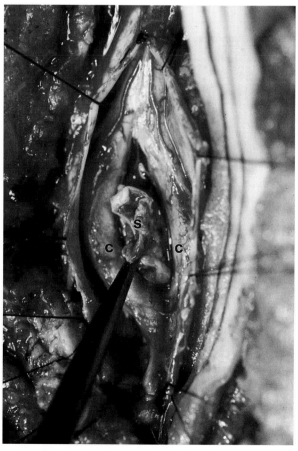

Generally speaking, in the 50% of patients in whom the dural tube is undivided,[17,33] clinical findings are rare and surgery is not indicated. In the remaining 50%, however, there is either complete or partial splitting of the dural sac by a fatty, fibrous, cartilaginous, or bony spur that causes tethering of the cord and results in clinical symptoms. Often the split is asymmetric, with one cord larger than the other. The larger cord may have a dilated central canal or a syrinx.

The cleft may be complete or incomplete, with the spur usually located at the caudal end of the cord division. Spurs tend to arise from the lamina; thus, if a partial spur is present, it will be seen posteriorly in the spinal canal. Rarely are spurs multiple, the split in the cord occurring generally between T9 and S1. In over 90% of cases the split will reunite inferior to the spur[45] (Fig. 9-20).

Often these bony spurs are difficult to identify at routine spinal radiography since many of the patients with diastematomyelia have severe segmentation anomalies of the vertebral bodies, such as butterfly vertebrae or hemivertebrae. These can result in severe scoliosis, which may also make the spur more difficult to see. Thus the diastematomyelia is also characterized by spina bifida at several levels.

When the spinal cord is perfectly duplicated, the term *diplomyelia* may be used. Each hemicord in diplomyelia has its own central canal, two anterior and two posterior nerve horns, and its own anterior spinal artery.

The embryologic theories to explain this interesting anomaly are multiple. The lesion has been produced experimentally in chick embryos[46] by placing a nonabsorbable shell in the spine. It may be that an adhesion or a persistent neurenteric canal blocks the normal cranial migration of the notochord, resulting in two hemicords and associated segmental anomalies of the spine[45] (Fig. 9-20). Other theories include failure of the neural plate to fuse in the dorsal midline, with incurving of the lateral portions of the plate to form two separate cords,[17,33] or a primary mesodermal abnormality that splits the neural plate.

The lesion affects primarily girls (80% to 95% of cases). Some 50% to 75% of patients have skin changes (e.g., lipoma, dimple, hemangioma, or nevus) overlying the site of the diastematomyelia.

In patients who are symptomatic 50% have orthopedic problems such as clubfoot deformity or muscle weakness and wasting.

In a series by Scatliff et al.[47] 23 of 25 patients had disparity in limb size, with the smaller extremity being on the same side as the smaller hemicord. With growth of the patient a traction myelopathy developed consisting of numbness of the legs as well as urinary and rectal dysfunction.[47]

Treatment is aimed at identifying the lesion early and performing surgery prior to progressive symptoms. If surgery is delayed, sensory and bladder dysfunction may not return to baseline.

Associated lesions include myelomeningocele (35%), hydromyelia (50%), tethered conus or thickened filum terminale, dermal sinus, lipoma, and myelodysplasia (Fig. 9-21).

Dorsal dermal sinus

The dorsal dermal sinus is a midline sinus tract, lined by epithelium, that extends inward from the skin surface for a variable distance. It may terminate in the subcutaneous tissues of the back or extend deeper to communicate with the conus or distal spinal cord (Fig. 9-22).

The dorsal dermal sinus is thought to arise from focal incomplete separation of cutaneous ectoderm from neural ectoderm. During the eighteenth week of gestation, when the spinal cord ascends relative to the spinal canal, this epithelium-lined tube may tether the cord and after birth allow seeding of bacteria from the skin to the tract, resulting in a local abscess or meningitis if the tract communicates with the intradural space. The epithelium lining the tract may also desquamate, producing a dermoid or epidermoid in 30% to 50% of cases.

The dermal sinus occurs most frequently in the sacrococcygeal region and at this site rarely communicates with the spinal canal. It may also be called a simple sacrococcygeal dimple. When it occurs above this level, however, usually in the lumbosacral region, it will often extend into the spinal canal or cord (Fig. 9-23).

The sinus is seen with equal frequency in boys and girls. A hyperpigmented patch, hairy nevus, or capillary angioma is usually associated with a skin dimple. Patients often present with infection (cutaneous or intraspinal abscess) (60%) or signs of cord or nerve root compression from an expanding dermoid or epidermoid.

Other associated anomalies are uncommon.

Experience with MRI to date suggests that, except for the areas of the tract lined by fat, the intraspinal portions of the tract may be poorly seen (Fig. 9-24). In a series of seven patients reported by Barkovich et al.,[48] five patients had associated epidermoids or dermoids that were seen but two had diffuse subarachnoid tumors that were missed. The authors suggested heavily T_1-weighted MR sequences in addition to either ultrasound or CT myelography.[48] Rindahl et al.[49] had two patients with infected sinus tracts seen on T_2-weighted images, presumably caused by infected edematous tissue.

Filum terminale

The filum terminale is the distalmost slender portion of the spinal cord that contains neural tissue. It continues as a long fibrous band adherent to the dorsal aspect of the first coccygeal vertebra.[50] The cranial portion is intradural, the caudal most fibrous portion extradural.

Text continued on p. 381.

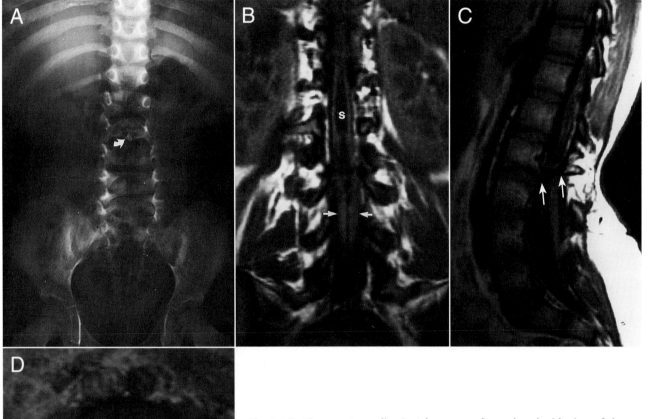

Fig. 9-20. Diastematomyelia. **A,** A bony spur *(arrow)* and widening of the lumbar interpediculate distance are evident on this AP radiograph. **B,** The coronal MR study demonstrates a syringohydromyelia *(a)* and splitting of the cord *(arrows).* **C,** The sagittal image shows that the spur extends ventrad to dorsad *(arrows).* **D,** The axial scan shows the two hemicords.

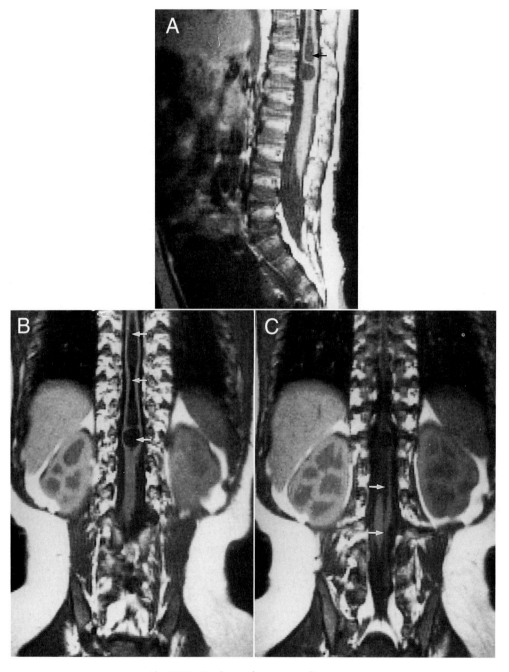

Fig. 9-21. For legend see opposite page.

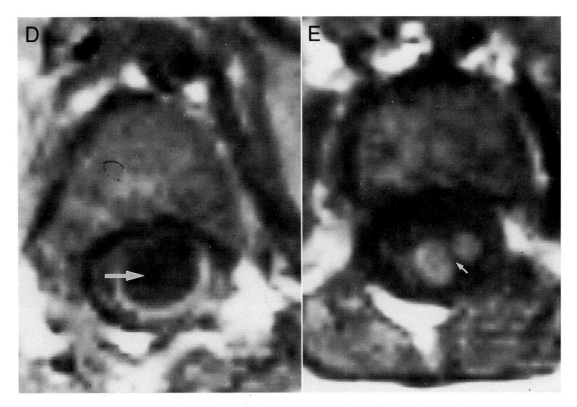

Fig. 9-21. Tethered spinal cord, syringohydromyelia, and diastematomyelia. **A,** A sagittal T$_1$-weighted spin-echo image demonstrates tethering of the cord at the L4 level. There is evidence of syringohydromyelia *(arrows).* **B** and **C,** Contiguous coronal sagittal T$_1$-weighted images through the thoracolumbar region. The central cystic dilation is well appreciated, as are the asymmetric hemicords below the level of the syringohydromyelia *(arrows).* The hemicords may be missed in the sagittal plane. **D** and **E,** Axial images through the syringohydromyelia superiorly (**D,** *arrow*) and diastematomyelia inferiorly (**E,** *arrow*). Note the asymmetric hemicords in **E** above the level of tethering.

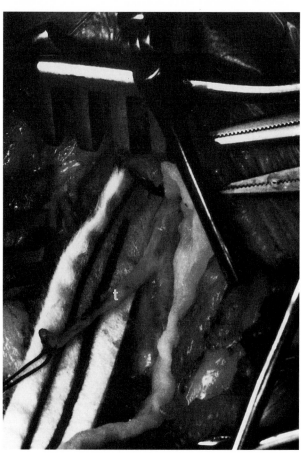

Fig. 9-22. Dermal sinus. This intraoperative photograph demonstrates a long sinus tract *(t)* that had extended from the skin to the spinal cord. (Courtesy Arno Fried, M.D., Providence.)

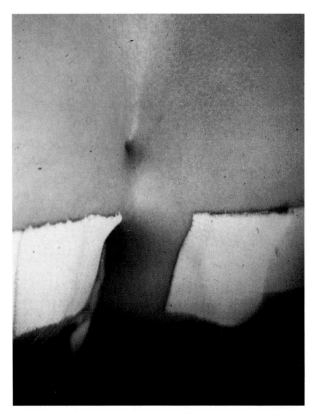

Fig. 9-23. Dermal sinus. Skin dimple in the lumbosacral region with a dermal sinus extending to the spinal cord. (Courtesy Arno Fried, M.D., Providence.)

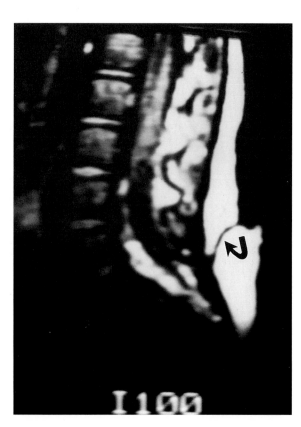

Fig. 9-24. Dermal sinus. This sagittal T_1 image demonstrates the sinus tract extending from a skin dimple to involve the cord in an infant. (Courtesy Arno Fried, M.D., Providence.)

Raghavan et al.[35] point out the importance of the filum terminale. The spinal cord itself is a "viscoelastic structure" that is secured and "buffered" by the dentate ligaments and filum terminale. The compliance of the normally thin filum protects the spinal cord from undue stretching. Thus, when the filum is thick or infiltrated with fat, its elasticity may be lost and the spinal cord will be stretched, resulting in ischemia or other metabolic changes that cause cell damage to the neurons.[35]

Fibrolipomas of the filum terminale. Fibrolipomas of the filum terminale are often seen as a normal variant, appearing on T$_1$-weighted images as an area of high signal intensity (Fig. 9-25). The conus is in normal position, and the patients are asymptomatic.

In one autopsy series[51] these tumors were found in 6% of patients, presumably with a normal spine; and in a series from Japan[52] a 0.24% incidence of fatty filum was shown (4 of 1691 patients with no clinical symptoms related to tethering). The latter authors proposed that this developmental anomaly, when isolated, may be without clinical significance. However, it also has been stated[14] that fibrolipomas may be associated with myelomeningoceles or the tight filum terminale syndrome and should be followed closely.

Tight filum terminale syndrome. In this syndrome the patient has a short thickened filum (normal measurements: ≤2 mm diameter at the L5-S1 level), a low-lying conus, and a clinical picture consisting of neurologic symptoms or orthopedic deformities.[35]

Patients may present with muscle atrophy or weakness and abnormal lower extremity reflexes. Bladder dysfunction, back pain, and radiculopathy are also noted, with symptoms worsening in the morning or after exercise.[14,17] Orthopedic deformities such as clubfoot may be seen. This anomaly is thought to result from an abnormal phase of retrogressive differentiation.

On MR the filum will demonstrate thickening with fibrous tissue (isointense to the cord). It may be difficult on sagittal images to differentiate the filum from distal nerve roots; axial images are usually necessary. Some authors[53] have proposed the term *neurofibrous structure* to describe the conus-thickened filum terminale unit when these structures can no longer be differentiated. The low-lying conus is best seen on sagittal T$_1$ images.

Intradural lipoma

The intradural lipoma is a localized collection of encapsulated fat enclosed within the dural sac.[14] Embryologically there may be premature separation of neuroectoderm from cutaneous ectoderm, allowing (1) paraaxial mesoderm to infiltrate the spinal cord and differentiate into fat, (2) a proliferation of native fat cells, or (3) embryonic ectoderm to overgrow and differentiate into fat cells.[54]

Intradural lipomas are not common, comprising less than 1% of primary intraspinal tumors. They lie on the surface of the cord and do not infiltrate the cord. They usually are subpial, although an estimated 50% will have

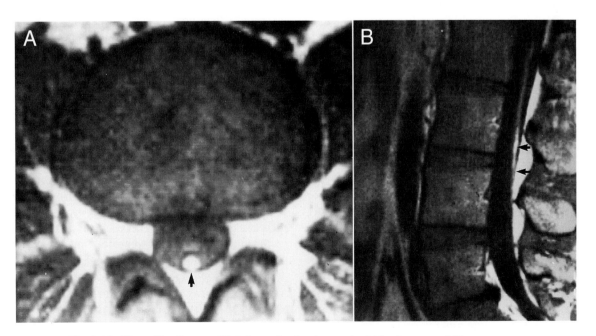

Fig. 9-25. Filum fibrolipoma. High-intensity fat *(arrows)* within the normal filum was an incidental finding on these T$_1$-weighted axial, **A,** and sagittal, **B,** images.

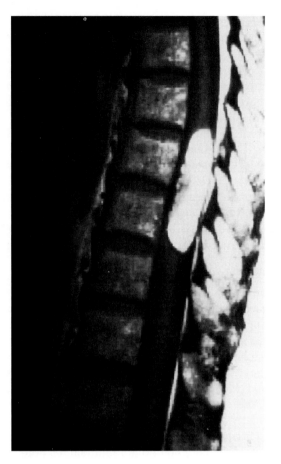

Fig. 9-26. Intradural lipoma. Note the localized collection of fat in the thoracic region on this T_1-weighted sagittal image.

an exophytic component above the pia but usually contained within the dura.

These lipomas are found anywhere along the cord though most commonly in the cervicothoracic region (Fig. 9-26). They are more common in males and are seen in children less than 5 years old and during middle age.

Clinical symptoms include slowly developing ascending spastic paresis without pain or radiculopathy.[55] The skin overlying the lipoma is normal. The spinal canal may be normal or widened at the site of the lipoma. Segmentation anomalies of the vertebrae are unusual. MRI findings consist of localized high signal within the thecal sac or spinal cord on T_1-weighted images.

Syringohydromyelia

Syringohydromyelia consists of a longitudinal cavitary lesion within the spinal cord surrounded by gliosis. Hydromyelia, which is an enlargement of just the central canal, and syringomyelia, an eccentric cavity in the cord parenchyma not involving the central canal, are im-

possible to differentiate in vivo; and distinguishing them premortem is irrelevant. Thus the term *syringohydromyelia* is used to encompass all these lesions.[4]

There are a number of fascinating theories to explain the development of syringohydromyelia: (1) obstruction of the fourth ventricular foramen forces CSF into the central canal, ultimately distending it[56]; (2) the normal cephalad flow of CSF from the spinal subarachnoid space is partially blocked from the intracranial spaces, causing a pressure differential that allows CSF to accumulate within the central canal[57]; and (3) craniospinal fluid pressure differentials force CSF from the spinal subarachnoid space into the central canal through the spinal cord.[58]

Syringohydromyelia is divided into a communicating type (indicating patency with the rest of the ventricular system) and a noncommunicating type (nonpatency).

In the communicating type there is generally an association with congenital or acquired lesions at the foramen magnum, most commonly Arnold Chiari I and II malformations. Since these patients often have a myelomeningocele, however, the enlarged central canal may be a primary developmental anomaly[33] (Fig. 9-21).

In the noncommunicating type it is postulated[59] that fluid enters through enlarged perivascular spaces, nerve roots, or macroscopic rents in the cord and becomes trapped within because of pressure differentials. Later the glial surface may secrete fluid.

Clinically patients with a syringohydromyelia will often have no symptoms until late adolescence or early adulthood. Children with myelomeningocele will have an extensive syringohydromyelia with few symptoms apparently related to it.[59]

In patients with posttraumatic syringohydromyelia the symptoms may not occur until years after the initial insult. Spinal cord tumors may also cause syringohydromyelia secondary to obstruction of the central canal. Typically the patient will have pain, often severe, with dissociated sensory loss (such that the sense of touch is preserved but temperature and pain discrimination is lost). This is often accompanied by weakness, muscle atrophy, dystrophic skin changes, and neuropathic joints. Symptoms can be unilateral or bilateral. The clinical course is sometimes unpredictable, with periods of stability marked by rapid decompensation. Again, the relationship of other coexisting conditions often makes it difficult to distinguish the role that syringohydromyelia plays relative to the patient's clinical deterioration.

Sagittal T_1-weighted spin-echo images with a slice thickness of 3 mm or less are the appropriate first step in evaluating syringohydromyelia. The region of the foramen magnum should be included (to evaluate for any associated Chiari malformation). Axial T_1-weighted spin-echo 5 mm thick sections should also be obtained. Syrinx cavities can be eccentric and may be missed on sagittal T_1 spin-echo images alone. Once identified, it is

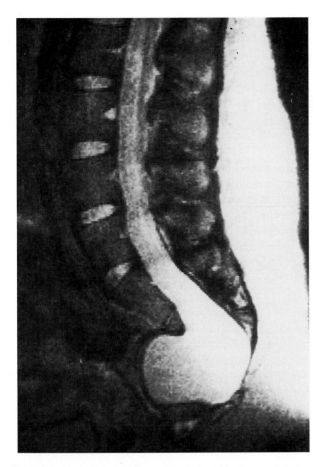

Fig. 9-27. Anterior sacral meningocele. This T_2-weighted sagittal image through the lumbosacral region demonstrates a low-intensity cystic mass anterior to the sacrum that communicates with the sacral CSF space.

important to evaluate the caudad and cephalad extent of the cavity. These are important data points for surgical treatment and for establishing a baseline prior to subsequent follow-up.

On T_1-weighted spin-echo images the fluid within the syrinx cavity will usually demonstrate a low signal intensity, but it can vary depending on the effect of CSF pulsations and the pulse sequence used. Increasing the TE and/or TR will increase the signal intensity of fluid within the cavity. Likewise, the addition of refocusing pulses to the sequence can increase the signal intensity by reducing the signal loss secondary to CSF pulsations. Long TR sequences may also demonstrate increased signal intensity in the tissue immediately surrounding the syrinx, most often at the caudal portion. This is thought to be related to microcystic or gliotic changes in the adjacent cord.[9]

Phase-contrast cine MR can provide useful information regarding the alterations of CSF signal intensity secondary to flow. Flow within a syrinx cavity has a sys-

tolic and diastolic component similar to that of the general CSF space.[59,60]

Gadolinium-enhanced images may be obtained to look for possible associated tumors as a cause of the syringohydromyelia, even in children with Chiari I malformation. A syringohydromyelia not associated with tumor will not enhance.

Meningocele

The simple posterior meningocele has been discussed. However, a meningocele may occur at other sites and have more typical clinical associations or presentations.

Meningoceles are an extension of the CSF-filled meningeal sac through a bony defect in the spine not associated with neural elements. In the thoracic region they involve the dura protruding through an enlarged neural foramen possibly into the extrapleural space. Neurofibromatosis is seen in 85% of patients with a thoracic meningocele.[9] In the lumbar region they may be idiopathic or associated with the Marfan syndrome or neurofibromatosis.

Anterior sacral meningoceles result from erosion or lack of development of the sacrum and coccyx, allowing the herniated ventral sac to present as a presacral mass (Fig. 9-27). Because such protrusion exerts pressure on the rectum, bladder, or sacral nerve roots, the patient usually has constipation, bladder dysfunction, low back pain or pressure, and/or sciatica—which also can occur in neurofibromatosis and the Marfan syndrome.

On MRI an associated tethering of the cord or a lipoma or dermoid may be demonstrated. A preoperative MR examination will often reveal the location of surrounding nerve roots and help in planning the surgery.

CAUDAL REGRESSION SYNDROME

Caudal regression syndrome is a spectrum of anomalies that includes absence of the lowermost spine, anal atresia, malformed external genitalia, renal abnormalities, and in the most severe forms fusion of the lower extremities (sirenomyelia).[9] In its mildest form there is absence just of the coccyx and patients are asymptomatic. Severe forms may include absence of the spine below T8. This anomaly is quite rare, occurring in 1 per 7500 births.[62] Approximately 16% of infants with caudal regression have diabetic mothers.[33]

The exact relationship of maternal diabetes to caudal regression syndrome, however, is not known although the role of insulin, sulfur-containing substances, and altered carbohydrate metabolism has been studied.[63] A similar condition can be induced in chickens by injections of insulin.

Barkovich et al.[64] postulate that at 3 weeks of gestation there is increased metabolic activity in the caudal end of the embryo along with earlier development of the

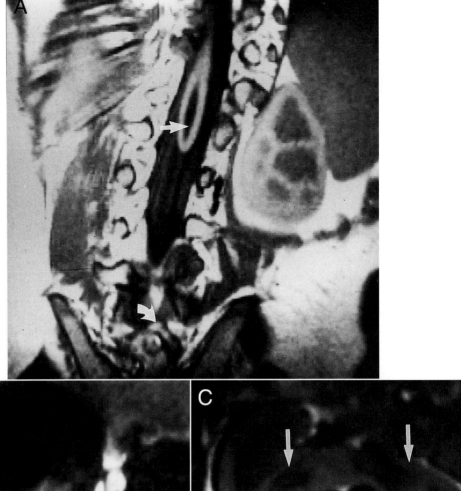

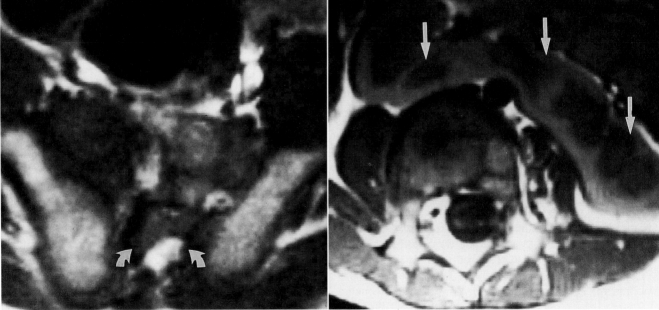

Fig. 9-28. Sacral agenesis. **A,** Coronal T$_1$-weighted spin-echo image through the lumbosacral region. Note the dilated distal central canal *(straight arrow)*, scoliosis, and absence of the sacrum *(curved arrow)*. **B,** An axial T$_1$-weighted spin-echo image through the ilia demonstrates absence of the sacrum *(curved arrows)*. **C,** Another axial T$_1$-weighted spin-echo image, through the upper lumbar region, shows mild deformity of the vertebral body and an associated horseshoe kidney *(arrows)*.

circulatory system to the caudal end of the ventral neural tube and notochord relative to the cranial end of the cord. Therefore focal delivery of a teratogenic substance, infection, or ischemia might cause this regional damage and result in the anomaly.[64]

There are three types of sacral agenesis, a less severe form of caudal regression, described by Smith[65] (Fig. 9-28): complete absence of the sacrum (with the ilia articulating with each other), subtotal sacrococcygeal agenesis (with absence of only caudal segments and a hemisacrum), and partial or total absence of sacral segments unilaterally. The triad of sacral agenesis, a presacral mass, and anorectal stenosis is known as the Currarino triad.[66]

Clinically patients have a range of deformities, from mild distal muscle weakness or deformities of the feet to complete paralysis and sensory loss of the lower extremities. Most patients have a neurogenic bladder. Renal aplasia or dysplasia and anal atresia are often present.

On plain films the degree of absence of the spinal column can be assessed. On CT and MRI there is often bony spinal canal stenosis immediately above the last intact vertebra. Stenosis of the canal may add to the patient's already severe neurologic deficit. Other associated bony and vertebral anomalies may be seen; and other dysraphisms (myelomeningocele, diastematomyelia, lipoma of the filum terminale, dermal sinus, intradural lipoma) may occur with caudal regression.[17]

On MRI, sagittal images demonstrate not only the vertebral body abnormalities but also a typical "wedge-shaped" appearance of the spinal cord terminus as described by Barkovich[9] (Fig. 9-29).

The distal cord may be tethered and tapered, particularly if associated with other dysraphisms.[9]

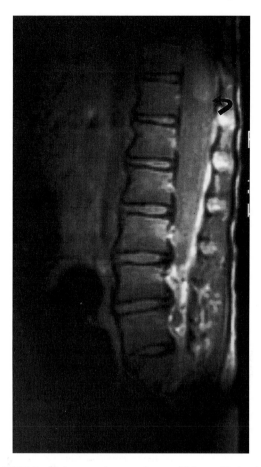

Fig. 9-29. Caudal regression syndrome. This sagittal spin density image demonstrates absence of much of the sacrum as well as a wedge-shaped termination of the spinal cord (arrow).

SPLIT NOTOCHORD SYNDROME

The split notochord syndrome encompasses a group of anomalies characterized by persistent communication of the gut, spine, and spinal cord posteriorly through the skin of the back. It is thought to be due to a lack of separation of the ventral endoderm from the ectoderm. The notochord, which develops between these two cell layers, must split or deviate around the adhesion. As the fetus grows, the "through and through" defect from gut to dorsal skin may persist, all or in part, and give rise to a variety of anomalies. The tract may become obliterated to form a cyst, diverticulum, fistula, sinus, or fibrous band.[17]

The lesions are classified according to their location of communication, either mediastinal or abdominal. They may be lined with gastric or small or large bowel mucosa. The most common lesion is the mediastinal dorsal enteric cyst, usually noted in infancy, in which the

child presents with respiratory difficulty or sagittally cleft vertebrae. It usually occurs (80%) in boys.

MRI is useful for demonstrating the diverticulum or cyst as well as the bony dysraphism. Sinus tracts and fistulae may be missed.

REFERENCES

1. Byrd S: Imaging of the spine in infants and children. *Curr Opin Radiol* 1990;2(6):885-894.
2. Gusnard DA, Zimmerman RA: Computed tomography versus magnetic resonance imaging of the pediatric central nervous system: techniques, indications, and examples. *Clin Pediatr* 1990;29(3):136-157.
3. Gower DJ: The pediatric spine: a view through clearer glasses. *J Child Neurol* 1990;5(1):2, 49.
4. Naidich TP, Doundoulakis SH, Poznanski AK: Intraspinal masses: efficacy of plain spine radiography. *Pediatr Neurosci* 1985;12:10-17.

5. Brunberg JA, DiPietro MA, Venes JL, et al: Intramedullary lesions of the pediatric spinal cord: correlation of findings from MR imaging, intraoperative sonography, surgery, and histologic study. *Radiology* 1991;181:573-579.

6. Nelson MD Jr, Bracchi M, Naidich TP, McLone DG: Natural history of repaired myelomeningocele. *Radiographics* 1988;8:695-706.

7. Naidich TP, Fernback SK, McLone DG, et al: Sonography of the caudal spine and back: congenital anomalies in children. *AJR* 1984;142:1229-1242.

8. Committee on Drugs, Section on Anesthesiology: Guidelines for the elective use of conscious sedation, deep sedation, and general anesthesia in pediatric patients. *Pediatrics* 1985;76:317-321.

9. Barkovich AJ: Techniques and methods in pediatric imaging. In Barkovich AJ (ed): *Pediatric neuroimaging,* New York, Raven, 1990, pp 1-4.

10. Strain JD, Campbell JB, Harvey LA, Foley LC: IV Nembutal: safe sedation for children undergoing CT. *AJR* 1988;151:975-979.

11. Fisher, DM: Sedation of pediatric patients: an anesthesiologist's perspective. *Radiology* 1990;175:613-615.

12. Bloomfield EL, Masaryk TJ, Caplin A, et al: Intravenous sedation for MR imaging of the brain and spine in children: pentobarbital versus Propofol. *Radiology* 1993;186:93-97.

13. Verbout AJ: *The development of the vertebral column,* New York, Springer, 1985, pp 1-2.

14. Barkovich AJ, Naidich JP: Congenital anomalies of the spine. In Barkovich AJ (ed): *Pediatric neuroimaging,* New York, Raven, 1990, pp 227-271.

15. Theiler K: *Vertebral malformations,* New York, Springer, 1988, pp 1-36.

16. Langman J: Human development, normal and abnormal. In *Medical embryology,* Baltimore, Williams & Wilkins, 1969, pp 54-68.

17. Byrd SE, Darling CF, McLone DG: Developmental disorders of the pediatric spine. In Modic MT (ed): Imaging of the spine, *Radiol Clin North Am* 1991;29(4):711-752.

18. O'Rahilly R, Benson DR: The development of the vertebral column. In Bradford DS, Hensinger RM (eds): *The pediatric spine,* New York, Thieme, 1985, pp 3-17.

19. Flannigan-Sprague BD, Modic MT: The pediatric spine: normal anatomy and spinal dysraphism. In Modic MT, Masaryk TJ, Ross JS (eds): *Magnetic resonance imaging of the spine,* Chicago, Year Book, 1988, pp 240-256.

20. Ho PSP, Yu S, Sether LA, et al: Progressive and regressive changes in the nucleus pulposus. I. The neonate, *Radiology* 1988;169:87-91.

21. Yu S, Haughton VM, Ho PSP, et al: Progressive and regressive changes in the nucleus pulposus. II. The adult, *Radiology* 1988;169:93-97.

22. Sarwar M: Imaging of the pediatric spine and its contents. *J Child Neurol* 1990;5(1):3-18.

23. Cohen MD: *Pediatric magnetic resonance imaging.* Philadelphia, Saunders, 1986, pp 81-82.

24. Peacock A: Observation on the post-natal structure of the intervertebral disc in man. *J Anat* 1952;86:162-179.

25. Schmorl G, Junghanns H: *The human spine in health and disease,* ed 2. New York, Grune & Stratton, 1971, pp 2-30.

26. Keyes DC, Compere EL: The normal and pathological physiology of the nucleus pulposus of the intervertebral disc. *J Bone Joint Surg [Am]* 1932;14:897-938.

27. Sze G, Baierl P, Bravo S: Evolution of the infant spinal column: evaluation with MR imaging. *Radiology* 1991;181:819-827.

28. Wilson DA, Prince JR: MR determination of the location of the normal conus medullaris throughout childhood. *AJR* 1989; 152:1029-1032.

29. James CCM, Lassman LP: Spinal dysraphism; spina bifida occulta. New York, Appleton, 1972, Chap 8.

30. Naidich TP, McLone DG: Congenital pathology of the spine and spinal cord. In Taveras JM, Ferrucci JT (eds): *Radiology: diagnosis, imaging, intervention.* Philadelphia, Lippincott, 1986, pp 1-23.

31. Carter CO: Clues to the aetiology of neural tube of neural tube malformations. [Abstract.] *Develop Med Child Neurol* 1974;16(suppl 32):3.

32. Balasubramaniam C, Laurent JP, McCluggage C, et al: Tethered cord syndrome after repair of meningomyelocele. *Childs Nerv Syst* 1990;6(4):208-211.

33. Brunberg JA, Latchaw RE, Kanal E, et al: Magnetic resonance imaging of spinal dysraphism. *Radiol Clin North Am* 1988;26(2):198-201.

34. Rubin JM, DiPietro MA: Spinal ultrasonography: intraoperative and pediatric applications. *Radiol Clin North Am* 1988;26(1):1-27.

35. Raghavan N, Barkovich AJ, Edwards M, Norman D: MR imaging in the tethered spinal cord syndrome. *AJR* 1989;152:843-852.

36. Levy L, DiChiro G, McCullough DC, et al: The fixed spinal cord: diagnosis with MR imaging. *Radiology* 1988;169:773-778.

37. Naidich TP, McLone DG, Mutluer S: A new understanding of dorsal dysraphism with lipoma (lipomyeloschisis): radiologic evaluation and surgical correction. *AJR* 1983;140:1065-1078.

38. Brophy JD, Sutton LN, Zimmerman RA, et al: Magnetic resonance imaging of lipomyelomeningocele and tethered cord. *Neurosurgery* 1989;25(3):336-340.

39. Taviere V, Brunelle F, Baraton J, et al: MRI study of lumbosacral lipoma in children. *Pediatr Radiol* 1989;19(5):316-320.

40. McLone DG, Naidich TP: Terminal myelocystocele. *Neurosurgery* 1985;16:36-43.

41. Lemire RJ, Loeser JD, Leech RW, et al: *Normal and abnormal development of the human nervous system.* Hagerstown Md, Harper & Row, 1975.

42. Naidich TP, Harwood-Nash DC, McLone DG: Radiology of spinal dysraphism. *Clin Neurosurg* 1983;30:341-365.

43. Anderson FM: Occult spinal dysraphism: diagnosis and management. *J Pediatr* 1968;73:163-177.

44. Vade A, Kennard D: Lipomeningomyelocystocele. *AJNR* 1987;8:375-377.

45. Castillo M: MRI of diastematomyelia. *MRI Decisions* 1991;5:12-17.

46. Rilliet B, Berney J, Schowing J, Kostli A: Experimental diastematomyelia in the chick embryo. Poster presentation, 21st Annual Meeting of the Swiss Societies for Experimental Biology, University of Fribourg, 1989.

47. Scatliff JH, Kendall BE, Kingsley DP, et al: Closed spinal dysraphism: analysis of clinical, radiological, and surgical findings in 104 consecutive patients. *AJR* 1989;152:1049-1057.

48. Barkovich AJ, Edwards MS, Cogen PH: MR evaluation of spinal dermal sinus tracts in children. *AJNR* 1991;12(1):123-129.

49. Rindahl MA, Colletti PM, Zee CS, et al: Magnetic resonance imaging of pediatric spinal dysraphism. *Magn Reson Imaging* 1989;7(2):217-224.

50. Sarwar M, Kier EL, Veraspongse C: *Development of the spine and spinal cord.* San Anselmo Calif, Clavadel, 1983.

51. Emery JL, Lendon RG: The local cord lesion in neurospinal dysraphism (meningomyelocele). *J Pathol* 1973;110:83-96.

52. Uchino A, Mori T, Ohno M: Thickened fatty filum terminale: MR imaging. *Neuroradiology* 1991;33:331-333.

53. Tortori-Donat P, Cama A, Rosa ML, et al: Occult spinal dysraphism: neuroradiological study. *Neuroradiology* 1990;31:512-522.

54. Naidich TP, McLone DG, Harwood-Nash DC: Spinal dysraphism. In Newton TH, Potts DG (eds): *Modern neuroradiology: computed tomography of the spine and spinal cord,* San Anselmo Calif, Clavadel, 1982, pp 299-353.

55. Giuffrè R: Intradural spinal lipomas: review of the literature (99 cases) and report of an additional case. *Acta Neurochir* 1966;14:69-95.

56. Gardner WJ: Hydrodynamic mechanism of syringomyelia: its relationship to myelocele. *J Neurol Neurosurg Psychiatry* 1965;28:247-259.

57. Williams B: On the pathogenesis of syringomyelia: a review. *J Royal Soc Med* 1980;73:798-806.

58. Ball MJ, Dayan AD: Pathogenesis of syringomyelia. Lancet 1972;2:799-801.

59. Enzmann DR, DeLaPaz RL, Rubin JB: *Magnetic resonance of the spine,* St Louis, Mosby, 1990, pp 540-567.

60. Feinberg DA, Mark AS: Human brain motion in cerebral spinal fluid circulation demonstrated with MR velocity imaging. *Radiology* 1987;163:793-799.

61. Banta JV, Nichols O: Sacral agenesis. *J Bone Joint Surg [Am]* 1969;51:693-703.

62. Källén B, Winberg J: Caudal mesoderm pattern of anomalies: from renal agenesis to sirenomelia. *Teratology* 1974;9:99-111.

63. Pang D, Hoffman HJ: Sacral agenesis with progressive neurologic defect. *Neurosurgery* 1980;7:118-126.

64. Barkovich AJ, Raghavan N, Chuang S, Peck WW: The wedge-shaped cord terminus: a radiographic sign of caudal regression. *AJNR* 1989;10:1223-1231.

65. Smith ED: *Congenital malformations of the rectum, anus, and genito-urinary tracts.* Edinburgh, Livingstone, 1963.

66. Riordan DS, O'Connell RR, Kirwan WO: Hereditary sacral agenesis with presacral mass and anorectal stenosis: the Currarino triad. *Br J Surg* 1991;78(5):536-538.

10

Cystic Lesions, Vascular Disorders, Demyelinating Disease, and Miscellaneous Topics

THOMAS J. MASARYK

INTRAMEDULLARY CYSTIC CAVITIES

Despite the minor variability in nomenclature as well as considerable debate surrounding the pathophysiology of intramedullary cystic cavities, magnetic resonance imaging has significantly facilitated the diagnosis, treatment, and understanding of these lesions.[1-11] The distinction between hydromyelia and syringomyelia was first articulated by Simon[12] in 1875. The term *hydromyelia* is reserved specifically to designate a cystic dilation of the ependyma-lined central canal of the spinal cord by cerebrospinal fluid. The term *syringomyelia* refers to the state characterized by the presence of glial-lined (central or eccentric), longitudinally oriented, CSF cavities within the spinal cord. Inasmuch as it is frequently difficult to distinguish between these two conditions, there has been a trend to combine the two terms *(syringohydromyelia)* or refer to them generically as "syrinx cavities." Such lesions may be idiopathic or occur in association with congenital malformations (e.g., Chiari), trauma, arachnoiditis, or intradural-intramedullary and intradural-extramedullary neoplasms. As might be expected from their varied etiology, these cavities are sporadic, but they are seen most frequently in young adults. Although they commonly involve the cervical and/or thoracic spinal cord, their precise clinical picture depends on the cross-sectional and vertical extent of cord destruction. Common presenting signs and symptoms include brachial amyotrophy with dissociative anesthesia in a "cape" or "vest" distribution. Paradoxically, pain is

a frequent symptom in syringomyelia. Deep tendon reflexes are commonly diminished or absent; Horner's syndrome may be present. Early diagnosis is important since early treatment has been associated with improved clinical outcome.[13]

Pathogenesis

Multiple theories have been offered to explain the pathophysiology that produces cystic cavitation of the spinal cord. Gardner[14] and Gardner and Angel[15] initially attempted to explain the mechanism behind syrinx cavities from their work in treating patients with a Chiari malformation. They maintained that in such patients normal CSF egress from the fourth ventricle is prevented by congenital obstruction of the foramina of Magendie and Luschka. As a result, systolic CSF pressure pulsations generated by the choroid plexus are transmitted to the central canal of the cord via the obex of the fourth ventricle. Thus the syrinx consists of a dilated central canal and/or diverticula of the central canal that extend by dissecting along the spinal cord fiber tracts. However attractive, this theory fails to explain such cavities in patients whose foramina of the fourth ventricle are patent, who have no hindbrain malformations, and in whom the syrinx and fourth ventricle do not communicate.[16-18]

Williams[19,20] modified the Gardner theory by considering intracranial and spinal venous and CSF pressure shifts. He maintained that coughing, sneezing, Valsalva maneuvers, etc. increase intraspinal venous distention,

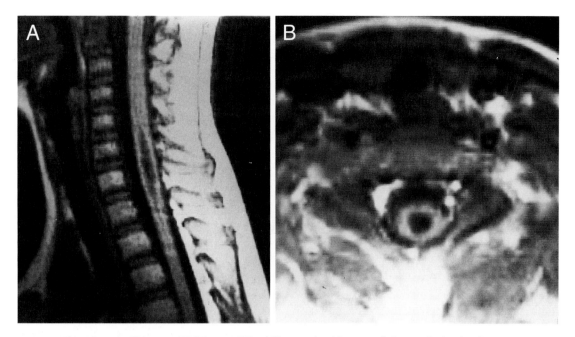

Fig. 10-1. A, 500 msec TR/17 msec TE midline sagittal image of the cervical spine in a patient with a simple syrinx cavity. The contents of the cavity are essentially isointense with CSF, and the cavity has smooth well-marginated borders. **B,** A 500 msec TR/17 msec TE axial image through the level of the syrinx.

thus raising intraspinal CSF pressures. In the presence of partial spinal block (e.g., at the foramen magnum in Chiari malformation) a ball-valve phenomenon exists. When CSF pressure is increased below the lesion, fluid is forced temporarily above the point of obstruction. When venous pressure returns to normal, however, CSF pressure remains elevated above the site of block, which then forces fluid into the central canal below the block until the pressures equalize. Such cavities involving the central canal were termed *communicating* syringomyelia (rather than hydromyelia) whereas those not connecting to the central canal were termed *noncommunicating* syringomyelia. Pulsations of the epidural venous plexus induced by changes in intraabdominal pressure were thought to produce shift ("slosh") that extended these cavities.[21] Experimental work by Hall et al.,[22] utilizing a canine model, supports these concepts, suggesting that a ventriculosyrinx valve effect initially inflates the syrinx during transient rises in intracranial pressure. Subsequent transmission of thoracic pressure changes to the subarachnoid space may compress the syrinx and result in the driving force that enlarges it.

These theories have been questioned on other grounds by Ball and Dayan.[16] They calculated the pulse pressure wave transmitted to the cord substance under the circumstances just described to be such that it would not likely produce cord cavitation. Instead, they maintained, CSF under pressure secondary to subarachnoid obstruction would track into the spinal cord by way of the Virchow-Robin spaces. Subsequently, small collections of CSF would coalesce to form larger syrinx cavities that might or might not connect to the central canal. Quencer et al.[23] have invoked an analogous theory to explain the development of syrinx cavities in patients with intradural-extramedullary neoplasms. They maintain that long-standing compression secondary to such mass lesions results in permanent enlargement or microcystic change of the perivascular space that predisposes to the development of syrinx cavities.

A similar mechanism for the development of syrinx cavities was subsequently proposed by Aboulker[24] and Aubin et al.,[25] who claimed that increased spinal CSF pressure forces CSF into the cord parenchyma along the posterior nerve rootlets.

Despite the lack of a comprehensive theory on the pathogenesis of spinal cord cystic cavities, a unifying theme among all the hypotheses put forth to date is the presence of dissecting and moving cerebrospinal fluid shifts. This is important because such CSF motion may have significant impact on the MRI appearance of the syrinx cavity.[9,10]

Magnetic Resonance
Anatomic evaluation

That MR is the safest, most efficient, and most sensitive diagnostic imaging examination for the detection of intramedullary cystic cavities is no longer questioned (Fig. 10-1). The majority of the literature on this subject describes examinations performed on patients with sagittal and/or axial short TR/short TE (T_1-weighted) spin-echo and sagittal long TR/long TE (T_2-weighted) spin-echo pulse sequences. Particular attention must be paid to the orientation of the phase and read gradients of such scans as well as to the number of Ky-steps to avoid truncation error (the Gibbs phenomenon), which may mimic syrinx cavities on sagittal images[26,27] (Fig. 10-2). The typical appearance of a simple syrinx is of a well-defined linear, crescentic, or ovoid area of low signal within the spinal cord on T_1-weighted images that parallels the signal intensity of CSF with progressively more T_2 weighting. As radiologists have become increasingly sophisticated with respect to determining the effect of CSF motion on MR images of the spine, low signal (flow-void) has been recognized as a frequent finding within syrinx cavities on T_2-weighted images.[9,10] Whether resolution of these motion-induced signal changes with surgical shunting of the syrinx cavities equates with a favorable clinical outcome will be decided on the basis of future long-term studies.

Other variations from the simple MR description of syrinx cavities just described arise with chronic cavities that may demonstrate (1) multiple loculi secondary to the presence of gliotic parenchymal bands and cord septa or

(2) variable signal intensities secondary to proteins present in solution (Fig. 10-3). Such circumstances can lead to problems with interpretation of the MR study, particularly with respect to the underlying etiology of the syrinx.[28,29] More specifically, difficulty may arise in two instances: (a) the exclusion of an underlying cavitary neoplasm from an otherwise idiopathic complicated syrinx and (b) the differentiation of posttraumatic myelomalacia from syringomyelia.

With respect to the first diagnostic dilemma, Williams et al.[29] found that although the appearance of a simple syrinx with distinct margins and signal intensity paralleling CSF correlated favorably with a nonneoplastic etiology there were few additional clues on the MR examination to distinguish atypical idiopathic, posttraumatic, or congenital cavities (Figs. 10-1 and 10-4). Areas of high-signal tissue within adjacent cord parenchyma on T_2-weighted images may appear as an ominous finding, but this can easily be explained on the basis of reactive gliosis and does not indicate the presence of an underlying tumor.[9,10] The use of intravenous paramagnetic contrast material may facilitate the distinction between neoplastic and nonneoplastic cord cavities in some instances when prominent focal enhancement reflects the presence of underlying tumor. Similarly, it has been suggested

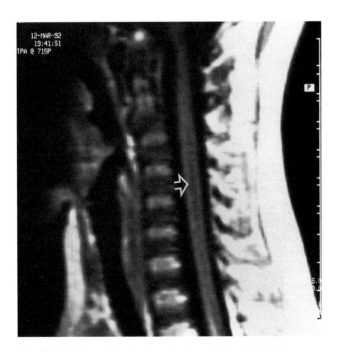

Fig. 10-2. This sagittal spin-echo image, TR 425/TE 15, demonstrates an area of low signal intensity within the central portion of the cord *(open arrow)* simulating a syrinx cavity. The acquisition matrix was 128 × 256, resulting in a Gibbs artifact (or "truncation error") that simulated the syrinx cavity.

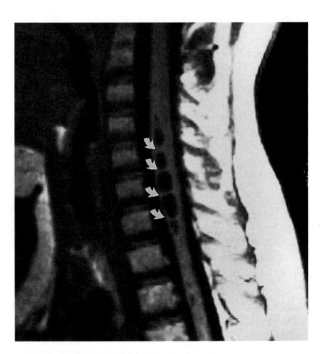

Fig. 10-3. This midline sagittal TR 500/TE 15 msec spin-echo scan shows a syrinx cavity within the lower aspects of the cervical cord. Multiple "gliotic bands," or parenchymal scarring, result in the multiloculated or septated appearance *(arrows)*. This is a common finding in benign syrinx cavities and does not indicate an underlying neoplasm.

that true benign syrinx cavities should demonstrate discernible CSF motion whereas intratumoral cavitations should not.

The distinction between posttraumatic myelomalacia and syringomyelia is usually less problematic. Both entities demonstrate long T_1 and T_2 relaxation times—that is, low signal on short TR/short TE images and high signal on long TR/long TE studies. If the signal intensity within the area of question closely parallels that of CSF on both T_1- and T_2-weighted scans, the lesion is probably a syrinx cavity.[11] Myelomalacia, however, while demonstrating low signal on T_1-weighted images, is isointense-hyperintense to the spinal cord on long TR/short TE images and less intense than CSF on long TR/long TE images. If motion-induced signal changes are present within a syrinx cavity, similar findings to those of myelomalacia may also be anticipated on long TR/long TE scans. Nevertheless, the distinction between myelomalacia and syringomyelia is still possible, through the use of axial gradient echo scans, which may demonstrate flow-induced signal changes in a syrinx cavity though not in an area of solid spinal cord tissue.[10]

Physiologic evaluation

As noted, CSF flow may alter the signal intensity and thus the typical appearance of syrinx cavities. It is also possible to quantify the normal and abnormal flow patterns of CSF within the ventricles, basal cisterns, and spinal subarachnoid spaces by utilizing MR flow measurement techniques (predominantly the phase-sensitive methods). Although these data are only now being accumulated, as might be surmised from the various theories proposed for the pathogenesis of spinal cord cysts they should provide useful information for diagnosis and treatment of such lesions.[30-36]

Quencer et al.[30] have accumulated significant experience utilizing a cardiac-gated, cine, phase-contrast technique for evaluating CSF flow velocities in the brain and spinal subarachnoid spaces. CSF motion was displayed as to-and-fro cephalocaudal movement that varied throughout the cardiac cycle. In the normal brain maximum CSF motion occurs 175 to 200 msec after the R wave, with outflow from the fourth ventricular foramina slightly preceding (by 100 to 150 msec) that through the aqueduct of Sylvius. Midway through the cardiac cycle the flow reverses in the aqueduct, becoming cephalad, followed by a quiescent period before the next systolic pulse. These observations suggest that supra- and infratentorial CSF flow is asynchronous. Despite some limitations due to partial volume effects, aqueduct flows in the caudal direction were measured in six normal volunteers and the velocities ranged from 3.7 to 7.6 mm per second. Flows through the area of the foramen of Magendie were measured, and the values ranged from 2.4 to 5.6 mm per second. Peak caudal velocity ranges of 7.8 to 38.1 mm

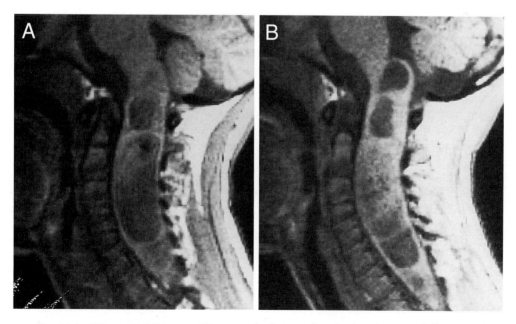

Fig. 10-4. 500 msec TR/17 msec TE parasagittal, **A,** and sagittal, **B,** images of the cervical spine in a patient with a complicated syrinx cavity. Note the heterogeneity of the cyst contents as well as the multiple septations throughout the cavity. The syrinx is poorly marginated and ill defined. Syrinxes such as these are difficult to distinguish from cavitary intramedullary neoplasms.

per second in the CSF cisterns anterior to the brain stem were also observed. The relatively wide variation in values reflects normal anatomic changes imposed on flow through the cisterns as well as individual variability. As in the brain, superior-inferior phase-sensitive flow maps in the spine are more responsive to CSF movement *(hyperintense, caudal; hypointense, rostral)* than to conventional imaging flow-related CSF signal changes.

Post et al.[31] have also demonstrated that caudal flow within the cervical subarachnoid space is most dramatic ventrally and begins 100 to 150 msec following the R wave; maximum velocity is, on average, reached 75 to 100 msec later (i.e., 175 to 250 msec after the R wave). Thereafter, flow decreases and then reverses so that cranial flow of CSF occurs later in the cardiac cycle (400 to 500 msec after the R wave). Normal peak CSF velocities in the anterior cervical subarachnoid space at C2 range from 10.9 to 52.4 mm per second. Itabashi et al.[33] reported peak CSF velocities in the cervical spine of 50 to 100 mm per second that increased when the neck was flexed and changed direction earlier with neck flexion. Enzmann et al.[32] found that in a normal population the highest CSF velocity in the cervical spine was at the C6 level because the canal area is smallest there.

Several normal thoracic and lumbar spines have also been investigated with this technique, and it has been observed[30] that maximum flow occurs later (300 to 400 msec after the R wave in the lumbar spine) in areas other than the cervical region and is slower (17 to 28 mm/sec in the lumbar spine).

Quencer et al.[30] have also implemented qualitative and quantitative cine CSF flow maps to investigate cystic abnormalities of the spine, both inside and outside the cord. Intramedullary cysts may show a flow void (reflecting areas of greater and/or faster flow) if there is pulsatile CSF within the cyst. Smaller intramedullary cystic lesions (less than two vertebral segments) may not show similar signal voids, either because of the small size of the cyst or because there are dense adhesions around the periphery of the residual cord that prevent expansion and contraction of the cord cyst.[34] Signal voids were commonly seen in congenital and large posttraumatic syrinx cavities,[35] and in benign cysts above intramedullary tumor (i.e., benign cystic dilation of the central canal), but not in cysts within neoplastic masses.[36] Additionally, these motion measurements may be most helpful in distinguishing posttraumatic myelomalacia from posttraumatic syrinx cavities.[30]

EXTRAMEDULLARY CYSTIC CAVITIES OF THE MENINGES

Unlike the intramedullary cysts, which are generally accepted under the unifying, generic heading of "syrinx," extramedullary cysts of the meninges have long been mired in a loosely defined confusing array of eponyms and synonyms. Nabors et al.[37] introduced a lucid, concise, and unambiguous classification system for these lesions that not only lends perspective and insight to the previous literature but also encompasses knowledge gained through modern spinal imaging modalities. Spinal meningeal cysts are congenital diverticula of the dural sac, nerve root sheaths, or arachnoid that according to this classification can be categorized into three major groups: extradural cysts without spinal nerve roots (type I), extradural cysts with spinal nerve roots (type II), and intradural cysts (type III).

Extradural meningeal cysts without nerve roots (type I) are dural diverticula that maintain contact with the thecal sac by a narrow ostium.[37] The term encompasses those lesions previously referred to as "extradural cysts, pouches, or diverticula" as well as "occult intrasacral meningoceles."[37,38] Type I meningeal cysts in the thoracic spine are found commonly in adolescents, arising from a dural pedicle near a dorsal nerve root, and are believed to be congenital[38-40] (Figs. 10-5 and 10-6). Sacral type I cysts are found in adults and are connected to the tip of the caudal thecal sac by a pedicle[40,41] (Fig. 10-7). Symptoms depend on the location of the lesion with respect to the cord and nerve roots and are usually of shorter duration for thoracic lesions.

Meningeal cysts with nerve roots (type II) are extradural lesions previously distinguished as (Tarlov) "perineural cysts" and "nerve root diverticula."[39,40,42] Although generally seen as multiple incidental lesions in the lumbosacral spine of adults, they will occasionally be the cause of radiculopathy and/or incontinence (Fig. 10-8). Despite the lack of a definable pedicle and ostium, both *type I* and *type II* cysts are suspected to produce pressure on adjacent structures and bone erosion via CSF pressure increases created by a valvelike mechanism.[43]

Type III meningeal cysts are intradural lesions most frequently found in the posterior subarachnoid space. Synonyms for these (primarily thoracic) lesions include "arachnoid diverticula" and "arachnoid cyst."[37,44-46] The cysts are usually lined by a single layer of normal arachnoidal cells and filled with CSF.[44,47-50] There may be an adjacent connective tissue stroma or fibrosis.[47,48] A variety of causes has been proposed to explain the pathogenesis of intradural arachnoid cysts.[47-51] Cysts dorsal to the spinal cord may arise congenitally from the septum posticum, the membrane dividing the midline dorsal subarachnoid space of the cervical and thoracic spinal canal (however, this does not explain lesions located anteriorly in the spinal canal)[37,44] (Fig. 10-8). Arachnoid cysts may also be formed as a result of arachnoidal adhesions caused by meningitis, instillation of drugs (especially certain pharmacologic preservatives), or spinal trauma.[44,49-52] The mechanism of cyst enlargement and the degree of communication with the subarachnoid

Text continued on p. 397.

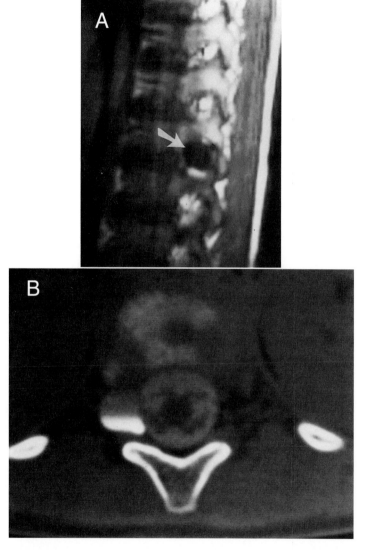

Fig. 10-5. A, This 500 msec TR/17 msec TE parasagittal image through the lower thoracic spine of an adolescent demonstrates a focal area of low signal intensity within the neural foramen *(arrow)*. The clinical suspicion was for a type I meningeal cyst. **B,** A type I meningeal cyst was confirmed by computed tomography after water-soluble myelography.

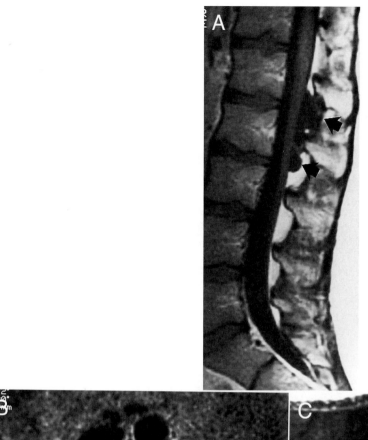

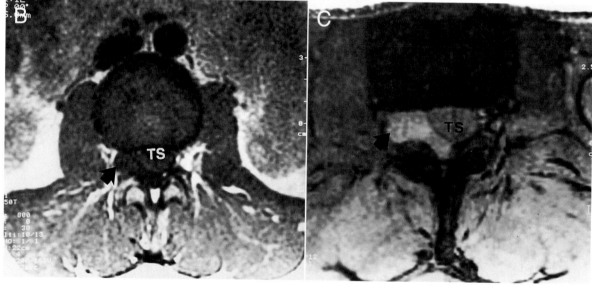

Fig. 10-6. **A** and **B,** Sagittal and axial T$_1$-weighted spin-echo images of the lumbar spine demonstrate posterolateral cystic collections *(solid arrows)* extending to the inferior aspects of the neural foramina (the exiting nerves lie at the upper aspects of the foramina) from the thecal sac *(TS).* **C,** An axial T$_1$-weighted low–flip angle gradient echo scan, likewise, shows these collections *(arrows),* which track CSF within the thecal sac on the sagittal and parasagittal T$_2$-weighted spin-echo studies, **D** and **E.** Confirmatory myelography, **F** and **G,** and a post-myelographic CT scan, **H,** demonstrate the presence of a type I meningeal cyst *(arrow).* (Courtesy Cathryn Powers, M.D., Ocala, Fla.)

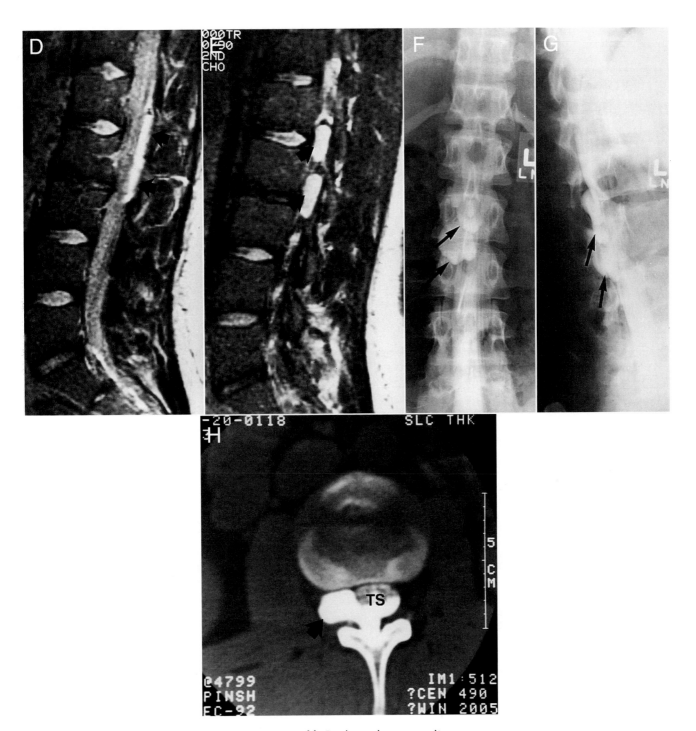

Fig. 10-6, cont'd. For legend see opposite page.

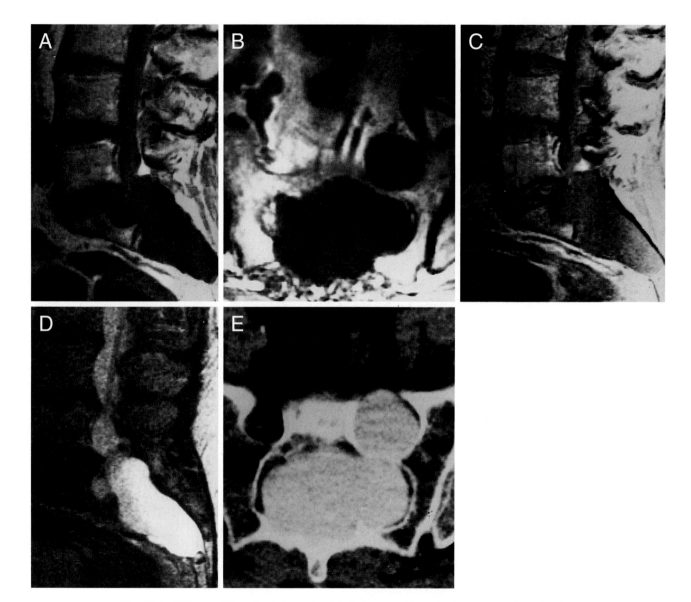

Fig. 10-7. 500 msec TE sagittal, **A,** and axial, **B,** images of a sacral type I cyst (previously referred to as an occult intrasacral meningocele). Note the large, low-signal, lytic process arising from the distal thecal sac and eroding the sacrum. **C,** A 2000 msec TR/30 msec TE sagittal image again shows a large cystic structure at the distal thecal sac eroding the sacrum. Its signal intensity parallels that of CSF within the thecal sac on this long TR/short TE study. **D,** A 2000 msec TR/120 msec TE sagittal image of the lumbosacral spine again demonstrates the large cystic mass, which parallels the signal intensity of CSF on this long TR/long TE study. **E,** Delayed high-resolution CT scan through the sacrum following water-soluble myelography. The cystic mass within the sacrum communicates with the thecal sac, as evidenced by the contrast material within it.

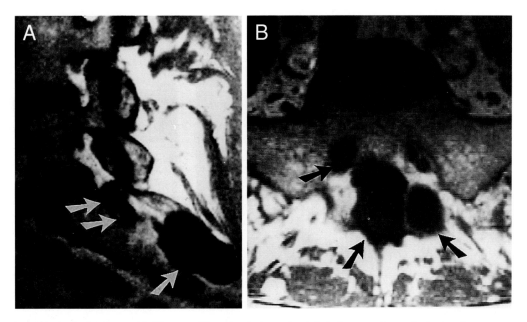

Fig. 10-8. 500 msec TR/17 msec TE sagittal, **A,** and axial, **B,** images through the lumbosacral spine demonstrate multiple small, low-signal, cystic areas *(arrows)* associated with various nerve root sleeves consistent with type II meningeal cysts (previously described as perineural cysts or nerve root diverticula).

space may be related to a one-way valve effect at the neck of the diverticulum.[53,54] Arachnoid cysts can be entirely asymptomatic or can produce neurologic symptoms by compressing the nerve roots or the spinal cord.[54a] When symptomatic, they typically present with signs suggesting posterior cord compression that may fluctuate with time.[55] Additionally, there may be rare cases of anteriorly located cervical intradural cysts.[56,57] Also not surprising in light of the proposed pathophysiology for syrinx cavities, there have been reports of associations between type III meningeal cysts and intramedullary syrinx cavities. Andrews et al.[58] discuss five such cases seen following trauma and/or surgery.

Magnetic Resonance Findings

Reports describing magnetic resonance findings in these lesions are few, but the imaging characteristics are by no means unexpected. Type I and type II lesions are typically anterior, posterior, or paraspinal, lying within or outside the vertebral canal, and produce parallel CSF signal intensities on all spin-echo pulse sequences (Figs.

10-5 to 10-8). Depending on the force of CSF motion within the cyst, and on the use of gating, even echos, or refocusing gradients in the T_2-weighted study, signal intensity of the cyst may vary slightly compared to CSF signal within the canal. Using flow-sensitive gradient echo studies, Davis et al.[54a] have reported that symptomatic cysts do not demonstrate CSF motion (indicative of free communication with the spinal subarachnoid space) whereas asymptomatic cysts do demonstrate such flow. Bone erosion (detectable as scalloping of the vertebral bodies or thinning of the pedicles) may be present. Type III cysts may be the most difficult to detect because they occur within the thecal sac and have very thin walls. They are often recognizable only by virtue of the mass effect and spinal cord deformity that they produce on T_1- and T_2-weighted spin-echo images[59,60] (Figs. 10-9 and 10-10). The "mass" should closely approximate the expected signal intensity of cerebrospinal fluid on all pulse sequences, although some signal loss from motion-induced dephasing within such cysts has been reported.[60]

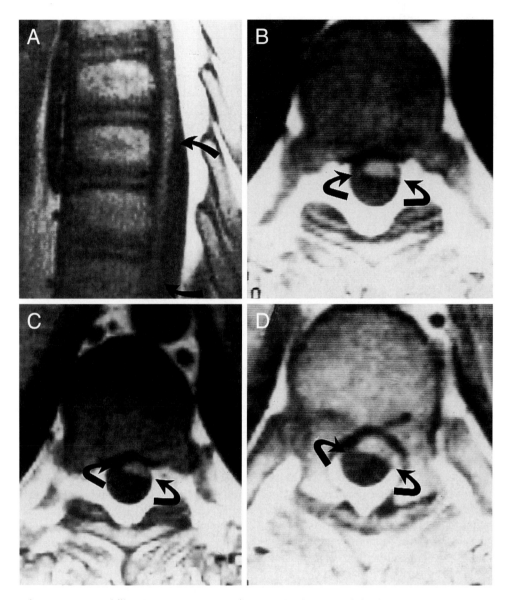

Fig. 10-9. A, A midline 600 msec TR/17 msec TE sagittal image of the lower thoracic spine in a young woman suggests that there is sudden and smooth tapering of the thoracic cord *(arrows)* despite an apparent widening of the adjacent CSF space. **B** to **D,** Serial 600 msec TR/17 msec TE rostrocaudal axial images through the midthoracic and lower thoracic spine demonstrate severe effacement and flattening of the posterior surface of the cord *(arrows)* despite an apparently "normal" appearance of the thecal sac. This case represents a surgically confirmed type III meningeal cyst (arachnoid cyst).

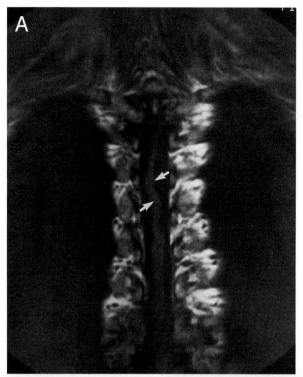

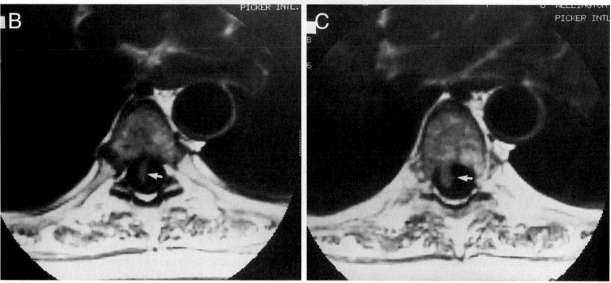

Fig. 10-10. A, A coronal and, **B** and **C,** two axial T$_1$-weighted spin-echo scans through the thoracic spine demonstrate severe distortion and compression of the cord bilaterally *(arrows)* with significant cord compression. The signal about the cord parenchyma attracts CSF on all pulse sequences, a finding suggestive of a CSF filled meningeal cyst.

Continued.

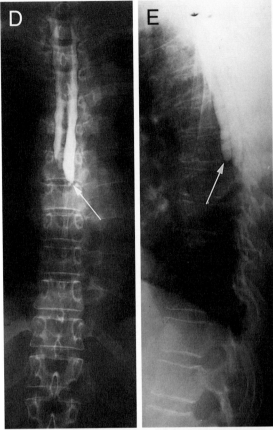

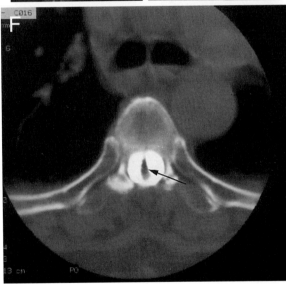

Fig. 10-10, cont'd. D and **E,** Frontal and lateral views of a water-soluble myelogram and, **F,** an axial view from a follow-up CT scan confirm the diagnosis of a type III meningeal cyst with significant posterolateral mass effect distorting the cord *(arrow)*.

VASCULAR DISEASES OF THE SPINE

Thirty-one pairs of segmental arteries (or the local equivalent, e.g., bronchial arteries) supply the spinal column and surrounding structures.[61-66] The bone, muscle, and connective tissues at each vertebral level (with the exception of the spinal cord) receive blood from the bilateral segmental arteries or their equivalents at the same and/or adjacent levels.[61-66] Branches of the segmental arteries extend posteriorly from the aorta, providing extraspinal arteries that supply muscle, bone (via the anterior central arteries), and nerve roots as well as intraspinal *radicular* branch arteries that supply bone and neural structures, including the meninges, epidural soft tissue structures, and spinal cord within the vertebral canal.[62-66] The radicular arteries are the first branches of the dorsal division of the segmental arteries or their equivalent. They enter the intervertebral foramina (as either single or multiple vessels) accompanying the emerging veins and spinal nerves. At this point the radicular arteries on each side of the vertebrae may divide into a triad of vessels: (1) the posterior central and (2) prelaminar arteries (to supply the bony vertebral body and posterior elements and spinal cord respectively) and (3) a radiculomedullary artery to the anterior spinal cord.[61-66] Radicular arteries have an ascending course with their segmental nerve roots whose obliquity increases from the cranial to caudal.[62-64] Therefore the levels of spinal cord supply are frequently not the same as those of the bone served by the same segmental trunk.

The blood supply to the spinal cord itself is based on three rostrocaudal arterial trunks, a single anterior spinal artery and paired posterior spinal arteries, which extend from the medulla oblongata to the conus medullaris, covering three major vascular territories or "zones"[61-64,67,68]: cervicothoracic, midthoracic, and thoracolumbar. Although these vertical arteries are usually continuous along the length of the cord, the anterior spinal artery is narrowest in the midthoracic region and widest in the cervical region.[69]

The number of anterior radiculomedullary arteries supplying the single anterior spinal artery rarely exceeds nine but has been reported to vary from 2 to 17. The artery of Adamkiewicz is the largest anterior medullary feeder and supplies the thoracolumbar region. It occurs on the left side in 80% of subjects and can arise anywhere between T5 and L4 (T9-L2 in 85%, T9-T11 in 75%, L1-L2 in 10%, and T5-T8 in 15%).[69] The anterior arterial trunk to the spinal cord is a centrifugal system formed by central arteries that arise from the anterior spinal artery, run horizontally in the central sulcus, and turn alternately to the right and to the left.[70,71] This centrifugal system supplies the central gray matter and an adjacent mantle of central white matter that includes the corticospinal tracts.[71]

The posterior medullary vessels (radiculomedullary arteries) supplying the paired posterior spinal arteries are more numerous, varying from 10 to 23.[72,73] The posterior spinal arteries run in the posterolateral sulcus and are also supplied by radicular arteries derived from segmental arteries or their regional equivalents (including the vertebral arteries and the posterior inferior cerebellar arteries). The posterior spinal vessels comprise an interconnected anastomotic plexus forming a centripetally oriented vascular territory with penetrating branches that supply one third to one half of the outer spinal cord.[74] In some cases the artery of Adamkiewicz supplies the entire lumbosacral cord, including the posterior spinal arteries.

Vascular Malformations

In the past, vascular malformations of the spine and spinal cord have been categorized according to etiology and histologic configuration, angiographic pattern and relationship to the vascular supply of the spinal cord, and macroscopic appearance at the time of surgery.[75-77] Unfortunately, this diversity of classification criteria resulted in a wide variety of complex and confusing nomenclature for a group of relatively rare lesions. It is hoped that this section represents a distillation of the seminal features of each malformation that are important to its diagnosis and management. Readers interested in additional information are referred to the articles by Rosenblum et al.,[78] Heros et al.,[79] and Oldfield and Doppman.[80]

Technically, vascular malformations of the spine and spinal cord are hemangiomas that can possess some neural tissue as an interstitial component whereas vascular tumors (i.e., hemangioblastomas) are not.[75] Similar to malformations in the brain, such lesions may be further subdivided into (1) arteriovenous malformations (AVMs) (both dural and parenchymal), (2) cavernous angiomas (hemangiomas), and (3) capillary telangiectasias. An exception to this is the venous angioma, which represents a distinct entity in the brain. With respect to the spine, the term *venous angioma* has been erroneously applied to radiculomeningeal (dural) AVMs. It is unclear whether venous angiomas exist as such in the spine and, if so, whether they are clinically significant or (like those in the brain) just normal variants of venous anatomy.

Arteriovenous Malformations

AVMs consist of a fistulous communication between an artery and a vein in the absence of an intervening capillary network. Of paramount importance to their pathophysiology, presenting signs and symptoms, diagnosis, and treatment is the location of the fistulous nidus with respect to the spinal cord and its vascular supply.[81] Con-

sequently these fistulae may be either intradural (intramedullary and extramedullary) or dural and are usually supplied by anterior radiculomedullary, posterior radiculomedullary, or radiculomeningeal arteries.[78] Of some clinical importance is the presence of posterior or lateral cutaneous angiomas at the same segmental level as the AVM in 12% to 21% of such patients.[82-84] These are often referred to as metameric malformations, indicating their common embryologic origin, and can, by simple inspection, be seen to denote the approximate level of the intraspinal portion of the malformation. In a review of their experience with 81 spinal vascular malformations, Rosenblum et al.[78] found 67% of cases to be intradural with the nidus meningeally located in 33%. Oldfield and Doppman[80] have suggested that as many as 85% of spinal vascular malformations may be dural.

Intradural (radiculomedullary) malformations

Previous classifications referred to *intradural-intramedullary* lesions as either juvenile or glomus malformations and *intradural-extramedullary* malformations as superficially placed direct A-V fistulae involving a radiculomedullary feeding artery. Among patients with intradural malformations (i.e., those fed by both anterior and posterior radiculomedullary vessels), there is an approximately equal distribution among patients of both sexes. Such lesions are believed to be congenital and are usually cervical or cervicothoracic, possessing a relatively large shunt volume fed by arteries that normally supply the cord.[78,79] Consequently they generally present earlier (before 50 years of age*), with symptoms of vascular steal (ischemia) or more commonly subarachnoid hemorrhage and/or hematomyelia.[78] Possibly because of their high-flow state, such lesions may be accompanied by arterial aneurysms (44%).[80] Although both lesions possess arterial supplies common to the spinal cord, the intramedullary lesions (often with anterior radiculomedullary supply) are embedded deep within the spinal cord and are extremely difficult to treat without grave risk of neurologic deficit. This is in contradistinction to the extramedullary lesions, which have the nidus located more superficially on the dorsal aspect of the cord and are thus more remedial to surgical resection.[85]

Experiences of Doppman et al.[85] and Di Chiro et al.[86] indicate that MR may be useful in detecting such lesions by its ability to reveal low-signal feeding and draining vessels within the spinal cord on T_2-weighted images through the so-called flow-void phenomenon. Additionally, sagittal and/or coronal T_1-weighted images may further characterize the malformation by revealing the low-

---

* In Rosenblum's series the mean age was 27 years.

signal nidus and enlarged anterior spinal artery of intramedullary lesions[85,86] (Figs. 10-11 and 10-12). With this constellation of findings, MR can distinguish such lesions from spinal hemangioblastomas—a task that may be difficult with myelography, computed tomography, or even angiography.[86] It is also possible to document the response to therapy of such lesions with MR by virtue of its ability to detect thrombosis through the absence of flow void.[85]

Dural (radiculomeningeal) malformations

Dural vascular malformations—long an enigmatic vascular spinal lesion—most frequently are recognized surgically and angiographically by the enlarged, arteriolized, slow-draining coronal veins of the spinal cord. These lesions have previously been referred to as *angioma racemosum venosum, malformation rétromédullaire, venous angioma,* or *long dorsal arteriovenous malformations.* Unlike their high-flow medullary coun-

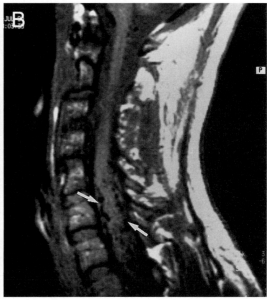

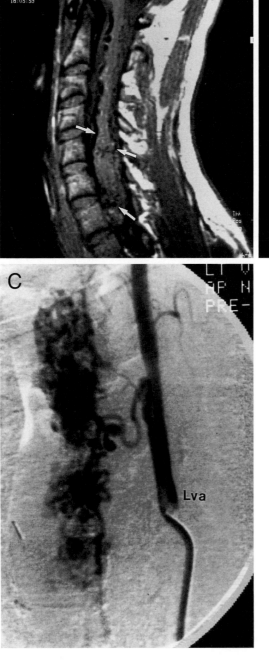

Fig. 10-11. A and **B,** Sagittal and parasagittal TR 500/TE 15 spin-echo images of the cervical spine demonstrate enlargement of the middle and lower cord with multiple serpentine areas of flow void *(arrows)* indicative of an intramedullary vascular malformation in a young man with an acute onset of quadriparesis following multiple episodes of subarachnoid hemorrhage. **C,** The single PA view of a left vertebral angiogram demonstrates a large radiculomedullary feeding artery extending to an extensive intramedullary arteriovenous malformation. Note the aneurysms on the feeding pedicle.

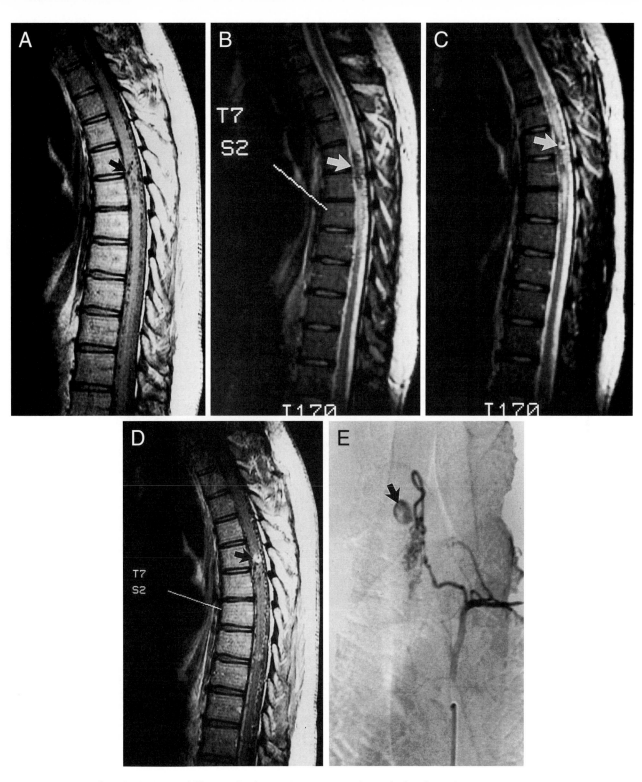

Fig. 10-12. A, A midline sagittal TR 500/TE 20 scan through the thoracic spine demonstrates multiple areas of flow void anterior and posterior to the cord above and below T5. At approximately the T5-6 level there are numerous flow voids within the parenchyma itself *(arrows).* **B** and **C,** Sagittal and parasagittal TR 2000/TE 80 scans through the thoracic spine again demonstrate a focal signal abnormality at T5-6 *(arrows)* with long tapering areas of high signal reflective of intramedullary edema extending above this lesion as well as a more proximate area of low signal about the lesion reflective of susceptibility artifact from hemosiderin-ferritin, probably the result of remote hemorrhage. **D,** A sagittal TR 500/TE 20 midline image through the thoracic spinal cord following gadolinium continues to show areas of flow void and enhancement anteriorly and posteriorly along the margins of the cord as well as a focal intramedullary area of enhancement *(arrow).* **E,** PA selective intercostal angiogram at T7 on the left. Note the intramedullary vascular malformation with a large aneurysm *(arrow)* on the major feeding vessel. This most likely represents the focal area of enhancement seen on the gadolinium-enhanced MR study.

Fig. 10-13. For legend see opposite page.

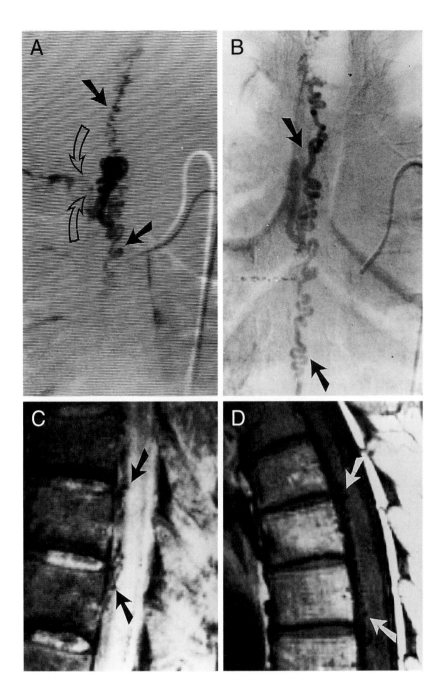

terparts, these lesions are believed to be acquired and are typically present in the thoracic and thoracolumbar spine of patients over age 50 (the large majority of whom are men).[75,76,78,80] Also the mode of presentation is quite different, commonly leading to a slowly progressive myelopathy with (typically) lower extremity paraparesis and bowel or bladder symptoms[78,80] that often are exacerbated by exertion; one report[87] even describes deterioration with menses. Rarely a sudden thrombophlebitis, the probable cause of a so-called Foix-Alajouanine syndrome, may produce rapid deterioration.[88,89] Originally termed *extramedullary*, these lesions came under serious scrutiny in 1974 when Aminoff et al.[90] argued that their

myelopathic symptoms were the product of intramedullary edema and ischemia secondary to raised venous back pressure within the varicosed coronal veins of the spinal cord. The dural site of arteriovenous shunting, however, remained to be discovered by Kendall and Logue[91] in 1977. Interestingly, the edema appears to cause symptoms initially in the most distal (dependent) portion of the spinal cord regardless of the level of the dural nidus. Indeed, numerous reports[92-95] describe lesions arising from feeding arteries in the internal iliac pedicles as well as cervicocerebral vessels, including posterior meningeal branches of the vertebral, middle meningeal, occipital, and ascending pharyngeal arteries,

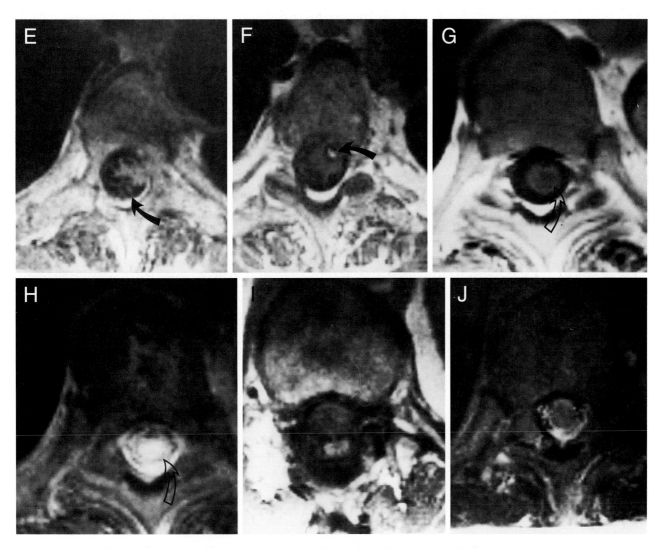

Fig. 10-13. A, An early angiogram from selective injection of the right T5 intercostal artery demonstrates washout of contrast from dural arteriovenous malformations *(open arrows)* and the lateral nerve root sleeve with diffuse opacification of the dilated coronal veins *(solid arrows).* **B,** A lateral venous film from the same T5 injection demonstrates slow opacification *(arrows)* of additional coronal veins along the cord. **C,** A midline 2000 msec TR/90 msec TE sagittal examination of the midthoracic spine depicts serpentine areas of low signal *(arrows)* outlined by high-signal CSF thought to represent intradural longitudinally oriented coronal veins. **D,** A 500 msec TR/17 msec TE midline sagittal image at approximately the same level shows small filling defects about the cord consistent with dilated coronal veins, but the defects are obviously not as conspicuous as those identified on the T_2-weighted image. **E** and **F,** 600 msec TR/17 msec TE axial images through the upper thoracic spine demonstrate the circumferentially oriented coronal veins with several small areas of high signal, possibly representing a thrombus *(arrows).* **G,** A 600 msec TR/17 msec TE axial image through the lower thoracic spine suggests an ill-defined area of low signal intensity within the cord *(arrow).* **H,** A 2000 msec TR/90 msec TE axial image at approximately the same level reveals high signal intensity within the cord at the same region where low signal intensity is identified on the T_1-weighted scan *(arrow).* These findings suggest intramedullary edema. **I** and **J,** T_1- and T_2-weighted axial scans through the lower thoracic spine following surgery for this radiculomeningeal vascular malformation demonstrate partial resolution of the intramedullary signal-intensity changes noted on the preoperative scans.

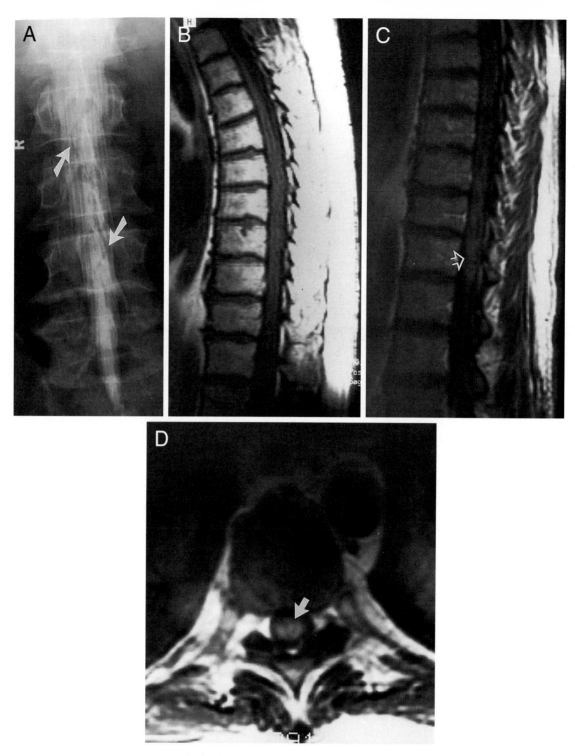

Fig. 10-14. A, AP view of a lumbar myelogram in an elderly man performed 2 years earlier before a second, unsuccessful, decompressive laminectomy at L5-S1. (Note the deformity of the distal thecal sac.) There is also the faint outline of a large draining vessel *(arrows).* **B,** A sagittal TR 500/TE 15 midline image through the thoracic spinal cord demonstrates generalized cord enlargement. **C,** The enhanced TR 500/TE 15 study demonstrates faint gadolinium enhancement within the distal conus medullaris *(arrow).* **D,** An axial study performed with TR 500/TE 15 at approximately the same level in the thoracolumbar region, likewise, shows intense enhancement following IV gadolinium *(arrow).* **E,** A TR 2000/TE 90 sagittal scan through the thoracolumbar spine again demonstrates generalized cord enlargement with central cord edema *(open arrow)* and small nodular areas of flow void along the dorsal aspect of the cord *(solid arrows).* **F** and **G,** Partially and completely subtracted views from the selective left internal iliac angiogram depict a single draining vessel (previously noted on the myelogram), indicated here by the *arrows,* that leads from the spinal cord along with numerous varicosed coronal veins. Surgical findings were a dural (radiculomeningeal) vascular malformation.

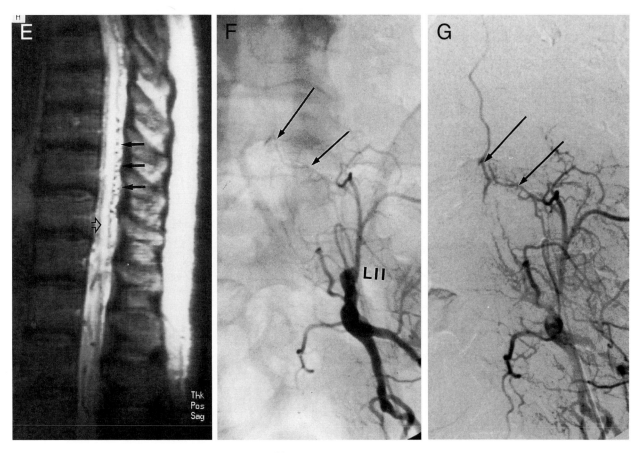

Fig. 10-14, cont'd. For legend see opposite page.

branches of the external carotid, and dural vessels arising at the carotid siphon. Successful treatment is often achieved by simple ligation of the dominant intradural draining veins as they depart the dural nidus.[96]

Magnetic resonance is unlikely to replace myelography and angiography in the evaluation of such lesions; however, it is important to recognize the MR findings in patients being evaluated for myelopathy since these lesions are potentially amenable to surgical relief. As are parenchymal AVMs of the spinal cord, draining vessels of these dural lesions are identified as serpentine areas of low signal within the spinal canal on sagittal T_2-weighted images.[97] Axial T_1- and T_2-weighted images locate the low-signal dilated coronal veins in their expected peripheral and circumferential location about the spinal cord[97] (Fig. 10-13). Occasionally higher-signal thrombi may be seen within these structures. Additionally, it is possible to appreciate the spinal cord edema first described by Aminoff et al.[90] in the lower spinal cord segments as areas of low signal on T_1-weighted images that progressively increase in signal with more T_2-weighting, despite the fact that the actual nidus may be

far removed from this region[97] (Figs. 10-14 and 10-15). These intramedullary signal derangements may reverse following successful treatment (Fig. 10-13). Furthermore, Terwey et al.[98] have described contrast enhancement within the ischemic segment of the distal cord (centrally) as well as more peripheral enhancement in the draining veins (Fig. 10-14) that was more conspicuous on delayed images (40 to 45 min) than on those acquired immediately after injection. Larsson et al.[99] have also described MR findings in patients suspected of having sustained venous spinal cord infarction secondary to a dural AVM, although in these patients the degree of cord enhancement appeared to be much greater. Such findings may mimic an intramedullary neoplasm during the acute phase, when there is often cord enlargement with variable enhancement; chronic cases may demonstrate cord atrophy.

Direct vertebral-venous fistulae

A unique type of fistula has been identified in which there is a single direct communication between the vertebral artery and the immediately adjacent foraminal

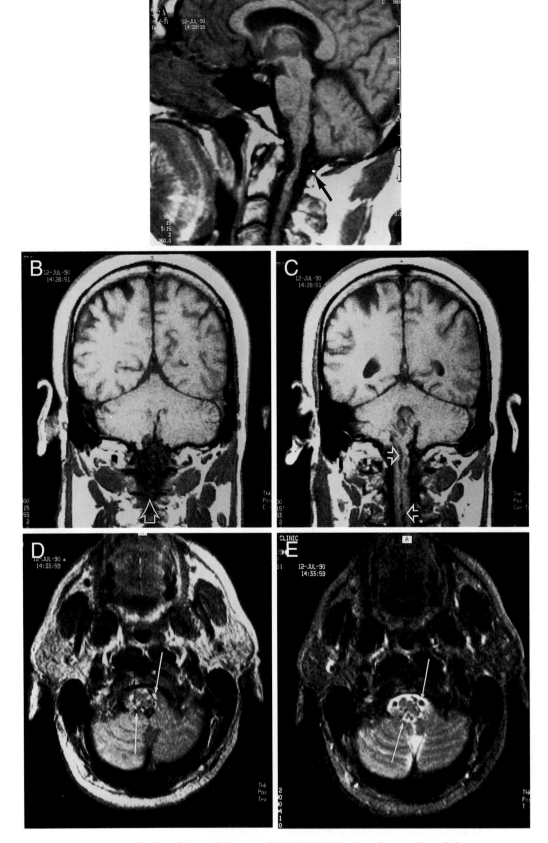

Fig. 10-15. A, Sagittal and, **B** and **C,** coronal TR 500/TE 15 spin-echo studies of the foramen magnum performed in a middle-aged man with lower extremity myelopathy demonstrate multiple serpentine areas of flow void in the region of the foramen *(solid arrow)* as well as more vertically oriented vessels within the cord *(open arrows).* **D** and **E,** TR 2000/TE 20 and 90 msec axial images through the cervicomedullary junction again show multiple areas of flow void (on the T$_2$-weighted scan) and flow-related enhancement as well as flow void on the long TR/short TE study *(arrows).* Note that the cord and brain parenchyma do not surround or contain an intramedullary "nidus" of abnormal vessels.

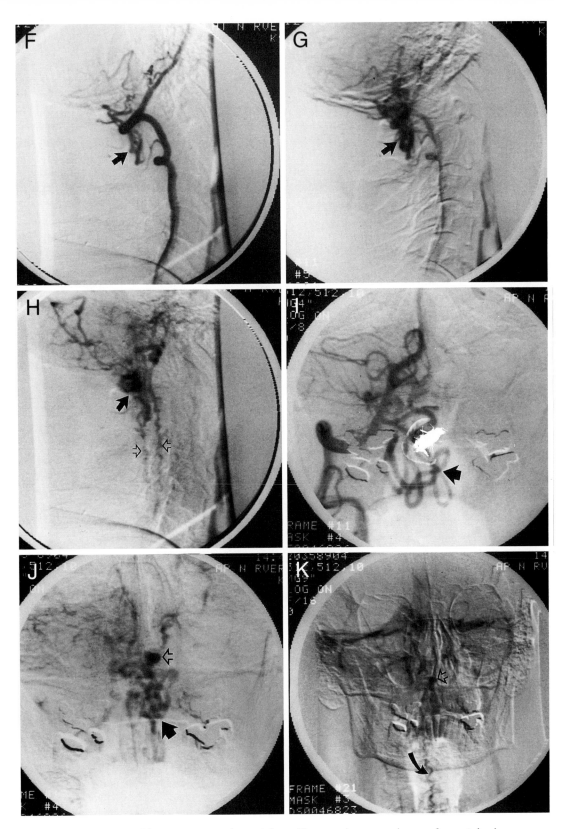

Fig. 10-15, cont'd. F to **H,** Lateral arterial, capillary, and venous phases of a vertebral angiogram demonstrate a prominent posterior meningeal artery arising from the right vertebral *(arrow)* and filling a vascular nidus along with the subsequent appearance of coronal perimedullary spinal veins *(open arrows)*. **I** to **K,** PA views of the same right vertebral angiogram in the arterial, capillary, and venous phases, likewise, showing prominent posterior meningeal vessels forming a dural nidus *(solid arrow)*. Note the varix near the cervicomedullary junction *(open arrow)* and the coronal draining veins on the delayed venous image *(curved arrow in* **K).**

and/or intradural veins. Many of these lesions are congenital, but acquired (e.g., traumatic or iatrogenic in association with anterior cervical diskectomy) fistulae have also been reported. Patients may be asymptomatic or present with either radiculopathy or myelopathy. The exact mechanism by which symptoms are produced is unclear, although local mass effect secondary to enlarged foraminal or intradural veins, a steal phenomenon, or ischemia secondary to venous hypertension is most frequently implicated. A similar type of lesion was described by Heros et al.[79] in which there was direct fistulous communication between the anterior spinal branch of a vertebral artery and a single medullary vein that drained cephalad to the posterior fossa.

Spin-echo MR studies typically demonstrate a unilaterally enlarged vertebral artery with multiple lobulated areas of flow void intra- and extradurally at the approximate level of the fistulous communication. Gradient echo studies may identify these same vessels with high signal on the basis of flow-related enhancement. Intradural vessels may demonstrate significant mass effect on the cervical spinal cord (Fig. 10-16).

Cavernous Hemangiomas

Cavernous hemangiomas are uncommon spinal vascular hemangiomas that consist of dilated endothelium-lined sinusoids separated by thin strands of fibrous tissue devoid of smooth muscle and elastic fibers.[100-102] They are histologically distinguished from capillary telangiectasias by their abundance of hemosiderin and the paucity of intervening normal neural tissue.[100-102] Histologic parallels and the reported presence of both lesions in the central nervous system of a single patient suggest that they are, in fact, representatives of a single entity.[100-105]

Cavernous angiomas, or cavernomas, are uncommon vascular malformations that may affect any part of the neuraxis but are generally seen intracranially. Whereas they have been estimated to represent 5% to 12% of all spinal vascular anomalies, most arise within the vertebral bodies and only occasionally extend into the extradural space.[101] Purely extradural or intradural-extramedullary lesions have been reported, but strictly intramedullary lesions are rare.[101,106-108] Grossly the intramedullary lesions are usually solitary and can be identified as a mulberry lesion or simply a discoloration of the cord substance. There are no abnormal leptomeningeal vessels. Cavernous angiomas are composed of multiple cysts containing old blood with dense fibrous walls and occasional calcification. The presence of a fibrous capsule may facilitate surgical excision.[109] Clinically the lesions may be asymptomatic, or may present with progressive paraparesis and sensory loss with pain that is difficult to distinguish from chronic progressive radiculomyelopathy or the Foix-Alajouanine syndrome.[110] Rarely a patient may present with acute subarachnoid hemorrhage or hematomyelia.[101]

The majority of spinal cavernous hemangiomas arise in the vertebral bodies with extension to the epidural space.[108] The MR appearance of these extradural lesions (high signal on T_1- and T_2-weighted images) is thought to be related to the presence of adipose and hematopoietic tissue[111] (Chapter 7). Fontaine et al.[112] have described the MR appearance of intramedullary cavernous hemangiomas. The lesions typically have a peripheral area of low signal on T_1- and T_2-weighted spin-echo images thought to be secondary to the abundant hemosiderin contained within them.[112] The central portion may have variable areas of increased and decreased signal secondary to the presence of calcifications and various forms of hemoglobin.[112] It should be remembered that the signal-intensity characteristics of hemoglobin and its breakdown products are variable depending on the concentration, magnetic field strength, and pulse sequence used[113,114] (Figs. 10-17 and 10-18). Although the MR appearance of capillary telangiectasia of the spinal cord has yet to be reported, one might logically presume it to be similar to that of cavernous angiomas but without the peripheral ring of hemosiderin.

SPINAL CORD HEMORRHAGE AND ISCHEMIA
Spontaneous Subarachnoid, Subdural, and Epidural Hemorrhage

Spinal subarachnoid hemorrhage is unusual, accounting for less than 1% of all cases of subarachnoid hemorrhage (SAH).[115] The most common cause appears to be an AVM of the cord.[116,117] Spinal arterial aneurysms alone have also been reported to cause spinal SAH and occur at a number of locations, most commonly the anterior spinal artery.[116,117] The artery of Adamkiewicz, the posterior spinal artery, and the cervical radicular arteries are other sites. Spinal tumors, especially in the region of the cauda equina and conus medullaris, are known to cause spinal SAH. Ependymoma is most frequently encountered.[118] Other entities, usually mechanical or hematologic in nature, such as extreme physical exertion or external trauma, have been reported[117,119] to cause spontaneous spinal SAH. Collagen vascular disorders, possibly related to associated coagulopathy, have also been associated with spontaneous SAH. Gundry and Heithoff[119a] have reported an association between lumbar disk herniations and anular tears with focal epidural hemorrhages.

Clinical presentation is usually heralded by acute back pain, which often radiates to the extremities or occasionally to the abdomen.[117] In rare cases of spontaneous epidural hematoma this may be clinically indistinguishable from acute disk herniation.[119a] With spontaneous SAH there may be a history of multiple similar episodes and a relative paucity of neurologic findings. Meningismus,

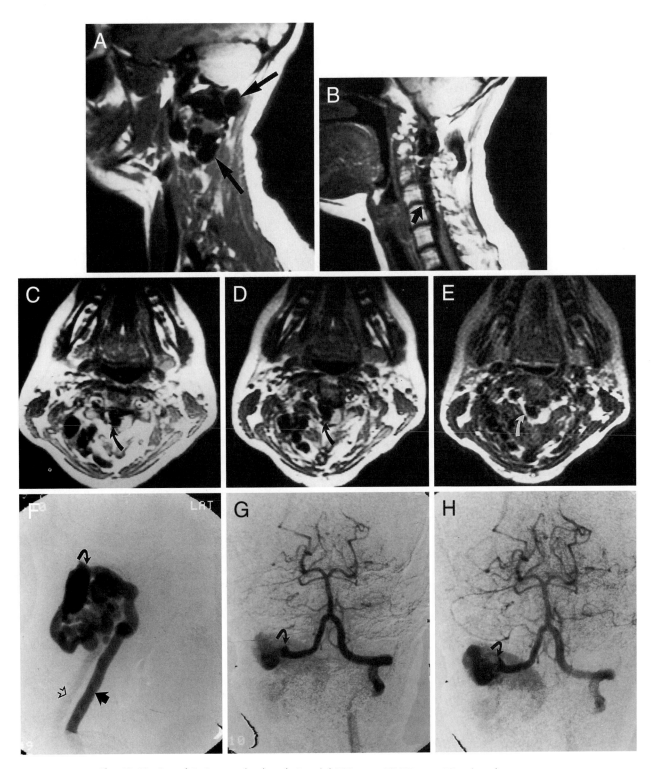

Fig. 10-16. A and **B,** Parasagittal and, **C,** axial 500 msec TR/17 msec TE spin-echo scans through the cervical spine demonstrate a large cluster of low-signal or flow-void regions near the foramen magnum. The parasagittal examinations show extraspinal vessels *(long arrows)* and an enlarged vertebral artery *(short arrow* in **B**). The axial study demonstrates that the suspected vessels compress the cervical spinal cord *(curved arrows).* **D** and **E,** 2000 msec TR/20 and 90 msec TE axial scans again show an intradural mass effect *(curved arrows).* **F** to **H,** Lateral and PA vertebral arteriograms demonstrate the vertebral artery *(straight solid arrow),* the draining vein *(open arrows),* and the site of fistulous communication *(curved arrow).*

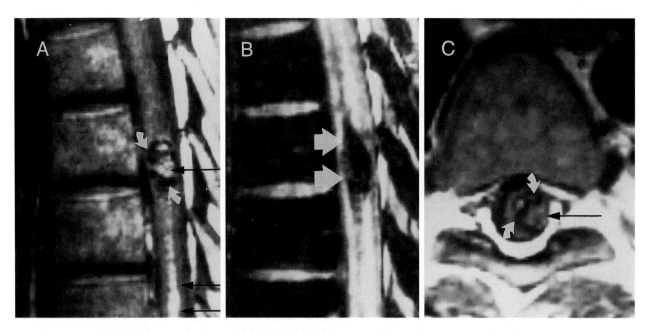

Fig. 10-17. A, A 500 msec TR/17 msec TE sagittal spin-echo scan through the lower thoracic spine demonstrates a histologically proved cavernous hemangioma, represented by the low-signal ring of hemosiderin *(curved white arrows),* surrounding a focal area of high signal intensity, representing methemoglobin. The long linear area of high signal beneath the lesion represents methemoglobin from recent hemorrhage *(long arrows).* **B,** A midline sagittal FISP 10-degree scan demonstrates the hemangioma as a large area of low signal *(white arrows)* because of the signal loss secondary to the magnetic susceptibility effect of blood breakdown products. **C,** An axial 500 msec TR/17 msec TE spin-echo scan through the hemangioma again shows the peripheral hemosiderin *(curved white arrows)* surrounding methemoglobin *(straight black arrow).*

with Brudzinski's and Kernig's signs, is often prominent; intracranial signs and symptoms of SAH are delayed and typically seen the more cephalic the source of bleeding.[120] Accurate diagnosis is important for distinguishing the source of hemorrhage from intracranial SAH and for recognizing possible cord compression.

In view of the paucity of blood vessels traversing the subdural space, it has been suggested[121,122] that spinal SAHs may originate in the more vascular subarachnoid space and dissect subdurally. Rader[123] has postulated that the vessels traversing the subarachnoid space are subjected to rapid intraluminal pressure increases transmitted from the intrathoracic and intraabdominal pressures. CSF pressure lags momentarily behind the intravascular pressure, and this leads to vessel rupture. In cases of epidural hematoma (which are rare), the suggestion has been made[119a] that they may result from tearing of epidural veins in the premembranous space between the vertebral body and posterior longitudinal ligament, with acute displacement of the anulus fibrosus.

The sensitivity of MR to blood may be variable and dependent on the field strength of the imager, the relative concentration and age of hemoglobin, the concentration of hemoglobin breakdown products, and the type of pulse sequence utilized. Existing reports[124] describe spin-echo pulse sequences as demonstrating abnormal areas of high signal (typically on T_1-weighted spin-echo scans) that reflect the paramagnetic effect of methemoglobin, which often distorts the normal tubular shape of the thecal sac. T_2-weighted scans may show low or high signal at the same location depending on whether the blood is acute, subacute, or chronic.[119a,124] Gradient echo scans should also demonstrate low signal on the basis of susceptibility artifact. It is important to search for ancillary findings (e.g., serpentine areas of flow void), which may suggest an underlying vascular anomaly. With respect to morphology, SAH will often spread and layer over a large area of the subarachnoid space whereas epidural hematomas are more focal and reminiscent of disk fragments (Fig. 10-19).

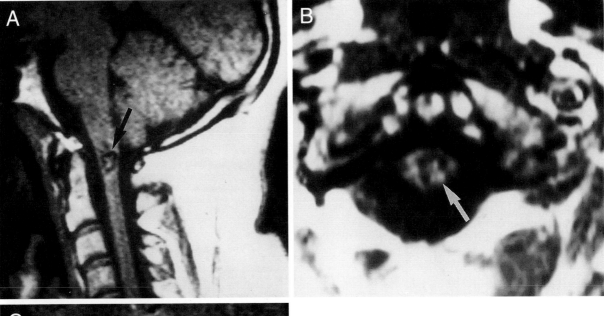

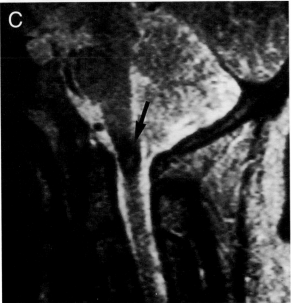

Fig. 10-18. A, A TR 500/TE 20 midline sagittal image through the cervicomedullary junction demonstrates a focal area of high signal intensity, representing the paramagnetic effect of methemoglobin, surrounded by an area of lower signal, reflecting susceptibility artifact secondary to hemosiderin-ferritin *(arrow)*. In the absence of significant flow void suggestive of a dural or intramedullary vascular malformation, these findings are suggestive of a cavernous angioma. **B,** An axial TR 500/TE 15 view through the upper cervical spine, likewise, demonstrates the lesion *(arrow)*. **C,** The TR 2000/TE 90 midline sagittal T_2-weighted scan also shows the lesion, although with a longer TE the susceptibility artifact is much more dramatic *(arrow)*.

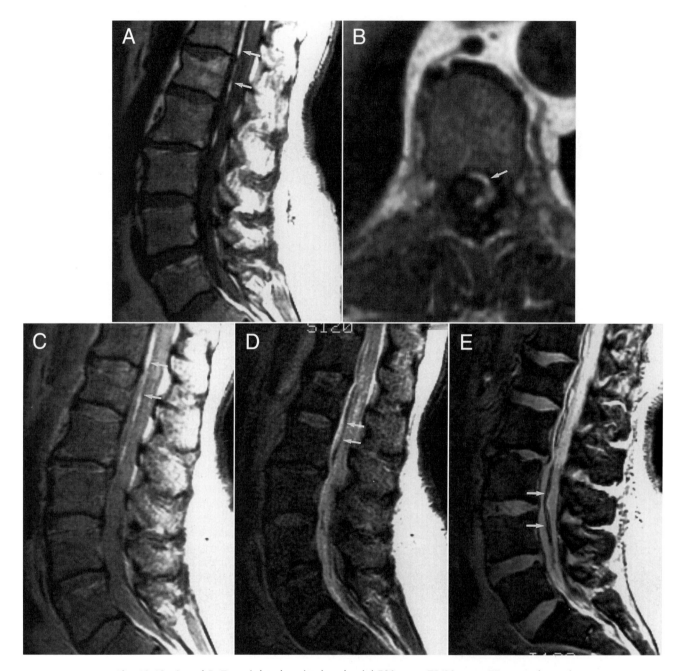

Fig. 10-19. A and **B,** T$_1$-weighted sagittal and axial 500 msec TR/20 msec TE scans through the lumbar spine demonstrate linear areas of high signal intensity anterolateral to the thecal sac (*arrows*) consistent with a paramagnetic effect of methemoglobin in a case of spontaneous subarachnoid hemorrhage. **C** and **D,** Spin density and T$_2$-weighted 200 msec TR/20 and 90 msec TE scans through the same region both show areas of paramagnetic susceptibility effect from subarachnoid blood (*arrows*). **E,** A sagittal gradient echo scan, likewise, demonstrates significant susceptibility artifact secondary to spontaneous subarachnoid hemorrhage (*arrows*).

Superficial Siderosis of the Spinal Cord

Superficial siderosis of the central nervous system is a rare disorder characterized by the deposition of hemosiderin in the leptomeninges and subpial tissues.[125] Symptoms are nonspecific and include cerebellar ataxia, hearing loss, myelopathy, and progressive dementia.[126] Before MRI, histopathologic confirmation was required for this diagnosis.[127]

Superficial siderosis is thought[125-127] to result from repeated or continuous hemorrhages into the subarachnoid spaces. In half the cases, autopsy has identified a potential source of bleeding (e.g., aneurysms, subdural hematomas, and brain or spinal angiomas or tumors).

The toxic effect of iron causes gliosis, demyelination, and nerve cell destruction.[128] The concentration of symptoms to the posterior fossa is believed to be related to accelerated ferritin biosynthesis in Bergmann glia.[126]

Typical MR findings are a low signal halo about the pial surface of the cerebellum, brain stem, and spinal cord caused by a susceptibility artifact resulting from the deposition of hemosiderin and ferritin.[129,130] This becomes more obvious on scans with longer echo times (i.e., T_2-weighted studies) because the susceptibility effect is directly related to TE. It is also more prominent on gradient echo scans because of the greater prominence of T_2^* with these acquisitions relative to spin-echo studies (Fig. 10-20).

Spinal Cord Infarction

The sources of arterial supply to the spinal cord are limited, and any pathologic process that compromises them can result in ischemia and/or infarction of the cord. Elderly patients with atherosclerosis, hypertension, and/or diabetes are thought to be at greater risk, typically presenting with acute-onset thoracic or thoracolumbar deficits of variable severity.[131,132] Most cases of spontaneous cord ischemia occur in patients with a thoracoabdominal aortic aneurysm; the presumed mechanism is occlusion of the intercostal artery, from which the anterior spinal artery arises. Dissecting thoracoabdominal aortic aneurysms, especially those with a left-sided false lumen, are associated with a higher incidence of spinal cord ischemia (because in 85% of the population the anterior spinal artery arises from the left lower intercostal vessels).[132] Additional possible etiologies for arterial infarction in such patients include hypotension, angiography, vertebral occlusion or dissection, syphilis, arteritis, sickle cell anemia, polycythemia, leukemia, spinal trauma, caisson disease, and disk herniation.[133]

Vandertop et al.[134] and Brown et al.[135] reported the MR findings in spinal cord infarction: cord enlargement with increased signal on the T_2-weighted spin-echo sequences. There was no evidence of paramagnetic effect to suggest the presence of hemorrhage. Three-year follow-up in the Vandertop patients showed cervical cord atrophy with high signal on the long TR/short TE sequence, presumably representing gliosis. Casselman et al.[136] reported a cervical cord infarct that had normal signal on T_1- and T_2-weighted sequences within 24 hours of the infarct. Follow-up imaging at 1 week in this case demonstrated normal signal on the T_1-weighted images, but increased signal on the T_2-weighted images (Fig. 10-21). There were enhancing lesions in the anterior portion of the cord following gadolinium administration.

Mawad et al.[132] attempted to correlate the pattern of MR signal derangement on multiecho T_2-weighted scans with neurologic deficit and to predict the outcome in 24 patients who had neurologic deficits following aortic surgery. They found that signal abnormalities started in the anterior horns of the gray matter and, with increasing severity of ischemia, spread posteriorly to involve the posterior horns. Ultimately, the ischemic changes and corresponding MR signal abnormalities extended laterally to the posterolateral funiculi of the spinal cord, including the crossed corticospinal tracts. In severe cases the whole cross section of the spinal cord was infarcted. They also stressed the need for axial double-echo MR studies in the diagnosis of spinal cord ischemia, since the geographic distribution of the signal abnormalities within the gray matter could not be accurately displayed on sagittal scans.

Yuh et al.[131] stressed the importance of ancillary findings outside the cord itself that could aid in the diagnosis of their series of 12 patients. Specifically they cited the absence of flow-void phenomena in the distal aorta caused by complete occlusion and the abnormal high bone marrow signal on T_2-weighted images in the anterior portion of the vertebral body. (Both were demonstrated best on the T_2-weighted images.) One of their three patients had a lesion involving predominantly the anterior half of one vertebra whereas the other two had multiple bone marrow lesions located near the endplate and/or deep medullary portions of several vertebrae. Abnormal bone marrow was demonstrated on the T_1-weighted image in only one of the three patients, in whom abnormal marrow was apparent on the T_2-weighted image. One patient had a 1-year follow-up MR study that demonstrated persistence of bone marrow findings with a reduction in lesion size and a typical triangular configuration both near the endplate and in the deep medullary portion of the vertebral body. These triangular areas may be the most vulnerable regions of the vertebral body during ischemia. Appropriate clinical history and associated ancillary findings help to distinguish this entity on MR from acute transverse myelitis.

Venous infarction of the spinal cord is an uncommon phenomenon, usually associated with dural arteriovenous (radiculomeningeal) vascular malformations and with hypercoaguable states and fibrocartilaginous emboli.[88,133,137] Presentation may differ from that of arte-

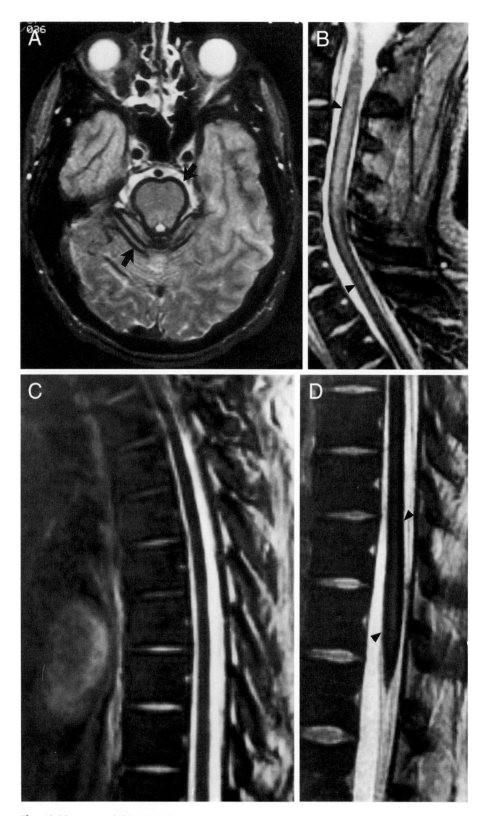

Fig. 10-20.   An axial TR 2000/TE 90 scan through the mesencephalon demonstrates significant low signal intensity about the pons, tectum, and folia of the cerebellum *(arrows)* consistent with a susceptibility artifact arising from superficial siderosis. **B** to **D,** Cervical, thoracic, and lumbar TR 100/TE 9 FISP gradient echo scans demonstrate the shape and contour of the spinal cord to be normal, although there is significant low signal intensity about the pial surface *(arrowheads),* reflective of superficial siderosis.

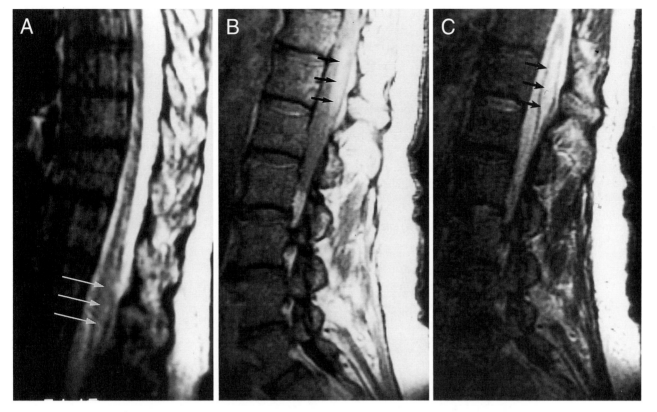

Fig. 10-21. A, Magnified view from a sagittal TR 2000/TE 90 localizing scan through the thoracic spine in a patient who became paraplegic following thoracoabdominal aneurysm surgery. There is high signal intensity within the distal conus medullaris *(arrows)*. **B** and **C,** Surface coil TR 2000/TE 20 and 90 images demonstrate high signal within the conus *(arrows)*, which is slightly enlarged. Taken with the clinical history, these findings are consistent with spinal cord infarction.

rial infarction as regards the underlying disease process, being often less abrupt with a stuttering clinical course. The imaging and clinical findings may be indistinguishable from those of intramedullary neoplasm, with prolongation of normal spinal cord T_1 and T_2 relaxation times, cord enlargement, and possibly peripheral enhancement. The findings are also identical to those associated with the entity termed *subacute necrotizing myelopathy*.[137]

DISEASES OF THE SPINAL CORD WHITE MATTER
Multiple Sclerosis

Multiple sclerosis is a clinically variable disease characterized by multifocal destruction of myelin in the optic nerves, brain, and spinal cord. It usually begins in the second to fifth decades, often manifesting with visual, sensory, and motor dysfunction.[138] Signs and symptoms characteristically wax and wane, though often with less improvement and greater disability as time

passes.[139] The prevalence of the disorder is higher in northern latitudes and among family members.[139,140] Emigrants from areas of high risk to areas of low risk have a lower incidence of the disease if they move before 15 years of age.[141,142] This familial and geographic tendency suggests a possible environmental factor(s). Infectious agents and/or autoimmune disorders have been postulated as possible mechanisms. Pathologically, macroscopic lesions range in size from 1 mm to several centimeters and are scattered throughout the white matter; those involving the spinal cord tend to be more elongated.[143] Histologic sections demonstrate perivenous breakdown of the myelin sheath with sparing of adjacent axons.[144,145] The plaques contain lymphocytes, plasma cells, and macrophages, which may contain myelin breakdown products.[144] Spinal cord involvement by multiple sclerosis often presents with weakness and/or paresthesias in one or more limbs, Lhermitte's signs, gait disturbance, and disorders of micturition. In association with optic nerve involvement, this syndrome has been referred to as "neuromyelitis optica" or Devic disease.[139]

Fig. 10-22. A and **B**, TR 2000/TE 20 midline sagittal and parasagittal scans through the cervical spinal cord demonstrate multiple small focal areas of high signal within the cord parenchyma reflective of demyelinating disease. **C** and **D**, TR 2000/TE 90 T_2-weighted sagittal and parasagittal scans, likewise, demonstrate plaques with high contrast although slight blurring secondary to the longer echo time. **E** and **F**, TR 600/TE 20 T_1-weighted sagittal and parasagittal scans following IV gadolinium show clear enhancement of all the lesion at C2 in the cervicomedullary junction. This was believed to reflect more active demyelinating disease.

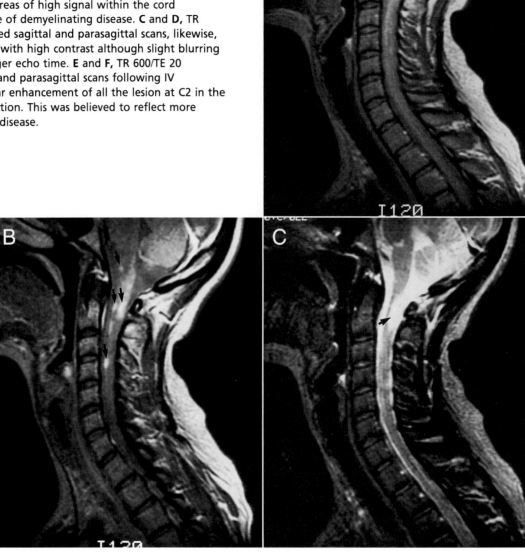

Primarily because of its variable presentation, criteria for the diagnosis of multiple sclerosis have been developed on the basis of clinical and paraclinical (e.g., neuroimaging or laboratory) evidence of CNS lesions.[146] Magnetic resonance imaging has been found[147,148] to be exquisitely sensitive to the presence of multiple sclerosis plaques involving the brain. The number and size of brain lesions detected by MR correlate well with the severity of disease.[149] The lesions are generally round or ovoid areas of low signal on T_1-weighted images that have increased signal on T_2-weighted scans, usually without mass effect. Whether these signal-intensity changes represent breakdown of the blood/brain barrier, destruction of the myelin sheath, or both may be a reflection of the acuteness of the lesion.[150] It has been proposed[151] that enhancement by paramagnetic contrast may reflect the level of clinical activity of a given lesion. Reports of MR imaging of multiple sclerosis plaques in the spinal cord are few, but they describe similar linear or elongated signal-intensity changes on spin-echo images[143,148] (Figs. 10-22 to 10-24). It must be noted that these reports have been limited to the cervical spinal cord

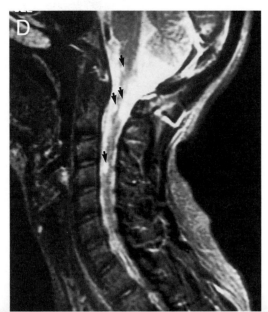

Fig. 10-22, cont'd.   For legend see opposite page.

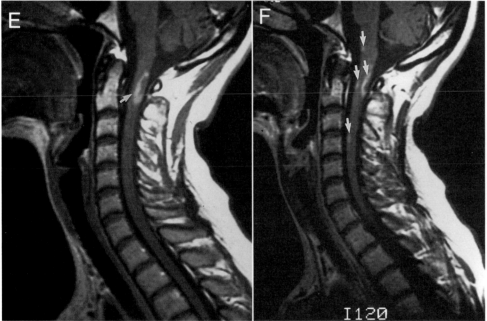

in patients examined with a head coil; the use of surface coils, cardiac gating, and even echo rephasing or refocusing gradients has undoubtedly improved the recognition of lesions below the foramen magnum. It must also be kept in mind that the MR evaluation of patients with signs and symptoms of demyelinating disease is useful not only for what it shows but also for what it does not.[139] Similar clinical presentation can be mimicked by brain stem gliomas, epidermoids of the fourth ventricle, meningiomas and arachnoid cysts of the foramen magnum, brain stem and spinal cord vascular malforma-

tions, a Chiari malformation, and cervical spondylosis.[139,152-159] Consequently, even a negative MR examination of the spine and foramen magnum supplies useful clinical information.

Acute Disseminated Encephalomyelitis

Acute disseminated encephalomyelitis (ADEM) is pathologically indistinguishable from multiple sclerosis (i.e., perivenous demyelination).[160] Clinically, however, it occurs as a predominantly monophasic illness in children that often is preceded or accompanied by a vi-

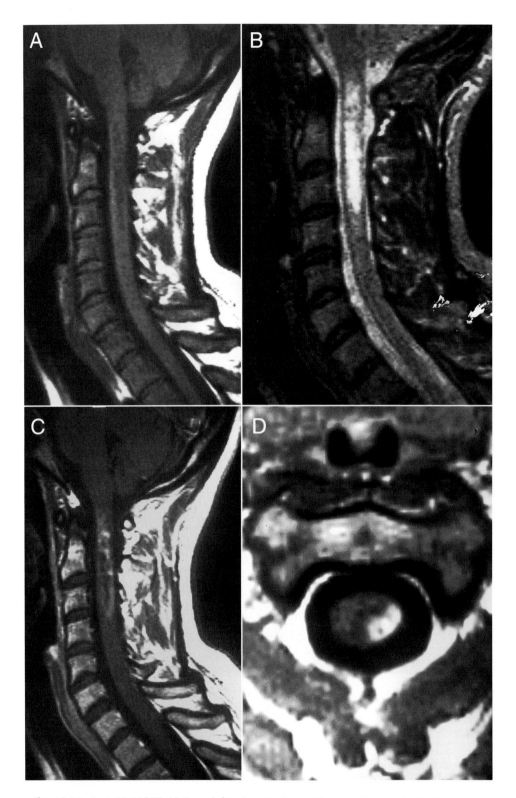

Fig. 10-23. A, A TR 500/TE 15 T_1-weighted sagittal scan through the cervical spine demonstrates mild enlargement from C1-2 through C3 with central low signal intensity within the cord parenchyma. **B,** A TR 2000/TE 90 midline sagittal T_2-weighted scan demonstrates the large area of abnormal high signal within the cord at the same location. **C** and **D,** Sagittal and axial TR 500/TE 15 gadolinium-enhanced images show irregular patchy enhancement from the foramen magnum through C3. Surgical findings confirmed the clinical diagnosis of acute demyelinating disease.

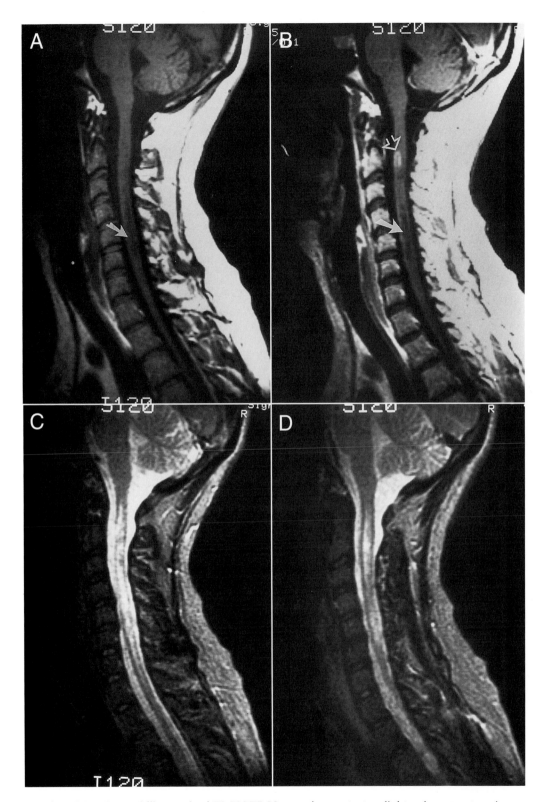

Fig. 10-24. A, A midline sagittal TR 500/TE 20 scan demonstrates slight enlargement and central low signal intensity within the spinal cord at C4 through C6 *(arrow).* **B,** A sagittal gadolinium-enhanced T_1-weighted scan shows the same area at C4 through C6 *(solid arrow)* as well as an additional enhancing lesion at C2 *(open arrow).* **C** and **D,** TR 2000/TE 90 T_2-weighted sagittal and parasagittal scans through the cervical cord reveal diffuse abnormal signal from the foramen magnum through the lower cervical segments. The diagnosis was demyelinating disease.

ral infection or immunization. Neurologic signs point toward multiple focal lesions of the brain, spinal cord, and optic nerves. Permanent neurologic deficits are not infrequent (particularly with spinal cord involvement), and the mortality rate is high.[161] Cases of relapsing ADEM are indistinguishable from those of multiple sclerosis.

Radiation Myelitis

Chronic progressive myelopathy following radiation therapy in the vicinity of the spinal cord is rare, estimated to be between 2% to 3% of cases.[162] Pallis et al.[163] recommend no more than 33 Gy over 42 days for more than 10 cm of the cord, and only 43 Gy to fields less than 10 cm. There is usually a latency period of at least 12 to 24 months (inversely related to dose) followed by the slow onset of dysesthesia and paresthesia at and below the site of therapy. Subsequently, corticospinal and/or spinothalamic tracts become involved. Pathologically there is a coagulation necrosis (involving the white matter to a greater extent than the gray matter) as well as hyaline thickening and thrombotic occlusion of arterioles.[164]

Magnetic resonance imaging will demonstrate abnormally high signal intensity of the vertebral bodies within the radiation port on T_1-weighted images secondary to replacement of normal hematopoietic elements by fat.[165] The spinal cord itself is also characterized by signal-intensity derangements, with abnormally low signal on T_1-weighted images and high signal on T_2-weighted studies over the affected area[166-168] (Fig. 10-25). Additionally there may be cord enlargement and possible areas of cord enhancement.[168]

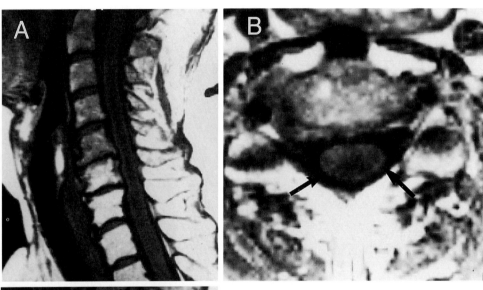

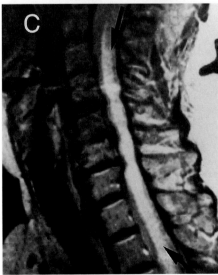

Fig. 10-25. A, A 500 msec TR/17 msec TE midline sagittal image of the cervical spine in a patient previously irradiated for metastatic carcinoma of the breast to the spine shows high signal in the lower cervical vertebral bodies and spinous processes consistent with the previous radiotherapy. Bony osteophytes can be seen at the C5-6 and C6-7 levels, along with an ill-defined decrease in signal from the central portion of the cervical cord. **B,** A 500 msec TR/17 msec TE axial image of the cervical cord confirms the abnormal low signal, mainly posteriorly *(arrows)*. **C,** A 2000 msec TR/60 msec TE midline sagittal image of the cervical spine again demonstrates the osteophytes. Note, however, the abnormal signal intensity throughout the cervical cord *(arrows)*, primarily within its central segment, extending well above the level of radiation. The presumptive diagnosis was radiation myelitis.

Acquired Immunodeficiency Syndrome Myelitis

Clinically, AIDS myelitis may be difficult to distinguish and diagnose from the previously reported, and highly variable, polyradiculoneuropathy seen in AIDS patients.[169,170] The latter can be described as (1) polyradiculopathy, (2) mononeuritis multiplex, (3) asymmetric distal sensory-motor type, and (4) distal, symmetric, sensory type.[169-172] The clinical course is highly variable; postulated etiologies include direct infection by the HIV I or herpes simplex virus.[169-172] Myelopathy in AIDS patients also may be due to mechanical cord compression (e.g., by a tumor or epidural abscess), direct viral infection (varicella-zoster, HIV I, herpes simplex), viral superinfection (CMV), or parainfectious demyelination.[169-172] Shabas et al.[173] have described the MR findings, which are indistinguishable from those of multiple sclerosis. Not surprisingly, Esposito et al.[174] have made similar observations in a patient with herpes zoster involving the spinal cord.

Adrenoleukodystrophy and Adrenomyeloneuropathy

Adrenoleukodystrophy (ALD) is a sex-linked recessive disorder of childhood characterized by CNS demyelination and adrenal insufficiency.[175] Phenotypes differ according to patterns of involvement of the central and peripheral nervous systems and the endocrine system. Childhood ALD appears in boys, usually between 4 and 8 years of age, in the form of behavioral disorders, dementia, and visual or hearing impairment. Adrenal insufficiency may follow CNS symptoms, with death usually occurring in several years.[175,176]

Adrenomyeloneuropathy (AMN) is manifested in young adult members of families affected by childhood ALD. It also is X-linked recessive and is the second most common form of the ALD-AMN complex.[175,177]

Neonatal ALD is the rarest form and is autosomal recessive.[175] Survival is limited; neonatal ALD has not been described in the same families as childhood ALD or AMN.

AMN commonly has its onset between the ages of 20 and 30 years, with progressive spastic paraplegia, peripheral neuropathy, and ataxia. Hypoadrenalism may be present. Female heterozygotes are usually asymptomatic; however, approximately 12% will be symptomatic, most often with a spastic paraparesis.[175,178] Excess very long-chain fatty acids (VLCFAs) are found in the Schwann cells and adrenocortical cells of affected individuals and heterozygotes.[175,178,179] Definitive diagnosis is made by gas-liquid chromatography of serum for elevated VLCFAs.[175] A peroxisomal enzymatic defect causing impairment of oxidation of VLCFAs may be the cause of ALD-AMN.[175]

Snyder et al.[180] have amassed 23 such cases, of which 30% manifested spinal cord disease on MR. Spinal cord disease in ALD may involve degeneration of the entire length of the corticospinal tracts, possibly from interruption of the tracts in the cerebral hemispheres. In AMN, loss of axons and myelin occurs throughout the lateral corticospinal, dorsal spinocerebellar, and gracile tracts.[181] These processes likely account for the findings by Snyder et al.[180] of diffuse spinal cord atrophy in heterozygotes recognized on MRI.[177]

SARCOIDOSIS

Sarcoidosis is a noncaseating chronic granulomatous disease that affects multiple organs, including the central nervous system (clinical manifestations involving the brain and spine reported in 5% of patients). Spinal cord involvement is relatively rare.[182,183] CNS involvement may include meningeal disease, cranial neuropathy, hypothalamic and pituitary dysfunction, and intra- and/or extraaxial masses.[184-187] Involvement of the hypothalamus and the pituitary stalk was considered characteristic of CNS sarcoidosis by Seltzer et al.[188] in conjunction with meningeal disease. Although response to therapy is variable, CNS involvement can (rarely) be fatal.

Manifestations of the disease on unenhanced and enhanced MR images of the brain and spine have been reported.[188-193] Nesbitt et al.[189] described generalized spinal cord enlargement with prolongation of T_1 and T_2 relaxation times in conjunction with patchy intramedullary enhancement that was virtually indistinguishable from intramedullary tumor. In their review of the literature they found 35% of cases with solely intramedullary involvement, 35% with leptomeningeal involvement, and 23% of cases with both (2% having extradural disease and 4% not specified). Several reports[188,189] have emphasized the sensitivity of MR imaging in detecting meningeal sarcoidosis. The detection of meningeal enhancement narrows the differential—including bacterial, viral, lymphomatous, and carcinomatous meningitis as well as en plaque meningioma. Many of these entities can be diagnosed by lumbar puncture. Seltzer et al.[188] also note that meningeal sarcoidosis has low signal intensity on the T_2-weighted images, which in many cases may reduce the imaging differential diagnosis to sarcoid versus meningioma. Confirmatory evidence in establishing the diagnosis can be obtained with chest radiographs, by the use of serum angiotensin converting enzyme (ACE) levels, or by performing a conjunctival, liver, transbronchial, or lymph node biopsy.

EXTRAMEDULLARY HEMATOPOIESIS

At birth hematopoietic activity is clearly concentrated in the bone marrow, with minimal residual liver activity.[194-197] Initially, all bone cavities are activated and blood production equals physiologic destruction. Hematopoietic stress at this stage can readily result in reactivation of extramedullary foci in the liver and spleen. Eventually hematopoietic marrow is found only in the vertebrae, ribs, sternum, bones of the skull, and proximal ends of the femora and humeri. During adult life the bone marrow space continues to expand, possibly by bone resorption. To maintain a stable production of blood elements, there is a gradual increase in the fatty-tissue components of all bone cavities.[194-197]

Hematopoietic stresses in later life can easily be met by expansion of active marrow into inactive bone marrow cavities. Extramedullary hematopoiesis (EMH) often reflects inappropriate rather than compensatory blood formation.[194,196] Ectopic marrow production has been observed in the liver, spleen, hila of the kidneys, thymus gland, adrenal glands, pleura, appendix, retroperitoneal space, and paraspinal region of the thorax. The phenomenon has also been described in a wide variety of pathologic conditions in which there is hyperplasia of blood-forming marrow: severe anemias of infancy and young children, pernicious anemias in relapse, and macrocytic and hemolytic states (e.g., hereditary spherocytosis and thalassemia). Marrow replacement in patients with osteosclerosis, invading tumor, Hodgkin's disease, leukemia, or lymphoma, and in cases of myelofibrosis, is also associated with ectopic foci of hematopoietic tissue.[194,196,198]

Cohnheim, as reported by Lyall[196] and others,[194,199] postulated the activation of quiescent rests of extramedullary hematopoietic elements. Others[200] have described the epidural extension of expanding adjacent marrow spaces. Compressive myelopathy from EMH has also been reported[199-211] in association with these diverse disorders. Most cases of EMH present with posterior mediastinal or extradural masses; and spinal cord compression is well documented, being first described by Gatto et al.[201] It is most commonly associated with long-standing congenital hemolytic anemias. In their report and review of the literature Heffez et al.[211] found that 88% of the patients were men. Symptoms lasted longer than a week in 90% of cases, and 91% demonstrated incomplete neurologic deficits. The clinical presentation may be an acute, but more commonly is a gradual, paraparesis.

In most cases the epidural block is midthoracic in location, likely reflecting the small size of the thoracic epidural space. Plain radiographs may demonstrate a thoracic mass but are rarely helpful in establishing the diagnosis of EMH.[212-214] Technetium–sulfur colloid bone marrow scanning has been used successfully to detect EMH. With CT, Long et al.[215] and Jackson and Burton[216] have described homogeneous, well-demarcated, soft tissue masses (usually in the paravertebral region),

confirming the absence of calcification and bone destruction. Mediastinal and abdominal paraaortic nodes may be enlarged, but hilar adenopathy is rare. Discrete subpleural masses may also be seen. Papavalisou et al.[217] reported five cases of tumorlike EMH causing spinal cord compression or back pain. Three of their patients were suffering from thalassemia major, one from sickle cell anemia, and one from thalassemia intermedia. CT findings included soft tissue masses in the epidural space of the spinal canal, spinal cord displacement, and involvement of the underlying bone. MRI studies showed masses compressing the spinal cord (Fig. 10-26). On T_1-weighted images there was a signal of slightly higher intensity than that of the adjacent abnormal marrow. CT suggested the diagnosis in four cases (in the fifth it was not performed) whereas MRI was positive in all five.

Treatment includes laminectomy and radiation therapy.

EPIDURAL LIPOMATOSIS

Abnormal fat deposition is a hallmark of exogenous or endogenous Cushing syndrome and Cushing disease.[218,219] This adipose tissue, abnormal in amount and location, is classically described[220] as occurring in a centripetal distribution that involves the trunk, face, and neck. Asymptomatic epidural lipomatosis is not uncommon in classic pituitary-dependent Cushing disease and is even more common in the ectopic adrenocorticotropic hormone (ACTH) syndrome.[219] It is part of the central or truncal lipomatosis associated with both exogenous and endogenous hypercortisolemia and is not related to the influence of other pituitary or adrenal hormones. Quint et al.[218] have reported such findings on MR in six symptomatic patients with Cushing syndrome, and Doppman[219] in asymptomatic patients with Cushing disease.

The increased accumulation of high-signal fat on T_1-weighted images is predominantly posterior and posterolateral within the spinal canal, displacing and compressing the thoracic spinal cord anteriorly. As noted, most symptomatic cases have occurred in patients with exogenous hypercortisolism. The absence of documented cases of cord compression in endogenous, as opposed to exogenous, hypercortisolism is probably related to the shorter duration and lesser severity of the hypercortisolism.[219] In the series and literature review of Quint et al.[218] the onset of symptoms ranged from 6 months to over 20 years after corticosteroid treatment was initiated. All patients had myelopathic or radicular symptoms. Doppman[219] noted that generalized muscular weakness due to myopathy and back pain due to vertebral osteoporosis are both common in patients with Cushing disease or syndrome and might mask the symptoms of mild cord compression. Additionally, most of the lesions reviewed by Quint et al.[218] were located in

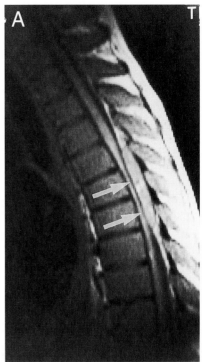

Fig. 10-26. A, A 500 msec TR/32 msec TE sagittal T$_1$-weighted image through the thoracic spine demonstrates a posteriorly placed epidural mass lesion compressing the cord. **B,** A 500 msec TR/32 msec TE T$_1$-weighted axial image through the thoracic spine also shows the paraspinal lesion as well as largely thickened ribs and subpleural soft tissue masses consistent with extramedullary hematopoiesis. Note the epidural component compressing the cord *(arrows).* **C,** A 500 msec TR/32 msec TE sagittal T$_1$-weighted scan 2 ½ weeks after radiotherapy to the thoracic spine demonstrates complete resolution of the cord compression.

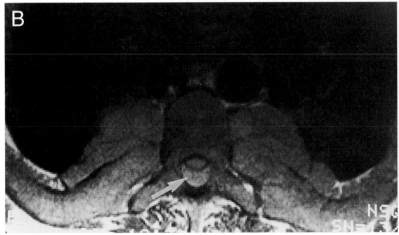

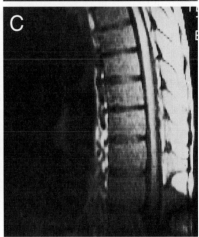

the thoracic region, although in four patients the increased spinal canal fat was localized to the lumbosacral junction region. Most patients are successfully treated surgically with decompressive laminectomy.

PAGET DISEASE

Osteitis deformans was first described by Sir James Paget in 1877 and continues to bear his name; however, the etiology of this common abnormality (3% of the population over 40 years) remains obscure.[221,222] Viral, autoimmune, and genetic factors have all been implicated in the genesis of Paget disease.[223] It may be a localized process involving one or more bones and is often discovered incidentally; less commonly it is more diffuse

and may produce extensive osseous deformity. The axial skeleton is commonly affected, with frequent involvement of the pelvis (40%), spine (75%), and skull (65%).[224,225] Local pain and tenderness are frequently present, and neurologic deficits (including motor weakness and incontinence) from spinal cord impingement may follow vertebral body compression fractures or bony expansion resulting from remodeling.[223,226,227]

The disease is characterized by abnormal remodeling of bone, which produces a characteristic pathologic and radiographic appearance with irregular bony fragments that are visualized as coarsened and enlarged osseous trabeculae.[223] Initially resorption of bony trabeculae predominates because of the intense osteoclastic activity. This is recognized on radiographs as the osteolytic form of the disease, which is particularly common in the skull, where it is termed *osteoporosis circumscripta*. Subsequently, abnormal bone remodeling can occur, which results in enlargement of bone and cortical thickening due to bone apposition on the periosteal and endosteal envelopes.[228] Increased external bone diameter with a thin cortex is caused by periosteal apposition with concomitant resorption along the endosteal envelope, leading to enlargement of the marrow cavity. Radiographic evidence of increased density or sclerosis of bone may be seen in both active and inactive stages of the disease.

The MR appearance of Paget disease reflects not only the changes of abnormal bone remodeling but also the attendant changes in the vertebral body marrow space[229] (Fig. 10-27). In the active phases of the disease the hematopoietic bone marrow is replaced by fibrous connective tissue with large numerous vascular channels.[230,231] In the inactive (osteosclerotic) phases the marrow may revert to normal. Cystlike lesions representing fat-filled marrow cavities can be present. Blood-filled sinusoids and cystic areas can appear radiographically as lucencies and have also been described in Paget disease.

Roberts et al.[229] have extensively described the MR appearance of Paget disease: cortical thickening is depicted as hypointense areas or areas of signal void on all pulse sequences; focal regions of signal within the normal void of cortical bone may follow the introduction of cellular or other marrow elements during remodeling; within the medullary canal, signal can be highly variable. They noted areas of decreased signal intensity on short TR/TE images, with increased intensity on long TR/TE images in three patients, which they believed might be due to fibrovascular change in the marrow in active Paget disease. Kelly et al.[232] have reported similar findings in association with osteoporosis circumscripta cranii. The presence of hypointensity on short TR/TE images and hyperintensity on long TR/TE images, however, is nonspecific and if associated with a new onset pain should prompt consideration of pathologic fracture or sarcomatous degeneration. In several patients described by Roberts et al.,[229] focal areas in the marrow had signal characteristics similar to those of fat but of much higher intensity and more homogeneous than normal fatty marrow (fat mixed with trabecular bone). In one patient a rectangular area of rarefaction containing fat in the posterior half of the vertebral body was seen. These may be reflective more of inactive disease.

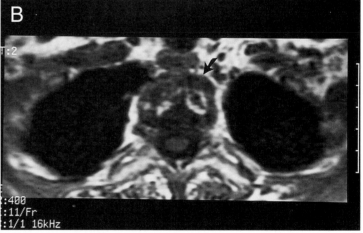

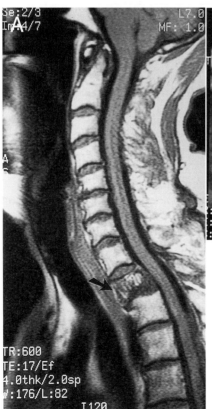

Fig. 10-27. A, A sagittal midline T$_1$-weighted scan (600 msec TR/17 msec TE) through the cervicothoracic junction demonstrates expansion of T2 with coarsening of the cortical and trabecular bone and increased focal areas of high signal reflecting increased marrow fat. **B,** An axial T$_1$-weighted scan through T2 again demonstrates increased thickening of cortical bone with focal areas of high signal intensity reflecting loculated fat within the remodeled marrow space.

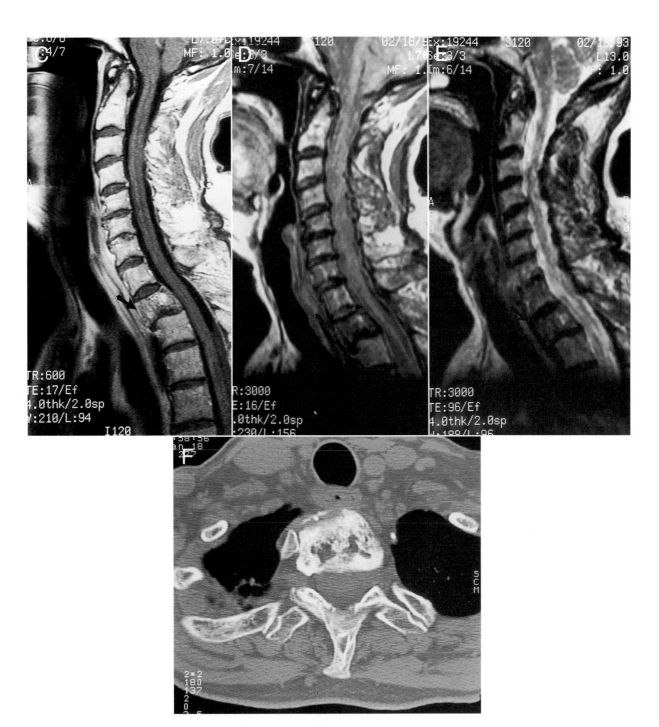

Fig. 10-27, cont'd. C, A sagittal T$_1$-weighted gadolinium-enhanced scan shows diffuse enhancement throughout the increased marrow space reflective of fibrovascular granulation tissue. **D** and **E,** T$_2$-weighted (3000 msec TR/16 and 96 msec TE) midline sagittal scans through the cervicothoracic spine likewise show expansion of T2 with an increase in cortical bone *(arrows)*. **F,** The axial CT scan with bone reconstruction confirms the presence of remodeled bone with multiple cystic loculations within the posterior elements as well as the vertebral body, consistent with Paget disease.

REFERENCES

1. DeLaPaz RL: Nuclear magnetic resonance (NMR) imaging of Arnold-Chiari type I malformation with hydromyelia. *J Comput Assist Tomogr* 1983;7:126-129.

2. Han JS, Kaufman B, El Yousef SJ, et al: NMR imaging of the spine. *AJNR* 1983;4:1151-1159.

3. Modic MT, Weinstein MA, Pavlicek W, et al: Nuclear magnetic resonance of the spine. *Radiology* 1983;148:757-762.

4. Yeates A, Brantzawadski M, Norman D, et al: Nuclear magnetic resonance imaging of syringomyelia. *AJNR* 1983;4:234-237.

5. Modic MT, Weinstein MA, Pavlicek W, et al: Magnetic resonance imaging of the cervical spine: techniques and clinical observations. *AJR* 1983;141:1129-1136.

6. Pojunas K, Williams AL, Daniels DL, Haughton VM: Syringomyelia and hydromyelia: magnetic resonance evaluation. *Radiology* 1984;153:679-683.

7. Kokmen E, Marsh WR, Baker HL: Magnetic resonance imaging in syringomyelia. *Neurosurgery* 1985;17:267-270.

8. Quencer RM, Sheldon JJ, Post MJD: Magnetic resonance imaging of the chronically injured cervical spinal cord. *AJNR* 1986;7:457-464.

9. Sherman JL, Barkovich AJ, Citrin CM: The MR appearance of syringomyelia: new observations. *AJR* 1987;148:381-391.

10. Enzmann DR, O'Donohue J, Rubin JB, et al: CSF pulsations within nonneoplastic spinal cord cysts. *AJR* 1987;149:149-157.

11. Castillo M, Quencer RM, Green BA, Montaluo BM: Syringomyelia as a consequence of compressive extramedullary lesions: postoperative clinical and radiological manifestations. *AJR* 1988;150:391-396.

12. Simon T: Über Syringomyelie und Geschwulstbildung im Rückenmark. *Arch Psychiatr Nervenkr* 1875;5:120-163.

13. Barbaro NM, Wilson C, Gutin PH, Edwards MSB: Surgical treatment of syringomyelia. Favorable results with syringoperitoneal shunting. *J Neurosurg* 1984;61:531-538.

14. Gardner WJ: Hydrodynamic mechanism of syringomyelia—its relationship to myelocele. *J Neurol Neurosurg Psychiatry* 1965;28:247-259.

15. Gardner LW, Angel J: The mechanism of syringomyelia and its surgical connection. *Clin Neurosurg* 1975;6:131-140.

16. Ball MJ, Dayan AD: Pathogenesis of syringomyelia. *Lancet* 1972;2:799-801.

17. Hughes JT: *Pathology of the spinal cord,* ed 2. Philadelphia, Saunders, 1978.

18. Feigin I, Ogata J, Buclzilovich G: Syringomyelia: the role of edema in its pathogenesis. *J Neuropathol Exp Neurol* 1971;30:216-232.

19. Williams B: The distending force in the production of "communicating syringomyelia." *Lancet* 1969;2:189-193.

20. Williams B: Current concepts in syringomyelia. *Br J Hosp Med* 1970;4:331-342.

21. Williams B: On the pathogenesis of syringomyelia: a review. *J R Soc Med* 1980;73:798-806.

22. Hall P, Turner M, Aichinger S, et al: Experimental syringomyelia. The relationship between intraventricular and intrasyrinx pressures. *J Neurosurg* 1980;52:812-817.

23. Quencer RM, El Gammal T, Cohen G: Syringomyelia associated with intradural extramedullary masses of the spinal canal. *AJNR* 1986;7:143-148.

24. Aboulker J: La syringomyelic et les liquides intrarachidiens. *Neurochirurgie* 1979;25(suppl 1):9-144.

25. Aubin ML, Lignanel J, Jardin Bar D: Computed tomography in 75 clinical cases or syringomyelia. *AJNR* 1981;2:199-204.

26. Bronskill MJ, McVeigh ER, Kucharczyk W, Henkelman RM: Syrinx-like artifacts on MR images of the spinal cord. *Radiology* 1988;166:485-488.

27. Levy LM, Di Chiro G, Brooks RA, et al: Spinal cord artifacts from truncation errors during MR imaging. *Radiology* 1988;166:479-483.

28. Rubin JM, Aisen AM, DiPietro MA: Ambiguities in MR imaging of tumoral cysts in the spinal cord. *J Comput Assist Tomogr* 1986;10:395-398.

29. Williams MW, Haughton VM, Pojunas KW, et al: Differentiation of intramedullary neoplasms and cysts by MR. *AJR* 1987;149:159-164.

30. Quencer RM, Post MJD, Hinks RS: Cine MR in the evaluation of normal and abnormal CSF flow: intracranial and intraspinal studies. *Neuroradiology* 1990;32:371-391.

31. Post MJD, Quencer RM, Hinks RS: Spinal CSF flow dynamics: its qualitative and quantitative evaluation by CINE-MR. ASNR, 1989.

32. Enzmann DR, Rubin J, Pelc N: Cine phase contrast maps of cervical cerebrospinal fluid motion. RSNA, 1989.

33. Itabashi T, Arai S, Kitahura H, et al: Quantitative analysis of cervical cerebrospinal fluid pulsation. RSNA, 1988.

34. Post MJD, Quencer RM, Green BA, et al: The role of cine-MR in the evaluation of the pulsatile characteristics of posttraumatic spinal cord cysts. ASNR, 1988.

35. Quencer RM: The injured spinal cord: evaluation with magnetic resonance and intraoperative sonography. *Radiol Clin North Am* 1988;26:1025-1045.

36. Post MJD, Quencer RM, Green BA, et al: Cine-MR imaging in determining the flow characteristics of CSF and blood in spinal and intracranial lesions. RSNA, 1988.

37. Nabors MW, Pait TG, Byrd EB, et al: Updated assessment and current classification of spinal meningeal cysts. *J Neurosurg* 1988;68:366-377.

38. Cloward RB: Congenital spinal extradural cysts: case report with review of literature. *Ann Surg* 1968;168:851-864.

39. Wilkins RH, Odom GL: Spinal extradural cysts. In Vinken PJ, Bruyn GW (eds): *Handbook of clinical neurology, tumors of the spine and spinal cord,* New York, Elsevier–North Holland, 1976, vol 20, pp 137-175.

40. Wilkins RH: Intraspinal cysts. In Wilkins RH, Rengacharry SS (eds): *Neurosurgery.* New York, McGraw-Hill, 1985, pp 2061-2070.

41. Lamas E, Lobato RD, Armor T: Occult intrasacral meningocele. *Surg Neurol* 1977;8:181-184.

42. Tarlov IM: Spinal perineurial and meningeal cysts. *J Neurol Neurosurg Psychiatry* 1970;33:833-843.

43. McCrum C, Williams B: Spinal extradural arachnoid pouches: report of two cases. *J Neurosurg* 1982;57:849-852.

44. Fortuna A, LaTorre E, Ciapetta P: Arachnoid diverticula: a unitary approach to spinal cysts communicating with the subarachnoid space. *Acta Neurochir* 1977;39:259-268.

45. Kendall BE, Valentine AR, Keis B: Spinal arachnoid cysts: clinical and radiological correlation with prognosis. *Neuroradiology* 1982;22:225-234.

46. Swamy KS, et al: Intraspinal arachnoid cysts. *Clin Neurol Neurosurg* 1984;86:143-148.

47. Chan RC, Thompson GB, Bratty PJA: Symptomatic anterior spinal arachnoid diverticulum. *Neurosurgery* 1985; 16:663-665.

48. Galzio RJ, Zenobii M, Lucantoni D, et al: Spinal intradural arachnoid cyst. *Surg Neurol* 1982;17:388-391.

49. Palmer JJ: Spinal arachnoid cysts: report of six cases. *J Neurosurg* 1974;41:728-735.

50. Teng P, Papatheodorou C: Spinal arachnoid diverticula. *Br J Radiol* 1966;39:249-254.

51. Zuccarello M, Powers G, Tobler WD, et al: Chronic posttraumatic lumbar intradural arachnoid cyst with cauda equina compression: case report. *Neurosurgery 1987; 29:* 636-638.

52. Sklar EM, Quencer RM, Green BA, et al: Complications of epidural anesthesia: MR appearance of abnormalities. *Radiology* 1991;181:549-554.

53. Gray L, Djang WT, Friedman AH: MR imaging of thoracic extradural arachnoid cysts. *J Comput Assist Tomogr* 1988; 12:646-648.

54. Spiegelmann R, Rappaport ZH, Sahar A: Spinal arachnoid cyst with unusual presentation: case report. *J Neurosurg* 1984;60:613-616.

54a. Davis SW, Levy LM, LeBihan DJ, et al: Sacral meningeal cysts: evaluation with MR imaging. *Radiology* 1993;187: 445-448.

55. Cilluffo JM, Gomez MR, Reese DF, et al: Idiopathic ("congenital") spinal arachnoid diverticula. *Mayo Clin Proc* 1981; 56:93-101.

56. Duncan A, Hoare RD: Spinal arachnoid cysts in children. *Radiology* 1978;126:432-439.

57. Hoffman GT: Cervical arachnoidal cyst: report of a 6-year-old Negro male with recovery from quadriplegia. *J Neurosurg* 1960;17:327-330.

58. Andrews BT, Weinstein PR, Rosenblum ML, Barbaro NM: Intradural arachnoid cysts of the spinal canal associated with intramedullary cysts. *J Neurosurg* 1988;68:544-549.

59. Gindre-Barrucand T, Charleux F, Turjman F, et al: Magnetic resonance imaging contribution to the diagnosis of spinal cord compression by a subdural arachnoid cyst. *Neuroradiology* 1991;33:87-89.

60. Sklar E, Quencer RM, Green BA, et al: Acquired spinal subarachnoid cysts: evaluation with MR, CT, myelography, and intraoperative sonography. *AJNR* 1989;10:1097-1104.

61. Di Chiro G: Angiography of obstructive vascular disease of the spinal cord. *Radiology* 1971;100:607-614.

62. Dommisse GF: The blood supply of the spinal cord. *J Bone Joint Surg [Br]* 1974;56:225-235.

63. Dommisse GF: The arteries, arterioles, and capillaries of the spinal cord: surgical guidelines in the prevention of postoperative paraplegia. *Ann R Coll Surg Engl* 1980;62:369-376.

64. Lasjaunias P, Berenstein A: *Surgical neuroangiography.* (Chapter 3. Functional vascular anatomy of brain, spinal cord, and spine.) New York, Springer, 1990, pp 40-55.

65. Parke WW: Applied anatomy of the spine. In Rothman RH, Simeone FA (eds): *The spine.* Philadelphia, Saunders, 1982, pp 18-51.

66. Willis TA: Nutrient arteries of the vertebral bodies. *J Bone Joint Surg [Am]* 1949;31:538-541.

67. Lazorthes G, Gouaze A, Zadeh JO, et al: Arterial vascularization of the spinal cord. *J Neurosurg* 1971;35:253-269.

68. Lazorthes G, Poulhes J, Bastide G, et al: La vascularisation artérielle de la moelle. *Neurochirurgie* 1958;4:3-19.

69. El-Toraei I, Juler G: Ischemic myelopathy. *Angiology* 1979;30:81-94.

70. Herren RY, Alexander L: Sulcal and intrinsic blood vessels of human spinal cord. *Arch Neurol Psychiatry* 1939;41:678-687.

71. Woollam DH, Millen JW: The arterial supply of the spinal cord and its significance. *J Neurol Neurosurg Psychiatry* 1955;18:97-102.

72. Hegedus K, Fekete I: Case report of infarction in the region of the posterior spinal arteries. *Eur Arch Psychiatry Neurol Sci* 1984;234:281-284.

73. Hughes JT: Thrombosis of the posterior spinal arteries: a complication of an intrathecal injection of phenol. *Neurology* 1970;20:659-664.

74. Gillilan L: The arterial blood supply of the human spinal cord. *J Comp Neurol* 1958;110:75-103.

75. Aminoff MJ: Introduction: the nature of spinal angiomas. In Aminoff MJ (ed): *Spinal angiomas.* Boston, Blackwell 1976, pp 1-4.

76. Doppman J, Di Chiro G, Ommaya AK: Arteriovenous malformations. In Doppman J, Di Chiro G, Ommaya AK (eds): *Selective arteriography of the spinal cord.* St Louis, Warren H Green, 1969, pp 59-124.

77. Teny P, Papatheodorou C: Myelography appearance of vascular anomalies of the spinal cord. *Br J Radiol* 1964; 37:358-366.

78. Rosenblum B, Oldfield EH, Doppman JL, Di Chiro G: Spinal arteriovenous malformations: a comparison of dural arteriovenous fistulas and intradural AVM's in 81 patients. *J Neurosurg* 1987;67:795-802.

79. Heros RC, Debrun GM, Ojemann RG, et al: Direct spinal arteriovenous fistula: a new type of spinal AVM. *J Neurosurg* 1986;64:134-139.

80. Oldfield EH, Doppman JL: Spinal arteriovenous malformations. *Clin Neurosurg* 1961;9:161-183.

81. Doppman JL, Di Chiro G, Oldfield EH: Origin of spinal arteriovenous malformation and normal cord vasculature from a common segmental artery: angiographic and therapeutic considerations. *Radiology* 1985;154:687-689.

82. Aminoff MJ: Associated lesions. In Aminoff MJ (ed): *Spinal angiomas.* Boston, Blackwell, 1976, pp 18-27.

83. Djindjian R: Neuroradiological examination of spinal cord angiomas. In Vinken PJ, Bruyn GW (eds): *Handbook of clinical neurology,* vol 12. New York, Elsevier–North Holland, 1972, pp 631-643.

84. Doppman JL, Wirth FP Jr, Di Chiro G, Ommaya AK: Value of cutaneous angiomas in the arteriographic localization of spinal-cord arteriovenous malformations. *N Engl J Med* 1969;281:1440-1444.

85. Doppman JL, Di Chiro G, Dwyer AJ, et al: Magnetic resonance imaging of spinal arteriovenous malformations. *J Neurosurg* 1987;66:830-834.

86. Di Chiro G, Doppman JL, Dwyer JL, et al: Tumors and arteriovenous malformations of the spinal cord: assessment using MR. *Radiology* 1985;156:689-697.

87. Kim D-I, Choi I-S, Berenstein A: A sacral dural arteriovenous fistula presenting with an intermittent myelopathy aggravated by menstruation. *J Neurosurg* 1991;75:947-949.

88. Wirth FP, Post KD, Di Chiro G, et al: Foix-Alajouanine disease: spontaneous thrombosis of a spinal cord arteriovenous malformation: a case report. *Neurology* 1970;20:1114-1118.

89. Crissuolo GR, Oldfield EH, Doppman JL: Reversible acute and subacute myelopathy in patients with dural arteriovenous fistulas. Foix-Alajouanine syndrome reconsidered. *J Neurosurg* 1989;70:354-359.

90. Aminoff MJ, Barnard RO, Logue V: The pathophysiology of spinal cord vascular malformations. *J Neurosci* 1974;23:255-263.

91. Kendall BE, Logue V: Spinal epidural angiomatous malformations draining into intrathecal veins. *Neuroradiology* 1977;13:181-189.

92. Stein SC, Ommaya AK, Doppman JL, Di Chiro G: Arteriovenous malformation of the cauda equina with arterial supply from branches of the internal iliac arteries. *J Neurosurg* 1972;36(5):649-651.

93. Wrobel CJ, Oldfield EH, Di Chiro G, et al: Myelopathy due to intracranial dural arteriovenous fistulas draining intrathecally into spinal medullary veins. *J Neurosurg* 1988;69:934-939.

94. Partington MD, Rufenacht DA, Marsh WR, Piepgras DG: Cranial and sacral dural arteriovenous fistulas as a cause of myelopathy. *J Neurosurg* 1992;76:615-622.

95. Gobin YP, Rogopoulos A, Aymard A, et al: Endovascular treatment of intracranial dural arteriovenous fistulas with spinal perimedullary venous drainage. *J Neurosurg* 1992;77:718-723.

96. Oldfield EH, DiChiro G, Quindlen EA, et al: Successful treatment of a group of spinal cord arteriovenous malformations by interruption of dural fistula. *J Neurosurg* 1983;59:1019-1030.

97. Masaryk TJ, Ross JS, Modic MT, et al: Radiculomeningeal vascular malformations of the spine: MR imaging. *Radiology* 1987;164:845-849.

98. Terwey B, Becker H, Thron AK, Vahldiek G: Gadolinium-DTPA enhanced MR imaging of spinal dural arteriovenous fistulas. *J Comput Assist Tomogr* 1989;13(1):30-37.

99. Larsson E-M, Desai P, Hardin CW, et al: Venous infarction of the spinal cord resulting from dural arteriovenous fistula: MR imaging findings. *AJNR* 1991;12:739-743.

100. Rubinstein LJ: Tumors and malformation of blood vessels. In Firminger HI (ed): *Tumors of the central nervous system.* Washington DC, Armed Forces Institute of Pathology, 1985, pp 235-256.

101. Jellinger K: Pathology of spinal vascular malformations and vascular tumors. In Pia HW, Djindjian R (eds): *Spinal angiomas: advances in diagnosis and therapy.* New York, Springer, 1978, pp 9-20.

102. McCormick WF: The pathology of vascular ("arteriovenous") malformations. *J Neurosurg* 1966;24:807-816.

103. Bicknell JM, Carlow TJ, Kornfield M: Familial cavernous angiomas. *Arch Neurol* 1978;35:746-749.

104. Heffner RR, Solitare GB: Hereditary hemorrhagic telangiectasia; neuropathological observations. *J Neurol Neurosurg Psychiatry* 1969;32:604-608.

105. McCormick WF, Hardman JM, Boulter TR: Vascular malformations ("angiomas") of the brain with special reference to those occurring in the posterior fossa. *J Neurosurg* 1968;28:241-251.

106. Padovani R, Tognetti F, Proietti D, et al: Extrathecal cavernous hemangioma. *Surg Neurol* 1982;118:475-476.

107. Richardson RR, Cerullo LJ: Spinal epidural cavernous hemangioma. *Surg Neurol* 1979;12:266-268.

108. Guthkelch AN: Hemangiomas involving the spinal epidural space. *J Neurol Neurosurg Psychiatry* 1948;11:199-210.

109. Zabramski JM, Spetzler RF, Sonntag VKH: Treatment of spinal cavernous angiomas. *J Neurosurg* 1988;69:476.

110. Cosgrove GR, Bertrand G, Fontaine S, et al: Cavernous angiomas of the spinal cord. *J Neurosurg* 1988;68:31-36.

111. Ross JS, Masaryk TJ, Modic MT, et al: Vertebral hemangiomas: MR imaging. *Radiology* 1987;165:165-169.

112. Fontaine S, Melanson D, Cosgrove R, Bertrand G: Cavernous hemangiomas of the spinal cord: MR imaging. *Radiology* 1988;166:839-841.

113. Gomori JM, Grossman RI, Goldberg RI, et al: Intracranial hematomas: imaging by high-field MR. *Radiology* 1985;157:87-93.

114. Edelman RR, Johnson K, Buxton R, et al: MR of hemorrhage: a new approach. *AJNR* 1986;7:751-756.

115. Walton JN: Subarachnoid haemorrhage of unusual aetiology. *Neurology* 1953;3:517-543.

116. Henson RA, Croft PB: Spontaneous spinal subarachnoid haemorrhage. *Q J Med* 1956;25:53-66.

117. Swann KW, Ropper AH, New PFJ, Poletti CE: Spontaneous spinal subarachnoid hemorrhage and subdural hematoma: report of two cases. *J Neurosurg* 1984;61:975-980.

118. Prieto A Jr, Cantu RC: Spinal subarachnoid hemorrhage associated with neurofibroma of the cauda equina: case report. *J Neurosurg* 1967;27:63-69.

119. Plotkin R, Ronthal M, Froman C: Spontaneous spinal subarachnoid haemorrhage: report of 3 cases. *J Neurosurg* 1966;25:443-446.

119a. Gundry CR, Heithoff KB: Epidural hematoma of the lumbar spine: 18 surgically confirmed cases. *Radiology* 1993; 187:427-431.

120. Jellinger K: Traumatic vascular disease of the spinal cord. In Vinken PJ, Bruyn GW (eds): Vascular diseases of the nervous system. II. *Handbook of clinical neurology,* vol 12. New York, Elsevier–North Holland, 1972, pp 556-630.

121. Vinters HV, Barnett HJ, Kaufmann JC: Subdural hematoma of the spinal cord and widespread subarachnoid hemorrhage complicating anticoagulant therapy. *Stroke* 1980;11:459-464.

122. Masdeu JC, Breuer AC, Schoene WC: Spinal subarachnoid hematomas: clue to a source of bleeding in traumatic lumbar puncture. *Neurology* 1979;29:872-876.

123. Rader JP: Chronic subdural hematoma of the spinal cord: report of a case. *N Engl J Med* 1955;253:374-376.

124. Levy JM: Spontaneous lumbar subdural hematoma. *AJNR* 1990;11:780-781.

125. Hughes JT, Oppenheimer DR: Superficial siderosis of the central nervous system; a report on nine cases with autopsy. *Acta Neuropathol* 1969;13:556-574.

126. Koeppen AH, Dentinger MP: Brain hemosiderin and superficial siderosis of the central nervous system. *J Neuropathol Exp Neurol* 1988;47:249-270.

127. Koeppen AHW, Barron KD: Superficial siderosis of the central nervous system. Histological, histochemical and chemical study. *J Neuropathol Exp Neurol* 1971;30:448-469.

128. Adams RD, Victor M: *Principles of neurology*. New York, McGraw-Hill, 1985, p 472.

129. Thulborn KR, Sorensen AG, Kowall NW, et al: The role of ferritin and hemosiderin in the MR appearance of cerebral hemorrhage: a histopathologic biochemical study in rats. *AJNR* 1990;11:291-297.

130. Gomori JM, Grossman RI, Bilaniuk LT, et al: High-field MR imaging of superficial siderosis of central nervous system. *J Comput Assist Tomogr* 1985;9(5):972-975.

131. Yuh WT, Marsh EE, Wang AK, et al: MR imaging of spinal cord and vertebral body infarction. *AJNR* 1992;13:145-154.

132. Mawad ME, Rivera V, Crawford S, et al: Spinal cord ischemia after resection of thoracoabdominal aortic aneurysm: MR findings in 24 patients. *AJNR* 1990;11:987-991.

133. Mikulis DJ, Ogilvy CS, McKee A, et al: Spinal cord infarction and fibrocartilaginous emboli. *AJNR* 1992;13:155-160.

134. Vandertop WP, Elderson A, van Gijn J, Valk J: Anterior spinal artery syndrome. *AJNR* 1991;12:505-506.

135. Brown E, Virapongse C, Gregorios JB: MR imaging of cervical spinal cord infarction. *J Comput Assist Tomogr* 1989;13:920-922.

136. Casselman JW, Jolie E, Dehaene I, et al: Gadolinium-enhanced MR imaging of infarction of the anterior spinal cord. *AJNR* 1991;12:561.

137. Mirich DR, Kucharczyk W, Keller MA, Deck J: Subacute necrotizing myelopathy: MR imaging in four pathologically proved cases. *AJNR* 1991;12:1077-1083.

138. McFarlin DE, McFarland HF: Multiple sclerosis. *N Engl J Med* 1982;307:1183-1188.

139. McAlpine D, Lumsden CE, Acheson ED: *Multiple sclerosis: a reappraisal*. London, Churchill Livingstone, 1972.

140. Kurtzke JF: Epidemiologic contributions to multiple sclerosis: an overview. *Neurology* 1980;30:61-79.

141. Dean G, Kurtzke JF: On the risk of multiple sclerosis according to age at immigration to South Africa. *Br Med J* 1971;3:725-729.

142. Alter M, Kahara E, Loewenson R: Migration and risk of multiple sclerosis. *Neurology* 1978;28:1089-1093.

143. Maravilla KR, Weinreb JC, Suss R, Nunnally RL: Magnetic resonance demonstration of multiple sclerosis plaques in the cervical cord. *AJNR* 1984;5:685-689.

144. Prineas JW, Wright RG: Macrophages, lymphocytes, and plasma cells in the perivascular compartment in chronic multiple sclerosis. *Lab Invest* 1978;38:409-421.

145. Prineas J: Pathology of the early lesion in multiple sclerosis. *Hum Pathol* 1975;6:531-554.

146. Poser CM, Paty DW, Scheinberg L, et al: New diagnostic criteria for multiple sclerosis: guidelines for research protocols. *Ann Neurol* 1983;13:227-231.

147. Bydder GM, Steiner RE, Young IR, et al: Clinical NMR imaging of the brain: 140 cases. *AJNR* 1982;3:459-480.

148. Sheldon JJ, Siddharthan R, Tobias J, et al: MR imaging of multiple sclerosis: comparison with clinical and CT examinations in 74 patients. *AJNR* 1985;6:683-690.

149. Edwards MK, Farlow MR, Stevens JC: Multiple sclerosis: MRI and clinical correlation. *AJNR* 1986;147:571-574.

150. Poser CM, Kleefield J, O'Reilly GV, Jolesz F: Neuroimaging and the lesion of multiple sclerosis. *AJNR* 1987;8:549-552.

151. Grossman RI, Gonzalez-Scarano F, Atlas SW, et al: Multiple sclerosis: gadolinium enhancement in MR imaging. *Radiology* 1986;161:721-725.

152. Sarkari NBS, Bickerstaff R: Relapses and remissions in brain stem tumors. *Br Med J* 1969;2:21-23.

153. Cohen J, Macrae D: Tumors in the region of the foramen magnum. *J Neurosurg* 1962;19:462-469.

154. Rosenbluth PR, Lichtenstein BW: Pearly tumor (epidermoid cholesteatoma) of the brain: clinicopathological study of two cases. *J Neurosurg* 1960;17:35-42.

155. Lehman RAW, Fieger HG: Arachnoid cyst producing recurrent neurological disturbances. *Surg Neurol* 1978;10:134-136.

156. Howe JR, Taren JH: Foramen magnum tumors: pitfalls in diagnosis. *JAMA* 1973;225:1061-1066.

157. Stahl SM, Johnson KP, Malamud N: The clinical and pathological spectrum of brainstem vascular malformations: long-term course simulates multiple sclerosis. *Arch Neurol* 1980;37:25-29.

158. Dhopesh VP, Weinstein JD: Spinal arteriovenous malformations simulating multiple sclerosis: importance of early diagnosis. *Dis Nerv Syst* 1977;38:848-851.

159. Banerji NK, Millar JHD: Chiari malformation presenting in adult life. *Brain* 1974;97:157-168.

160. Lumsden CE: The neuropathology of multiple sclerosis. In Vinken PJ, Bruyn GW (eds): *Handbook of clinical neurology,* New York, Elsevier–North Holland, 1979, vol 9, p 305.

161. Miller HG, Stanton JB, Gibbons JL: Acute disseminated encephalomyelitis and related syndrome. *Br Med J* 1957;1:668-672.

162. Palmer JJ: Radiation myelopathy. *Brain* 1972;95:109-122.

163. Pallis C, Louis C, Morgan RL: Radiation myelopathy. *Brain* 1961;84:460-479.

164. Burns RJ, Jones AN, Robertson JS: Pathology of radiation myelopathy. *J Neurol Neurosurg Psychiatry* 1972;35:888-898.

165. Ramsey RG, Zacharias CE: MR imaging of the spine after radiation therapy: easily recognizable effects. *AJR* 1985;144:1131-1135.

166. Wang PY, Shen WC: Magnetic resonance imaging in two patients with radiation myelopathy. *J Formosan Med Assoc* 1991;190:583-585.

167. Zwieg G, Russell EJ: Radiation myelopathy of the cervical spinal cord: MR findings. *AJNR* 1990;11:188-190.

168. Wang PY, Shen WC, Jan JS: MR imaging in radiation myelopathy. *AJNR* 1992;13:1049-1055.

169. Snider WD, Simpson DM, Nielsen S, et al: Neurological complications of acquired immunodeficiency syndrome: analysis of 50 patients. *Ann Neurol* 1983;14:403-418.

170. Ho DD, Rota TR, Schooley RT, et al: Isolation of HTLV-III from cerebrospinal fluid and neural tissues of patients with neurologic syndromes related to acquired immunodeficiency syndrome. *N Engl J Med* 1985;313:1493-1497.

171. Britton CB, Miller JR. Neurologic complications in acquired immunodeficiency syndrome (AIDS). *Neurol Clin* 1984;2(2):315-335.

172. Levy RM, Bredesen DE, Rosenblum ML: Neurological manifestations of the acquired immunodeficiency syndrome (AIDS): experience at UCSF and review of the literature. *J Neurosurg* 1985;62:475-479.

173. Shabas D, Gerard G, Cunha B, et al: MR imaging of AIDS myelitis. *AJNR* 1989;10:S51-S52.

174. Esposito MB, Arrington JA, Murtaugh FR, et al: MR of the spinal cord in patients with herpes zoster. *AJNR* 1993;14:203-204.

175. Moser HW, Moser AE, Singh I, O'Neill BP: Adrenoleukodystrophy: survey of 303 cases: biochemistry, diagnosis, and therapy. *Ann Neurol* 1984;16:628-641.

176. Davis LE, Snyder RD, Orth DN, et al: Adrenoleukodystrophy and adrenomyeloneuropathy associated with partial adrenal insufficiency in three generations of a kindred. *Am J Med* 1979;66:342-347.

177. Griffin JW, Goren E, Schaumburg HH, et al: Adrenomyeloneuropathy: a probable variant of adrenoleukodystrophy. I. Clinical and endocrinologic aspects. *Neurology* 1977;27:1107-1113.

178. O'Neill BP, Moser HW, Saxena KM, Marmion LC: Adrenoleukodystrophy: clinical and biochemical manifestations in carriers. *Neurology* 1984;34:798-801.

179. Powers JM, Schaumburg HH: Adrenoleukodystrophy: similar ultrastructural changes in adrenal cortical cells and Schwann cells. *Arch Neurol* 1974;30:406-408.

180. Snyder RD, King JN, Keck GM, Orrison WW: MR imaging of the spinal cord in 23 subjects with ALD-AMN complex. *AJNR* 1991;12:1095-1098.

181. Schaumburg HH, Powers JM, Raine CS, et al: Adrenomyeloneuropathy: a probable variant of adrenoleukodystrophy. II. General pathologic, neuropathologic, and biochemical aspects. *Neurology* 1977;27:1114-1119.

182. Banerjee T, Hunt WE: Spinal cord sarcoidosis: case report. *J Neurosurg* 1972;36:490-493.

183. Caroscio JT, Yahr MD: Progressive myelopathy due to sarcoid. *Clin Neurol Neurosurg* 1980;82:217-222.

184. Delaney P: Neurologic manifestations in sarcoidosis: review of the literature, with a report of 23 cases. *Ann Intern Med* 1977;87:336-345.

185. Matthews WB: Neurologic manifestations of sarcoidosis. In Asbury AK, McKhann GM, McDonald WI (eds): *Diseases of the nervous system: clinical neurobiology.* London, Heinemann, 1986, pp 1563-1570.

186. Kendall BE, Tatler GLV: Radiological findings in neurosarcoidosis. *Br J Radiol* 1978;51:81-92.

187. Leeds NE, Zimmerman RD, Elkin CM, et al: Neurosarcoidosis of the brain and meninges. *Semin Roentgenol* 1985;20:387-392.

188. Seltzer S, Mark AS, Atlas SW: CNS sarcoidosis: evaluation with contrast-enhanced MR imaging. *AJNR* 1991;12:1227-1233.

189. Nesbit GM, Miller GM, Baker HL Jr, et al: Spinal cord sarcoidosis: a new finding at MR imaging with Gd-DTPA enhancement. *Radiology* 1987;173:839-843.

190. Hayes WS, Sherman JL, Stern BJ, et al: MR and CT evaluation of intracranial sarcoidosis. *AJR* 1987;149:1043-1049.

191. Miller DH, Kendall BE, Barter S, et al: Magnetic resonance imaging in central nervous system sarcoidosis. *Neurology* 1988;38:378-383.

192. Martin CA, Murali R, Trasi SS: Spinal cord sarcoidosis. *J Neurosurg* 1984;61:981-982.

193. Greco A, Steiner RE: Magnetic resonance imaging in neurosarcoidosis. *Magn Reson Imaging* 1987;5:15-21.

194. Erslev AJ: Medullary and extramedullary blood formation. *Clin Orthop* 1967;52:25-36.

195. Gilmour JR: Normal haemopoiesis in intra-uterine and neonatal life. *J Pathol Bacteriol* 1941;52:25-55.

196. Lyall A: massive extramedullary bone-marrow formation in a case of pernicious anaemia. *J Pathol Bacteriol* 1935;41:469-472.

197. Ward HP, Block MH: The natural history of agnogenic myeloid metaplasia (AMM) and a critical evaluation of its relationship with the myeloproliferative syndrome. *Medicine* 1971;50:357-411.

198. Glew RH, Haese WH, McIntyre PA: Myeloid metaplasia with myelofibrosis: the clinical spectrum of extramedullary hematopoiesis and tumor formation. *Johns Hopkins Med J* 1973;132:253-270.

199. Appleby A, Batson GA, Lassman LP, et al: Spinal cord compression by extramedullary haematopoiesis in myelosclerosis. *J Neurol Neurosurg Psychiatry* 1964;27:313-316.

200. Luyendijk W, Went L, Schaad HDG: Spinal cord compression due to extramedullary hematopoiesis in homozygous thalassemia: case report. *J Neurosurg* 1975;42:212-216.

201. Gatto I, Terrana V, Biondi L: Compressione sul midollo spinale da proliferazione di midollo osseo nello spazio epidurale in soggetto affetto da malattia di Cooley splenectomizzato. *Haematologica* 1954;38:61-75.

202. Ammoumi AA, Sher JH, Schmelka D: Spinal cord compression by extramedullary hemopoietic tissue in sickle cell anemia: case report. *J Neurosurg* 1975;43:483-485.

203. Bree RL, Neiman HL, Hodak JA, et al: Extramedullary hematopoiesis in the spinal epidural space. *J Can Assoc Radiol* 1974;25:297-299.

204. Cauthen JC, McLaurin LP, Foster MT, et al: Spinal cord compression secondary to extramedullary hematopoiesis in two brothers: report of two cases. *J Neurosurg* 1968;29:529-531.

205. Close AS, Taira Y, Cleveland DA: Spinal cord compression due to extramedullary hematopoiesis. *Ann Intern Med* 1958;48:421-427.

206. Cromwell LD, Kerber C: Spinal cord compression by extramedullary hematopoiesis in agnogenic myeloid metaplasia. *Radiology* 1978;128:118.

207. Cross JN, Morgan OS, Gibbs WN, et al: Spinal cord compression in thalassaemia. *J Neurol Neurosurg Psychiatry* 1977;40:1120-1122.

208. Oustwani MB, Kurtides ES, Christ M, et al: Spinal cord compression with paraplegia in myelofibrosis. *Arch Neurol* 1980;37:389-390.

209. Rutgers MJ, van der Lugt PJ, van Turnhout JM: Spinal cord compression by extramedullary hemopoietic tissue in pyruvate-kinase-deficiency–caused hemolytic anemia. *Neurology* 1979;29:510-513.

210. Rice GPA, Assis LJP, Barr RM, et al: Extramedullary hematopoiesis and spinal cord compression complicating polycythemia rubra vera. *Ann Neurol* 1980;7:81-84.

211. Heffez DS, Sawaya R, Udvarhelyi GB, Mann R: Spinal epidural extramedullary hematopoiesis with cord compression in a patient with refractory sideroblastic anemia: case report. *J Neurosurg* 1982;57:399-406.

212. Papavasiliou CG: Tumor simulating intrathoracic extramedullary hemopoiesis. Clinical and roentgenologic considerations. *AJR* 1965;93:695-702.

213. Ross P, Logan W: Roentgen findings in extramedullary hematopoiesis. *AJR* 1969;106:604-613.

214. Lowman RM, Bloor CM, Newcomb AW: Roentgen manifestations of thoracic extramedullary hematopoiesis. *Dis Chest* 1963;44:154-162.

215. Long JA, Doppman JL, Nienhuis AW: Computed tomographic studies of thoracic extramedullary haematopoiesis. *J Comput Assist Tomogr* 1980;4:67-70.

216. Jackson A, Burton IE: Retroperitoneal mass and spinal cord compression due to extramedullary haemopoiesis in polycythaemia rubra vera. *Br J Radiol* 1989;62:944-947.

217. Papavasiliou C, Gouliamos A, Vlahos L, et al: CT and MRI of symptomatic spinal involvement by extramedullary haemopoiesis. *Clin Radiol* 1990;42:91-92.

218. Quint DJ, Boulos RS, Sanders WP, et al: Epidural lipomatosis. *Radiology* 1988;169:485-490.

219. Doppman JL: Epidural lipomatosis. *Radiology* 1989;171(2):581-582.

220. Plotz CM, Knowltor AI, Ragan C: The natural history of Cushing's syndrome. *Am J Med* 1952;13:597-614.

221. Paget J: On a form of chronic inflammation of bones (osteitis deformans). *Med Chir Trans* 1877;60:37.

222. Schmorl G: Ueber osteitis deformans Paget. *Virchows Arch* 1932;283:694.

223. Resnick D, Niwayama G: Paget's disease. In Resnick D, Niwayama G (eds): *Diagnosis of bone and joint disorders,* ed 2. Philadelphia, Saunders, 1987, pp 2127-2170.

224. Collins DH: Paget's disease of bone: incidence and subclinical forms. *Lancet* 1956;271:51-57.

225. Dickson DD, Camp JD, Ghormley RK: Osteitis deformans: Paget's disease of the bone. *Radiology* 1945;44:449-470.

226. Zlatkin MB, Lander PH, Hadjipavlou AG, Levine JS: Paget disease of the spine: CT with clinical correlation. *Radiology* 1986;160:155-159.

227. Schmidek HH: Neurologic and neurosurgical sequelae of Paget's disease of bone. *Clin Orthop* 1977;127:70-77.

228. Lander PH, Hadjipavlou AG: A dynamic classification of Paget's disease. *J Bone Joint Surg [Br]* 1986;68:431-438.

229. Roberts MC, Kressel HY, Fallon MD, et al: Paget disease: MR imaging findings. *Radiology* 1989;173:341-345.

230. Dalinka MK, Aronchick JM, Haddad JG: Paget's disease. *Orthop Clin North Am* 1973;4:3-19.

231. Singer FR: *Paget's disease of bone.* New York, Plenum Medical, 1977, pp 44-48.

232. Kelly JK, Denier JE, Wilner HI, et al: MR imaging of lytic changes in Paget disease of the calvarium. *J Comput Assist Tomogr* 1989;13:27-29.

233. Kaufmann GA, Sunderam M, McDonald DJ: Magnetic resonance imaging in symptomatic Paget's disease. *Skeletal Radiol* 1991;20:413-418.

Index